Practical Ultrasonography in Obstetrics and Gynecology

Taizhu Yang • Hong Luo
Editors

Practical Ultrasonography in Obstetrics and Gynecology

Chemical Industry Press Co., Ltd.

Springer

Editors
Taizhu Yang
Department of Ultrasonography
West China Second University Hospital
Sichuan University
Chengdu, China

Hong Luo
Department of Ultrasonography
West China Second University Hospital
Sichuan University
Chengdu, China

ISBN 978-981-16-4476-4 ISBN 978-981-16-4477-1 (eBook)
https://doi.org/10.1007/978-981-16-4477-1

Jointly published with Chemical Industry Press
The print edition is not for sale in China (Mainland). Customers from China (Mainland) please order the print book from: Chemical Industry Press.

This Springer imprint is published by the registered company Springer Nature Singapore Pte Ltd.
The registered company address is: 152 Beach Road, #21-01/04 Gateway East, Singapore 189721, Singapore

Preface

Translated by Feiran Liu

It is universally acknowledged that ultrasound examination plays a vital role in obstetrics and gynecology clinical practice. The rapid development of ultrasound technology broadens and deepens its clinical application. At the same time, the requirements for ultrasound diagnosis in obstetrics and gynecology are much higher. The diagnostic risk of obstetrics and gynecology ultrasound is high, especially in obstetrics. The requirements by doctors for ultrasound diagnoses prompt sonographers to improve and strengthen their ultrasound knowledge, scanning skills, picture recognition ability, and related obstetrics and gynecology clinical knowledge.

In our daily work, the questions put forward by medical students and training staff from the ultrasound department of elementary healthcare affiliations are not sophisticated theoretical ones but urgent practical problems met in daily clinical work, which include how to handle the ultrasound machine to get the best image and how to identify normal and abnormal images and then differentiate kinds of abnormal images to make the correct diagnosis. Therefore, it is necessary to write this obstetrics and gynecology ultrasound book with great practicality to solve confusion faced by medical students, residents, and intermediate doctors, and that is why we have written this book.

West China Women's and Children's Hospital is the largest hospital specializing in obstetrics and gynecology and pediatrics in the south-west of China. The number of its outpatients is almost 600,000 per year, and the number of operations performed is 10,000 per year. Notably, the number of ultrasound examination cases is more than 100,000 per year, which makes it possible for us to summarize variable cases and clinical data.

The content of this book, covering various aspects of obstetrics and gynecology ultrasonography, is illustrated with images, focusing on practicality. With more than 400,000 words in total, it included more than 500 cases of typical ultrasound images with a clear note. At the same time, this book summarized concise theories of common diseases and normal and abnormal diagnoses related to pregnancy. We also noted key points of differential diagnosis, as well as experience and lessons learned in daily work. Except for ultrasound diagnosis of common diseases of obstetrics and gynecology, we also summarize a comprehensive introduction to the application of ultrasound technology in obstetrics and gynecology. Based on the practicality and popularity of the knowledge, we also shed some light on the progress of ultrasound technology in obstetrics and gynecology. The attached video will provide you with vivid and intuitive examples of basic operation skills of obstetrics and gynecology ultrasonography.

After the first edition of *Practical Ultrasonography in Obstetrics and Gynecology* was published in 2006, it has been received with favor and welcomed by sonographers and readers. Based on the rapid development of practice and theory of ultrasound in obstetrics and gynecology, we update and revise the contents of this book to meet the needs in the work of ultrasonic diagnosis in obstetrics and gynecology and the demand from readers and the press in 2017. Following international practice, we make some revision, but the content and the form are consistent with the first edition. Except for some correction of inaccuracy in the original edition, we also added some new content. The amendments are as follows.

1. Focus on practice as in the original edition.
2. More attention has been paid to the cases and practical theory. Chapter one and chapter two were combined in the original edition. The section on uterine hypertrophy has been removed. The content of combined application of ultrasound and hysteroscopy has been edited and the chapter has been renamed "The application of endoscopic ultrasonography."
3. The following content in the corresponding chapter has been added: nuchal translucency in early pregnancy; fetal facial and thoracic malformation; vasa previa; abnormality of umbilical cord insertion site; CT and MRI examination of the neonatal head; three-vessel view of fetal heart; fetal cardiac functional score; intravenous contrast echocardiography; salpingography; and pelvic floor ultrasound.
4. More attention has been paid to the quality of pictures. Nearly 300 pictures have been replaced or updated.

This book is written and revised by Taizhu Yang, Hong Luo, Qi Zhu, Fan Yang, Jiao Chen, Yu Tian, Houqing Pang, Min He, Hong Xu, Ying Tang, Nan Guo, Bo Zang, and others. Special thanks for Jia Yuan who has done much work for collection of the images and editing of this book.

By all means, due to the limited time and the ability of authors, there might be some mistakes. We would appreciate if you figure it out and inform us. Also, we dedicate this book to the people who helped and encouraged us.

Chengdu, China Taizhu Yang

Contents

Editorial Board

Editor-in-Chief

Taizhu Yang Department of Ultrasonography, West China Second University Hospital, Sichuan University, Chengdu, China

Hong Luo Department of Ultrasonography, West China Second University Hospital, Sichuan University, Chengdu, China

Vice-Editor-in-Chief

Qi Zhu Department of Ultrasonography, West China Second University Hospital, Sichuan University, Chengdu, China

Fan Yang Department of Ultrasonography, West China Second University Hospital, Sichuan University, Chengdu, China

Members of the Board

Bo Zhang Department of Ultrasonography, West China Second University Hospital, Sichuan University, Chengdu, China

Hong Xu Department of Ultrasonography, West China Second University Hospital, Sichuan University, Chengdu, China

Houqing Pang Department of Ultrasonography, West China Second University Hospital, Sichuan University, Chengdu, China

Jiao Chen Department of Ultrasonography, West China Second University Hospital, Sichuan University, Chengdu, China

Min He Department of Ultrasonography, West China Second University Hospital, Sichuan University, Chengdu, China

Nan Guo Department of Ultrasonography, West China Second University Hospital, Sichuan University, Chengdu, China

Ying Tang Department of Ultrasonography, West China Second University Hospital, Sichuan University, Chengdu, China

Yu Tian Department of Ultrasonography, West China Second University Hospital, Sichuan University, Chengdu, China

Translators

Taizhu Yang Department of Ultrasonography, West China Second University Hospital, Sichuan University, Chengdu, China

Hong Luo Department of Ultrasonography, West China Second University Hospital, Sichuan University, Chengdu, China

Fan Yang Department of Ultrasonography, West China Second University Hospital, Sichuan University, Chengdu, China

Qiubo Lv Department of Obstetrics and Gynecology, Beijing Hospital, National Center of Gerontology, Beijing, China

Miaoqian Wang Department of Obstetrics and Gynecology, Beijing Hospital, National Center of Gerontology, Beijing, China

Qian Hu Department of Obstetrics and Gynecology, Beijing Hospital, National Center of Gerontology, Beijing, China

Tiantian Ye Department of Ultrasound, Beijing Luhe Hospital, Affiliated to Capital Medical University, Beijing, China

Mingchun Zhi Department of Obstetrics and Gynecology, Beijing Hospital, National Center of Gerontology, Beijing, China

Linlin Ma Department of Obstetrics and Gynecology, Beijing Hospital, National Center of Gerontology, Beijing, China

Feiran Liu Department of Obstetrics and Gynecology, Beijing Shijitan Hospital, Beijing, China

Clinical Basis of Diagnosis Ultrasound in Obstetrics and Gynecology

1

Taizhu Yang, Hong Luo, Bo Zhang, and Min He

1.1 Physics and Technology of Diagnostic Ultrasound

1.1.1 Basic Physics of Ultrasonic Wave

Ultrasonic wave, a special type of sound wave, belongs to elastic mechanical wave. Particles in the transfer medium move back and forth in the horizontal direction and produce alternative rarefaction waves and compression waves. Sound travels away in a longitudinal waveform.

1.1.1.1 Frequency of the Ultrasonic Wave

The acoustic frequency range of human hearing is limited from 20 to 20,000 Hz. Ultrasound is a sound with a frequency higher than 20,000 Hz. In general, ultrasound frequencies used for clinical applications range from 2 to 10 MHz.

1.1.1.2 The Relation between Wavelength and Frequency

The period is the time to complete a single cycle. The frequency of the wave is defined as the number of vibration periods of the sound per second. The wavelength, λ, is the distance between corresponding points per period. Frequency and wavelength are related inversely. Higher the frequency, the shorter the wavelength.

The following equation is the relationship between frequency and wavelength:

$$c = \lambda f \text{ or } \lambda = c/f$$

c—acoustic velocity,
f—frequency,
λ—wavelength.

1.1.1.3 Acoustic Velocity

Acoustic velocity is used to describe the distance that sound travels in a unit of time. Propagation velocity of the sound varies in different media: fastest in the solid, followed by liquid, and slowest in the gas. Propagation velocity of soft tissue in the body is about 1540 m/sec, similar to that in the liquid (1500 m/sec). The general difference in the acoustic velocity among different parts of soft tissues in the body is about 5%. Consequently, the measuring error of ultrasound is around 5%.

1.1.1.4 Acoustic Intensity

Acoustic intensity is defined as the power distributed in a unit of area, measured in W/cm^2. Usually, the acoustic output of diagnostic ultrasound is less than 100 mW/cm^2. Acoustic intensity for fetal use should be as low as possible, so does the examining time.

1.1.2 Physical Basis of Ultrasonic Imaging

1.1.2.1 Acoustic Impedance and Ultrasonic Imaging

The acoustic impedance varies in tissues with different densities. The interfaces will reflect the incident sound energy when the acoustic impedance difference between interfaces is larger than 1%. There is a positive correlation between echogenicity and acoustic impedance difference. Echoes with different intensities create various imaging (Table 1.1).

1.1.2.2 Attenuation of Ultrasonic Energy in the Body

1. The tissues with enormous water represent less attenuation and more transmission. When compared with

This chapter was translated by **Miaoqian Wang** and **Qiubo Lv**.
Department of Obstetrics and Gynecology, Beijing Hospital, National Center of Gerontology, Beijing, China.

T. Yang (✉) · H. Luo · B. Zhang · M. He
Department of Ultrasonography, West China Second University Hospital, Sichuan University, Chengdu, China

T. Yang, H. Luo (eds.), *Practical Ultrasonography in Obstetrics and Gynecology*,
https://doi.org/10.1007/978-981-16-4477-1_1

Table 1.1 Reflection type of the tissues

Echo	Acoustic impedance difference	Type of tissues
Extremely hyperechoic	Extremely large	Gas-tissue interface (bowel/lung), which goes against further traveling
Hyperechoic	Large	Tissues with enormous calcium or fibration (bone/calcification/stone/scar)
Relative hyperechoic	Relatively large	Solid heterogeneous tissues, fibroplasia, vessel wall, renal collective system
Medium	Small	Solid homogeneous tissues (uterus/ovary/liver/spleen/renal cortex/muscle)
Hypoecho	Very small	Tissues with uniform density (renal pyramids/certain cancers)
Anechoic	None	Blood/amniotic fluid/urine/cystic fluid/bile/transudate

surrounding tissues, they have reduced internal acoustic energy with posterior enhancement. Among the liquid media, cyst fluid, urine, and amniotic fluid transmit the largest amount of acoustic energy, followed by bile and blood.

2. Shadowing is visible when the tissue with enormous calcium or fibration attenuates more acoustic energy than the surrounding tissues. Bones, calculus, and the calcification of tissues represent hyperechoic with posterior shadow.

1.1.3 Ultrasonography Technology

1.1.3.1 B-mode Ultrasound

The echo is expressed in the form of light spots. Images of a certain depth and width can be obtained under multi-beam scanning. The intensity of the reflected echo, which was used to be expressed by the brightness of light spots, is indicated now by the gray-scale value. The more gray-scale variations, the better display. Ultrasonic imaging under different probes is in various shapes, such as rectangular, curvilinear, and fan shaped.

Transabdominal Ultrasonography

In gynecological and obstetrical applications, transabdominal ultrasound is frequently used. In a linear array transducer, the elements are arranged in a line, while the elements of a curved transducer are arranged in an arc shape. The curved transducer is more frequently utilized in transabdominal ultrasound, with a frequency of 3–5 MHz and numerous elements of 128–256. In a curved array transducer, elements transmit and receive sound waves in sequence, producing a frame of tomographic image in arc shape. Transabdominal ultrasound can display in real time, with a scanning frame of 16–18 frames per second.

Transvaginal Ultrasonography

The vaginal probe is small and its elements are placed in the front of the handle, which can be placed into the vagina to show the uterus, ovary, and other targets in the near-field.

High-frequency fan-shaped ultrasound (5–10 MHz) is often used to obtain higher definition images.

1.1.3.2 M-Mode Ultrasound Imaging

Based on the 2D imaging, move the M-mode sampling line to the ROI, collect the signals of the structures that are threaded by the echo, and display the dynamic curve. M-mode ultrasound is mainly used to analyze fetal heart activity because of its strong space–time relationship.

1.1.3.3 Doppler Ultrasound

All the Doppler ultrasonic instruments have a 2D ultrasound, color Doppler, and spectral Doppler.

Color Doppler Velocity (CDV)

Choose the color Doppler mode, move the sampling to the ROI, and encode the received Doppler signals.

1. Different colors indicate different directions of blood flow. The color red represents a positive frequency shift, indicating that the blood travels toward the transducer. Blue is assigned to present a negative frequency shift, indicating that the blood travels oppositely to the probe.
2. The brightness of the color stands for the magnitude of velocity. Typically, the brighter the color, the higher the velocity; the darker the color, the lower the velocity.
3. The color green indicates a large dispersion of the blood flow, representing turbulence.
4. Primary colors – red, green, and blue – can be mixed to form other colors. Red and blue are combined to produce purple, red and green to produce yellow, blue and green to produce cyan. When three primary colors are mixed in equal parts, white will be presented.

Color Doppler Energy (CDE)

Power Doppler is based on the intensity of ultrasonic signals scattered by the red blood cells, relating to the blood flow. Power Doppler is irrelevant to the direction or velocity of the blood flow. The blood flow is designed to display in a single color, without red (positive), blue (negative), or multi-color presentation. Power Doppler is more sensitive and has an advantage over color Doppler to show low-speed blood flow. Also, power Doppler is much less angle-dependent, contributing to a better display of the vessels. The image, with strong background noise, shows no information of the flow direction or velocity and fails to distinguish between vein and artery.

Spectral Doppler

The fast Fourier transform (FFT) algorithm is used to compute the Doppler spectrum. The complex signals received by the probe are transformed into simple frequency and amplitude signals to compose a spectral image. This image can be used to analyze the blood flow direction, velocity, dispersibility, and changes over time.

The ordinate (Y-axis) represents the velocity-frequency shift, and the abscissa (X-axis) represents time. The bandwidth reflects the dispersibility of the blood flow. In the case of laminar flow, the velocity is consistent, with narrow bandwidth. Whereas, in the turbulence cases, the velocity is varied, with large dispersion and wide bandwidth. The amplitude of the Doppler signal, signal on the Z-axis, is encoded as the spectrum's gray scale. High amplitude presents a high gray scale and high brightness, indicating a large number of erythrocytes. Those with low amplitude have a low gray scale and low brightness, indicating less red blood cells.

Spectral Doppler is divided into pulsed Doppler (PW) and continuous Doppler (CW). PW transmits and receives Doppler signals with a single chip, which can accurately locate and sample. CW has dual chips, one of which emits an ultrasonic wave, and the other receives the Doppler signal, which is used to detect high-speed blood flow.

Hemodynamics

General Parameters and Measurement

Peak systolic velocity, PSV(Vs, Vmax): measure at the highest point of the systolic phase of the spectrum.

End diastolic velocity, EDV(Vd, Vmin): measure at the lowest point of the diastolic phase of the spectrum.

Mean velocity (Vmean, Vm) and velocity time integral (VTI): trace along the blood flow spectrum, then the mean velocity and VTI can be obtained.

Hemodynamic Parameters

Resistance index, RI: reflects the resistance of the blood flow.

$$\mathrm{RI} = \frac{V_s - V_d}{Vs} \quad (\text{normal value}: 0.7 \pm 0.05)$$

Pulse index, PI: reflects the elasticity and compliance of the blood vessels.

$$\mathrm{PI} = \frac{V_s - V_d}{Vm} \quad (\text{normal value}: 1 - 1.5)$$

S/D (Vs/Vd): the ratio of the PSV to the EDV, and the normal value is 3:1.

PI, RI, S/D, the ratios of velocity parameters, are not affected by the exploration angle, which is of great value in evaluating the resistance of blood vessels and perfusion of tissues and organs.

1.1.3.4 3D Ultrasound Imaging

A series of 2-D sectional image information is collected and displayed as a 3-D image after digital processing by a professional computer.

1. 3-D reconstruction: place the 3-D probe on the lower abdomen and obtain a series of related 2-D images for further 3-D reconstruction. The image is intuitive, which has a strong 3-D sense.
2. Real-time 3-D imaging: place the real-time volumetric 3-D probe on the lower abdomen, and the electronic phase-controlled vibration probe scan automatically to obtain real-time 3-D images.

See Chap. 8 for the application of 3-D ultrasound imaging technology in obstetrics and gynecology.

1.2 Ultrasonic Anatomy and Physiology of Female Pelvic Cavity

1.2.1 Anatomy and Ultrasonic Imaging of Pelvic Cavity

1.2.1.1 Pelvic Structures

The pelvis is a ring-shaped bony structure, consisting of sacrum, coccyx, two hip bones, hip joints, and ligament. The anterior part of the pelvic cavity is mainly the bladder and urethra. The middle part is the uterus, cervix, and vagina, and the fallopian tubes and ovaries are on the two sides. The posterior part is the rectouterine pouch (Douglas cavity) and rectum. The blood vessels in the pelvis mainly include the internal iliac arteries and veins, external iliac arteries and veins, and branches. The pouches, formed by the bladder, uterus, rectum, and the peritoneum continuation between the pelvic wall, include the rectouterine pouch and the vesicouterine pouch. The rectouterine pouch is the lowest point of the female peritoneal cavity, where the exudate, bleeding, and empyema in the peritoneal cavity often accumulate (Fig. 1.1).

1.2.1.2 Female Internal Genitalia

The female internal genitalia include vagina, uterus, fallopian tubes, and ovaries. The fallopian tube and ovary are often called adnexa (Fig. 1.2).

The Vagina

1. Anatomy of the vagina
   (a) Vagina is a muscular duct, 10 to 12 cm long.

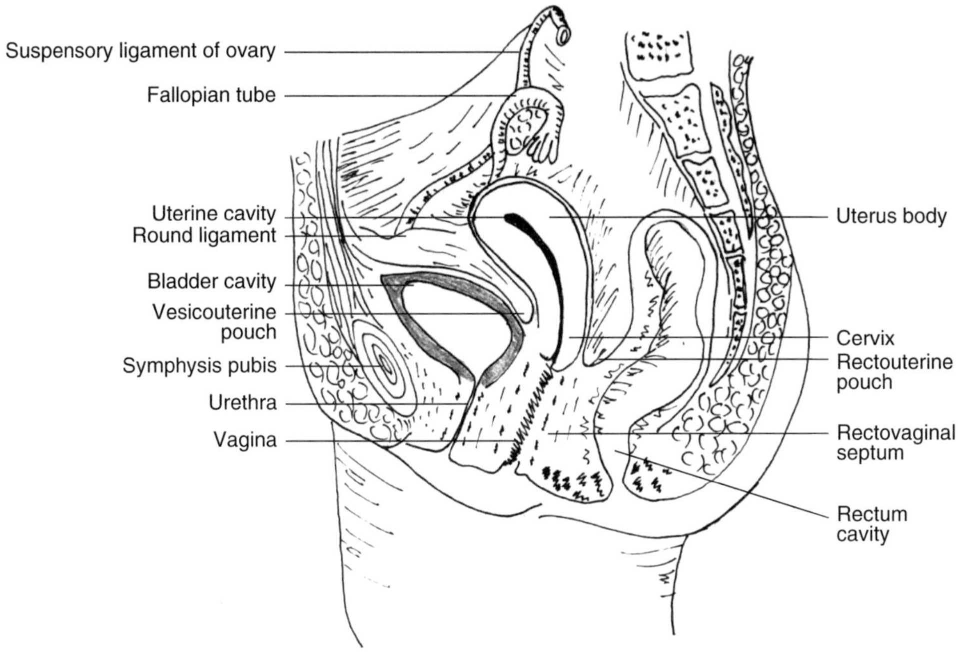

Fig. 1.1 Sagittal view of female pelvic cavity

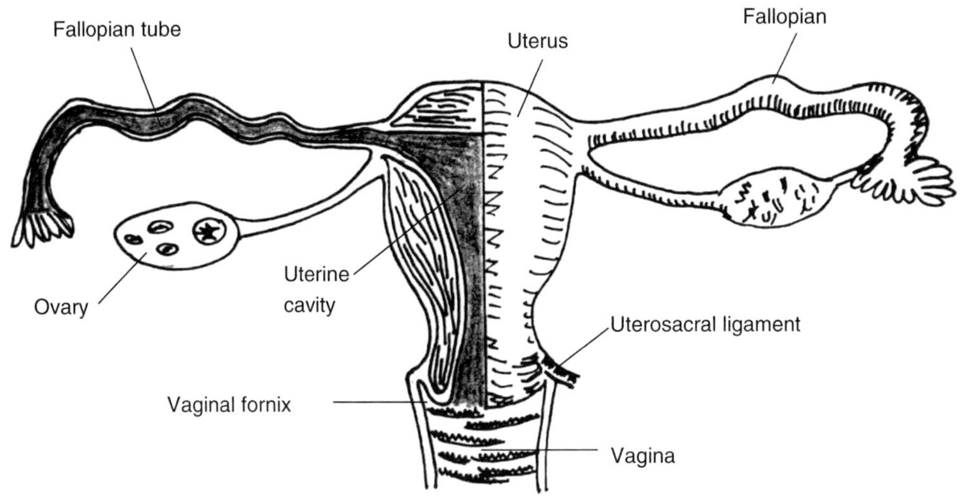

Fig. 1.2 Female internal genitalia

(b) The anterior wall is adjacent to the bladder and urethra, and the posterior wall is adjacent to the rectum.
(c) The vaginal fornix is formed between the vaginal wall and the cervix, which can be divided into anterior and posterior fornix and two lateral fornixes. The posterior fornix is deep, and the rectouterine pouch is above its back.
(d) Normally, the anterior and posterior walls of the vagina lie in contact, and the vagina and cervix are connected at an acute angle.

2. Normal ultrasonic image
   (a) The longitudinal view shows that the anterior and posterior walls of the vagina are closed to each other, and the center is the vaginal cavity. A small amount of gas is visible in the vaginal cavity, shown as a thin hyperechoic line by ultrasound, called the vaginal gas line. According to the presence of the vaginal gas line, it can be judged as having a vaginal cavity (Fig. 1.3).
   (b) The vaginal wall is a thin hypoechoic structure. The thickness of the anterior and posterior vaginal walls is shown via the filled bladder and the inflated rectum.
   (c) On the transverse view vagina is a short horizontal hypoechoic structure, and the hyperechoic horizontal line in the center of the vagina is the vaginal cavity.
   (d) The tissue between the bladder and the vaginal cavity is the vaginal-bladder diazoma, and that between the rectum and the vaginal cavity is the rectal-vaginal diazoma.

Uterus (UT)

1. Anatomy of the uterus

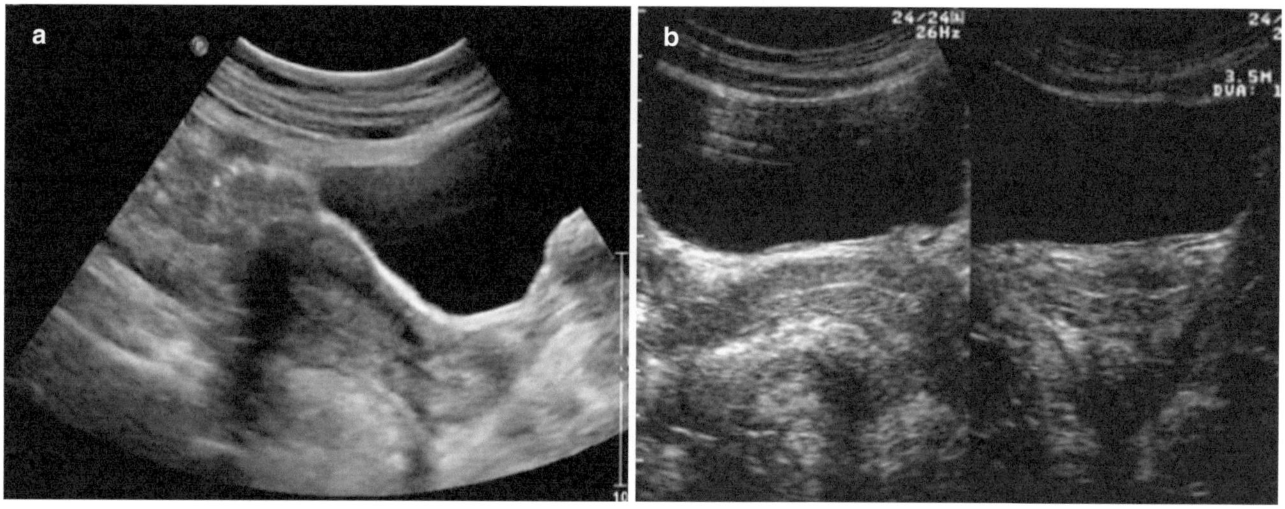

Fig. 1.3 Image of the uterus and vaginal gas line. (**a**). The longitudinal view shows the vaginal gas line; (**b**). The longitudinal and transverse view of the vagina

(a) The size of uterus, which is in an inverted pear shape, changes with age. The length of the neonatal uterus is 2.5–3.0 cm. The adult uterus is 7–8 cm long, 4–5 cm wide, 2–3 cm thick, and weighs about 50 g. The uterine volume of menopausal women becomes smaller.
(b) The upper part of the uterus is wider, and the bulge is called the fundus. The uterine horns are the two sides of the uterine fundus. The lower part of the uterus is narrow and cylindrical, called the cervix. The cervix of an adult woman is about 3 cm long, and the cervical canal is spindle-shaped.
(c) The uterine body wall is composed of serous layer, muscular layer and mucosal layer, namely endometrium. The myometrium is the thickest layer, which is about 0.8 cm thick in non-pregnant adult women. The uterine cavity is in a triangular shape, which is wider at the top and narrows at the bottom, and its volume is about 5 ml (Fig. 1.4).
(d) In different periods of growth, the length ratio of the uterine body to cervix is different. It is 1:2 in infancy, 1:1 in adolescence, and 2:l in adulthood.
(e) The isthmus of the uterus is a narrow portion of the junction between the uterus and the cervix and is the part between the histologic internal os of the cervix and the anatomical internal os. During non-pregnancy, the length is about 1.0 cm, and up to 10 cm in the third trimester.
(f) Uterine ligaments, including broad ligament, round ligament, main ligament, and uterosacral ligament, maintain the position of the uterus. Usually, the uterus is slightly anteversion, flexion, and easily affected by the body position, bladder filling degree, rectum, and abdominal pressure.

2. Normal uterine sonogram
   (a) Longitudinal view: the anterior or horizontal uterus is inverted pear-shaped, with a smooth and clear outline. The serous layer is hyperechoic surrounding the myometrium, and the muscular layer is uniform and moderate isoecho. The endometrium is in a linear echo. The endometrium is an essential marker for identifying the location of the uterus and lesions. When the normal anatomical structure of pelvic cavity changes due to pelvic surgery, tumors or pathological changes, and inflammatory adhesions, it is vital to find the endometrium for judging the position of the uterus and the relationship between the lesion and the uterus. There is a slight depression in the lower part of the anterior uterine wall, which is the isthmus' location and the internal os of the uterus. The uterine position can be identified by observing the angle between the uterus and the cervix or by the relationship between the uterine fundus and the bladder. The endometrium's thickness and shape vary with the menstrual cycle (Figs. 1.5 and 1.6).
   (b) Transverse view: The bottom of the uterus is triangular, the horn of the uterus protrudes like a beak, and the body is oval. In the center of the uterus, the endometrium can be seen in a Chinese character "—" shape (Fig. 1.7).
   (c) The cervix is mainly composed of connective tissue. The echo is slightly stronger and denser than the uterine body. It is fusiform and hyperechoic in the longitudinal view and ring-shaped and hyperechoic in the transverse view (Fig. 1.8).
3. Measure the uterine size: Through a moderately filled bladder, measure the length and anteroposterior diameter

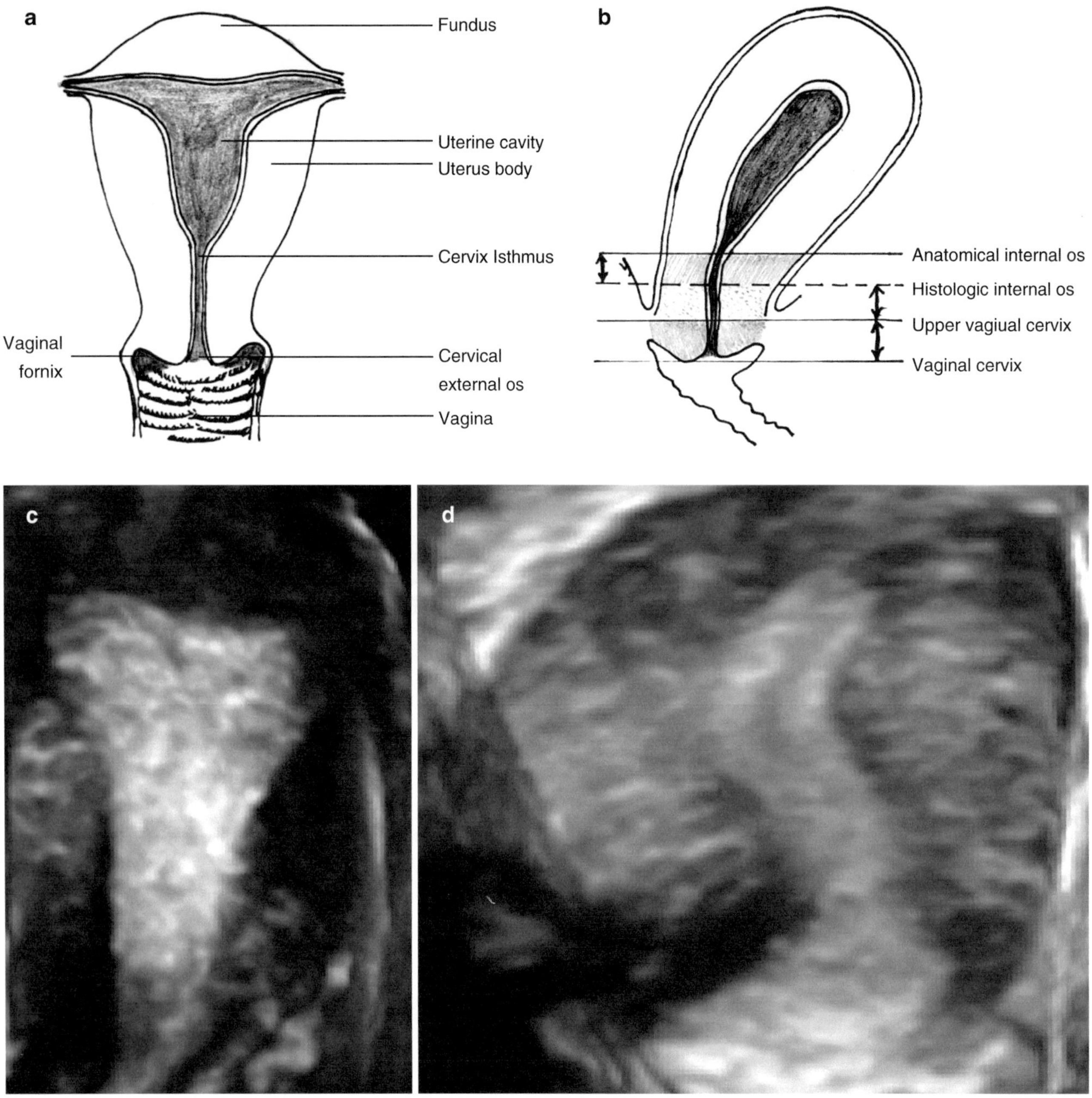

Fig. 1.4 Anatomy of the uterus. (**a**). Coronal view of the uterus; (**b**). Sagittal view of the uterus; (**c**). Coronal view of uterus (3-D ultrasound); (**d**). Sagittal view of uterus (3-D ultrasound)

of the uterine body on the longitudinal view, and measure the transverse diameter on the transverse view. The length and diameter of the cervix are measured on the longitudinal view, and the transverse diameter is measured on the transverse view. The reference values for ultrasonic measurement of the normal adult uterus are: 5.5–7.5 cm in length, 3.0–4.0 cm in anteroposterior diameter, 4.5–5.5 cm in transverse diameter, and 2.5–3.0 cm in cervix length. The uterine diameter in multiparous women can increase by 1.2 cm. The adolescent uterine body is about the same length as the cervix, and the uterine body is about twice the length of the cervix during fertility. Among the elderly, it becomes 1:1 (Figs. 1.9 and 1.10, normal values are shown in Table 1.2).

4. Cyclically change and sonographic appearance of the endometrium
   (a) Proliferative phase: The endometrium is composed of a zona functionalis and basalis layer. The basalis layer of the endometrium is echogenic, but the functional layer is hypoechoic. From the fifth to 14th day

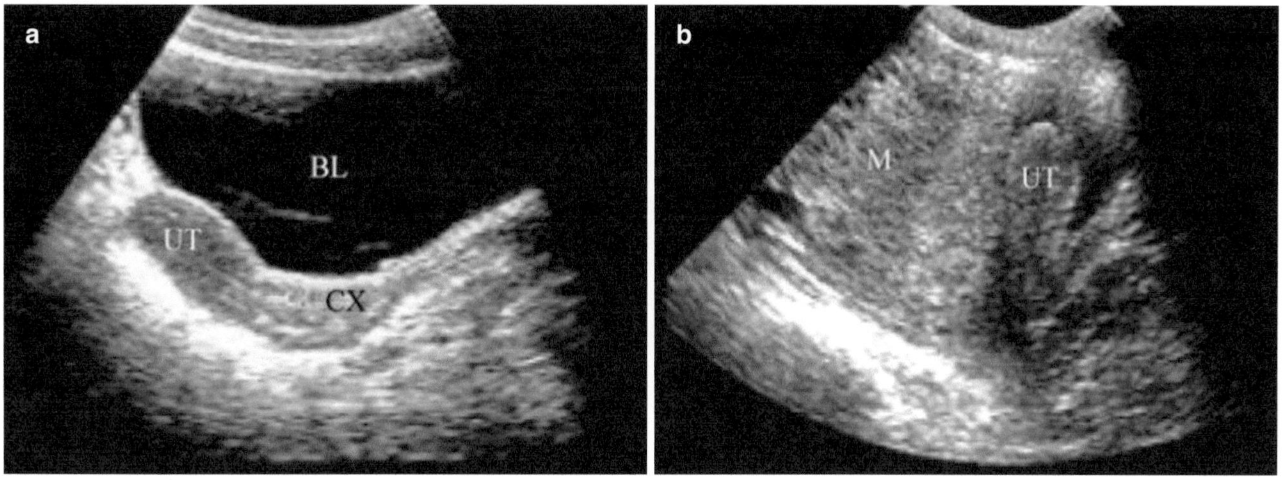

Fig. 1.5 The relationship between the mass and the endometrium. (**a**). Sagittal view of the uterus, the endometrium is linear and centered. The serous layer is hyperechoic surrounding the myometrium; (**b**). The uterus is compressed with displayed endometrium, indicating that the mass is outside the uterus

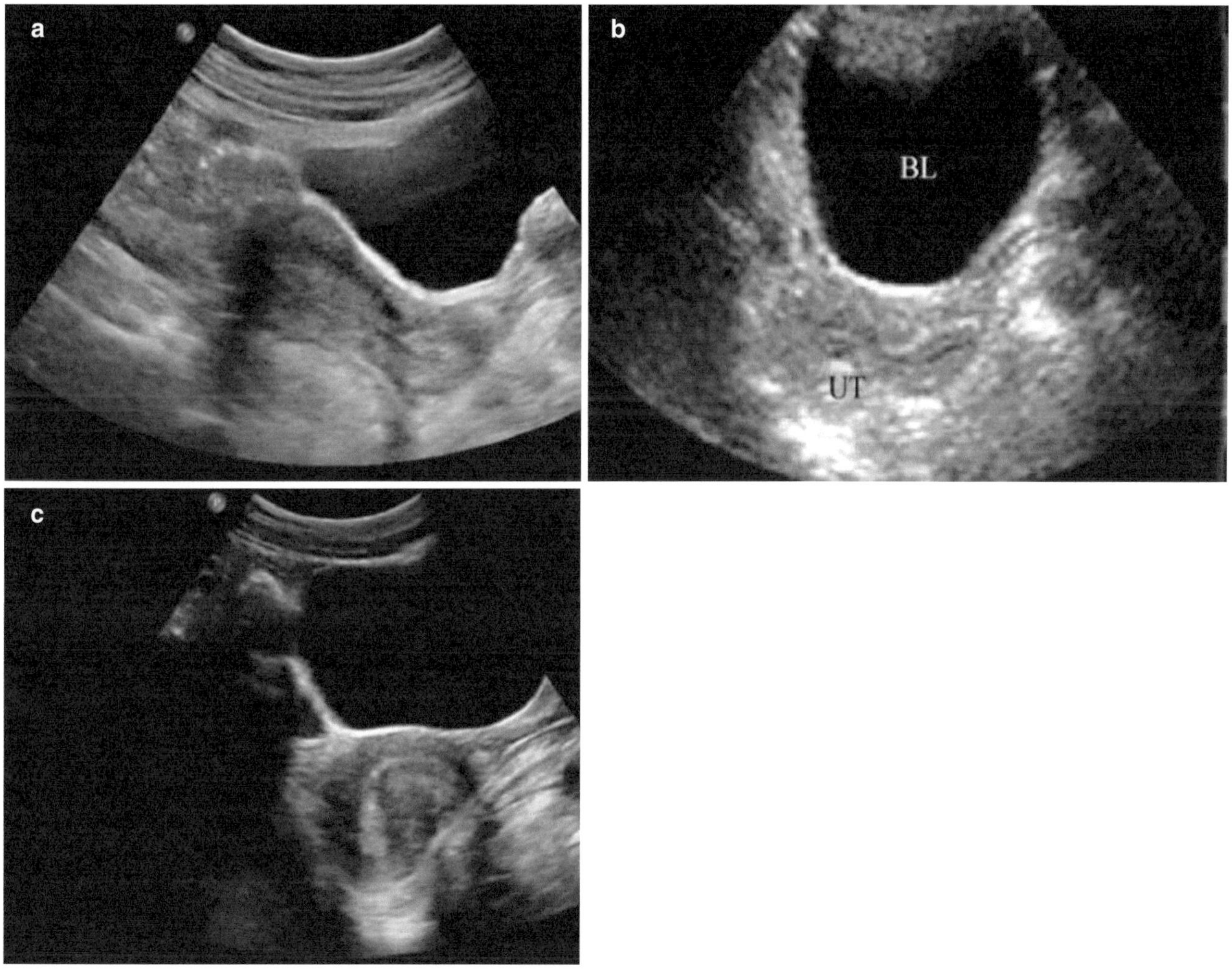

Fig. 1.6 Uterine position. (**a**). Sagittal view of the anterior uterus; (**b**). Horizontal uterus; (**c**). Posterior uterus: the uterine body is located behind the cervix

of the menstrual cycle, the endometrium begins to proliferate as a result of estrogen effects. From early to mid-hyperplasia, the endometrium appears as a hyperechoic line; in late hyperplasia, the endometrial echo is slightly thickened and hyperechoic, with a thickness of 2–4 mm (Fig. 1.11).

(b) Secretory phase From the 15th to 28th day of the menstrual cycle, under the influence of ovarian hormones, the functional layer increases in thickness. In early secretion, the thickness of the endometrium is 5–6 mm, fusiform and hypoechoic, surrounded by subendometrial halo. Throughout the mid to the late secretory phase, the endometrium measures up to 7–10 mm, representing a hyperechoic ellipse, and the surrounding subendometrial halo widens.

(c) Menstrual phase: from the first to fourth day of the menstrual cycle, the ovarian hormone decreases, the endometrium falls off, and menstruation comes. Ultrasonic image shows that the uterine cavity line is not clear, the echo of the endometrium is heterogeneous, and small anechoic areas may be seen.

(d) Measurement of the endometrium: Measure the junction boundary of the endometrium and myometrium and calculate the whole or 1/2 of the whole endometrial thickness. Transvaginal ultrasound can clearly show the thickness and shape changes of the endometrium during the menstrual cycle. For patients who are not suitable for transvaginal examination, the bladder is required to be moderately filled before transabdominal ultrasound examination.

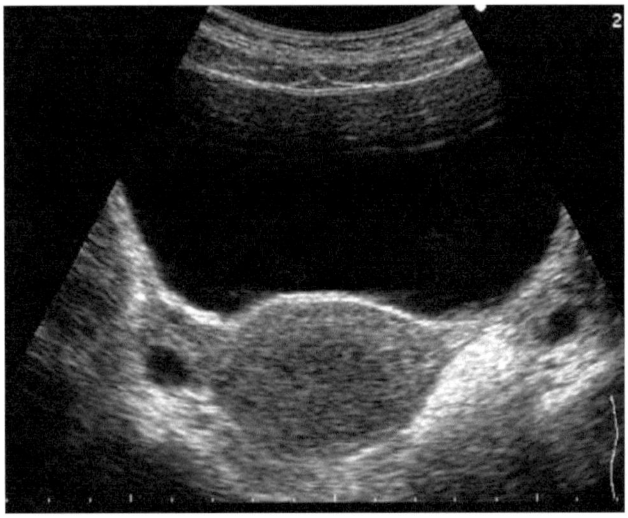

Fig. 1.7 Transverse view image of the uterus

Oviduct

1. The anatomy of the fallopian tube: it is a pair of slender and curved tubular muscular organs, with a total length of 8–14 cm. The proximal extremity of the fallopian tube is connected to the uterine horn, and the distal extremity is free, close to the ovary. The oviduct is divided into the interstitial, isthmus, ampulla, and funnel (Fig. 1.12).
2. Sonogram of the fallopian tube: Normally, the fallopian tube is not visible. When there is a fallopian tube disease or ascites in the pelvic cavity, ultrasound can show the fallopian tube or fallopian tube lesion floating in the ascites. In the diagnosis of fallopian tube diseases, transvaginal ultrasonography is superior to transabdominal ultrasonography (Fig. 1.13).

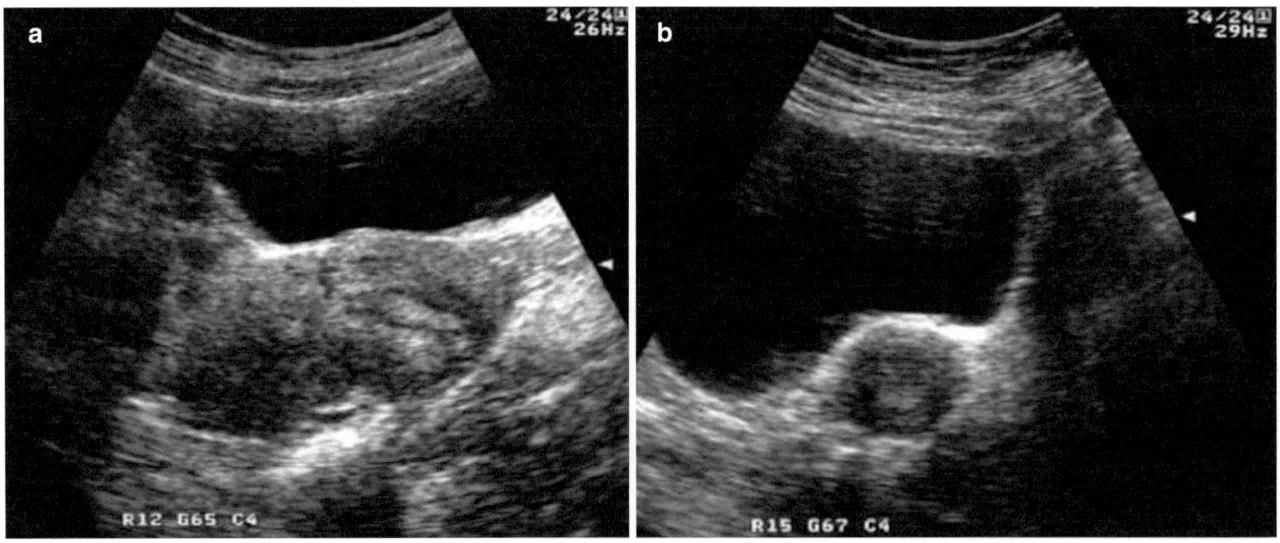

Fig. 1.8 The longitudinal and transverse view of the cervix. (**a**). The longitudinal view shows a fusiform hyperechoic cervix; (**b**). Transverse view, a ring-shaped hyperechoic cervix

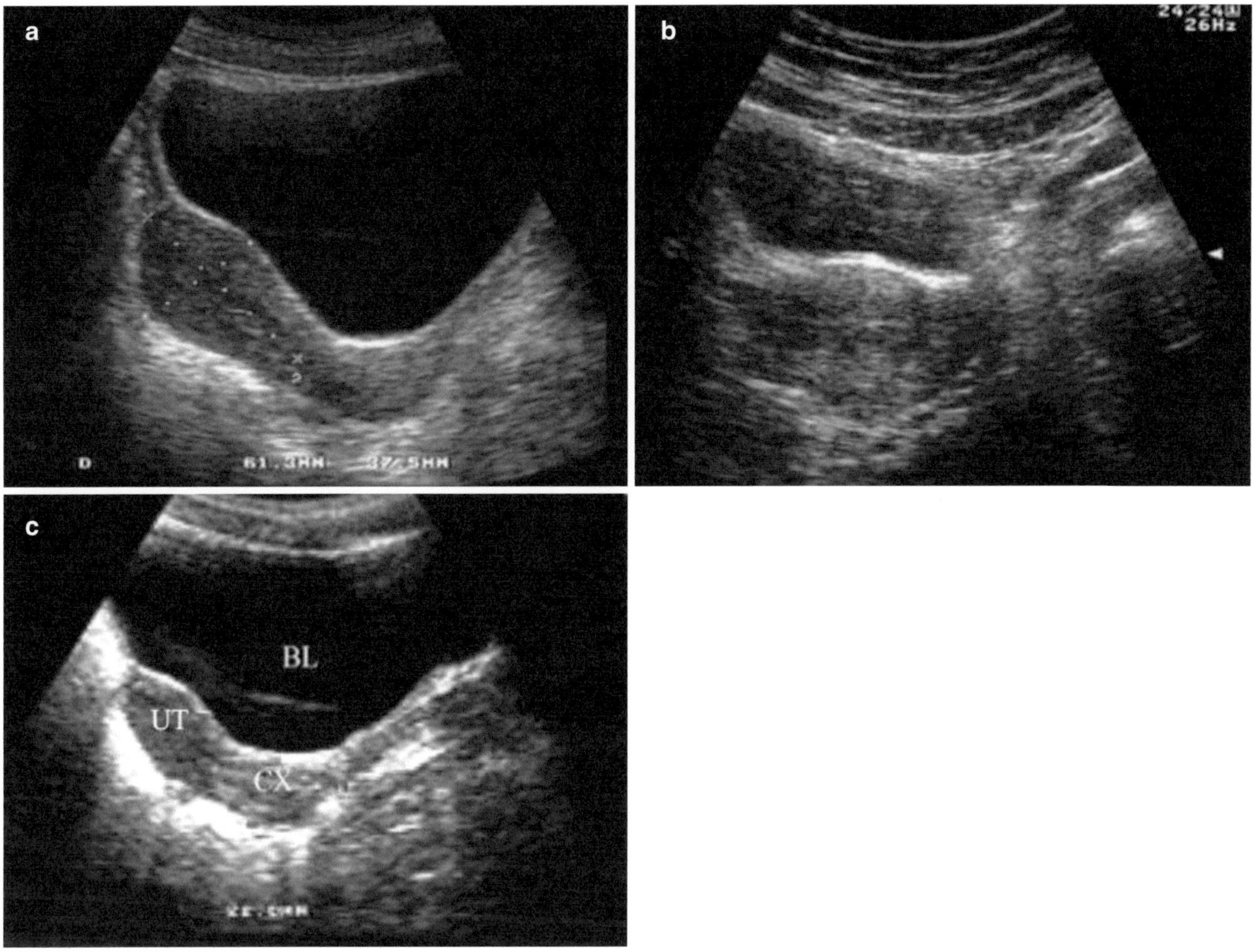

Fig. 1.9 Measurement of the uterus. (**a**). Longitudinal view of the uterus: the distance from the uterine fundus serous layer to the cervical ostium is the long diameter; the maximum thickness vertical to the longitudinal diameter of the uterus is the anteroposterior diameter; (**b**). The transverse diameter of the uterus: The left to right diameter of the oval uterus, measured at the lower edge of the uterine horn on the transverse view, is the transverse diameter; (**c**). The cervical length refers to the distance between the external os and internal os of the cervix, and cervical diameter is the maximum anteroposterior diameter perpendicular to the cervical length

Ovary

Anatomy of Ovary

1. The ovary is located in the pelvic cavity, behind the fallopian tube, one on the left sides of the uterus and the other on the right. The ovary is oval and is connected to the posterior layer of the broad ligament.
2. The dense connective tissue in the surface of the ovary is called the tunica albuginea. The ovarian tissue under the tunica albuginea is divided into cortex and medulla. There are tens of thousands of primordial follicles and dense connective tissue in the cortex. The medulla contains loose connective tissue, abundant blood vessels, nerves, lymphatic vessels, and a small amount of smooth muscle fibers. No follicles exit in the medulla.
3. The shape and size of the ovaries are age-related. The ovary in adult women weighs 5–6 g, and the volume is less than 6 ml. The ovarian volume is less than 1 ml before 2 years old, 2 ml before 12 years old, and reaches 6 ml in the ovulation phase in women of childbearing age. After menopause, the ovaries shrink and become smaller and harder. The length, width, and thickness of the ovary are about 0.5 cm, respectively. Prior to puberty, the surface of the ovary is smooth, which contains multiple follicles. Ovulation since puberty results in an uneven ovarian surface.

Ovarian Physiology

1. Development and maturation of the follicle: all the oocytes in the ovary are formed in the embryonic stage. In every menstrual cycle since puberty, more than 10 follicles, about 5 mm in diameter, begin to grow under the influence of follicle-stimulating hormone (FSH). If the FSH receptor is sufficient, the follicle will synthesize enough estrogen, which acts synergistically with growth

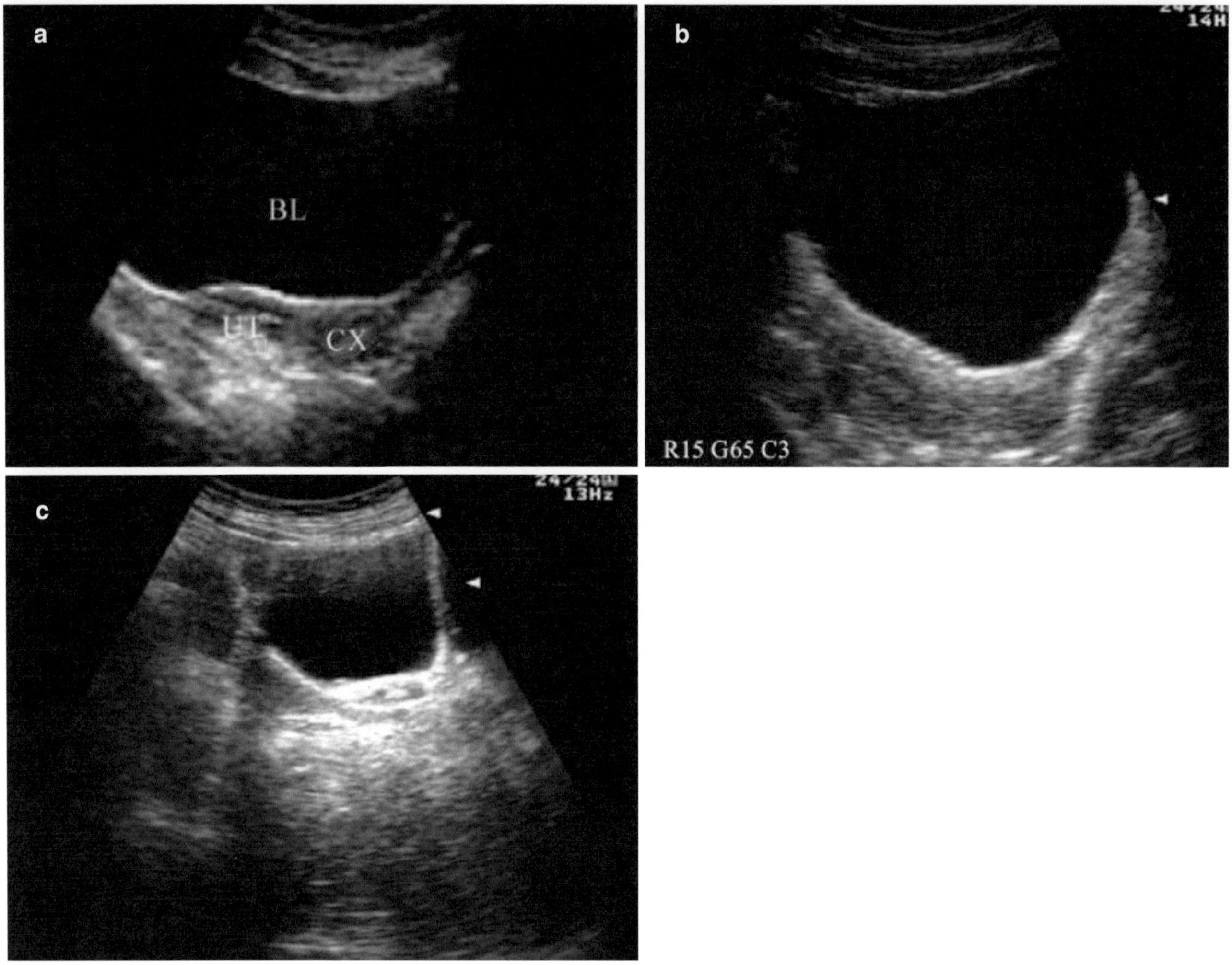

Fig. 1.10 Ratio of the uterine body to cervix length in different periods. (**a**). Ratio of the uterine body to cervix length is 1:1 in adolescence, (**b**). 2:1 in adulthood; (**c**). 1:1 in menopause

Table 1.2 Uterine size in adulthood in Sichuan province

	(cm, $\bar{x} \pm s$)			
	Nulliparous women		Multiparous women	
Items	Size of the uterus	95% confidence interval	Size of the uterus	95% confidence interval
Length of the uterine body	4.97 ± 0.62	3.80–6.21	5.35 ± 0.65	4.13–6.61
Anteroposterior diameter of the uterine body	3.48 ± 0.38	2.73–4.22	3.80 ± 0.36	3.10–4.56
Transverse diameter of the uterus	4.60 ± 0.56	2.54–5.70	4.96 ± 0.52	3.92–6.11
Length of the uterine cavity	3.75 ± 0.52	2.76–4.82	4.00 ± 0.55	2.94–5.14
Transverse diameter of the uterine cavity	2.73 ± 0.45	1.81–3.63	2.96 ± 0.51	2.00–4.42
Cervical length	2.64 ± 0.43	1.85–3.52	2.78 ± 0.42	2.62–3.60
Anteroposterior diameter of the cervix	2.62 ± 0.32	2.01–3.34	2.93 ± 0.40	2.17–3.70

Note: the data is from the West China Second University Hospital, Sichuan University

factor to stimulating further follicle development. Generally, only one growing follicle matures and reaches 18–20 mm in diameter during each menstrual cycle.

2. Ovulation: mature follicles secrete lots of estradiol and little progesterone. Under the stimulation of estrogen, luteinizing hormone (LH) and FSH are secreted in a peak form. The oocyte is discharged when the mature follicle ruptures, and the follicular fluid flows into the pelvic cavity.
3. Luteal phase: The mature follicle collapses after ovulation, the blood vessel in the theca ruptures, and the blood flows into the cavity and forms hematoma, called Corpus

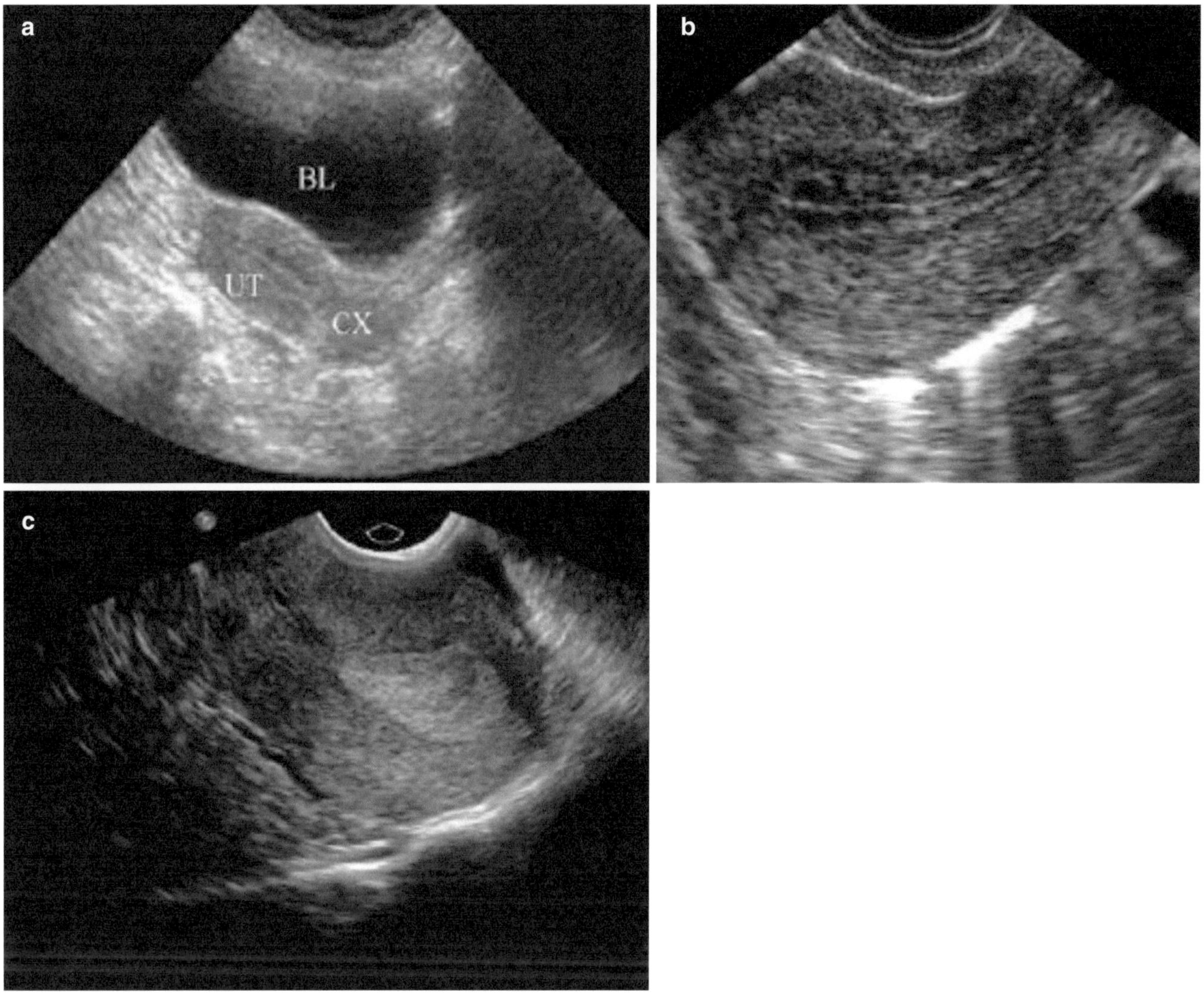

Fig. 1.11 Cyclically change of endometrium. (**a**). In the early phase of hyperplasia, the endometrium shows a hyperechoic line; (**b**). In hyperplasia, the endometrium is hyperechoic and strip-shaped; (**c**). In the secretory phase, the endometrium shows hyperechoic in a fusiform shape

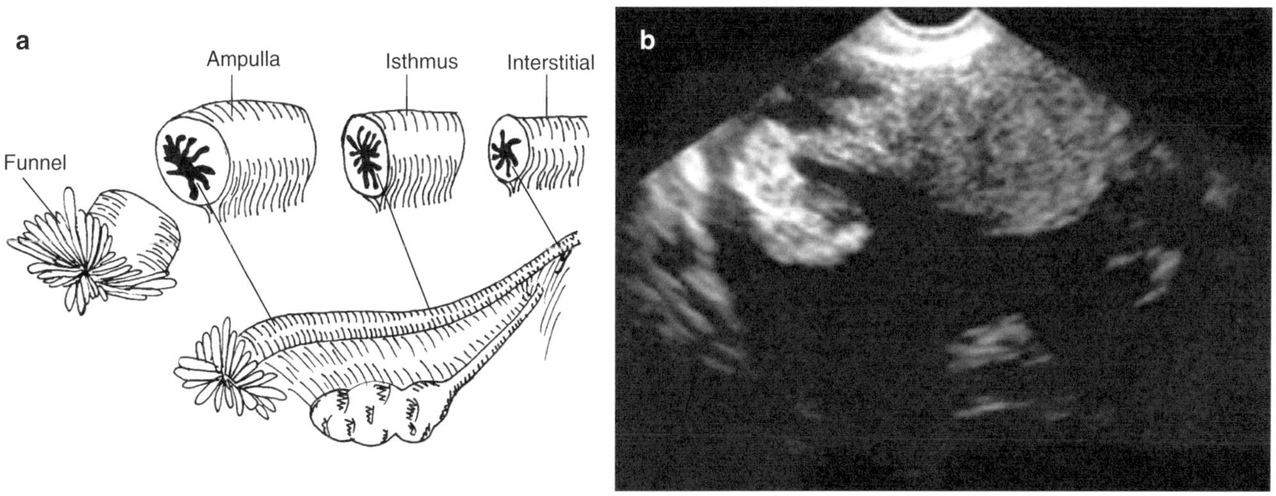

Fig. 1.12 The fallopian tube. (**a**). Composition of the fallopian tube and transverse view image; (**b**). Sonogram of the fallopian tube

hemorrhagicum. The rupture of the follicle wall is quickly closed by fibrin and repaired. The granulosa cells and endometrial cells of the follicle wall invade inward, forming the corpus luteum together with surrounding outer follicular membranes, and begin to secrete progesterone. After ovulation, progesterone secretion of the corpus luteum increases gradually, reaching the peak at day 7–8 after ovulation, then decreases slowly to the level in the follicular phase when menstruation comes. The life span of the corpus luteum is about 2 weeks. After 6–8 days of degeneration, cells of the corpus luteum degenerates, and the tissue is fibrotic and scar-like, which is called the corpus albicans (Fig. 1.14).

Sonogram of the Ovary

1. The ovaries are located on both sides of the uterus, near the bottom of the uterus. The sonogram shows that the ovary is solid elliptical tissue. The ovarian size is about 4 cm × 3 cm × 1 cm in childbearing women. The ovary appears attenuated and hypoechoic, and the follicle is round and anechoic. The two ovaries are slightly different in size, varying with age and menstrual cycle (Fig. 1.15).

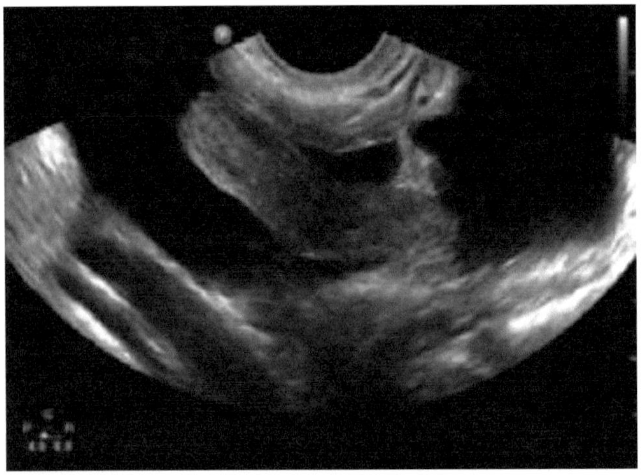

Fig. 1.13 Sonogram of the fallopian tube sonogram shows the fallopian tube floating in the ascites

The two ovaries are oval, with a clear boundary. The echo is slightly higher than that of the uterus. Small follicles are visible.

2. The ovary is connected to the uterus by the ovarian ligament, with a large degree of mobility and unfixed position. During an ultrasonic examination, pay attention to the scanning range, looking above and behind or far away from the uterus. The ovarian position variation and obvious intestinal gas interference affect the display rate of the ovary. The internal iliac vessels are anatomical markers for finding ovaries (Fig. 1.16).
3. Measure the ovarian length and anteroposterior diameter on the maximum long axis section of the ovary and measure its width on the transverse view.
4. The size of the follicle changes with the menstrual cycle in childbearing age. Ultrasound can observe the ovarian changes in the follicular phase, ovulatory phase, and luteal phase during the normal menstrual cycle (Fig. 1.17).

Adjacent Organs

1. Bladder and ureter
   (a) The bladder (BL) is located in front of the uterus and the upper part of the vagina and is divided into the bladder top, bladder bottom, bladder body, and neck of the bladder. There are no obvious boundaries among these parts. A closed urachus in the front center of the bladder is visible, and ureters are inserted on both sides of the back.
   (b) The ureters start from the renal pelvis, travel down the peritoneum, enter the pelvis, cross the uterine artery at the point 2 cm next to the cervix, and then enter the bladder. The total length of the ureters is about 25 cm.
   (c) The distended bladder represents a clear outline and smooth and continuous inner wall. The cavity filled with urine is an anechoic area. The bladder shape in females is affected by the degree of distention and by sonography view. Color Doppler flow imaging shows the urine spray phenomenon (Figs. 1.18 and 1.19).
   (d) Usually, ureter is not visible via ultrasound. According to its anatomical position, scan from bot-

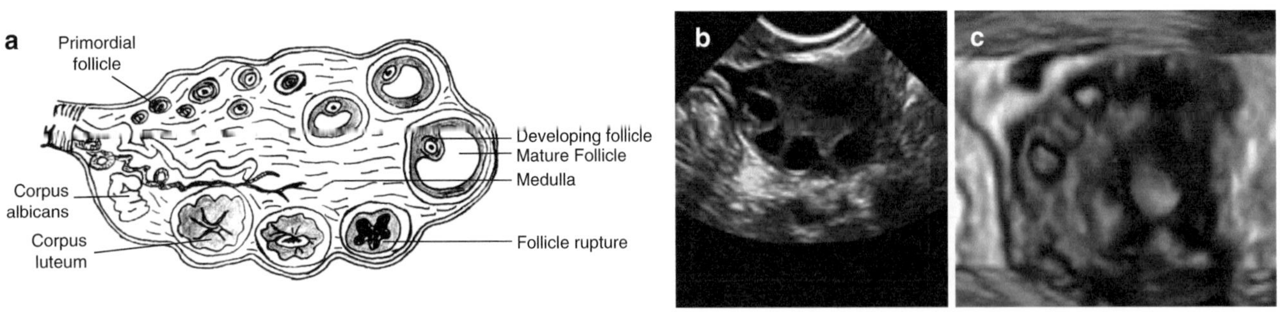

Fig. 1.14 Ovaries. (**a**). Ovarian structure and follicular diagram of each phase; (**b**). 2-D and 3-D ultrasound images of the ovary

tom to top through the distended bladder, and a tubular anechoic ureter is shown above the level of the vagina, lying posterior to the ovary and anterior to the internal iliac arteries and veins.

2. Pelvic Intestinal tract
   (a) The intestinal tract in the pelvic cavity is cloud-like hyperechoic due to inflation, accompanied by posterior shadows. Intestinal peristalsis is visible.

The pelvic organs cannot be displayed by transabdominal scanning if the bladder is not moderately distended. The intestinal tract can be pushed away by the distended bladder, then the pelvic organs and part of the intestinal tract could be shown clearly (Figs. 1.20 and 1.21).

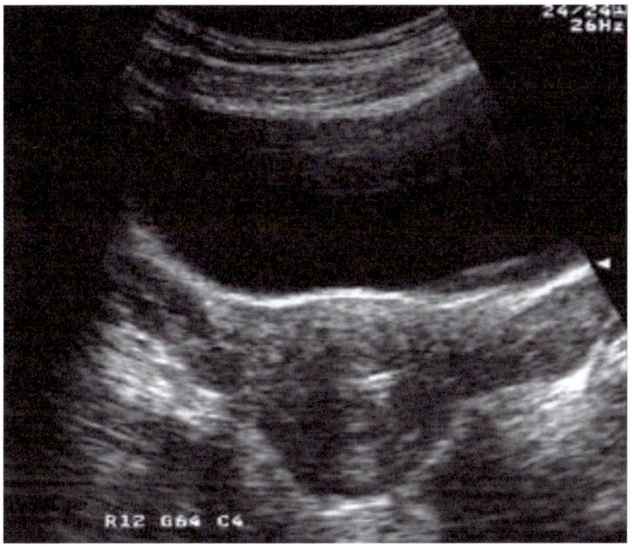

Fig. 1.15 Sonogram of the ovary

   (b) During the pelvic examination, pay attention to identify the solid or mixed ovarian tumors from the fecal and gas echoes in the rectum. If it is difficult to identify, thorough defecation or enema will be required before recheck.

3. Muscles in the pelvis
   (a) Iliopsoas muscle is located on both sides of the pelvis, displayed by the oblique view from the abdominal midline to the hip. They appear hypoechoic long-bands on the longitudinal view, and two hypoechoic ellipses on both sides of the bladder on the transverse view (Fig. 1.22).
   (b) Iliac fossa triangle: the iliac fossa triangle is composed of abdominal wall, iliopsoas muscle, and floating intestine. Usually, this triangle is full of intestinal tubes. When there is bleeding or fluid accumulation in the abdominal cavity, a liquid dark area appears in this triangle (Fig. 1.23).

1.2.2 Blood Vessels and Color Doppler Sonography of Female Pelvic Cavity

1. The internal iliac artery provides the main arterial supply to the pelvic organs via multiple branches (Fig. 1.24).
2. The uterine artery originates from the anterior trunk of the internal iliac artery, at the point about 2 cm outside the cervix, crosses the end of the ureter anteriorly to the lateral uterine margin, and divides into two branches before reaching the upper cervical vagina. The smaller branch travels downward and supplies the cervix and the upper vagina. The main branch of the uterine artery ascends in a tortuous course lateral to the uterus in the broad ligament, supplying the uterus, ovary, and fallopian tube.

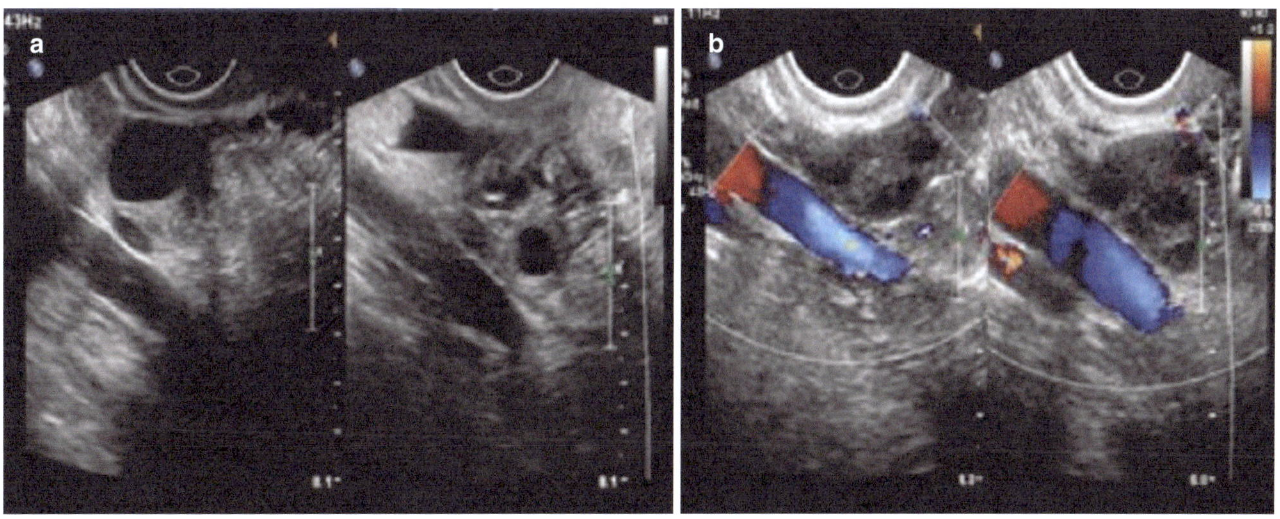

Fig. 1.16 Relationship between ovary and internal iliac vessels. (**a**). 2-D images of the ovary and internal iliac vessels; (**b**). Color Doppler flow images of ovary and internal iliac vessels

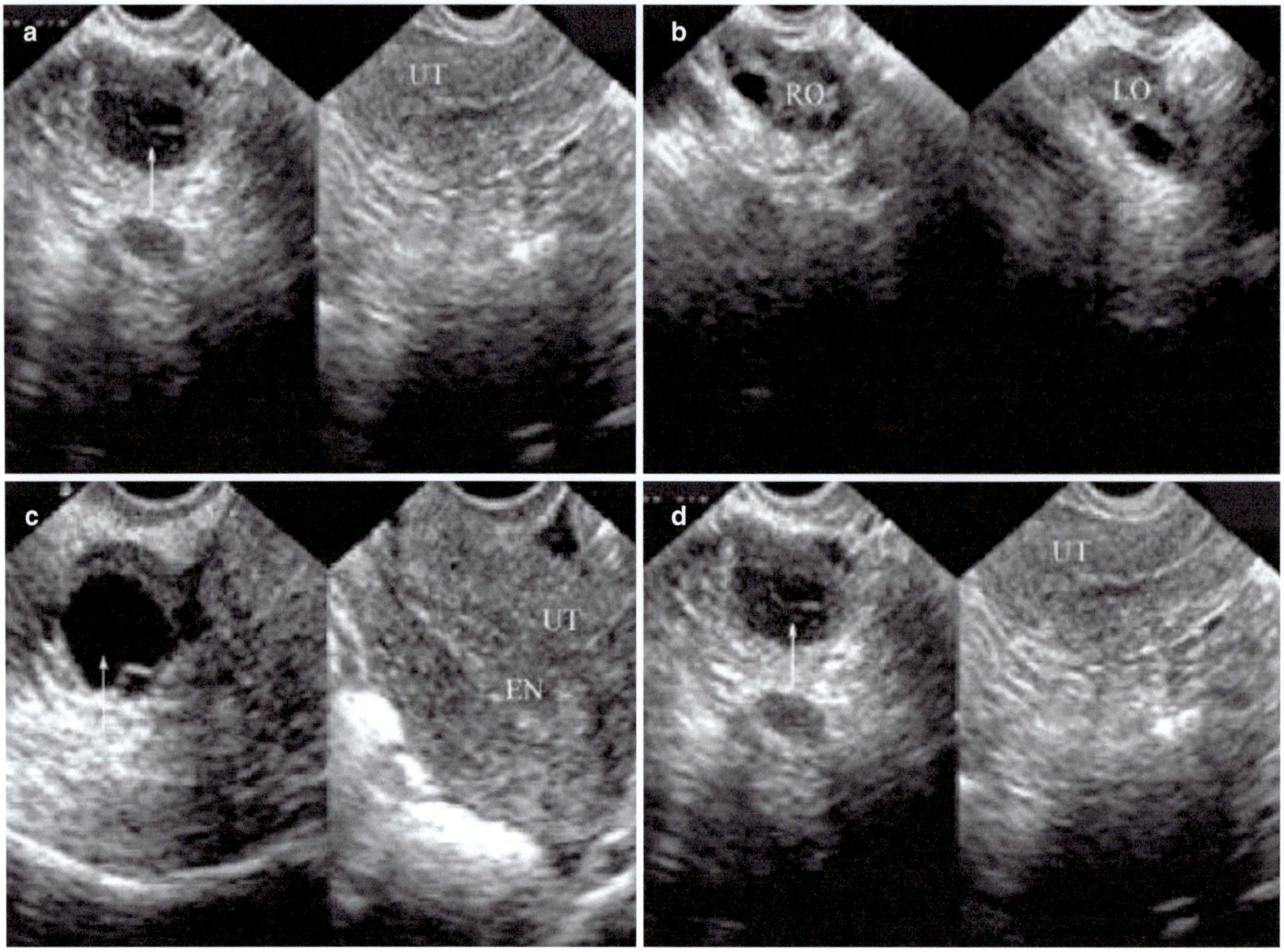

Fig. 1.17 The ovary in the follicular phase, ovulatory phase, and luteal phase during the normal menstrual cycle. (**a**). During a follicular development period, 5–10 developing follicles are visible; (**b**). Pre-ovulation phase: the follicle, reaching 14 mm in diameter, is likely to mature, which is defined as the dominant follicle (arrow); (**c**). Follicle maturation phase: The follicle is more than 18 mm in diameter, 20–25 mm in average, and moves to the surface of the ovary; (**d**). Luteal phase: the corpus luteum is formed after ovulation, hypoechoic, with a slightly thicker wall and irregular edge. Some weak dot echo can be seen inside the cyst

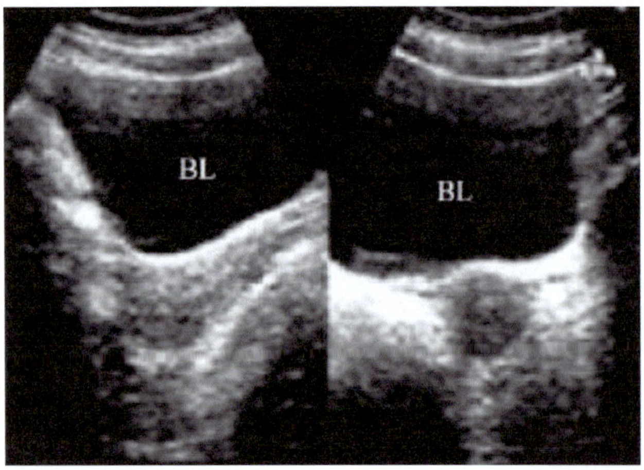

Fig. 1.18 Sagittal and transverse view of the distended bladder

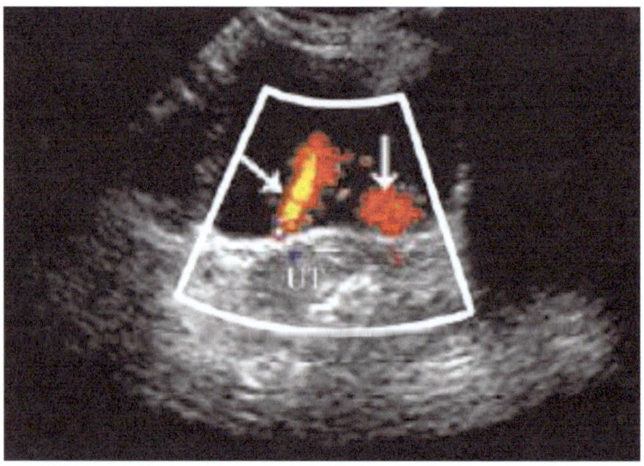

Fig. 1.19 Urine spray (arrow) in the trigone area of the bladder

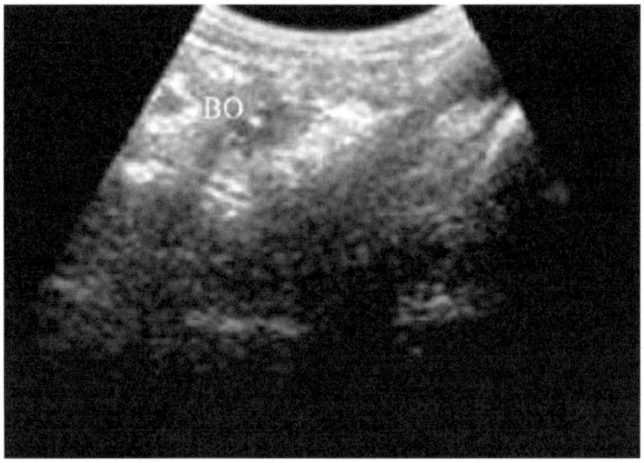

Fig. 1.20 Sonogram of an empty bladder. The pelvis is filled with intestine

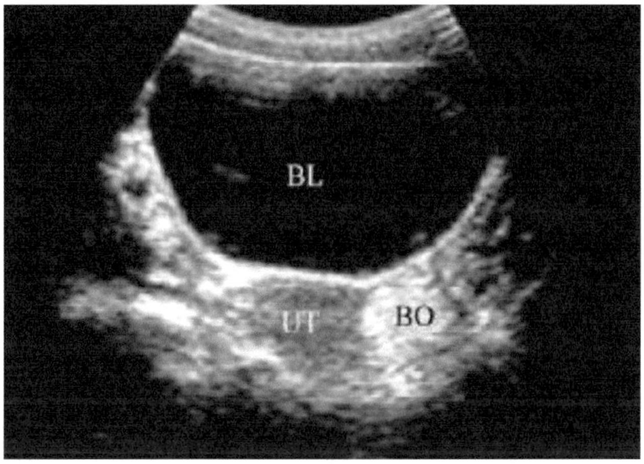

Fig. 1.21 Sonogram of the filled bladder, part of the intestinal tract is visible

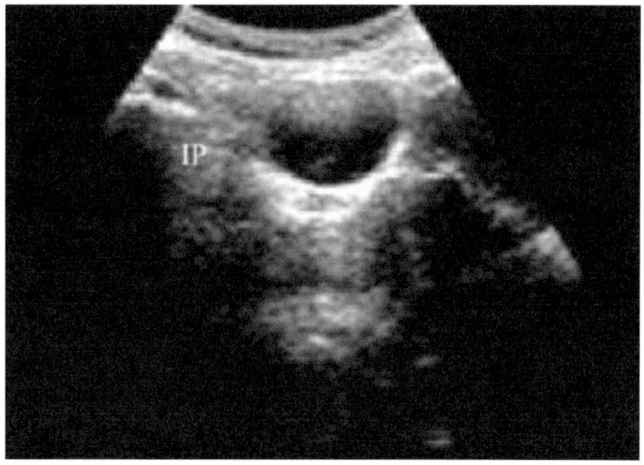

Fig. 1.22 Iliopsoas muscles located on both sides of the uterus

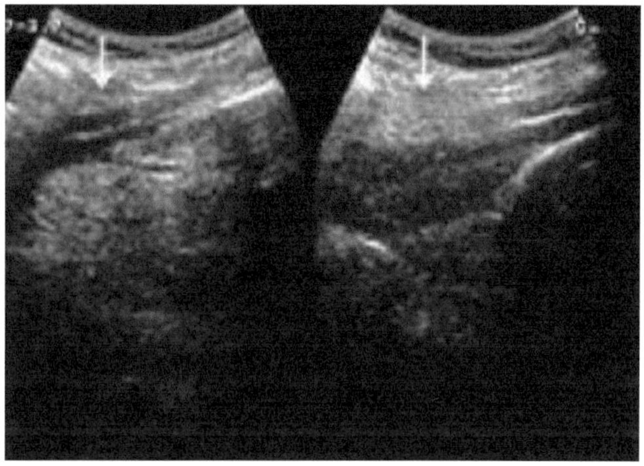

Fig. 1.23 Bilateral iliac fossa triangles

Fig. 1.24 Diagram of female pelvic blood supply

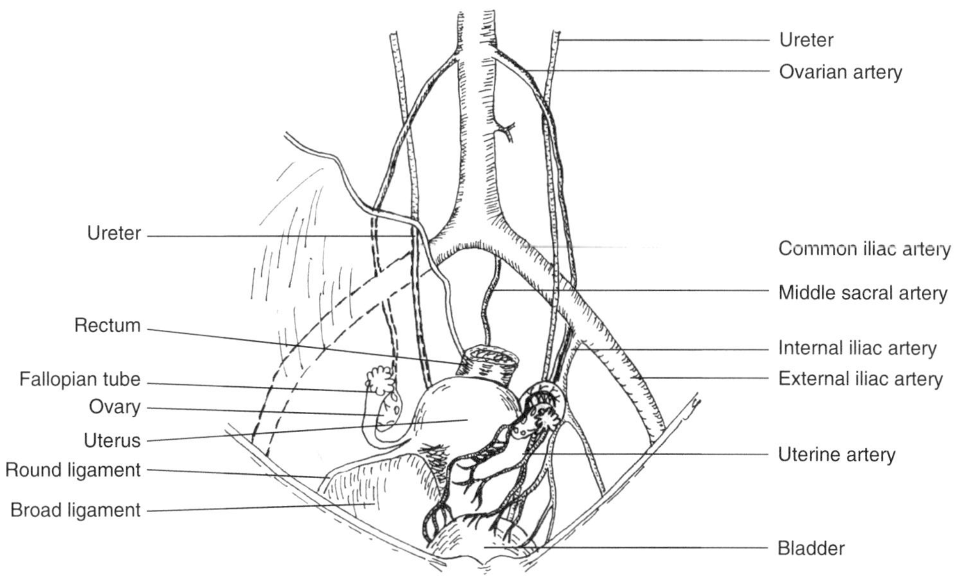

3. The uterine artery branches pierce the uterine myometrium and divide into arcuate arteries and spiral arteries to supply the uterine muscle and endometrium.
4. The uterine venous plexus accompanies the arcuate artery and circulates in the uterine myometrium.

1.2.2.1 Doppler Characteristics of the Internal Iliac Artery and Vein

1. The systolic spectrum of internal iliac artery is positive, with lower resistance.

Sometimes, small humplike spectrums are visible at the end of diastole.

2. The iliac vein, accompanied by the internal iliac artery, has no pulsatile features, and the waveform fluctuates with the breathing. The blood flow direction is opposite to the adjacent artery (Figs. 1.25 and 1.26).

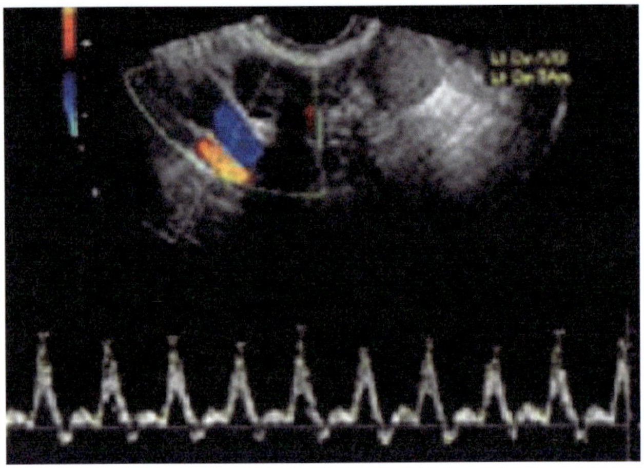

Fig. 1.25 Color Doppler flow image and spectrum of the internal iliac artery

1.2.2.2 Color Blood Flow Imaging of Uterine Artery

1. Place the interest box 2 cm away from the cervix for oblique or longitudinal scanning to show the uterine artery.
2. The blood flow in the uterine muscle is circular or punctate. The closer to the serosa, the more blood flow signal. The uterine spiral artery is challenging to display during non-pregnancy. In early pregnancy, the spiral artery presents punctate blood flow around the gestational sac, with low resistance (Figs. 1.27 and 1.28).

1.2.2.3 Doppler Ultrasound Characteristics of Uterine Artery

1. During the non-pregnant state and early pregnancy, the color Doppler spectrum of the uterine artery demonstrates a sharp systolic peak, decreased diastolic velocity, and early diastolic notch. With the change of the menstrual cycle, the resistance index (RI), pulsatility index (PI), and other related parameters of the uterine artery and branches change accordingly. The RI and PI values increase ($RI = 0.88 \pm 0.1$, $PI = 1.8 \pm 0.4$) during the late secretion and menstrual phase; keep intermediate in the proliferative phase; and decrease in the early and mid-secretion phase (Fig. 1.29).
2. During the second trimester of pregnancy, the uterine artery gradually thickens, resulting in a further decrease in blood flow resistance. The resistance index gradually decreases, changing from the high-resistance waveform pattern to the low-resistance waveform (Fig. 1.30).
3. The uterine artery and branches are challenging to display after menopause.

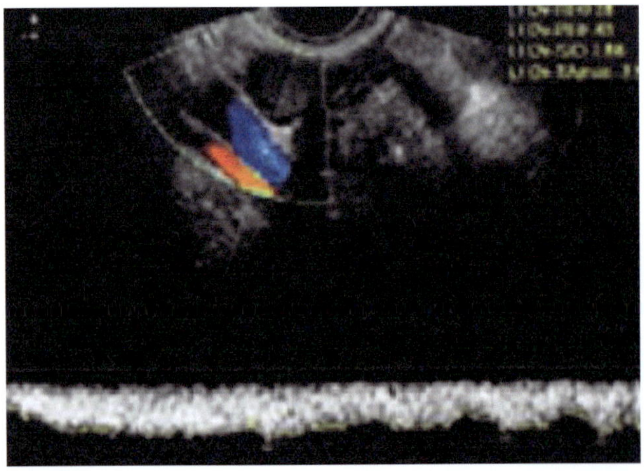

Fig. 1.26 Color Doppler flow image and spectrum of the internal iliac vein

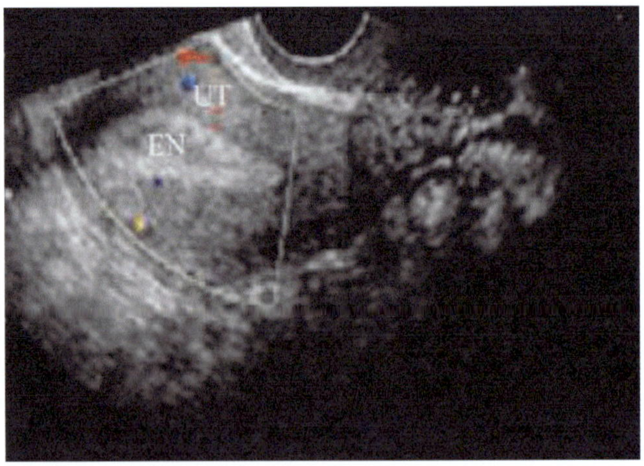

Fig. 1.27 Color blood flow imaging of uterine muscle

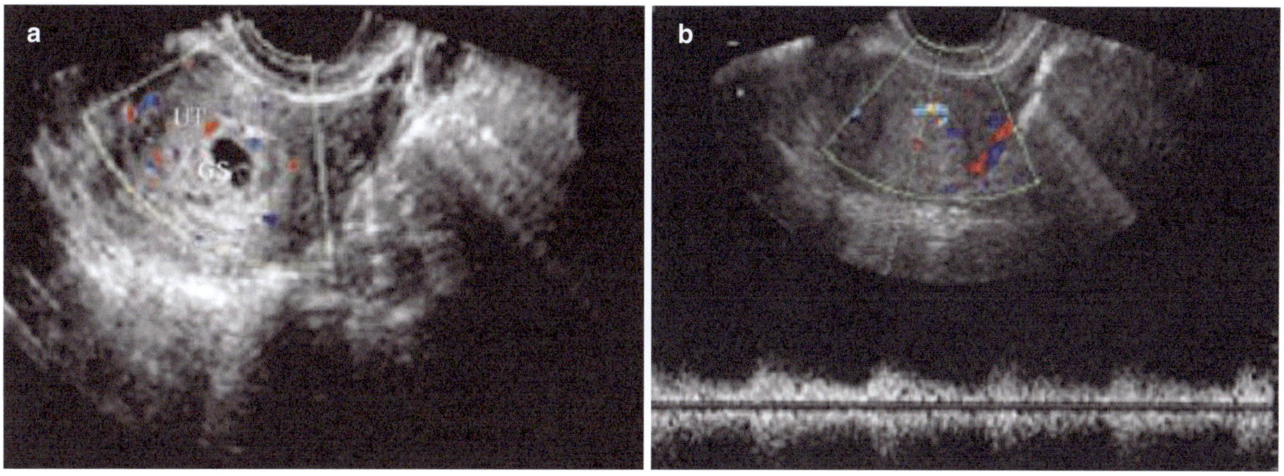

Fig. 1.28 Color flow imaging and spectrum of trophoblast around gestational sac. (**a**). Color blood flow signal of trophoblast; (**b**). Blood flow spectrum of trophoblast, with a low-resistance waveform

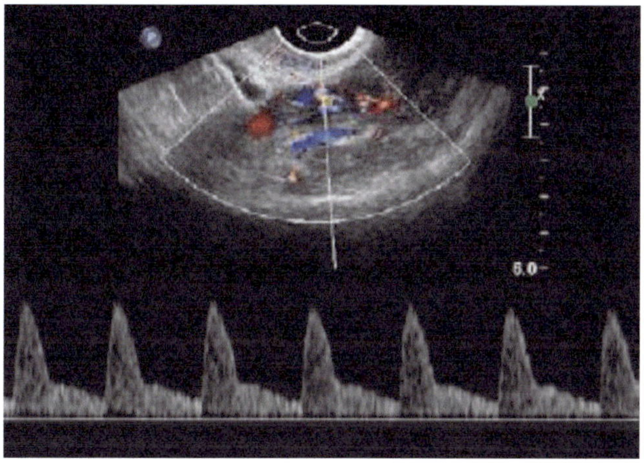

Fig. 1.29 Color Doppler spectrum of the uterine artery during the non-pregnant period

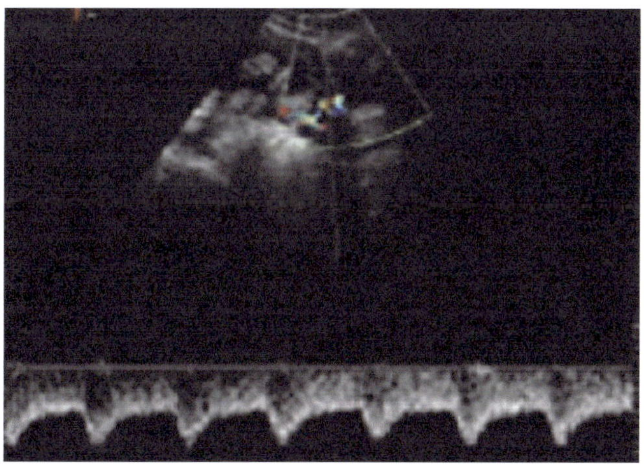

Fig. 1.30 Color Doppler spectrum of the uterine artery during pregnancy

1.2.2.4 Doppler Ultrasound Characteristics of Ovarian Arteries

1. The ovarian artery originates from the abdominal aorta, descends to the pelvis along with the anterior psoas muscle, crosses the ureter and the lower common iliac artery, and enters the ovarian hilum through the mesentery. The left side ovarian artery may originate from the left renal artery. The fallopian tube is supplied by ovarian arteria branches in the mesentery of the fallopian tube. The end of ovarian arteria branches anastomoses with the uterine artery's ovarian branch near the uterine horn. The ovaries have a dual blood supply system.
2. The detection of ovarian blood vessels is affected by the ultrasound instrument's sensitivity, the scanning method, and the operator's professionalism.
3. Color Doppler can display the blood vessels coming from the ovarian hilum and the ovarian blood signals distributed in a star or radial pattern (Fig. 1.31).
4. Color blood flow and spectrum Doppler examination can reflect ovarian function. The spectrum of the main ovarian artery branch presents a high-resistance waveform, indicating that the ovary is not functional or inactive. It is challenging to detect ovarian blood flow signals after menopause because of the decreasing ovarian function and reducing blood vessels in the ovary (Fig. 1.32).

1.3 Ultrasonic Examination and Scanning Method in Obstetrics and Gynecology

The main ultrasound examination methods in obstetrics and gynecology are transabdominal scanning, transvaginal scanning, transrectal scanning, transperineal scanning, and transcavitary scanning.

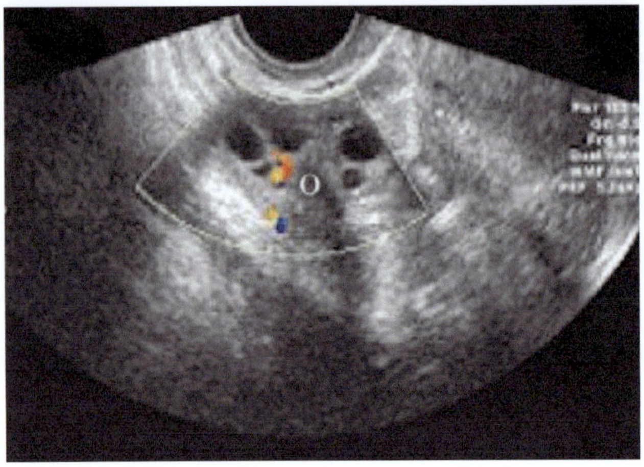

Fig. 1.31 Color Doppler flow image of the ovary

1.3.1 Transabdominal Scanning

Transabdominal scanning (TAS) is the most commonly used ultrasound method in obstetrics and gynecology, applicable to all women who need pelvic ultrasound examination. The frequency of probe used in TAS is 3.5–5.0 MHz, and the convex vibration electronic probe is preferred. TAS provides a wider field of view and flexible operation angle and plane, which is conducive to the overall display of pelvic viscera and adjacent organs.

1. Preparation before TAS.

Except for the women with normal condition in mid to late pregnancy, the bladder of the examinee is required to be appropriately filled before TAS.

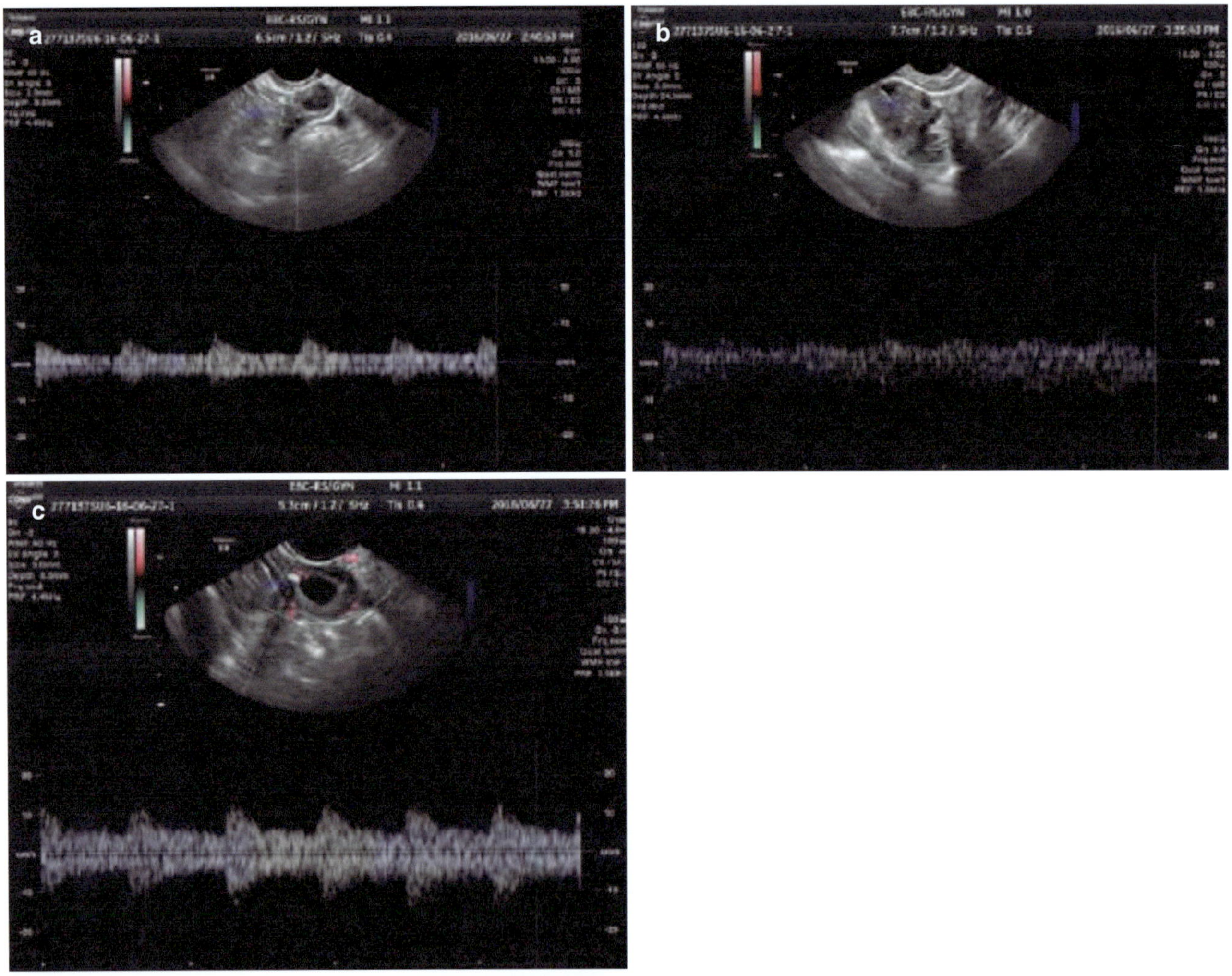

Fig. 1.32 Ovarian color blood flow imaging and spectrum during the physiological phases. (**a**). Menstrual phase: spectrum with low amplitude and high resistance; (**b**). Follicular phase: the spectrum of internal ovarian artery is parabolic, and the RI value is about 0.5; (**c**). Luteal phase: the formation of corpus luteum vessels and blood flow resistance is related to pregnancy

2. The purpose of bladder distention.

The urine in the moderately filled bladder is used as a liquid medium to form an acoustic window, which can push the intestine that covers the pelvic organs away, which can avoid intestinal gas interference, and which can contribute to better present the posterior pelvic organs' morphology and outline. For suspected cervical insufficiency or bleeding caused by placenta previa in mid-late pregnancy, a filled bladder is required to present the lower segment of uterus, the cervical structure, and the relationship between the lower placental edge and the internal cervical os clearly.

3. Methods and standards for filling the bladder.
   (a) Require the patient to drink 500–700 ml water in an hour, and TAS can be performed until the patient has obvious micturition desire.
   (b) Catheterization: For patients with emergencies, renal insufficiency, elderly, or unable to drink plenty of water in a short period or hold urine, insert urinary catheters under routine disinfection and inject 300–500 ml of sterile saline.
4. The influence of bladder filling degree on TAS. If the bladder is insufficiently filled or empty, the pelvic organs fail to completely display. Furthermore, because of the intestinal gas interference, the pelvic organs cannot be displayed at all, causing missed diagnosis or misdiagnosis. The overfilling bladder may compress the uterus to make it smaller, affecting the measurement accuracy. Some pelvic masses may be pushed out of the pelvis, leading to missed diagnosis (Fig. 1.33).
5. Scanning method.

The patient takes the supine position. Place the probe on the surface of the abdominal wall between the umbilicus and the pubic symphysis, and smear some couplant locally. Firstly, show the mid-sagittal view of the uterus using longitudinal scanning. In this view, the echo of the uterine endometrium and the cervical endometrial echo are displayed on the same sagittal view. Observe the morphology and contour of the uterus, cervix, and endometrium and the echo of the uterine three-layer structure, and measure the anteroposterior diameter, length of the uterus, and endometrial thickness on this section. Then, choose the midsagittal view of the uterus as the center, slide the probe slowly to each side of the uterus and change the scanning angle to observe whether the echo of the uterus and the pelvic sidewalls on each side is abnormal. Rotate the probe by 90 degrees, change to a transverse scan continuously, and sweep upward and downward. Observe the uterine cavity and echo of the anterior and posterior walls on each transverse section, and measure the transverse diameter of the uterus. The ovaries can be scanned longitudinally, horizontally, and diagonally. The scanning angle of the probe is changed during the scanning to display the lesions in the ovary and pelvis more clearly and obtain the best image for diagnosis.

1.3.2 Transvaginal Scanning

Transvaginal scanning (TVS) is an essential method of ultrasound examination in obstetrics and gynecology, which has become a routine method for pelvic ultrasound examination of married women. Choose a transvaginal probe with a frequency of 5.0–7.5 MHz or 5.0–9.0 MHz. Due to the high frequency of transvaginal probe, the scanning approach is closer to the pelvic organs, contributing to a clear display of

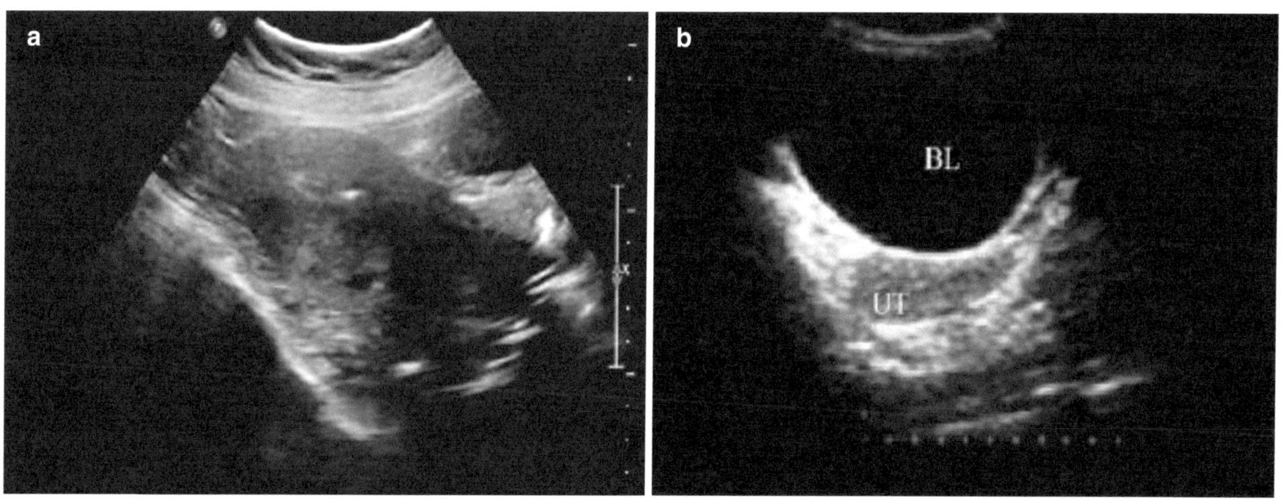

Fig. 1.33 The influence of bladder filling degree on TAS. (**a**). Insufficiently filled bladder. The uterus and ovaries are not clearly showed. (**b**). Overfilling bladder. The uterus is compressed

the tiny structure of the uterus, ovaries, and pelvic masses, so as to obtain sufficient and accurate information and improve the diagnostic accuracy of pelvic diseases.

1.3.2.1 Preparation before Examination

The patient should empty the bladder before the examination. TVS should be arranged in a particular ultrasound exam room, satisfying the conditions for pelvic examination in obstetrics and gynecology. Disposable pads, sterilized rubber condoms, and perineum disinfectants are required.

1.3.2.2 Scanning Method

The patient took the lithotomy position. Put a small amount of couplant inside the sterilized condom and place over the disinfected vaginal probe. Insert the vaginal probe into the vagina gently until the top of the probe reaches the vaginal fornix or cervix, and the probe is generally placed in the posterior vaginal fornix. First, find the standard mid-sagittal view of the uterus: the echo of the uterine endometrium and the cervical endometrium are displayed on the same sagittal view. Then identify the position of the uterus. The excessive anteverted or retroverted uterus may affect the display of the standard sagittal view. Adjust the depth of the probe into the vagina and the angle between the scanning beam and the uterus to obtain a relatively standard image. In this section, observe the condition of the cervix, endometrium, uterine cavity, and myometrium, and measure the anteroposterior diameter, length of the uterus, and endometrial thickness. When it is changeling to obtain satisfied sagittal images of the uterus, apply pressure on the examinee's pubic symphysis with the sonologist's non-scanning hand to make the uterus steady and close to the probe. The handle of the vaginal probe can also be adjusted to make the image more complete and clear. Then rotate the probe to scan the transverse section, measure the transverse diameter of the uterus, and observe the morphology and echo of uterine walls on each side and the uterine cavity. Finally, rotate the probe and slide to the left and right sides of the uterus, using the iliac blood vessels as markers, and find the bilateral ovaries. Measure the ovarian size, observe the shape of the ovary and the structural characteristics of the peripheral mass. Pay attention to distinguish the relationship between the masses and ovaries, and note whether there is fluid or other abnormalities in the rectouterine pouch.

1.3.2.3 Contraindications of TVS

For patients with sizeable pelvic mass or pregnant for more than 3 months, TVS fails to provide entire information of the uterus and mass due to the limitation of high frequency, limited penetration, and focusing depth. TVS is not suitable for unmarried women, patients with an imperforate hymen, and vaginal malformation that cannot place a vaginal probe.

1.3.3 Transrectal Scanning

Transrectal scanning (TRS) requires a special rectal probe. TRS is often used to diagnose malformation of rectum, sigmoid colon, prostate, and other diseases, and acts as an auxiliary way of ultrasound examination in gynecology and obstetrics. It is mainly used to examine the pelvic viscera of unmarried women, elderly patients with severe vaginal atrophy, or patients with vaginal stenosis or severe vaginal malformation caused by vaginal surgery or radiotherapy.

1.3.4 Transperineal Scanning

Transperineal scanning (TPS), placing the probe at the vulva area of women, can eliminate the intestinal gas interference and the attenuation of abdominal fat without a filled bladder. TPS is used to observe female pelvic floor structure and obtain a satisfactory display of cervical lesions, vaginal mass, urinary tract micro-lesions, etc. Pay attention to placing the sterilized condom over the vaginal probe.

1.3.5 Transcavitary Scanning

The probe for transcavitary scanning is a special probe 2–7 mm in diameter, with a frequency in the range of 7.5–20 MHz. Transcavitary scanning is mainly used to observe the tiny pathological lesions of the uterine cavity and myometrium, which is not widely used.

1.3.6 Key Points of Ultrasound Examination in Obstetrics and Gynecology

1. TAS of the pelvis.
   (a) The bladder of the examinee should be appropriately filled before TAS. Patients usually take the supine position. Rotate and slide the probe or combine several scanning techniques.
   (b) On the sagittal section of the uterus, observe the morphology and contour of the uterus, cervix, and endometrium, and measure the anteroposterior diameter, length of the uterus, and endometrial thickness. Observe the uterine body and fundus and measure the transverse diameter of the uterus on the transverse section. Observe the echo characteristics of the myometrium through various sections.
   (c) Measure the ovarian length and anteroposterior diameter on the maximum long axis section of the ovary, and measure its width on the transverse view. Observe the size, morphology, and echo of the ovary. It is recommended to measure the size of the follicle

and record the number when the diameter of the ovarian follicle is more than 1 cm.

(d) The combined scanning method is used in the ultrasound scanning of the fetus in the middle and late pregnancy. Change the scanning technique constantly with the fetal position and movement during the examination, to show the structure and morphology of the fetal surface and internal organs. Prenatal ultrasound scan of the fetus should be carried out in accordance with the prenatal ultrasound grading requirements: general, routine, systematic, and targeted.

2. TVS It is required to empty the bladder before TVS. The examinee should take the lithotomy position. Select a special vaginal probe and pay attention to sterilization and isolation of the vaginal probe during operation.

1.4 Reading and Writing of Sonogram in Obstetrics and Gynecology

1.4.1 Reading Methods of the Sonogram

1.4.1.1 Reading Method of TAS Sonogram

The Sagittal Plane (SP)

When the patient takes the supine position, the left side of the sonogram on the monitor represents the cranial direction of the subject--the uterine bottom, the right side represents the caudal direction--the cervix and vagina, the upper part is the anterior abdominal wall and bladder, and the lower part is the posterior pelvic wall and rectum.

The Transverse Plane (TP)

When the patient takes the supine position scanned in the transverse plane (TP), the left side of the image on the monitor is the left adnexa, and the right side is the right adnexa.

1.4.1.2 Reading Methods of TVS Pelvic Sonogram

The Sagittal View

According to the personal habits of the operator on the sagittal view, set the orientation of the image to display the uterus and adnexa superiorly or inferiorly on the screen.

Reading methods of TVS sonogram:

1. When the uterus and adnexa are displayed inferiorly on the screen, the upper part (near field) of the ultrasound image represents the cranial direction of the subject–the uterus and its bottom, the lower part (far-field) represents the caudal direction --the cervix and vagina, the left side represents the posterior pelvic wall and rectum, and the right side represents the anterior pelvic wall and bladder.
2. When the uterus and adnexa are displayed superiorly on the screen, the upper part of the ultrasound image represents the caudal direction of the subject–the cervix, the lower part represents the cranial direction–the uterus and its bottom, the left side of the sonogram represents the anterior pelvic wall and bladder, and the right side represents the posterior pelvic wall and rectum.

The Transverse Section

The transverse section of the uterus is displayed by rotating the probe until the beam is perpendicular to the axis of the uterus. The right side of the sonogram represents the right uterine wall and right adnexa, and the left side represents the left uterine wall and left adnexa. The scanning direction of the probe determines the position of the left and right adnexa.

1.4.1.3 Orientation Recognition of Fetal Sonogram

According to the relationship between the longitudinal axis of the pregnant women and that of the fetus, as well as the relationship between the fetal presentation and the pelvis of pregnant women, we can identify the fetal position and orientation.

1.4.2 Writing Methods and Requirements of an Ultrasonic Report in Obstetrics and Gynecology

The ultrasonic report is the conclusion of one examination, the clinical basis for diagnosis, and the evidence for informing the examinee of the ultrasonic examination with words or images as well. The report in gynecology and obstetrics mainly includes three parts: general items, examination findings (description), and diagnosis opinions.

1.4.2.1 The General Items

Complete the items according to the general items of the report. If necessary, add the instrument model, probe frequency, scanning method, etc.

1.4.2.2 Examination Findings

Analyze comprehensively and make a detailed and objective description after obtaining several ultrasound images by various scanning methods. It mainly includes the morphology, structure, size, location, and echo characteristics of the examined organs, as well as the relationship with the surrounding organs. When necessary, the important negative image features of relevant organs should also be described for differential diagnosis.

1.4.2.3 The Diagnosis Opinions

The diagnosis opinions should be brief to indicate the location and nature of the lesions. The principle of ultrasonic diagnosis is to point out the location and physical property. For the diseases that can be diagnosed from the image, we can directly prompt the definitive diagnosis or possible diagnosis of disease; for the diseases that cannot be determined from the image, it is not suitable to prompt the diagnosis of disease directly. In patients with multiple disease changes, the definitive diagnosis should be given priority. Generally, it is not appropriate to make a pathological diagnosis directly.

The designated superior doctor should review the ultrasonic report written by the refresher doctor or technician and sign before official releasing. The ultrasonic report should be neat, clear, and easy to understand, avoiding altering and typos. No false ultrasonic report is allowed in any case.

1.5 Notices for Ultrasound Examination in Obstetrics and Gynecology

1. The operation should be standardized, skilled, and pay attention to the scanning ways and methods of obstetrics and gynecology ultrasound. Interventional ultrasound and intracavitary ultrasound must strictly follow the asepsis principle to prevent infection. Make sure there are no mistakes in the prevention of complications and emergency preparation during operation. Interventional ultrasound diagnosis or treatment should be carried out in a special ultrasound intervention room.
2. Explain the necessity of examination, possible results and uncomfortable reactions or complications to the patients before the patients undertake intracavitary ultrasound, interventional ultrasound or treatment, and some special ultrasound diagnoses. The examinations can only be carried out after obtaining the understanding and agreement of the patients and their families, and the patients are requested to sign the relevant informed consent forms.
3. The ultrasonic report should be written thoughtfully, and the ultrasonic diagnostic results should be objective and authentic. For diseases or structures that cannot be judged by ultrasonic images, it is advisable to just make a description of the image rather than report a speculative diagnosis of diseases.

Suggested Reading

1. Society of Diagnostic Medical Sonographers. Sonography examination guidelines. 2nd ed. Plano: SDMS; 2006.
2. American Institute of Ultrasound in Medicine. Guidelines for cleaning and preparing endocavitary ultrasound transducers between patients. AIUM official statement. Laurel: AIUM; 2014.
3. American Institute of Ultrasound in Medicine. Official statement as low as reasonably achievable (ALARA) principle. Laurel: AIUM; 2014.
4. Shortliff EH, Cimino JJ. Biomedical informatics: computer applications in health care and biomedicine. 4th ed. New York: Springer; 2014.
5. Hacker NF, Moore JG. Essentials of obstetrics and gynecology. Philadelphia: WB Saunders; 1986.
6. Hansman M, Hackeloer BJ, Staudach A. Ultrasound diagnosis in obstetrics and gynecology. Berlin: Springer-Verlag; 1985.
7. American Institute of Ultrasound in Medicine. Guidelines for performance of the antepartum obstetrical ultrasound examination. Laurel: AIUM; 2007.

2 Application of Diagnostic Ultrasound in the Perinatal Period

Taizhu Yang, Ying Tang, Yu Tian, Bo Zhang, Hong Luo, Qi Zhu, and Houqing Pang

2.1 Changes of the Uterus During Pregnancy

During pregnancy, with the participation of hormones produced by the placenta and the influence of neuroendocrine, the maternal uterus will undergo a series of anatomical and physiological changes to meet the needs of the fetal growth and development.

2.1.1 The Uterus

2.1.1.1 The Volume and Size

The uterus undergoes a gradual increase in volume and size, and becomes softer during pregnancy. The uterus is about 7 cm × 5 cm × 3 cm in non-pregnancy period and rises to 35 cm × 25 cm × 22 cm at term.

The volume of the uterine cavity is about 10 ml or less in the non-pregnancy period, which increases over hundreds of times at term (nearly 5000 ml).

2.1.1.2 The Thickness of the Myometrium

The thickness of the myometrium is about 1 cm in non-pregnancy, 2.0–2.5 cm in the second trimester, and then becomes thinner from 1.0 to 1.5 cm at term.

2.1.1.3 The Morphology and Blood Flow of Uterine Arteries

The uterine artery twists in non-pregnancy and turns to be straight at term to meet the increasing need for blood flow in the placenta villous space. A 4 to six-fold increase in uterine blood flow is observed at term (450–650 ml per minute), of which the muscle layer accounts for about 5%, the uterine decidual layer accounts for 10% to 15%, and the placenta accounts for the most part (80% to 85%). However, uterine blood flow is significantly reduced during contraction.

2.1.2 Isthmus Uteri

Isthmus is the narrowest portion of the uterus, which is located between the uterine body and cervix, and becomes soft during pregnancy. It is just 1 cm in length in non-pregnancy. After 12 weeks of gestation, it gradually stretches and becomes thinner, and expands as a part of the uterine cavity, thereby forming the lower segment of the uterus. It gradually stretches to 7 to 10 cm in labor and becomes part of the soft birth canal.

2.1.3 Cervix

The length of the cervix tube is 2 to 3 cm before labor, and that of primipara was slightly longer than that of the multipara. After the onset of labor, with muscle at the level of internal ostium pulling upward, the cervix gradually shortens until it disappears. The changes are mediated through the coordinated effects of regular uterine contractions, fetal presentation, and anterior amniotic fluid sac.

This chapter was translated by Qian Hu, Tiantian Ye, and Miaoqian Wang.

Department of Obstetrics and Gynecology, Beijing Hospital, National Center of Gerontology, Beijing, China.
Department of Ultrasound, Beijing Luhe Hospital, Affiliated to Capital MedicalUniversity, Beijing, China.

T. Yang (✉) · Y. Tang · Y. Tian · B. Zhang · H. Luo · Q. Zhu · H. Pang
Department of Ultrasonography, West China Second University Hospital, Sichuan University, Chengdu, China

T. Yang, H. Luo (eds.), *Practical Ultrasonography in Obstetrics and Gynecology*,
https://doi.org/10.1007/978-981-16-4477-1_2

2.2 Embryonic and Fetal Developmental Characteristics

The mature oocyte is discharged from the ovary then into the fallopian tube and combines with sperm in the ampulla of the fallopian tubes. This process is defined as fertilization. The combined new cell, i.e., the zygote, divides to produce a solid cell mass named a morula. These cells continue to divide and increase, accompanied by the emergency of intercellular spaces between morula cells, and then coalesce to form the blastocele. Then the formation of blastocyst is complete. Trophoblasts of the blastocyst participates in the formation of embryonic accessory structures, while a part of inner cell mass develops into the embryo. Depending on the movement of the cilia and the muscle fibers of the fallopian tube, the fertilized ovum divides repeatedly as it gradually travels to the uterus and reaches the endometrial cavity 4–5 days after fertilization. The process of invasion of blastocyst to the endometrium is called implantation. It takes 7–8 days from fertilization to implantation. The implantation site usually locates in the posterior or anterior wall of the upper portion of the uterus. If the blastocyst implants near the cervix where the placenta will grow later, it is called placenta previa. When the blastocyst implants outside the body cavity of the uterus, it is called ectopic pregnancy, or called extrauterine pregnancy as an old saying.

Embryo development is a continuous process that proceeds through cell division and differentiation step by step, including fertilization, cleavage, implantation, ovigerm stage, embryo stage, and fetus stage.

The development of the embryo and the fetus takes four weeks (28 days) as a gestational month or a gestational age unit. The menstrual age is commonly the used gestational age in clinical practice, which is calculated from the first day of the woman's last menstrual period to the day the fetus and its appendages are discharged from the mother. The whole process is about 40 weeks on average (equivalent to 38 weeks of fertilized age). A full-term pregnancy is 280 days.

In the first eight weeks of pregnancy the living is called an embryo, and the formation and differentiation of main organs have completed at end of this stage. From the ninth week of gestation, the embryo has a human-like morphological trait, which is called a fetus. The first trimester is before the 13th week of pregnancy. After that, each organ develops further until it matures (Table 2.1).

2.3 Diagnostic Ultrasound of Normal Pregnancy

Since ultrasound has been used in obstetrics, with the rapid development of the ultrasound technique, clinicians can dynamically monitor the whole process of fetal growth in each stage and evaluate whether the morphological structures of fetal systems and organs are normal. According to the biological measurement of multiple parameters, ultrasound can accurately estimate fetal age and pulmonary maturity and evaluate the development of the fetus in the uterus. As a necessary method for obstetrics, prenatal ultrasound screening for fetal

Table 2.1 Length, weight, and characteristics during development of the fetus

Gestational age (week)	Length	Weight	Developmental characteristics and ultrasonic image characteristics
The end of the 8th week			The eyes, ears, nose, and mouth can be distinguished. It is initially humanoid, with early heart formation and pulsation seen by ultrasound. The crown-rump length can be measured
The end of the 12th week	9 cm	14 g	The external genitalia has developed, and the fetal fingers (toes) can be distinguished. The limbs are active. Ultrasound can display the skeletal system and scan the upper and lower limbs in sections
The end of the 16th week	16 cm	110 g	The sex of the fetus can be distinguished. Fetal respiratory movement began to appear, and some pregnant women could feel fetal movement. Ultrasound can observe the fetal head, intracranial structure, spine, trunk, maxillofacial, limb bone, stomach bubble, and bladder
The end of the 20th week	25 cm	320 g	Begin to swallow and urinate. Fetal heart sounds can be heard from the abdominal wall of pregnant women. A clear outline of fetal kidney appears
The end of the 24th week	30 cm	630 g	After 16 weeks of gestation, it can observe all fetal organs by ultrasound. 18th–26th week is the best period for fetal malformation screening
The end of the 28th week	35 cm	1000 g	Testicles drop gradually
The end of the 32th week	40 cm	1700 g	
The end of the 36th week	45 cm	2500 g	
The end of the 40th week	50 cm	3000 g	

growth anomalies and fetal anomalies is becoming an essential part of prenatal diagnosis. One or more times of ultrasonic scanning is needed for almost every pregnant woman during pregnancy. In recent years, image quality has been dramatically improved with the development of ultrasonic technology. The application of high-frequency vaginal probe becomes part of a first-trimester screening program for fetal abnormality. It shows excellent value in the field of Obstetrics and possesses essential clinical value in improving the quality of fetal life and reducing perinatal mortality.

2.3.1 Basic Concepts

1. Pregnancy is the process in which the embryo and the fetus develop in the mother's uterus. The fertilization of oocyte is the beginning of pregnancy, while the expulsion of the fetus and its appendages from the mother is the termination of pregnancy. Clinically, the process of pregnancy is divided into three stages: It is called the first trimester before the end of the 12th week of pregnancy, the second trimester which is from the 13th to the 27th week, and the third trimester after the 28th week.
2. The fetus undergoes embryonic and fetal development in the uterine cavity of the mother, and each organ completes differentiation and further maturation. The formation of fetal appendages, including placenta, amniotic fluid, and umbilical cord, ensure the connection between the fetus and the mother, as well as the growth and development of the fetus.
3. The clinical diagnosis of pregnancy is mainly based on a history of amenorrhea with morning sickness, cervical and uterine softening, and a bluish discoloration of the cervix. Human chorionic gonadotrophin (HCG) can be detected in either the mother's blood or urine. The abdominal size of pregnant women gradually increases in the second and third trimesters; also, maternal weight, fundal height, and abdominal circumference of pregnant women keep increasing with gestational age in the prenatal examination. The fetal heartbeat is visible from the 12th week of pregnancy, with an average of 120 to 160 times per minute.
4. From the 11th week of pregnancy until delivery, it is vital to monitor fetal growth and development in the uterus and evaluate the morphology and structure of fetal organs, placenta, amniotic fluid, and umbilical cord.
5. During 11 to 14 weeks of gestation, ultrasound is carried out to screen for aneuploidy chromosomal abnormalities, adverse outcomes through assessing the thickness of fetal nuchal translucency and nasal bone and detect fetal structural abnormality by observing morphological structure.
6. Most fetal anomalies can be identified during 18 to 26 weeks of gestation, which is the best time to observe whether the fetal development is normal. Multiparameter bio measurement using ultrasound is useful to predict gestational age and assess fetal growth. Moreover, ultrasound can also accurately determine fetal lie, fetal presentation, fetal position, and heart activity. By detecting the blood flow spectrum of the fetal umbilical artery and uterine artery, color Doppler flow imaging and spectral Doppler can reflect the blood flow of the placenta indirectly. The detection of uterine artery blood flow has clinical value in predicting the occurrence of pregnancy-induced hypertension (PIH).

2.3.2 Ultrasound Diagnosis

2.3.2.1 First Trimester

1. The changes of uterus and the appearance of gestational sac

With transabdominal ultrasound, the uterus is enlarged and swollen. The gestational sac is visible in the uterine cavity about six weeks after the last menstruation. Under transvaginal ultrasound, the gestational sac can be detected as early as 30 to 35 days after conception (Fig. 2.1).

2. Characteristics of the gestational sac.

The gestational sac (GS) is a round or oval anechoic area, and the decidual layers around the sac appear as a hyperechoic ring. The size of the gestational sac is becoming enlarged with the increase of menopause days. After 12 to 13 weeks, the chorion fuses with decidua, and the gestational sac is invisible by ultrasound (Figs. 2.2 and 2.3).

3. The yolk sac. Yolk sac (YS) is located inside the gestational sac. The image is characterized by a ring-shaped hyperechoic structure with an anechoic center. At 5 to 6 weeks after the last menstrual period, a yolk sac, 3 to 8 mm in diameter, is visible under transvaginal ultrasound, earlier than the embryo. The embryo is smaller than the initial yolk sac. The yolk sac is a vital sign to confirm intrauterine pregnancy. The appearance time, the size, and shape of the yolk sac are closely related to the outcome of early pregnancy. The excessive large or small yolk sac and strange echo, are indicative of an abnormal early pregnancy. The appearance of the yolk sac is useful in distinguishing an intrauterine pregnancy from a pseudogestational sac in ectopic pregnancy, and it disappears after the tenth gestational week (Figs. 2.4 and 2.5).
4. Embryo The embryo is first identified as the thickening part adjacent to the yolk sac. Under transvaginal ultrasound, a primitive embryonic heartbeat is identifiable when the embryo is more than 2 mm in length. Most of the fetal heartbeat is visible at the sixth week of pregnancy, and the embryonic growth rate is about 1 mm/d. After

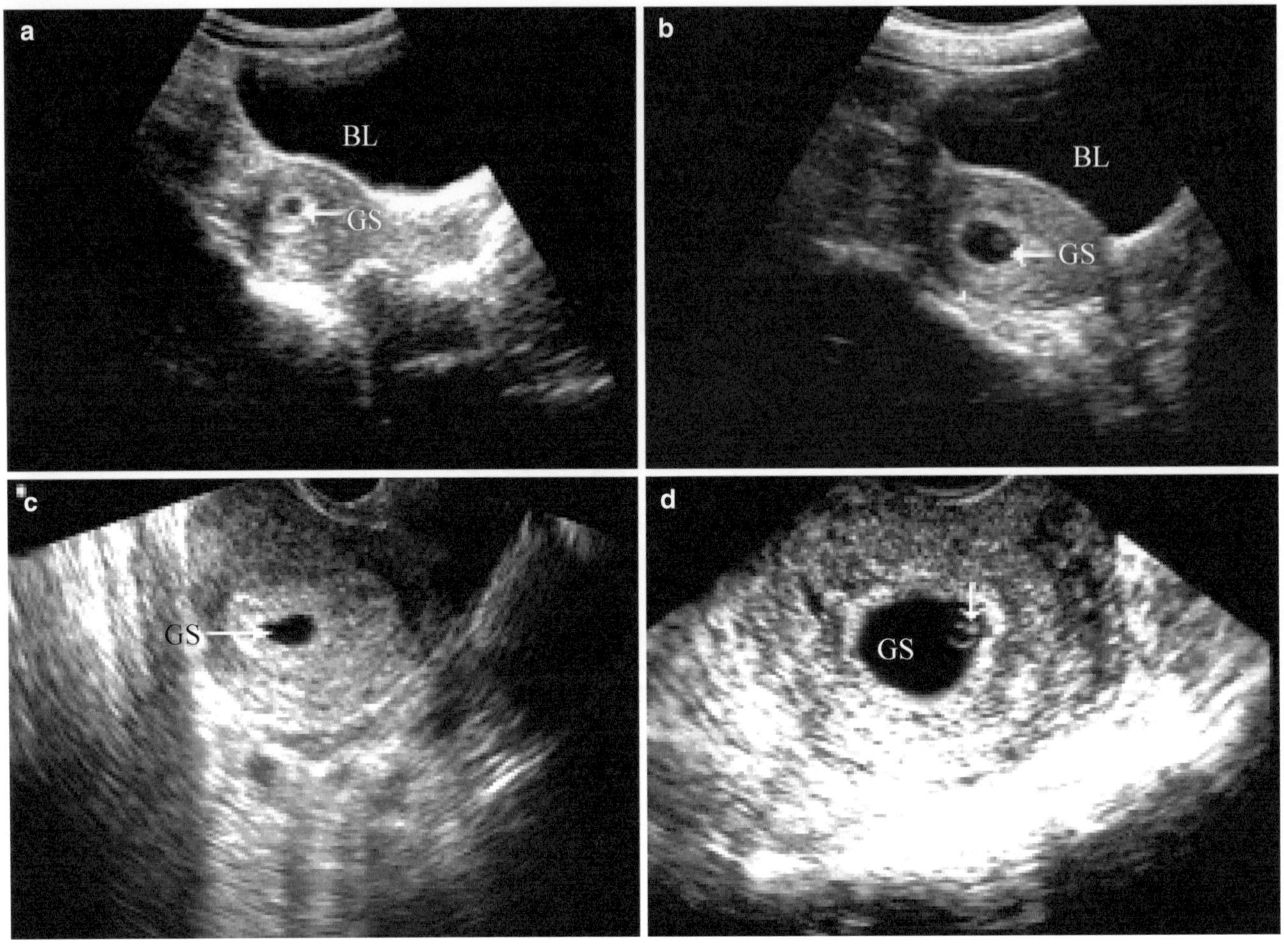

Fig. 2.1 Transabdominal/transvaginal ultrasound images in early pregnancy. (**a**). Transabdominal scan, a tiny intrauterine gestational sac on day 38 of gestation; (**b**). Swollen uterus and an intrauterine gestational sac on day 42 of gestation; (**c**). Transvaginal scan, a tiny intrauterine gestational sac on day 33 of gestation; (**d**). On 44 days of pregnancy, the thickening part adjacent to the yolk sac is the early embryo

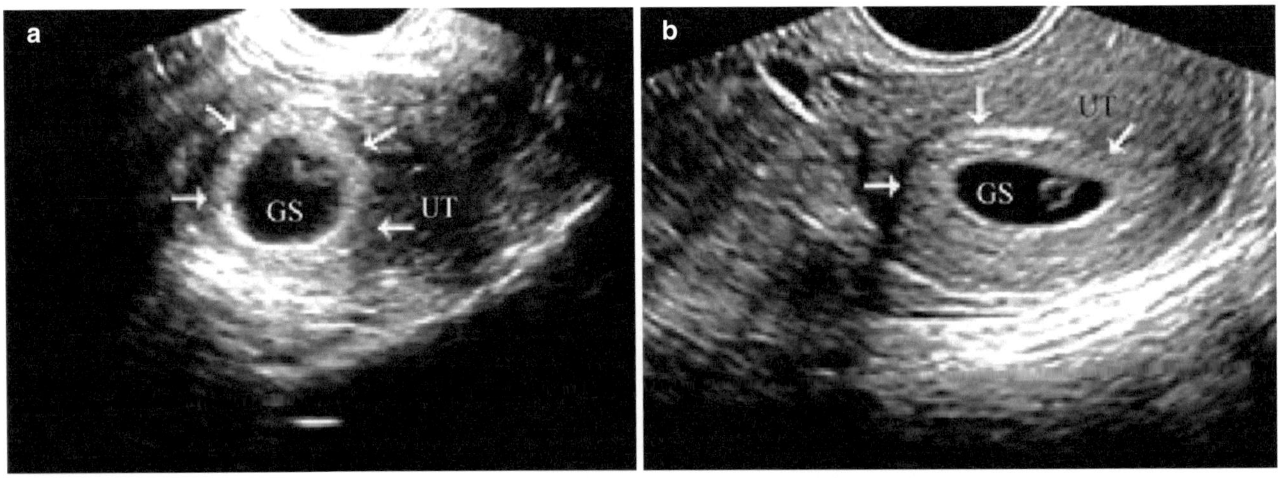

Fig. 2.2 Characteristics of the gestational sac. (**a**). The round gestational sac and the hyperechogenic decidua around the sac on day 38 of gestation; (**b**). The oval gestational sac and the hyperechogenic decidua around the sac on day 42 of gestation

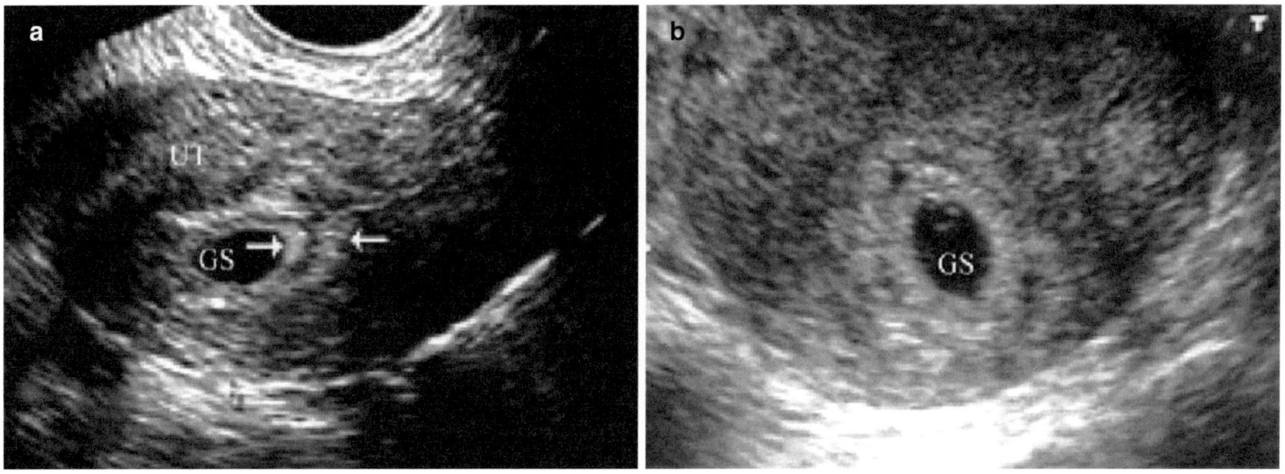

Fig. 2.3 The double-ring sign of the gestational sac. (**a, b**): On days 35 and 37 of gestation, the gestational sac presents a "double-ring sign"

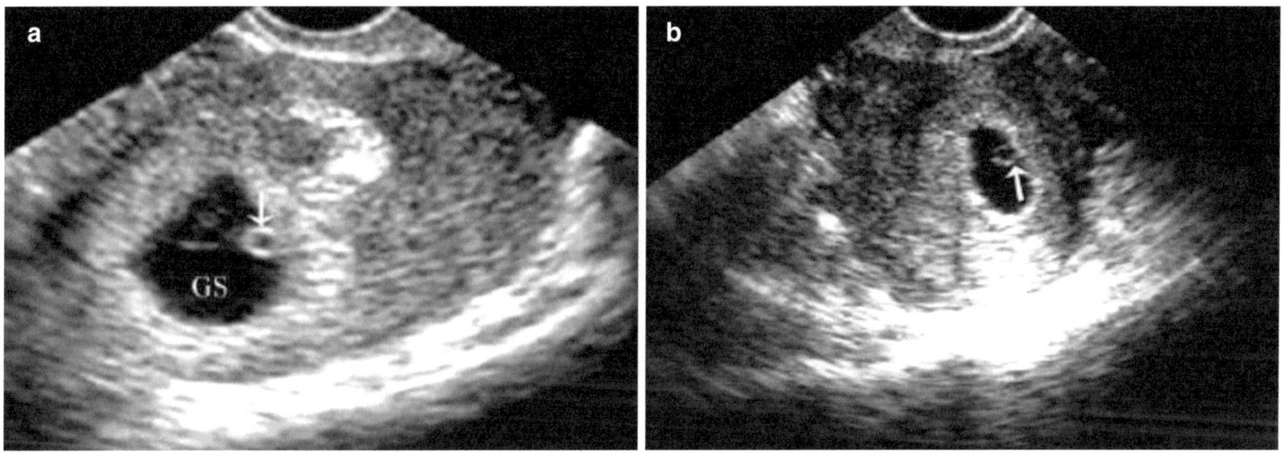

Fig. 2.4 Yolk sac in early pregnancy. (**a**). Forty eight-day pregnancy, a ring-shaped hyperechoic normal yolk sac; (**b**). The yolk sac appeared prior to the embryo

6.5 weeks of gestation, the embryo grows up gradually. At the eighth week of gestation, the embryo is in human shape, and the fetal limb buds are hyperechoic. The intrauterine pregnancy can be confirmed as long as the embryo in the gestational sac, and primitive cardiac pulsation is visualized (Figs. 2.6 and 2.7).

5. The Placenta After about 9 weeks of pregnancy, a crescent-shaped hyperechoic placenta can be clearly showed via ultrasound (Fig. 2.8).

On day 83 of gestation, the placenta has formed and presents in a crescent-shaped structure.

6. The amniotic sac.

With the increase of gestational age, the amniotic sac (AS) adheres closely to the chorion followed by their fusion. AS, which is filled with amniotic fluid, provides an important environment for fetal survival.

7. Estimation of gestational trimester ① Gestational sac measurement: gestational age (week) = the maximum diameter of gestational sac +3 (Fig. 2.9). ② Measurement of fetal crown rump length (CRL): CRL (cm) + 6.5 = gestational age (week)(a simple estimation method) (Fig. 2.10).

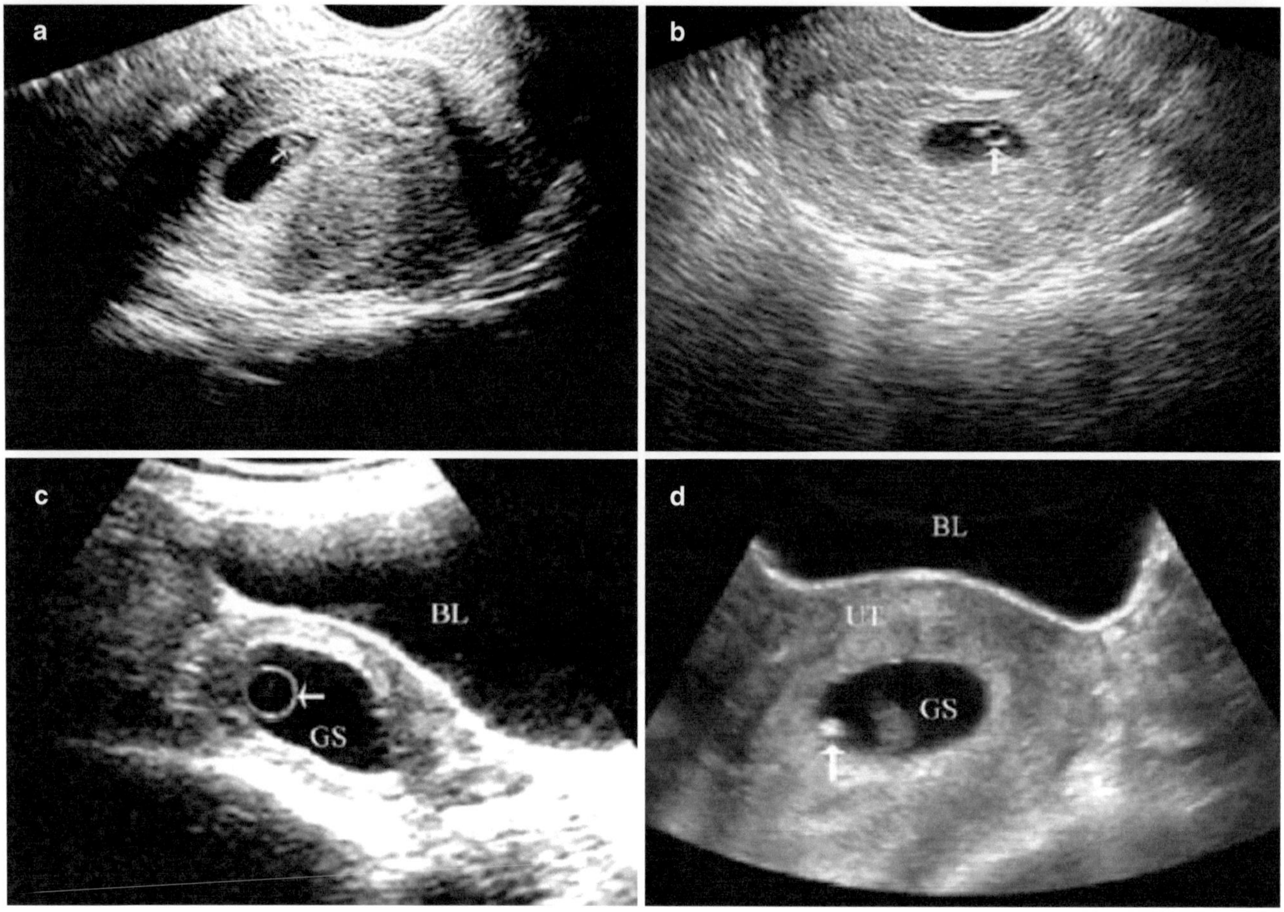

Fig. 2.5 Abnormal yolk sac in early pregnancy. (**a**). Fifty-day pregnancy, a very small yolk sac without an embryo; (**b**). Forty eight-day pregnancy, an irregular-shaped yolk sac without an embryo; (**c**). Fifty six-day pregnancy, an enlarged yolk sac without an embryo; (**d**). Fifty-day pregnancy, a calcified yolk sac and an embryo without cardiac pulsation

The measurement: When the fetus is naturally extended, measure the distance from the cephalic skin's outer edge to the fetal rump's outer edge. When CRL is less than 84 mm, CRL is recommended to calculate the gestational age. Still, when CRL is more than 84 mm, the head circumference (HC) is more accurate for estimating gestation age than the biparietal diameter (BPD).

8. Nuchal Translucency.

Nuchal Translucency (NT) refers to the fluid-filled space at the back of the fetal neck. The NT value increases with the gestational age (Table 2.2). In 11 to 13 + 6 weeks of gestation when the fetal CRL is in 45 to 84 mm, measure the NT when the fetus is in a naturally extended state on the midsagittal view. Enlarge the image to show only the fetal head, neck, and upper thorax in the picture, and then measure the distance perpendicular to the NT anechoic area at the widest part of NT. The horizontal line of the calipers should not be placed in the transparent area, but be overlapped with the hyperechoic edges exactly. Measure more than two times and record the maximum value. Multiple pregnancies require special considerations, especially for chorionicity. For measuring fetal NT, operators need to complete specialized training and certification, and have appropriate capacities for ultrasound instruments and corresponding management (Fig. 2.11).

9. Nasal Bone (NB): Nasal bone can be observed after 11 weeks. When the fetus is in a natural stretching state on the midsagittal view, enlarge the image to show only the fetal head, neck, and upper thorax in the picture. The nose root, nose tip, and nose bone present as three echogenic lines. The thicker line in the bottom, which is more echogenic than the skin line echo, represents the nasal bone (Figs. 2.12 and 2.13).

10. Essential structure screening in the first trimester.

Enlarge the screening site of the fetus to account for more than one-third of the screen. After 10 weeks of gestation, the fetal skull shows a hyperechoic ring under ultrasound. After

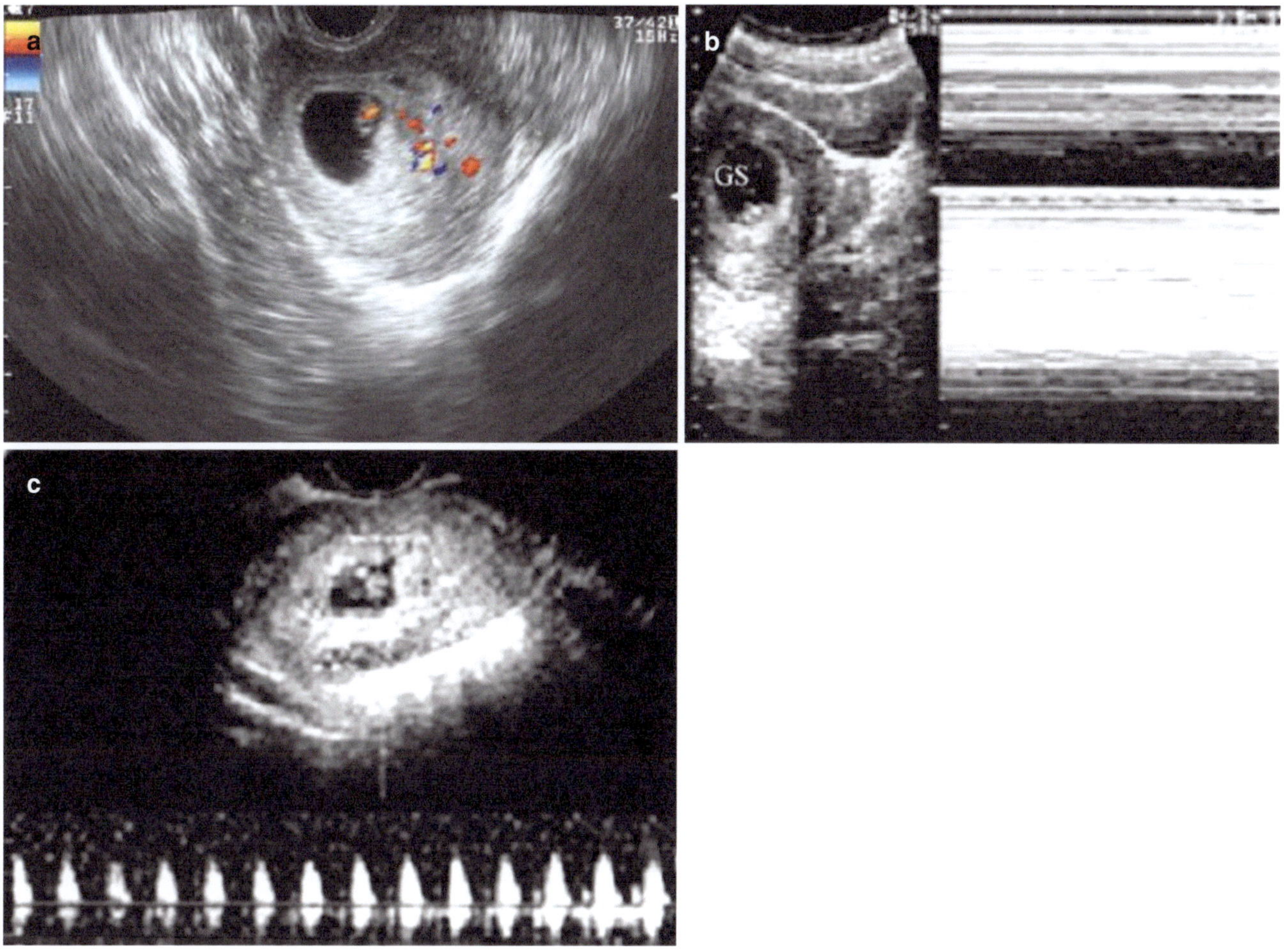

Fig. 2.6 Cardiac activity of the embryo in early pregnancy. (**a**). 46-day pregnancy, color Doppler image shows the primitive embryonic cardiac pulsation; (**b**). M-mode scan shows the primitive cardiac pulsation of the embryo; (**c**). Spectral Doppler image shows the fetal heart pulsation with a single peak wave

12 weeks, the brain midline, choroid plexuses, lateral ventricle, thalamus, and cerebellar hemisphere can be clearly shown on the transverse view of the fetal brain. Some structures of the brain, such as corpus callosum and cerebellum, are not fully grown in the first trimester and cannot be accurately evaluated. After 10 weeks of gestation, ultrasound shows the spinal canal and the parallel bead-like hyperechoic spine. The sacrococcygeal vertebral body completes ossification at about 18 weeks. Observe the vertebral arrangement and integrity of the vertebrae and the surface skin. After 12 weeks of gestation, observe the four-chamber view through the transverse view of fetal thorax, and confirm the location of the fetal heart and cardiothoracic ratio. After 11 weeks of gestation, the fetal stomach is visible in most of the fetuses. The fetal stomach locates on the left side of the abdominal cavity, and the liver on the right side. The normal ultrasound appearances of the fetal kidney are slightly hypoechoic, fava bean-shaped, and located near the spine. On the view of umbilical cord insertion into the anterior abdominal wall, confirm the integrity of the abdominal wall and the position where the umbilical cord inserts. A physiological umbilical hernia can be observed at 11 weeks of gestation, so the diagnosis of omphalocele should be made after 12 weeks. After 11 weeks of pregnancy, note the number of umbilicus artery, and the location and size of the fetal bladder in the transverse view of the bladder. Moreover, primary ossification centers of the long bones are visible at nine weeks of gestation, and the hands and feet can be identified at 11 weeks (Fig. 2.14).

2.3.2.2 The Second- and Third-Trimester Pregnancy

Ultrasound Images of the Fetal Head

Transverse view scanning is mainly used. The fetal head increases to be an oval and echo-reflective hyperechoic ring during the pregnancy.

Fetal brain structure is becoming apparent, and the structures including septum pellucidum, ventriculus system, thalamus, brain midline, choroid plexus, cerebellum, and cisterna

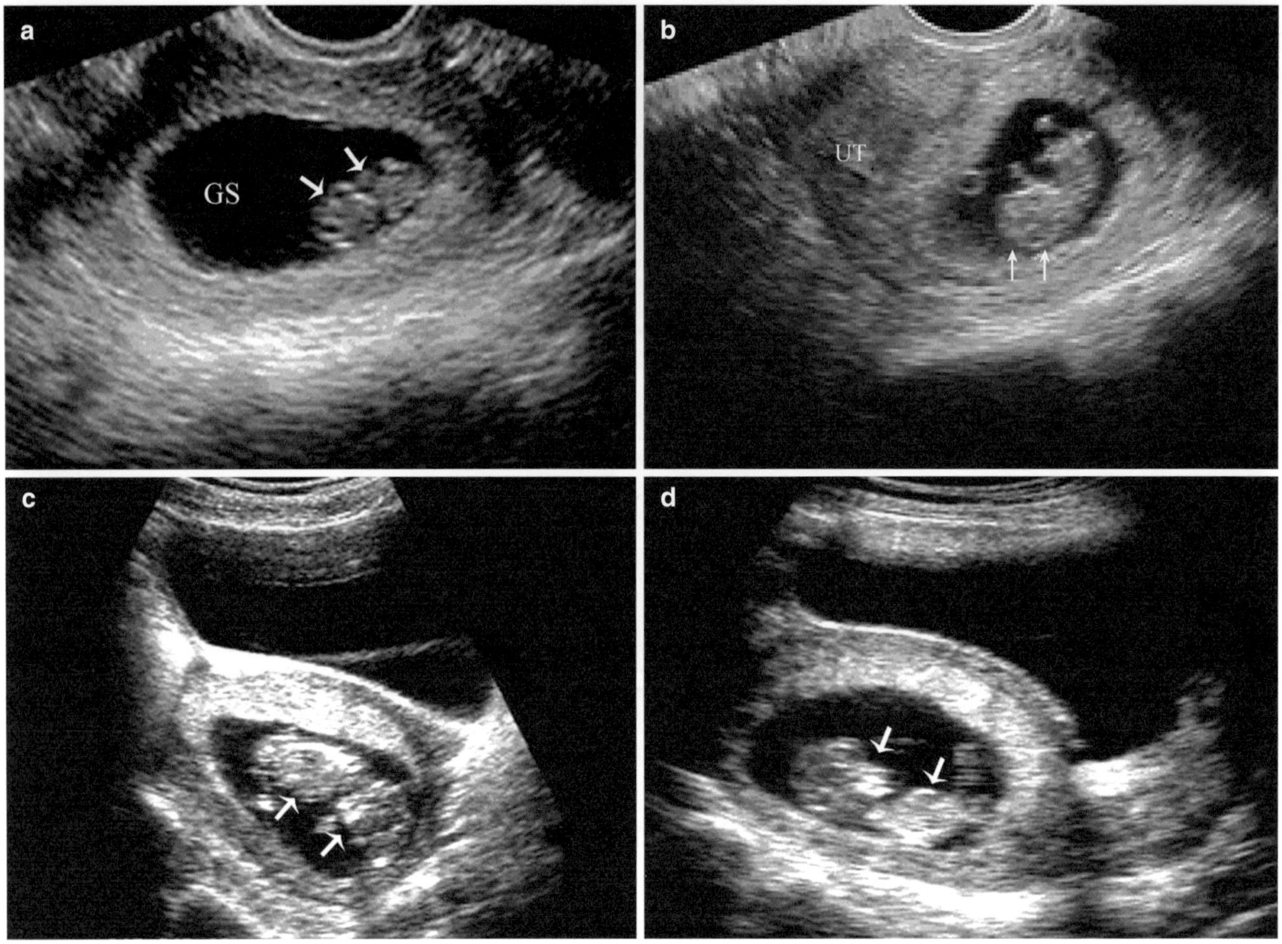

Fig. 2.7 Images of the embryo in early pregnancy. (**a**). On day 48 of gestation, an embryo in the uterus; (**b**). On day 56 of gestation, the intrauterine embryo in human shape; (**c**). On day 66 of gestation, the head, trunk, and limb buds of the embryo are visible; (**d**). On day 82 of gestation, the head, trunk, and limbs can be identified obviously

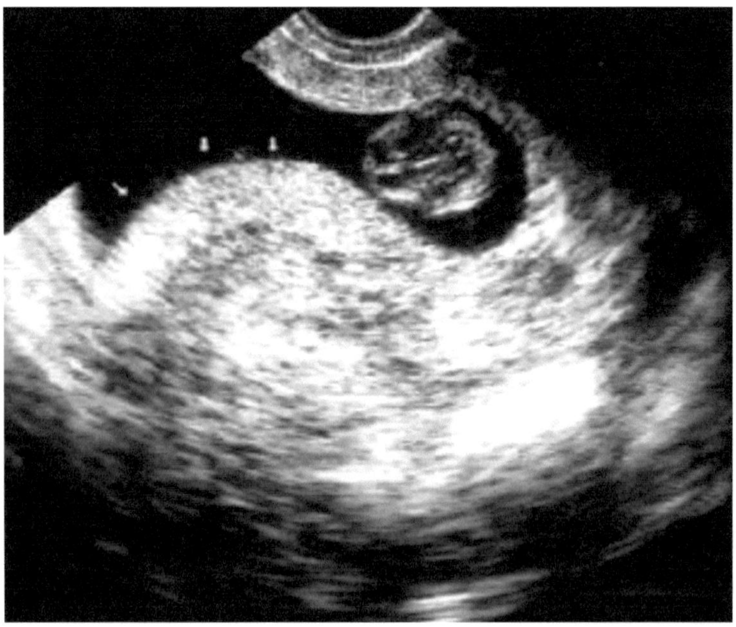

Fig. 2.8 Placenta in early pregnancy

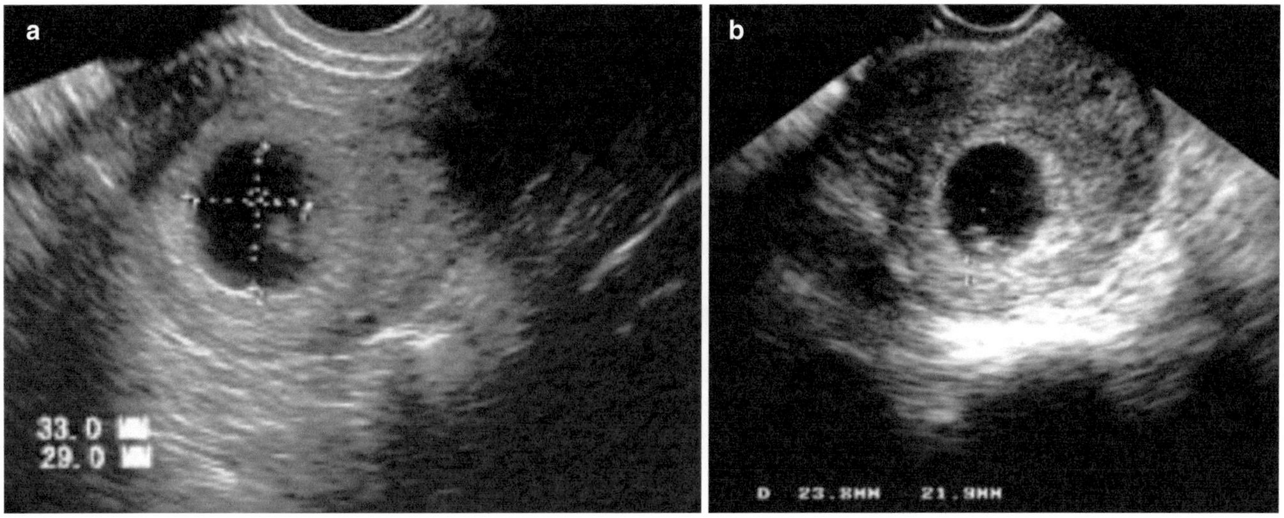

Fig. 2.9 Measurement of the gestational sac. (**a**). Sagittal image of the uterus, measurement of the length, and anteroposterior diameters of the gestational sac; (**b**). Transverse section of the uterus, measurement of the left to the right diameter of the gestational sac

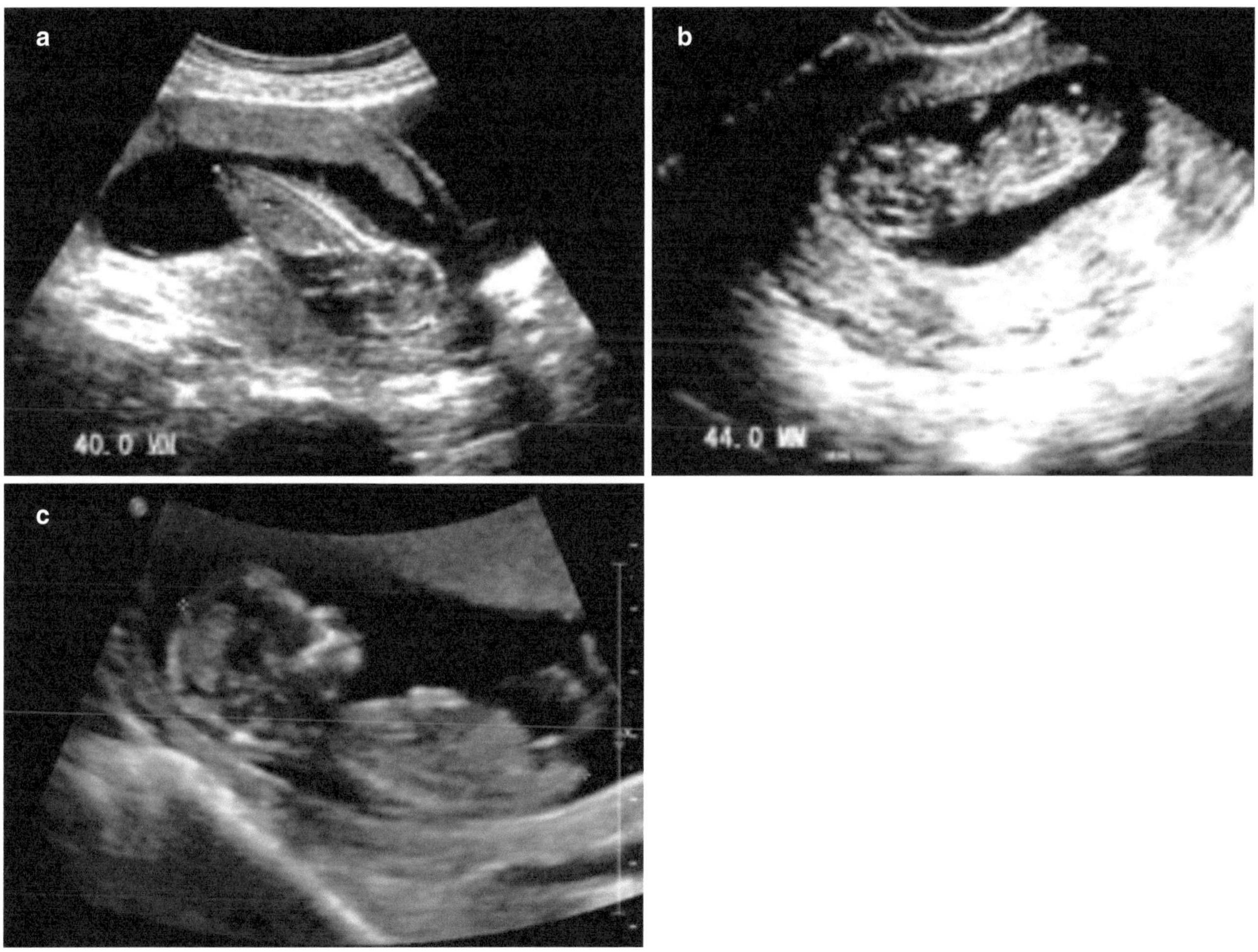

Fig. 2.10 Measurement of CRL. (**a**). The fetal length on day 66 of gestation; (**b**). Fetal CRL on day 74 of gestation; (**c**). Fetal CRL at 13 weeks of gestation

Table 2.2 NT and NB value of normal fetuses during 11 to 14 weeks of gestation

	NT			NB		
Gestation (week)	n (number)	*X*(mm)	*SD*(mm)	n(number)	*X*(mm)	*SD*(mm)
11	1252	0.995	0.333	329	1.969	0.474
12	2435	1.189	0.358	656	2.003	0.465
13	2227	1.331	0.371	564	1.995	0.458
14	1043	1.378	0.396	255	2.048	0.486

Note: The data are from the West China Second Hospital of Sichuan University

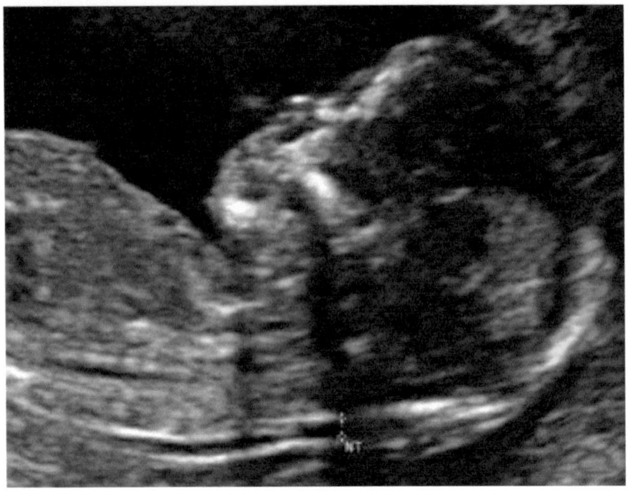

Fig. 2.11 Fetal NT. Measurement of NT at 12 + 3 weeks of gestation

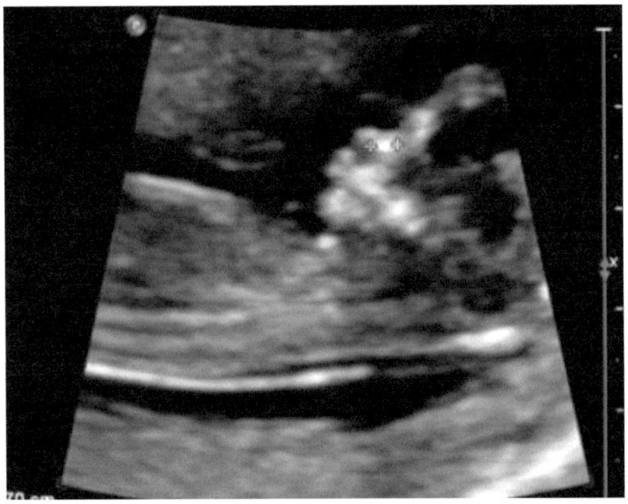

Fig. 2.12 Fetal nasal bone. Measurement of NB at 12 + 3 weeks of gestation

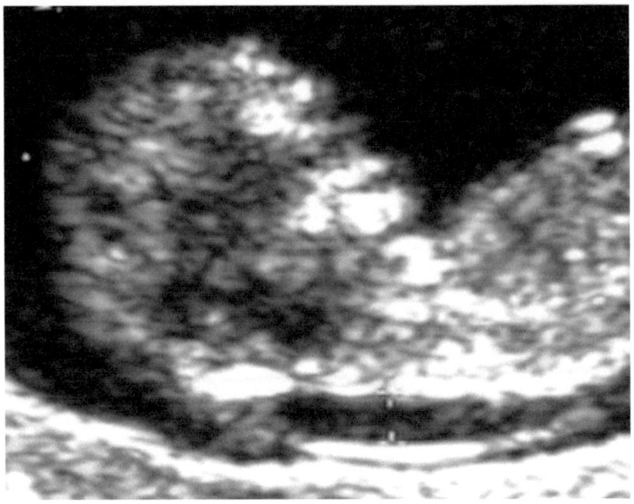

Fig. 2.13 Abnormal echo of fetal nasal bone. Thickened fetal NT with absent nasal bone at 12 + 6 weeks of gestation.

magna can be observed. Color Doppler flow shows the cerebral vessels of the fetus (Figs. 2.15 and 2.16).

Ultrasound Image of the Fetal Face

After 11 weeks of gestation, the fetal maxillofacial bones are gradually visible. Under appropriate scanning angle in the context of amniotic fluid, fetal eyes, nose, lips, philtrum, face, upper alveolar bone, lower alveolar bone, ears, scalp, and hair can be observed through a systematic evaluation in the coronal and sagittal views (Fig. 2.17).

Images of the Fetal Spine

The hyperechoic vertebrae show regular "string-bead" in parallel arrangement on sagittal view. The sacrococcygeal region slightly tilts backward and expands in the lumbar section. The vertebrae distribute as a triangle on a trans-

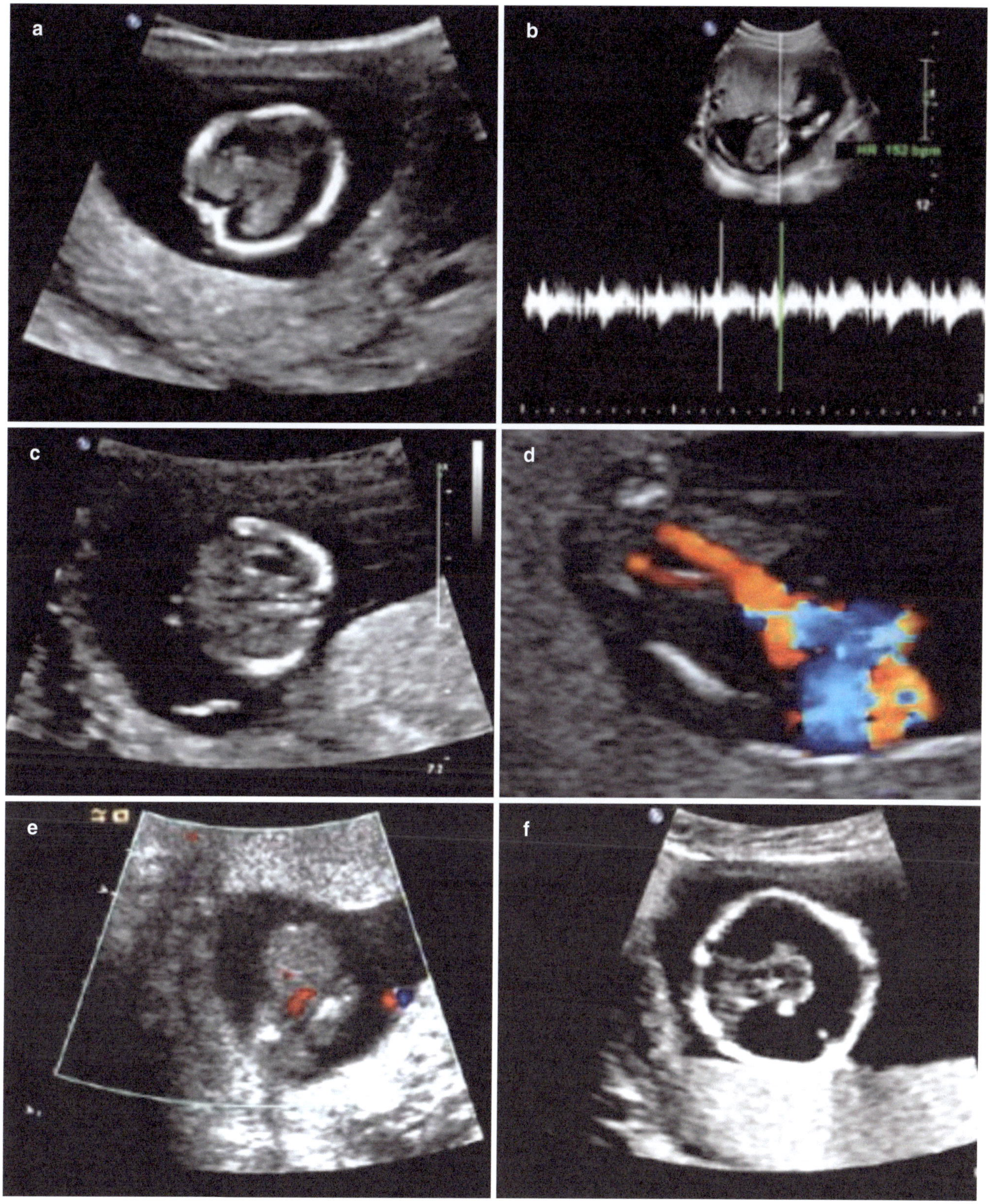

Fig. 2.14 Screening of essential structures in early pregnancy. (**a**). Transverse view of the fetal head at 13 weeks of gestation; (**b**). Transverse view of fetal chest: spectrum Doppler of fetal tricuspid valves; (**c**). Transverse view of the fetal stomach in abdominal level; (**d**). Transverse view of fetal bladder showing bilateral umbilical arteries; (**e**). Fetal omphalocele at 13 weeks of gestation, showing the umbilical cord inserting into the abdominal cavity on one side of the bulging area; (**f**). Holoprosencephaly at 13 weeks of pregnancy; (**g**). Fetal lower limbs at 12 weeks of gestation; (**h**). Fetal upper limbs at 12 weeks of gestation

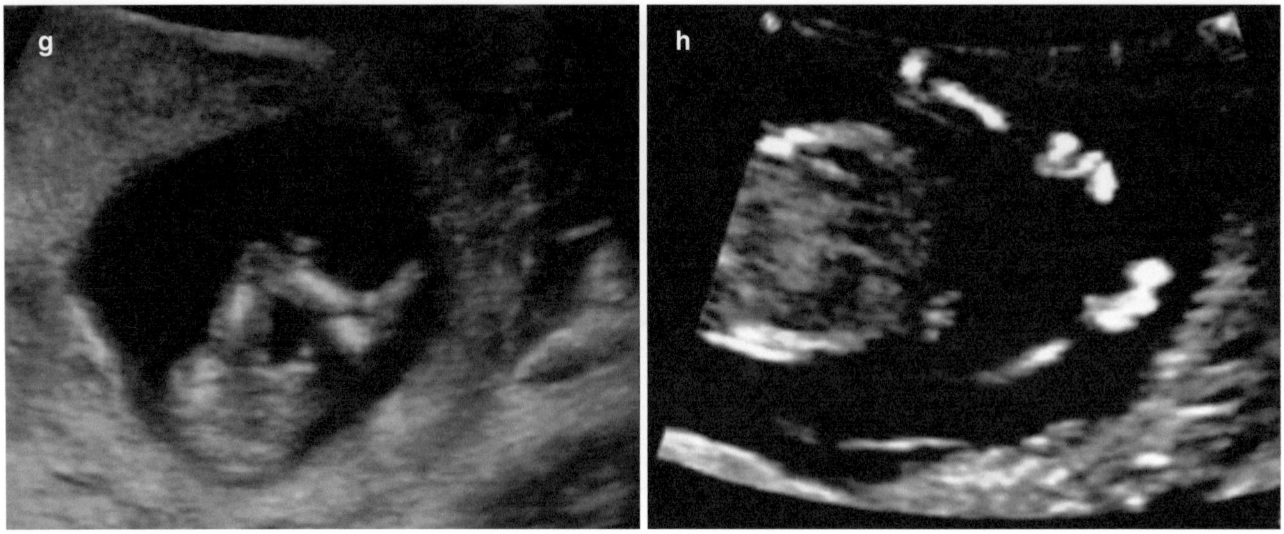

Fig. 2.14 (continued)

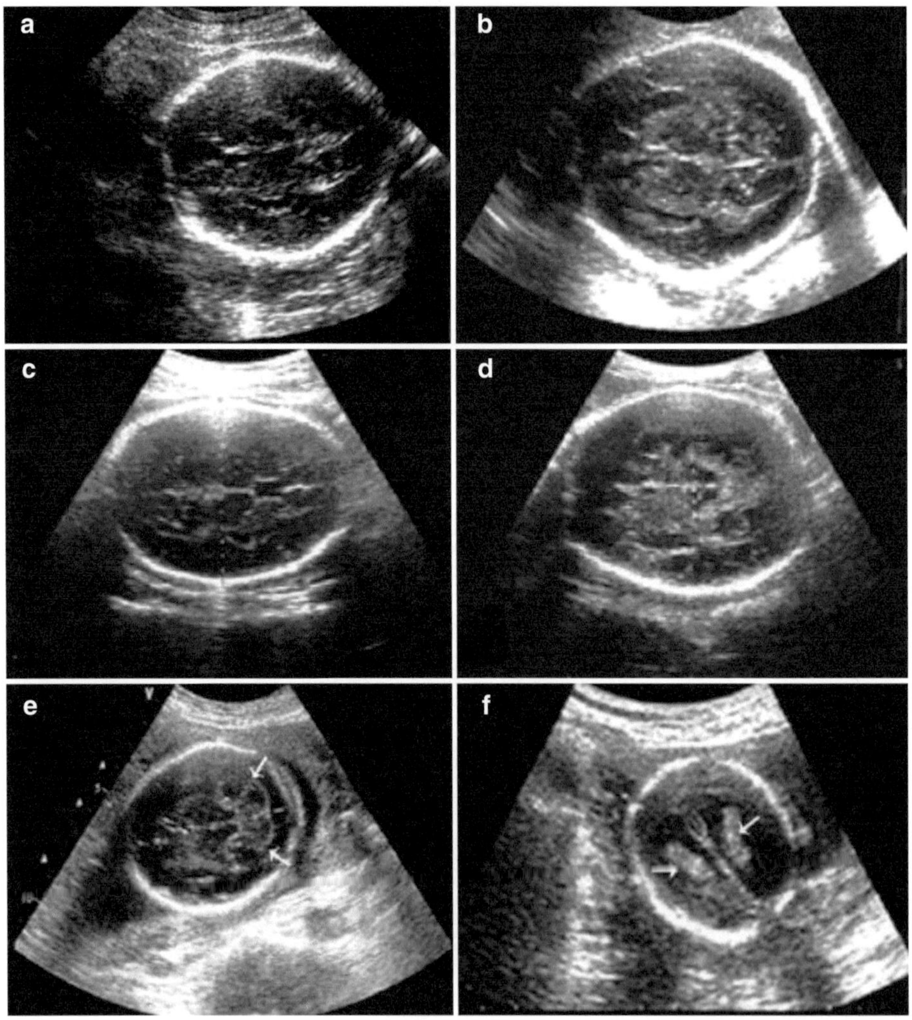

Fig. 2.15 Fetal head. (**a**). Transverse view of the fetal head presenting hyperechoic ring structure; (**b**). Transverse view of the fetal head showing fetal brain structure: midline and thalamus; (**c**). Transverse view of the fetal head presenting the complete and smooth ring echoic structure. The septum pellucidum and thalamus are showed; (**d**). Transverse view of fetal head showing anterior horns of the lateral ventricles; (**e**). Transverse view of fetal head showing cerebellum; (**f**). Intracranial choroid plexus of the fetus; (**g**). The lateral ventricle of the fetus

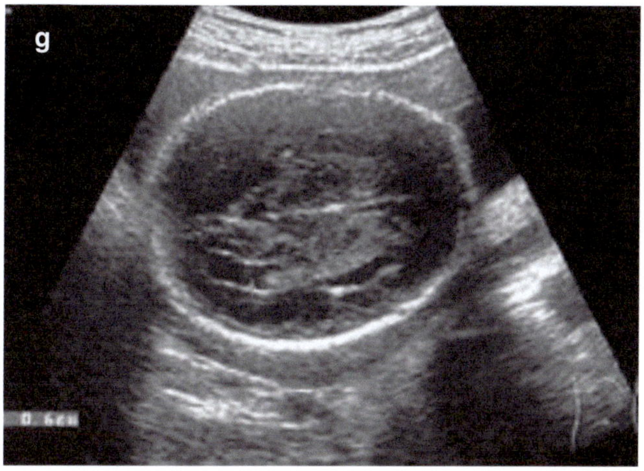

Fig. 2.15 (continued)

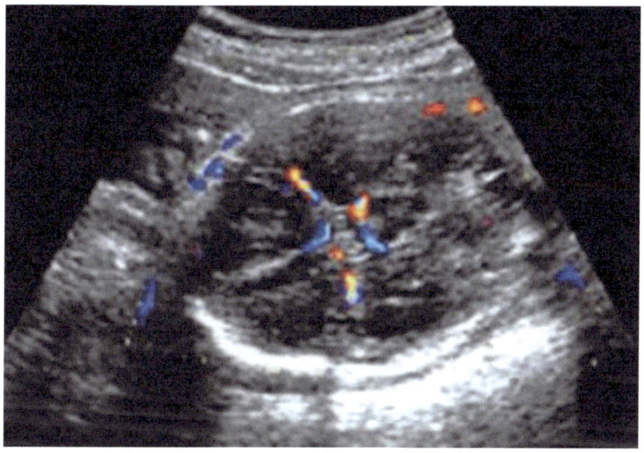

Fig. 2.16 Fetal intracerebral vessels. The cranial base view of Fetal Willis artery ring

verse view, and the spinal canal is visible as strip-like anechoic area. The centrum is the ossification center of the vertebral body. On the coronal view, the spine appears as three parallel hyperechoic lines near the ventral side (Figs. 2.18 and 2.19).

Ultrasound Images of Fetal Thorax

The fetal chest cavity is composed of spine, ribs, and sternum. Main organs in the fetal chest are the heart, large blood vessels, trachea, lungs, esophagus, and so on. The heart located in the left chest cavity, with the apex pointing to the left. The left and right ventricles and atria are of the same size. Multiple hyperechoic ribs in an oblique arrangement are visible after 11 to 12 weeks of gestation. During the third trimester, the echo of fetal ribs is becoming visualized. The fetal lung is of moderate echo with a smooth edge in the second and third trimesters. It does not squeeze the heart and is clearly displayed with the liquid background (Figs. 2.20 and 2.21).

Images of the Fetal Abdomen

The liver, located in the right upper fetal abdomen, presents homogeneous isoecho (as shown in the Fig. 2.22). The fetal umbilical vein inserts into the abdominal cavity in the midline of the fetal abdominal wall. It divides into two branches, one joins the portal system to the liver substance and the other connects to the inferior vena cava through the ductus venous. The umbilical cord inserts into the abdominal wall, as shown in the Fig. 2.22. The gallbladder, in the same view with the umbilical vein, is visible after 24 weeks of gestation. The fetal stomach is anechoic in the left side of the abdominal cavity (as shown in the Fig. 2.22). After 20 weeks of pregnancy, digestive tract malformation should be considered if there is an absent fetal stomach combined with hydramnios, and repeated examination should be carried out 30 to 45 minutes later. Multiple anechoic bowel loops are evident in the fetal abdominal cavity during the second and third trimesters of pregnancy (as shown in the Fig. 2.22). With the development of a pregnancy, meconium thickens, followed by gradually increased bowel echo (Fig. 2.22).

Images of Fetal Genitourinary Tract

After 16 weeks of pregnancy, the fetal kidneys are visible by the longitudinal and transverse view of transabdominal ultrasound. Fetal kidneys, showing as a circular or ovoid-shaped hypoecho, located lateral to the fetal spine. Echo of the renal capsule and collecting system is enhanced. The fetal bladder is a round cystic structure, the size of which varies during dynamic observation. After 16 to 18 weeks of gestation, fetal gender can be identified (Figs.2.23 and 2.24).

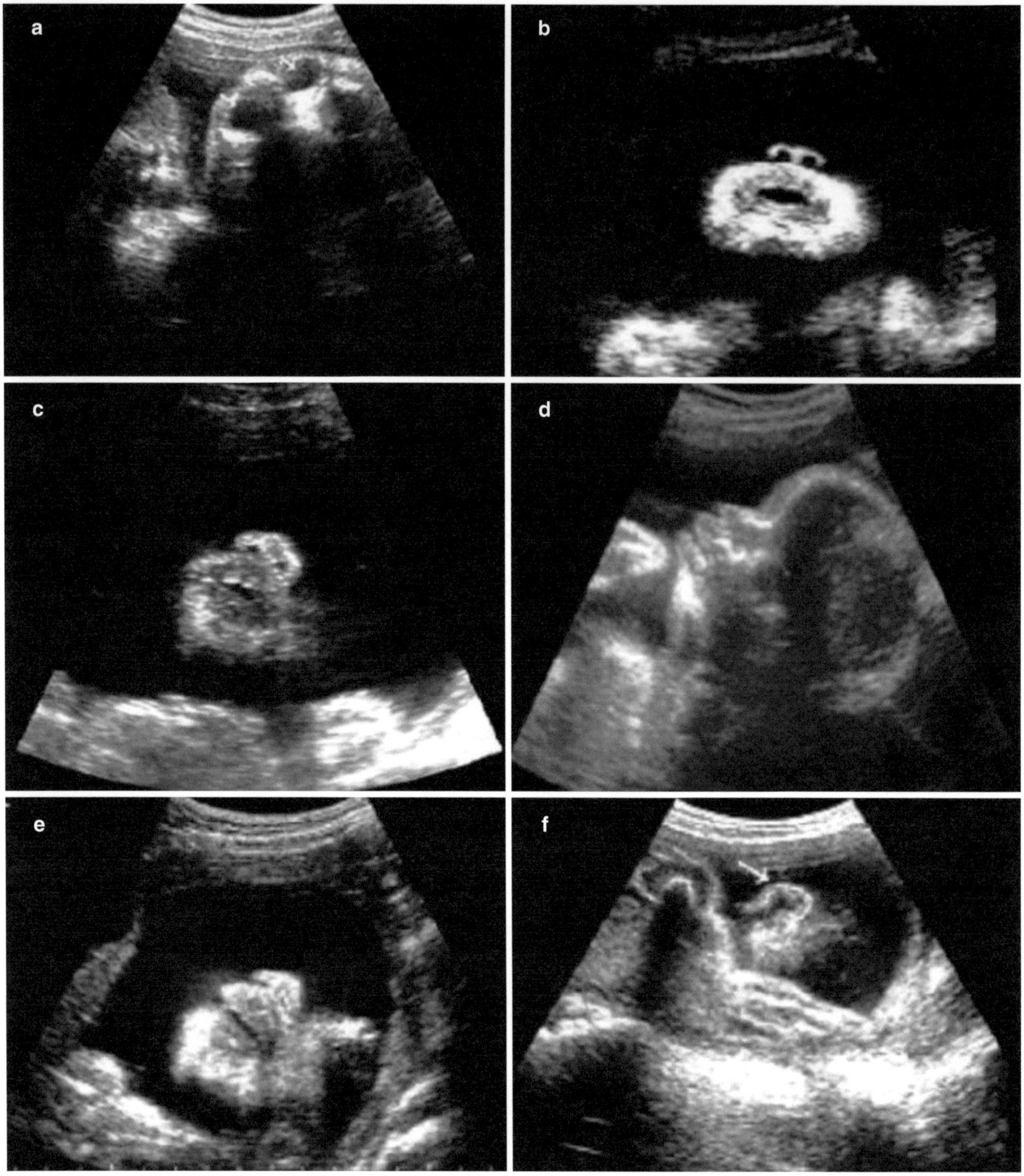

Fig. 2.17 Fetal maxillofacial region. (**a**). Image of fetal orbits; (**b**). 2-D image of fetal mandible, mouth, and nostrils; (**c**). Image of fetal nose and mouth; (**d**). Sagittal view of the fetal face; (**e**). Image of the fetal face; (**f**). Image of one fetal ear

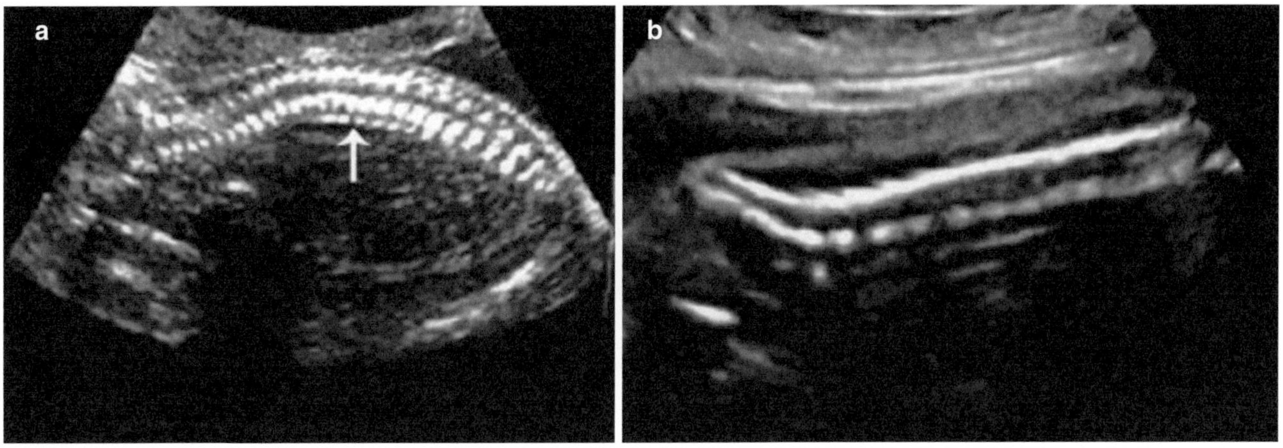

Fig. 2.18 Fetal spine. (**a, b**). Full view of the fetal spine, vertebrae are arranged regularly, the spinal canal presents strip-like anechoic area, and the spine has natural physiological curvature

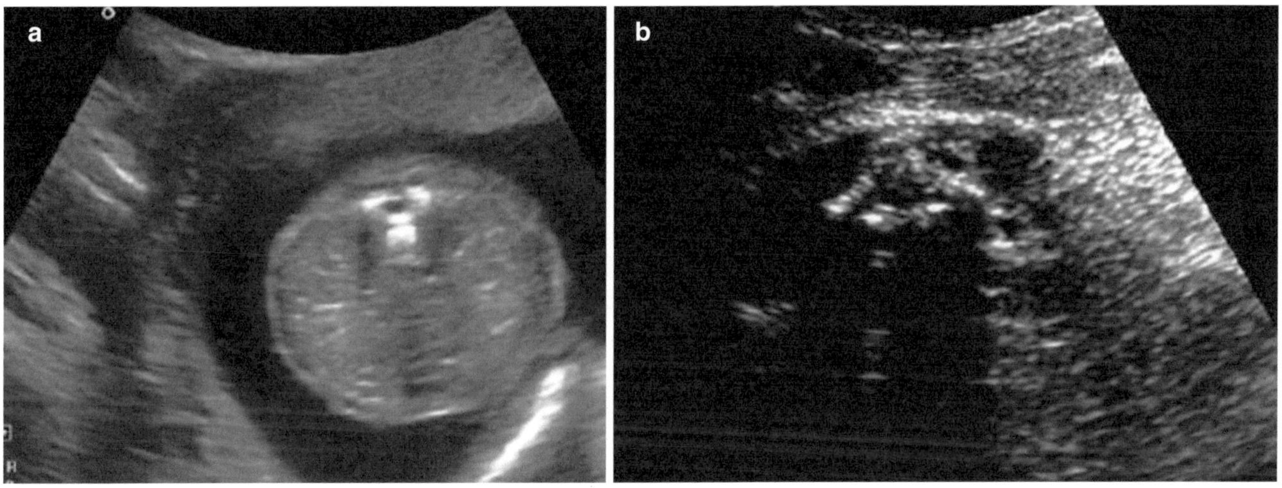

Fig. 2.19 Transverse view of fetal spine. (**a, b**). The vertebrae distribute as a triangle on transverse view of fetal spine

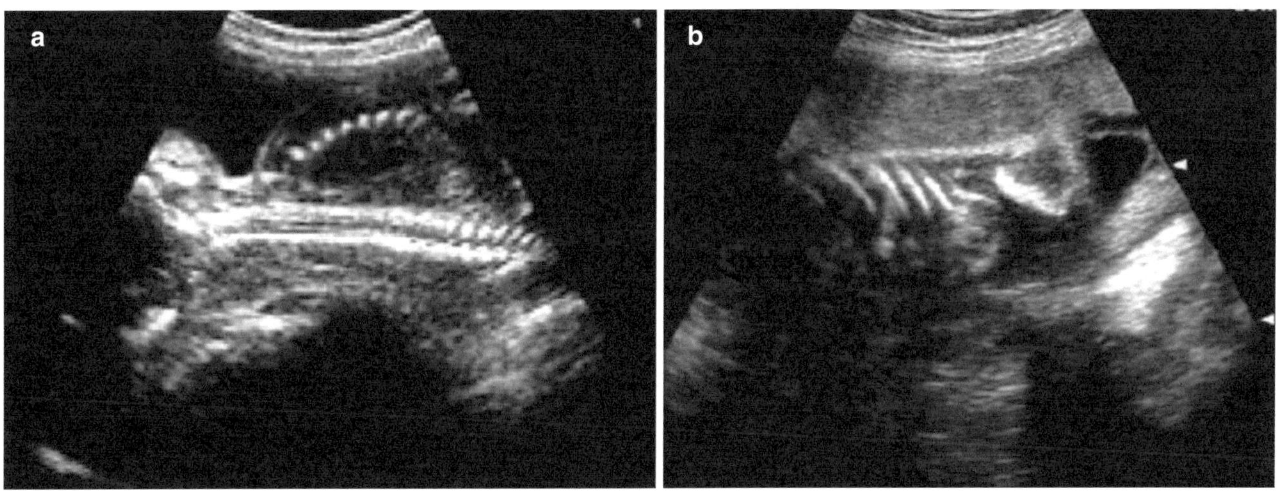

Fig. 2.20 Fetal ribs. (**a**). Transverse view of fetal ribs; (**b**). Sagittal view of fetal ribs

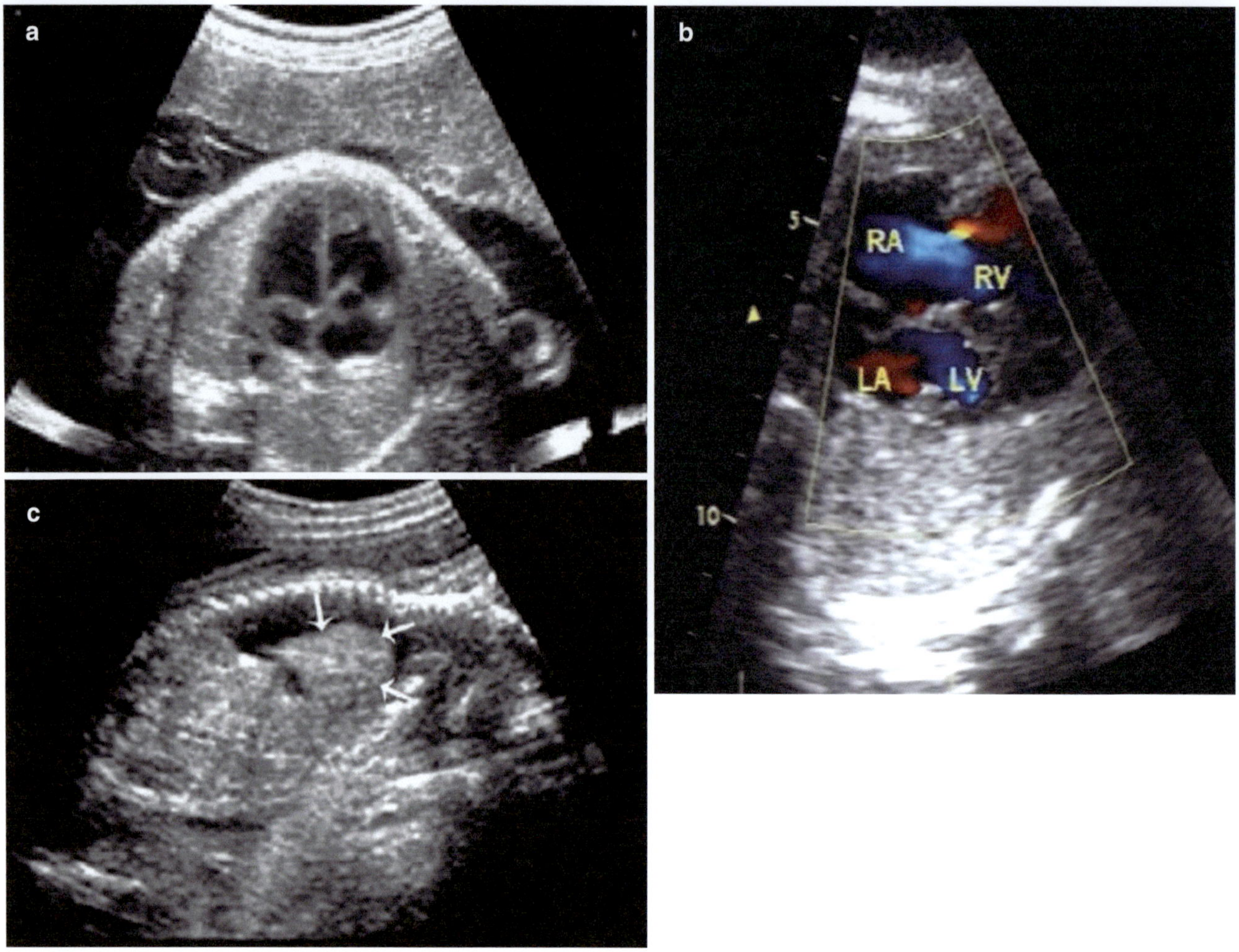

Fig. 2.21 Fetal thorax. (**a**). The Transverse view of the fetal thorax showing the heart; (**b**). Blood flow of fetal heart chambers; (**c**). The sagittal view of the fetal thorax showing hyperechoic fetal lung, which can be clearly shown with a pleural effusion

Images of Fetal Limbs and Fetal Movements

With the progress of the pregnancy, the echo of fetal bones is gradually enhancing, accompanied by posterior attenuation. Because of the amniotic fluid surrounding the fetus, the second trimester is the best period for observing fetal limbs and their movements. During the third trimester, it is difficult to display the fetal limbs due to the impact of fetal growth, fetal position, amniotic fluid, and other factors. After 28 weeks of gestation, a small oval mass echo which is identified by visualizing the distal femur is the femoral epiphysis. The appearance of skeletal epiphyseal ossification centers is conductive to estimate gestational age (Figs. 2.25 and 2.26).

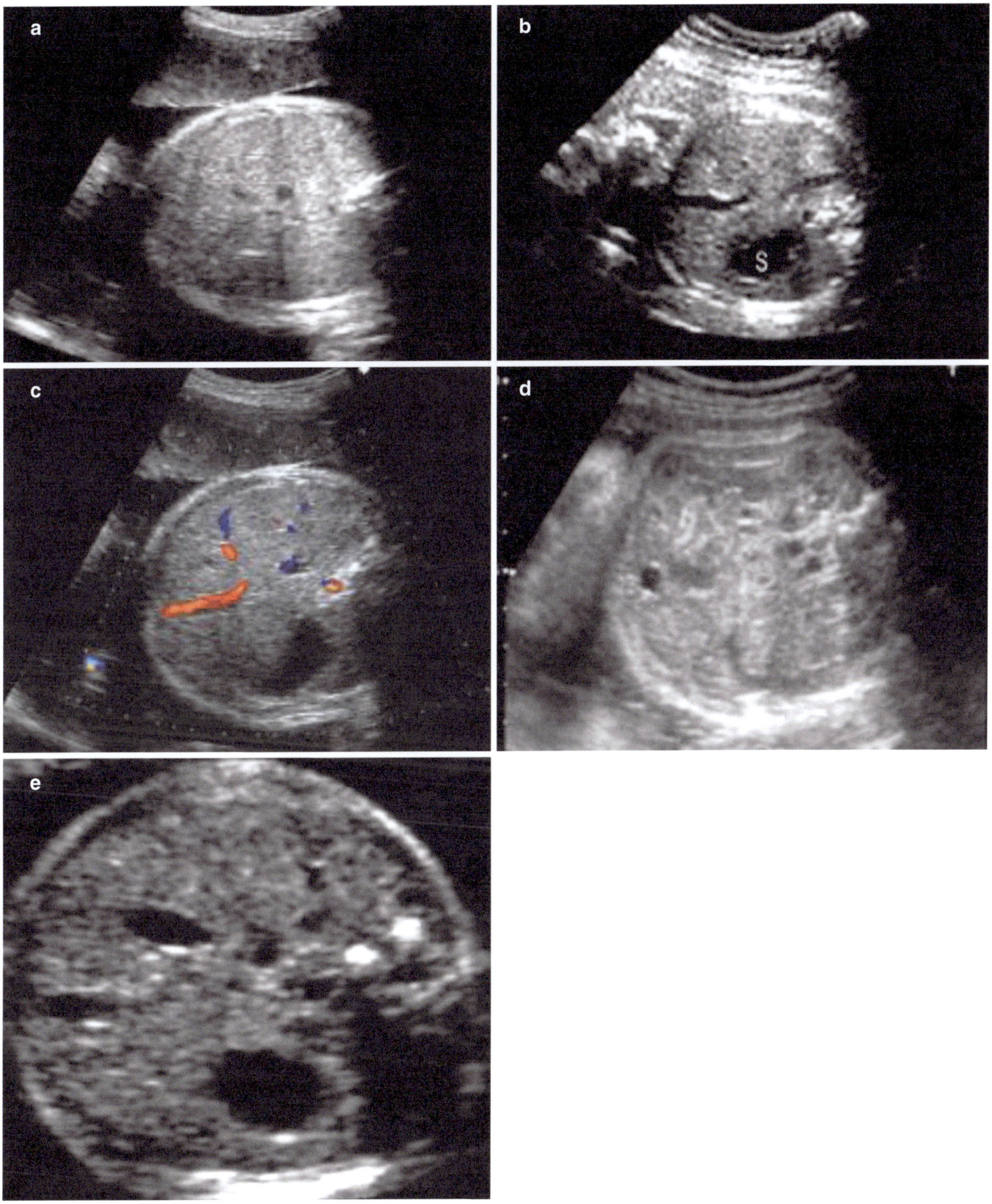

Fig. 2.22 Fetal abdominal cavity. (**a**). Homogeneous isoechoic fetal liver locates in the right upper abdominal cavity; (**b**). A horn-shaped or oval anechoic fetal stomach in the left upper abdomen; (**c**). Fetal intra-hepatic arteries; (**d**). Hyperechoic bowels in the abdominal cavity; (**e**). Fetal gallbladder

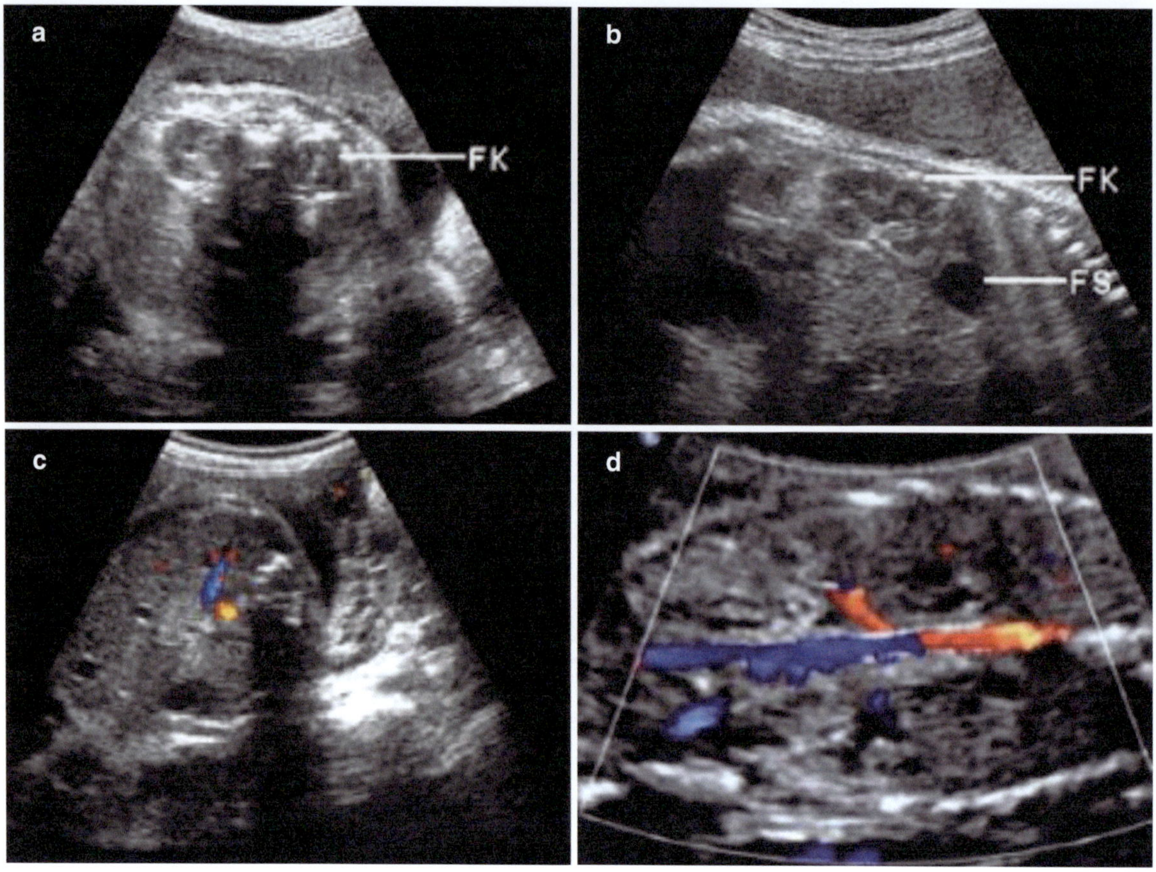

Fig. 2.23 Fetal kidney. (**a**). Transverse view of fetal abdomen showing the renal capsule, medulla, and pelvis; (**b**). Sagittal view of fetal abdomen showing oval fetal kidney on the side of spine; and (**c, d**). Transverse and Sagittal images showing the blood flow of fetal kidney

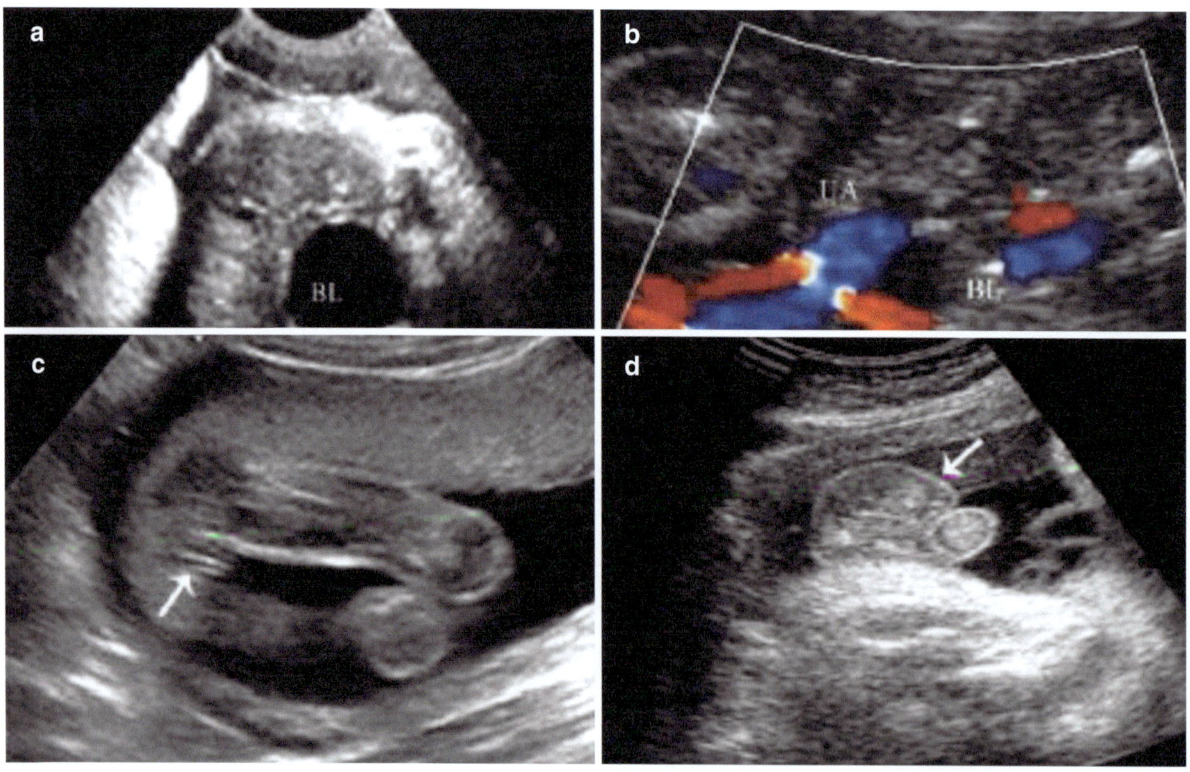

Fig. 2.24 Fetal bladder and genitalia. (**a, b**). Sagittal and transverse images of the lower abdomen show a circular anechoic bladder; (**c**). Axial image of female genitalia in a fetus shows the labia majora on both sides; (**d**). Image of male genitalia shows the scrotum, the penis, and the testicles on both sides clearly

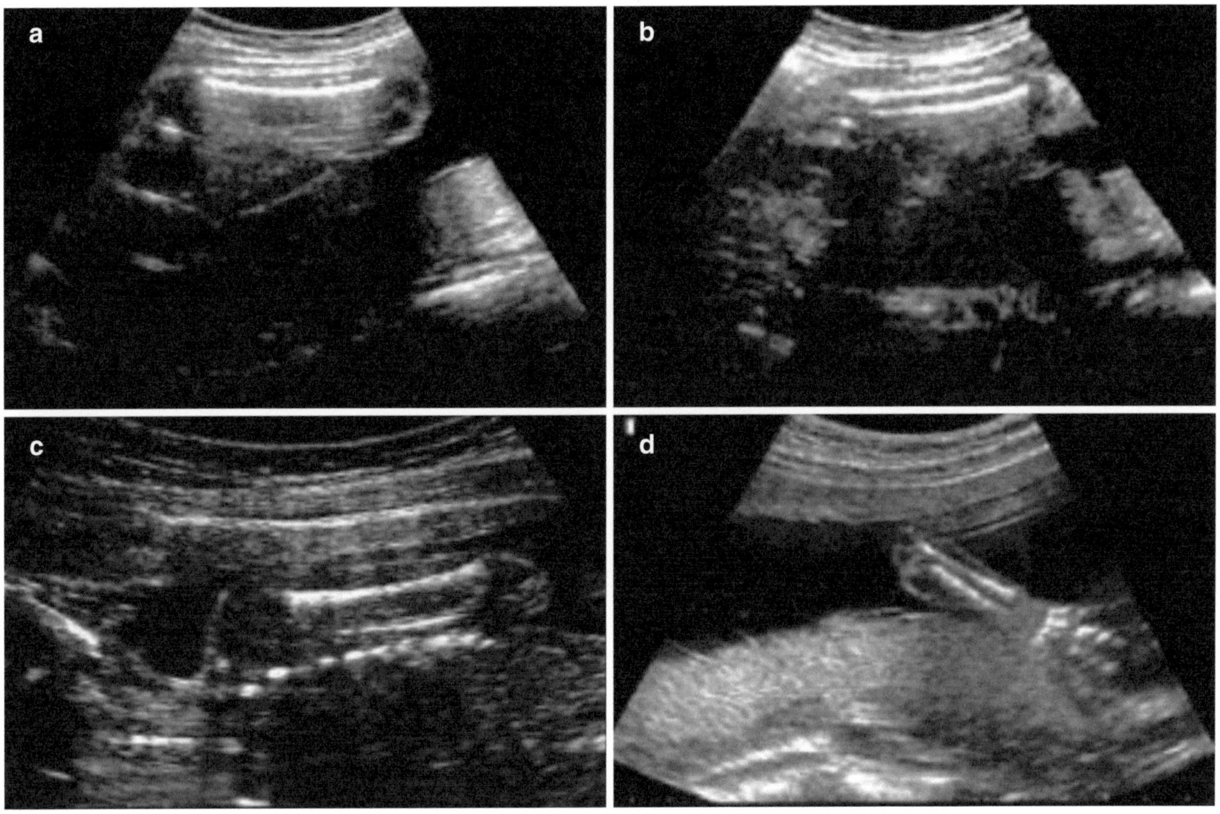

Fig. 2.25 Fetal limbs. (**a**). Longitudinal view of fetal femur; (**b**). Sagittal view of fetal tibia and fibula; (**c**). Sagittal view of fetal humerus; (**d**). Sagittal view of fetal ulna, radius, and metacarpus

2.3.2.3 Fetal Appurtenances

Placenta

The placenta is the organ that plays a crucial role in exchanging substances. As a combination of the embryonic and maternal tissues, it is composed of the amnion, lobule chorion, and decidua basalis. The placenta at term is circular or oval, 16 to 20 cm in diameter, and 1 to 3 cm in thickness (generally no more than 5 cm). The placenta is divided into the fetal side and maternal side. The arteries and veins of the umbilical cord radially distribute from the attachment of the umbilical cord to the placental (Fig. 2.27).

Fetal side of the placenta is covered with a smooth amniotic membrane, which presents as a thin strip-like hyperechoic. In contrast, the echo of the maternal side of the placenta is close to that of the myometrium. And the hypoechoic retroplacental space, composed of uterine vessels, can be visualized between posterior placenta and myometrium. The placental parenchyma appears as uniform and intermediate echo (Fig. 2.28).

Usually, the placenta is attached to anywhere of the uterine wall, including anterior, posterior, left lateral, right lateral, or fundal. The placenta substance in the first and second trimesters shows uniform moderate echo. During the second and third trimesters, the placenta can be divided into grades 0, I, II, and III according to the characteristics of the ultrasound image, which can be helpful to evaluate the maturity of the placenta (Figs.2.29 and 2.30).

Amniotic Fluid

Amniotic fluid is an essential environment for fetal growth, which protects the fetus and mother. The amount of amniotic fluid is sufficient in the second trimester and then decreased gradually. The amount of amniotic fluid significantly reduced in post-term pregnancy. The amniotic fluid shows anechoic areas for its excellent sound transmission. In the third trimester, moderate-echo particles are scattered in the amniotic fluid (Fig. 2.31).

There are two methods to estimate the amniotic fluid with the use of ultrasound techniques: one is to measure

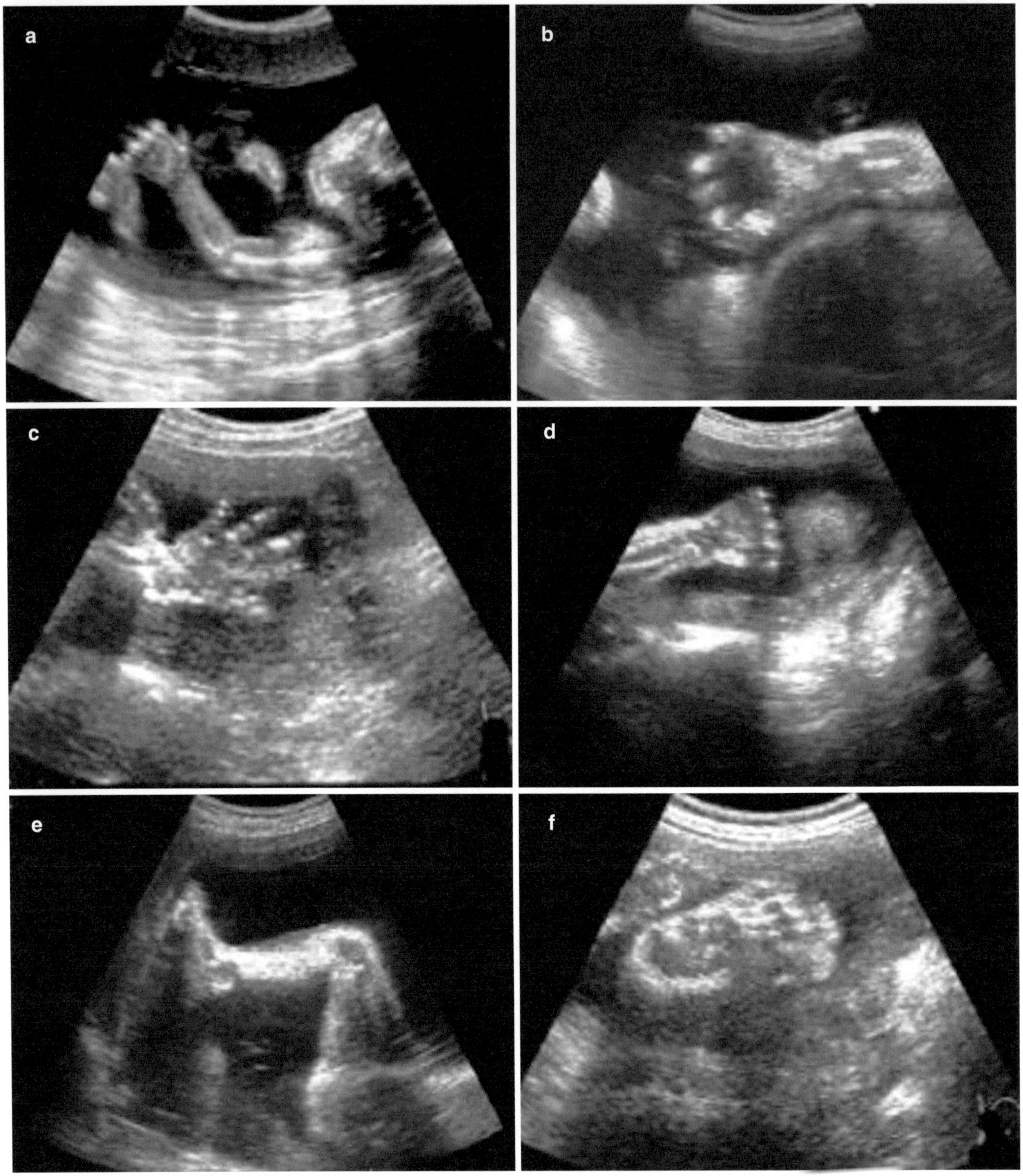

Fig. 2.26 Fetal movements. (**a to d**). The upper extremity and various positions of hand; (**e to g**). The lower extremity and different views of foot; (**h**). Fetal sucking its hand in the uterus

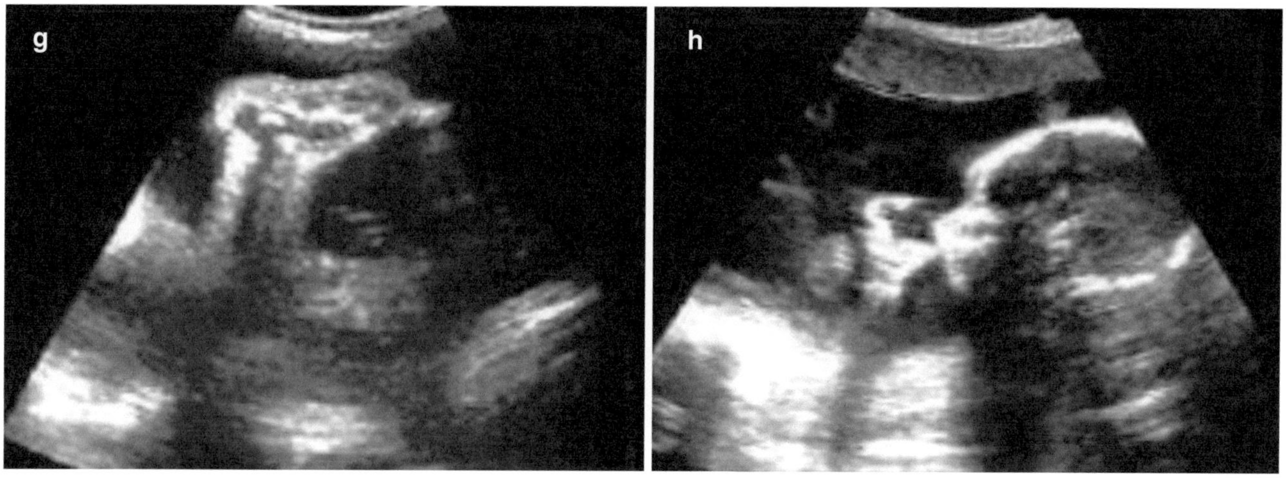

Fig. 2.26 (continued)

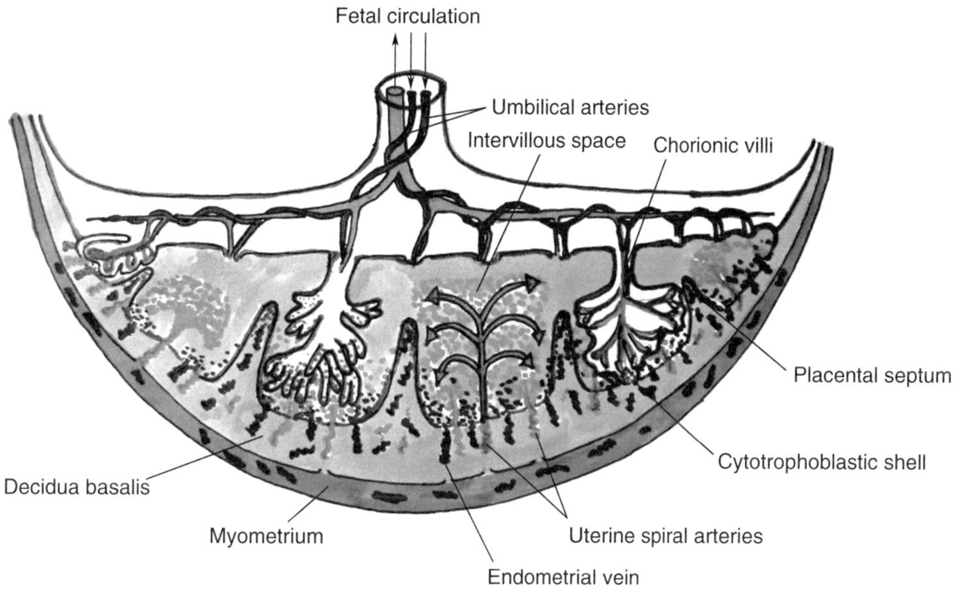

Fig. 2.27 Schematic representation of placenta

the deepest vertical pocket (DVP), the other is to measure the amniotic fluid index (AFI). To measure the depth of amniotic fluid, we should assess a pocket of a maximal depth of amniotic fluid and take the average value after repeated measurements. Measurement of amniotic fluid index (AFI): with the maternal midline and horizontal line through the umbilicus as the limits, the abdomen of pregnant women is divided into four quadrants: the upper left quadrant, the lower left quadrant, the upper right quadrant, and the lower right quadrant. Measure the maximum vertical depth of amniotic fluid in each of the uterine quadrants and sum up. The DVP ranges from 2 cm to 8 cm, and the normal range for AFI is 5 to 20 cm (Fig. 2.32).

Umbilical Cord

The umbilical cord is a strip-like tissue that connects the fetus and the placenta, which is vital for oxygen exchange, nutrients supply, and metabolites elimination between the mother and the fetus. One side of the cord is inserted into the umbilical ring of the fetal abdominal wall, the other is attached to the fetal side placenta. The cord contains one

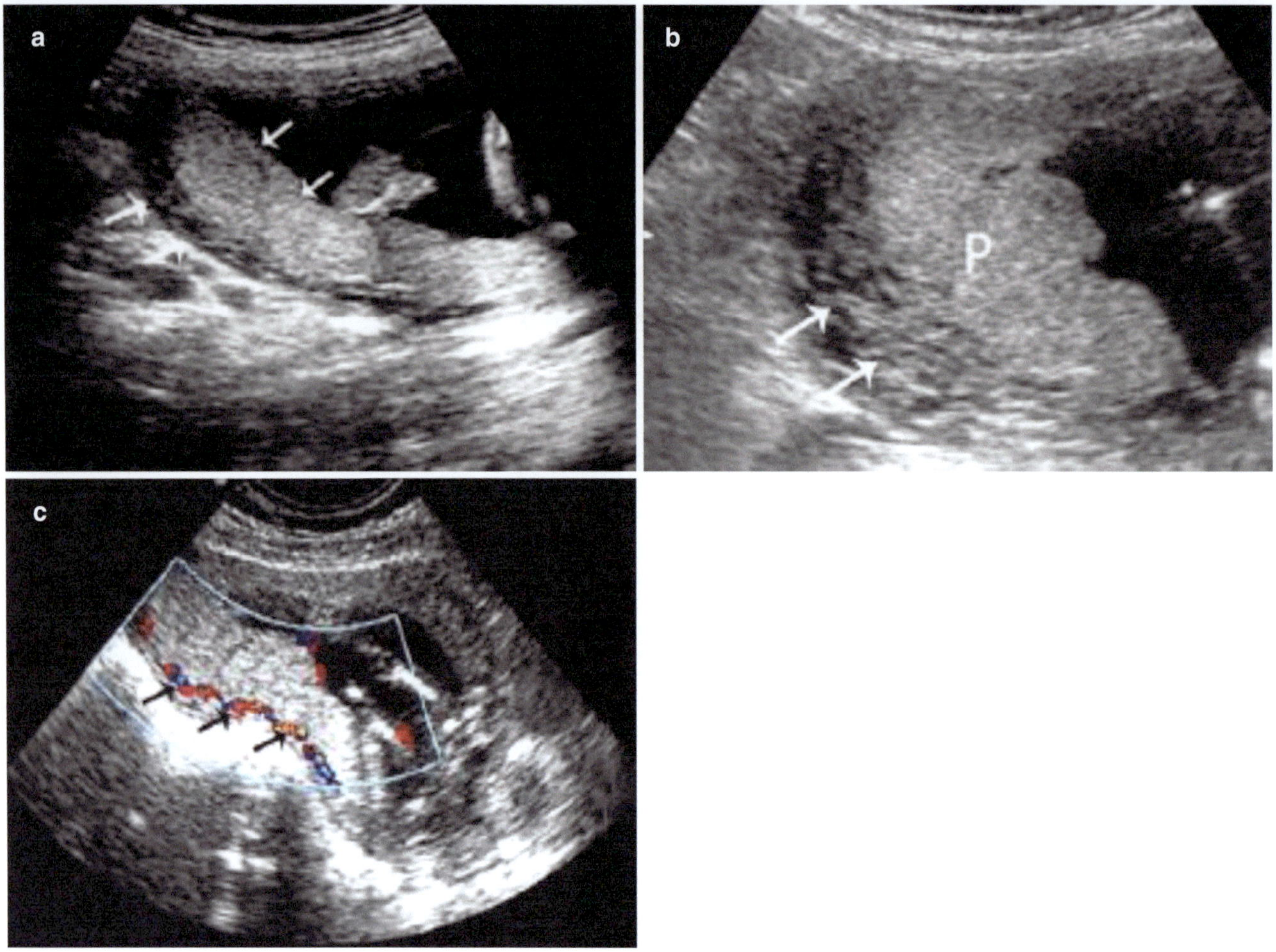

Fig. 2.28 Normal placenta. (**a**). Maternal side, parenchyma, and fetal side of the placenta; (**b**). Vena plexus in the retroplacental space appears hypoechoic; (**c**). The retroplacental space blood flow is shown by color Doppler ultrasound

umbilical vein and two arteries. Under ultrasound, the umbilical cord shows a twisted, alternating bright-dark echogenic structure, floating in amniotic fluid. The color Doppler shows a red and blue strip-like echo. Spectrum Doppler is utilized to analyze the spectrum of the umbilical artery and vein (Fig. 2.33).

2.3.2.4 Special Tips

1. During the ultrasound examination, we should confirm the gestational age and measure multiple parameters to evaluate whether the fetus is consistent with the gestational age.
2. The primary order of ultrasound scans in first, second, and third pregnancy is the fetal head, spine, trunk, internal organs, extremities, and appendages.
3. Detect fetal abnormalities at 11 to 13 + 6 weeks and 18 to 26 weeks, and repeated examination is recommended if necessary. The following fetal malformations should be prenatally diagnosed: anencephaly, encephalocele, spina bifida aperta, chest, and abdominal wall defects with the abnormal placement of internal organs, single cavity heart, and fatal achondroplasia.

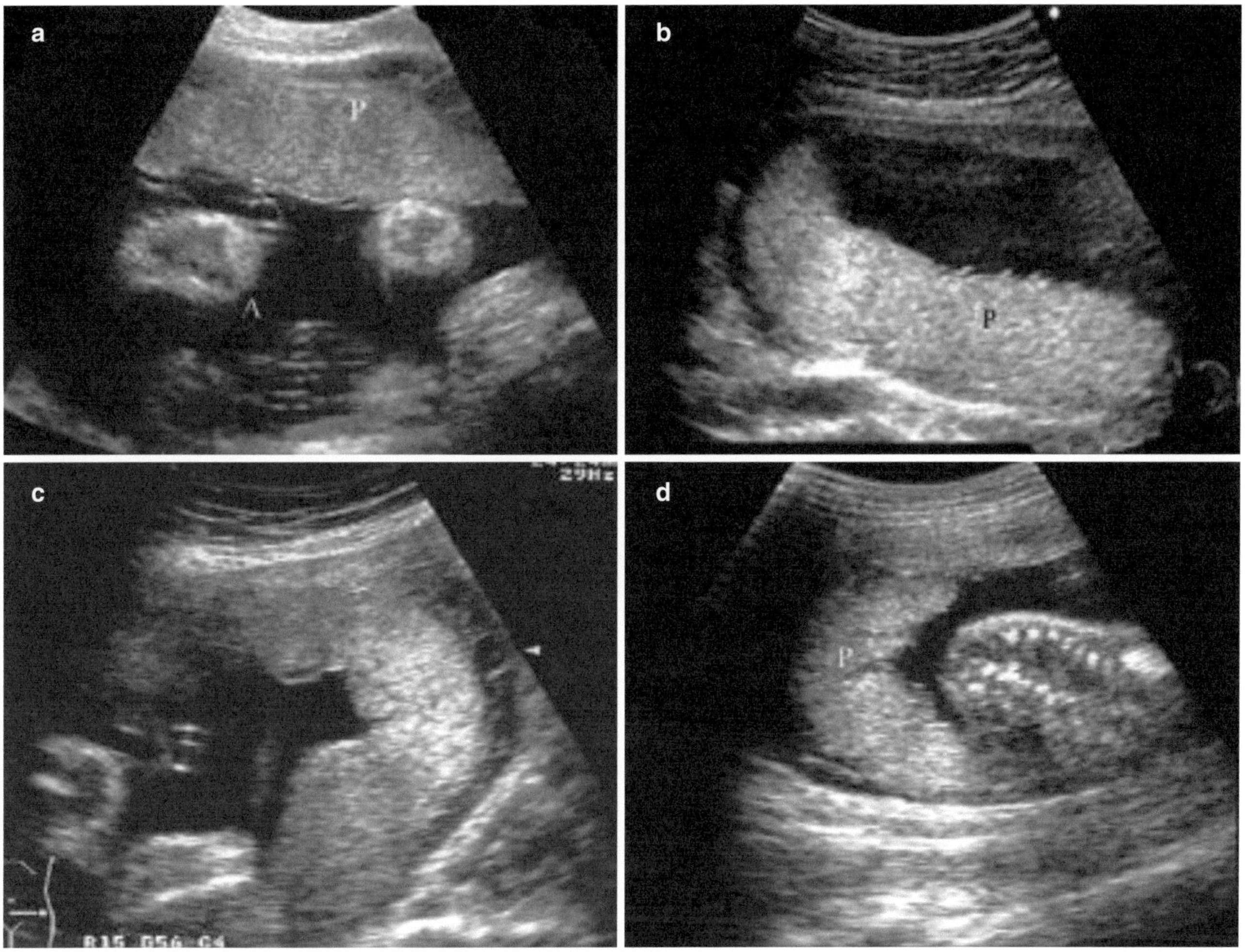

Fig. 2.29 Placental attachment. (**a**). Placenta is attached to the anterior wall of uterus; (**b**). Placenta is attached to the posterior wall of uterus; (**c**). Placenta is attached to the lateral wall of uterus; (**d**). Placenta is attached to the fundus of uterus

4. Early abortion with hematocele in uterine cavity should be distinguished from pseudogestational sac of ectopic pregnancy, twin pregnancy, intrauterine hematocele or effusion (Fig. 2.34).
5. During the second trimester, the placenta may be low-lying and partially or entirely covering the cervix, which requires dynamic observation. It is not appropriate to diagnose placenta previa too early.
6. When measuring the depth of amniotic fluid, the probe should be perpendicular to the uterine amniotic cavity, try to avoid the fetal limbs, and reduce the pressure on the abdominal wall of the pregnant woman.

2.3.2.5 Ultrasonic Bio-Parameter Evaluation of Fetal Development in the Second and Third Trimesters

After 12 weeks of pregnancy, all fetal systems develop rapidly. Real-time ultrasound can clearly display the morphological structure of each organ and its physiological activity. From the second trimester of gestation, measure the anatomic structures to detect fetal malformation as early as possible. Some standard biometric parameters are used to estimate fetal growth and gestational age by ultrasound, include biparietal diameter, head circumference, abdominal circumference, and femur length. When there is abnormal

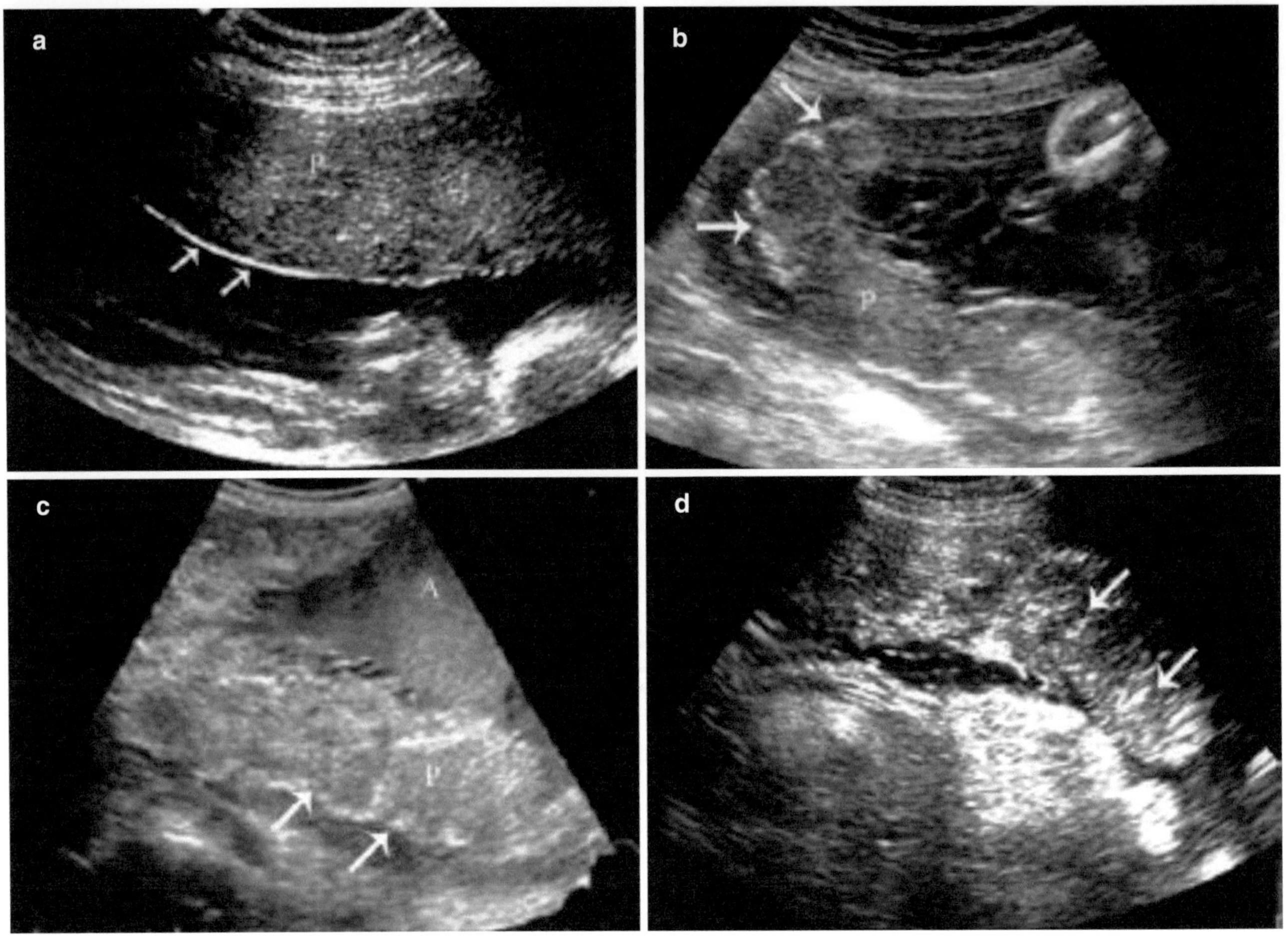

Fig. 2.30 Grading of placental maturity. (**a**). Grade 0 placenta, the chorionic plate showing as a bright, straight line, placenta substance presents uniform homogeneous echo, and the basal layer is not apparent; (**b**). Grade I placenta, chorionic plate surface is not smooth, and the echo of placenta substance is uniform, with a few hyperechoic spots on the maternal side of the placenta; (**c**). Grade II placenta, indentations along the chorionic plate extend to the placenta, which has not reached the basal layer. The echo of granules in the substance becomes thicker, and the hyperechoic strip area can be observed in the basal layer; (**d**). Grade III placenta, Indentations of the chorionic plate extend to the basal layer. The placenta lobules present as multiple isoechoic rings, and the blood pool in the central portion shows anechoic areas. The cellulose and calcium in the lobule space are hyperechoic. Thickened and highly reflective granule in placental substance is visible. The lobules integrate with the basal layer, without a distinctive boundary

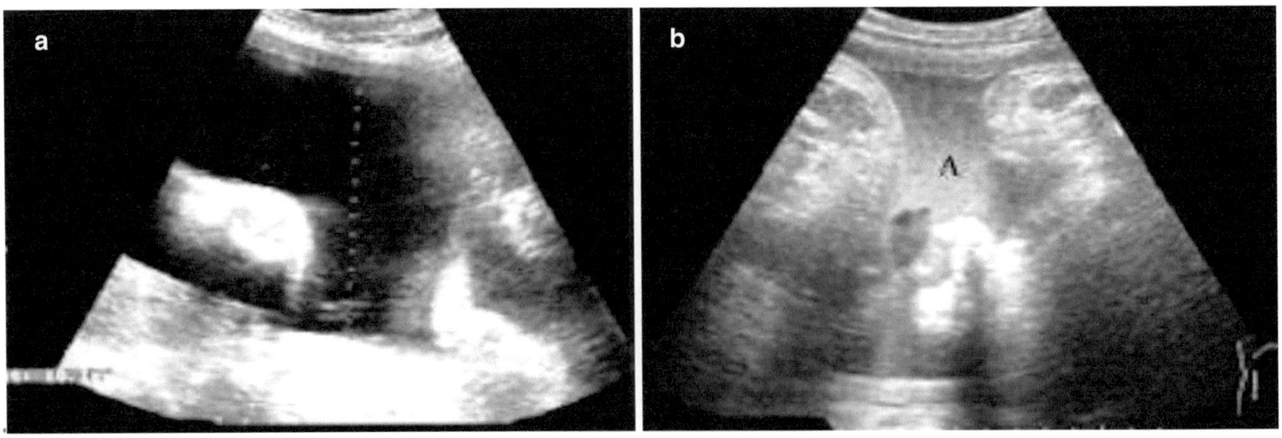

Fig. 2.31 Amniotic fluid. (**a**). The anechoic amniotic fluid with good sound transmission in the first and second trimester; (**b**). The amniotic fluid with scattered echogenic dots in the third trimester

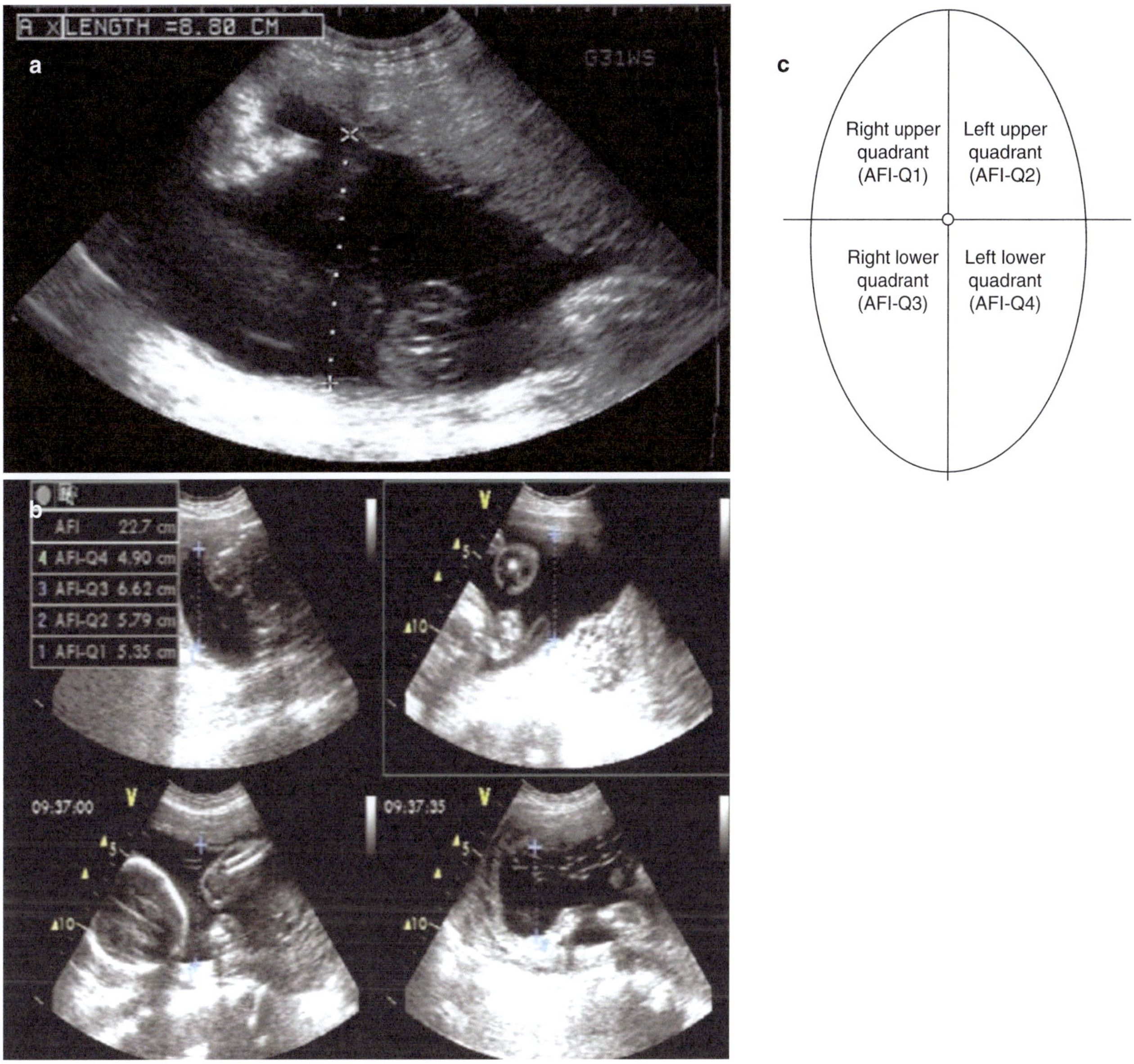

Fig. 2.32 Measurement of amniotic fluid. (**a**). Measurement of AFV should be performed in the vertical dimension, avoiding the fetal parts; (**b**). Schematic diagram of AFI measurement; (**c**). Measure the amniotic fluid of all the quadrants and sum up to obtain the AFI [Right upper quadrant(AFI-Q1); Left upper quadrant (AFI-Q2); Right lower quadrant(AFI-Q3); Left lower quadrant(AFI-Q4)]

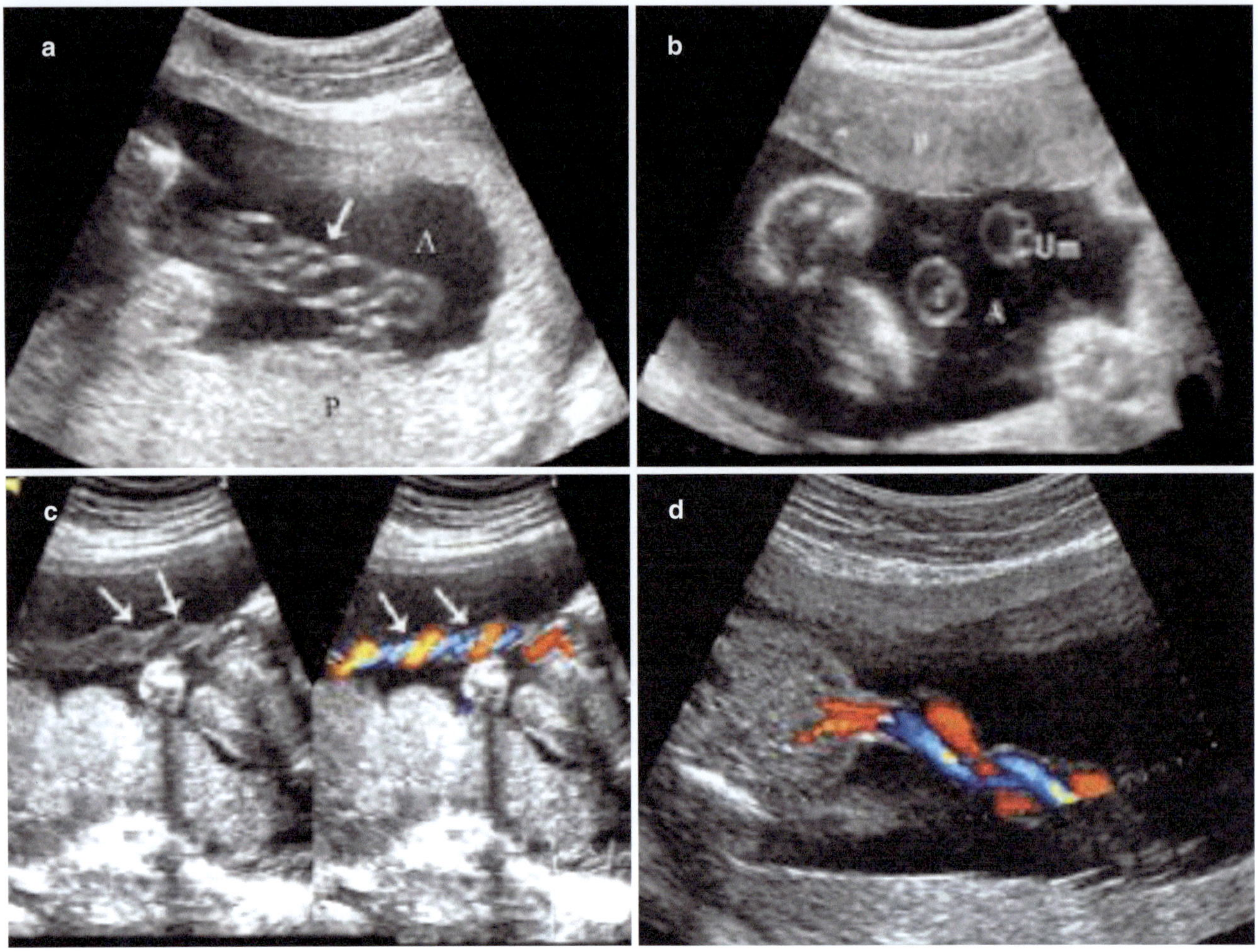

Fig. 2.33 Umbilical cord. (**a**). 2-D ultrasound shows the chain-like umbilical cord in amniotic fluid; (**b**). Transverse view of the umbilical cord distributed as a triangle; (**c**). The blood flow of the umbilical arteries and vein; (**d**). The umbilical cord originates from the umbilical ring of the fetal abdominal wall

development, the transverse cerebellum diameter, chest circumference, subcutaneous tissue, and other limb bones can be measured as well.

Estimation of Gestational Age by Ultrasound

1. Measurement of Biparietal Diameter

Biparietal diameter (BPD) is one of the basic prenatal examination biometers assessed by ultrasound. BPD should be measured on an axial plane at the level of thalami, where the calvaria presents as an oval ring, and the septum pellucidum, symmetrical thalamus, intermittently midline falx, the third ventricle, and other structures are visible. There are three methods to measure the BPD: ① from the outer edge of the fetal calvarial wall to the outer edge of the contralateral side; ② from the outer edge of the fetal calvarial wall in the near field to the inner edge of the contralateral side; ③ the distance between the two sides of the calvarial wall (Fig. 2.35).

2. Measurement of head circumference

Head circumference (HC) measurement can reflect the growth of the fetal head more accurately. When there is a nonstandard shape of fetal head, HC is used in conjunction with the BPD. The HC is measured on the same view as the

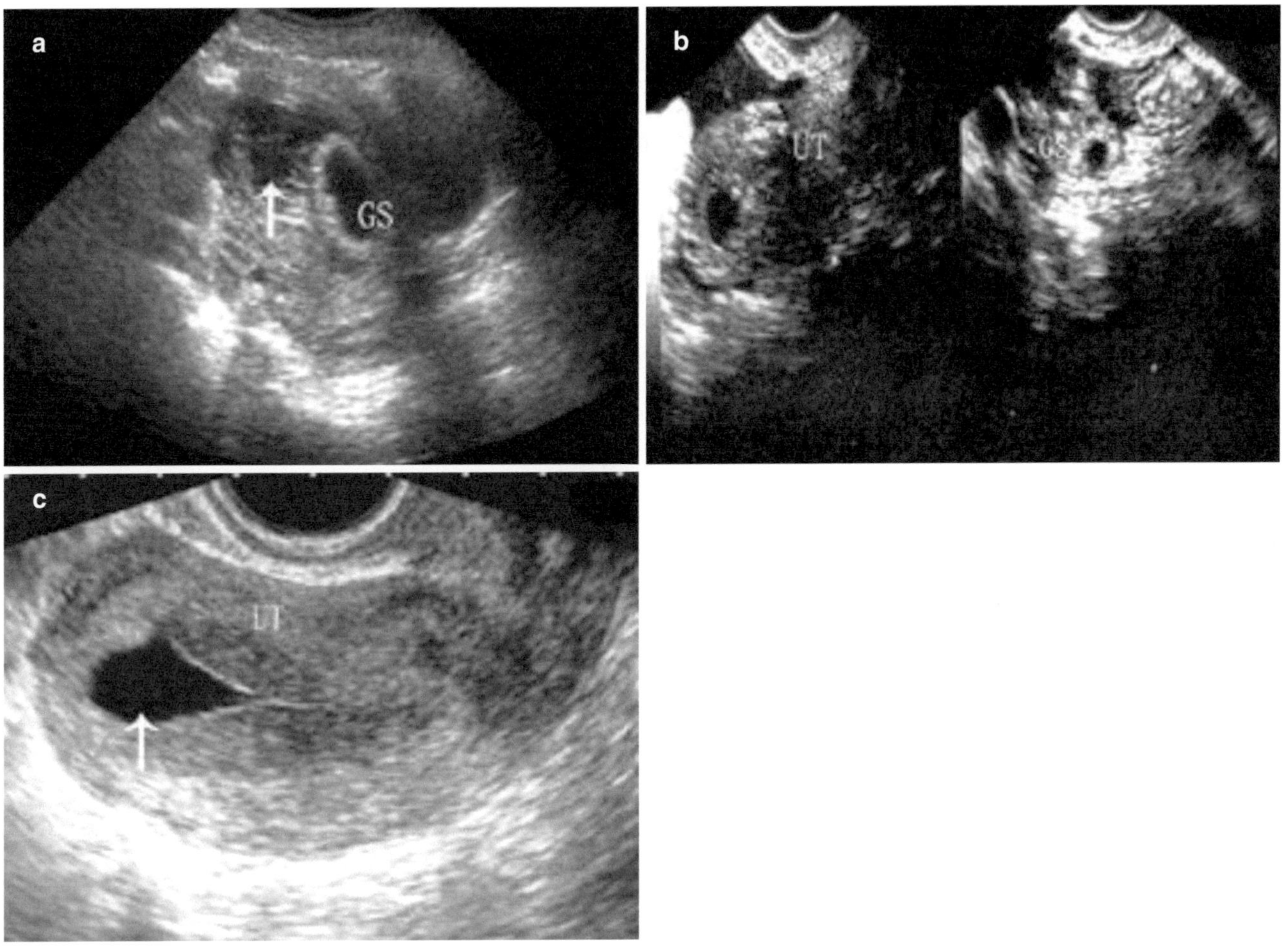

Fig. 2.34 Ultrasonographic features and differential diagnosis of uterine hematocele in early pregnancy. (**a**). Forty-five days after the last menstrual period, an embryo with a heartbeat in the gestational sac, accompanied by hematometra; (**b**). 36 days after the last menstrual period, the gestational sac-like echolucent area in the uterine cavity, without embryo inside. The decidual reaction is not obvious. The echo of the gestational sac, about 0.8 cm in diameter, is visible in the right adnexal area. The decidual reaction is obvious, and HCG was positive. (**c**). The intracavitary fluid is visible

BPD. Use the peripheral trace function button of the ultrasonic instrument to trace along the outer edge of the calvarium, and the HC value can be automatically obtained. Alternatively, it can be measured from the anteroposterior diameter (A) and transverse diameter (B) of the calvarium on the standard view of the skull. The calculation formula of HC is HC = (A + B) *1.57 (Fig. 2.36).

3. Measurement of abdominal circumference

The measurement of the abdominal circumference (AC) is mostly used in the third trimester. During late pregnancy, the growth rate of AC gradually exceeds that of HC, due to the development of internal organs and the increase of subcutaneous fat. Therefore, the abdominal circumference is considered to be the best indicator for assessing fetal growth and estimating body weight in late pregnancy. When measuring the AC, take a transverse image of the fetal abdomen, which is circular or oval, at the level of the stomach bubble. The portal vein is in the front, and the spine is visible in a transverse view. The measurements include skin and subcutaneous fat. The measurement method is the same as that of HC. The calculation formula for AC is AC = (A + B) × 1.57 (Fig. 2.37).

Calculation: Choose the ellipse function button of the ultrasonic instrument to trace over the outer edge of the abdominal wall, then the value of AC is obtained.

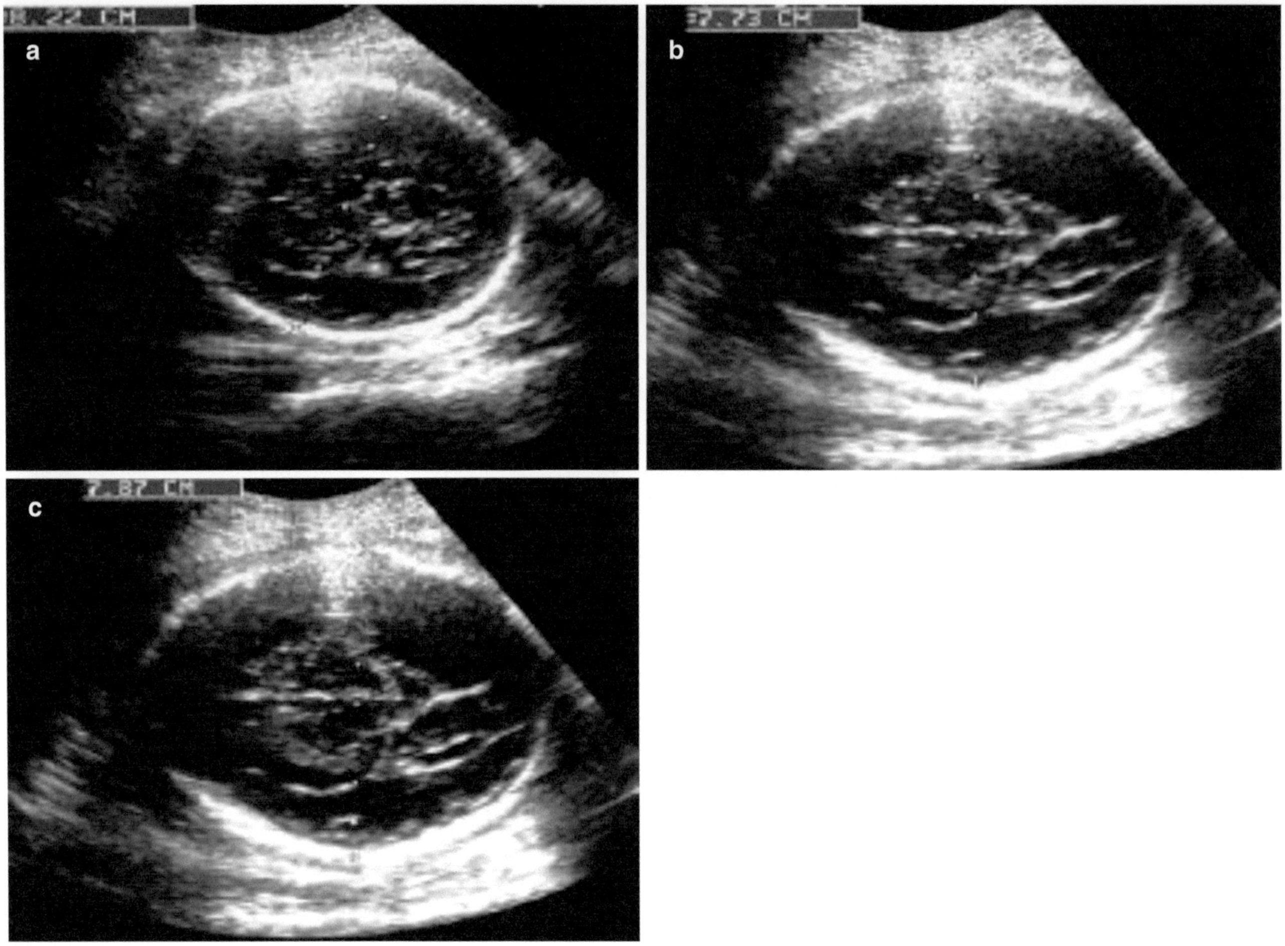

Fig. 2.35 Measurement of BPD. (**a**). The first method for BPD measurement: from the outer edge of fetal calvarial wall to the contralateral outer edge; (**b**). The second approach for BPD measurement: from the outer edge of the skull to the contralateral medial edge; (**c**). The third approach for BPD measurement: distance between the midpoints of the calvarial wall on both sides

4. Measurement of femur length

The length of the femur is relatively easy to measure, and its accuracy is similar to that of BPD. It is also one of the basic biometric parameters under prenatal ultrasound. When measuring the femur, hold the probe and scan down the fetal spine longitudinally to the sacrum, showing the transverse view of one femur, and then slowly rotate the probe to display the long axis of the whole femur. The beam must be perpendicular to the long axis of the femur, and the distance between the proximal apex of the femur and the midpoint of the distal slope is measured (Fig. 2.38).

The normal values of fetal BPD, chest circumference, AC, FL, and FL/AC at 19 to 42 gestational weeks are shown in Tables 2.3 and 2.4.

Estimation of Fetal Weight

Measure fetal bio-parameters by prenatal ultrasound to estimate the fetal weight, which is of great clinical significance for the diagnosis of threatened preterm delivery, intrauterine fetal growth retardation, giant fetus, and post-term pregnancy. The prediction of prenatal fetal weight is helpful for obstetricians to judge the survival rate of the fetus, to propose treatment protocol and to determine the delivery time and mode.

Up to now, many calculation methods and formulas for estimating fetal weight by ultrasonic measurement have been reported. The relationship between fetal weight and birth weight by single parameter measurement is analyzed in our hospital. This study conducted 115 cases from 38 to 41 weeks of gestation without any complications. Multiple parameters

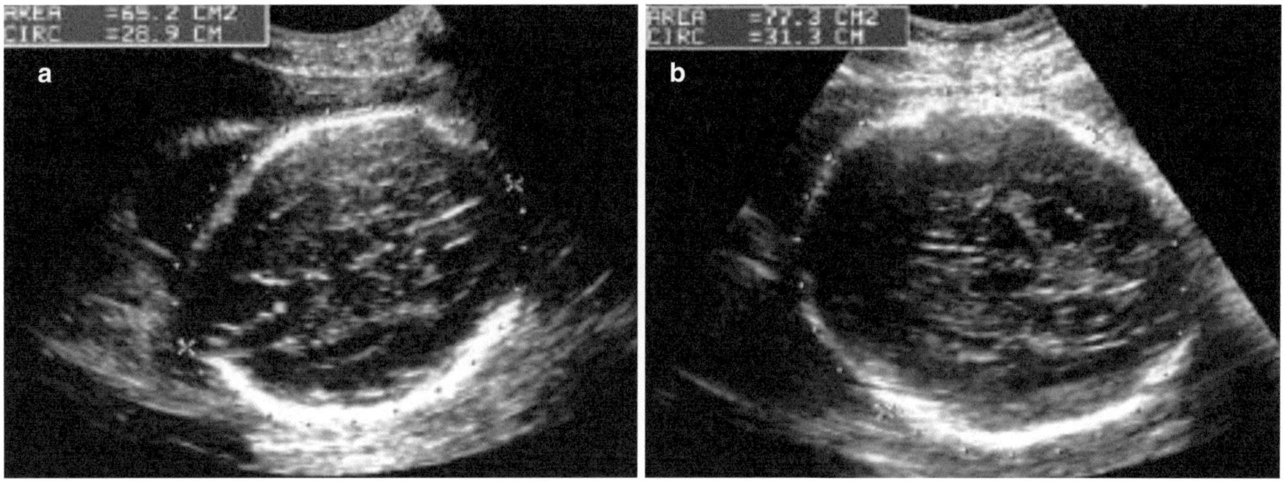

Fig. 2.36 Measurement of fetal head. (**a**). The first approach for HC measurement: trace along the outer perimeter of the calvarium with trace function button; (**b**). The second approach: HC = (A + B) × 1.57

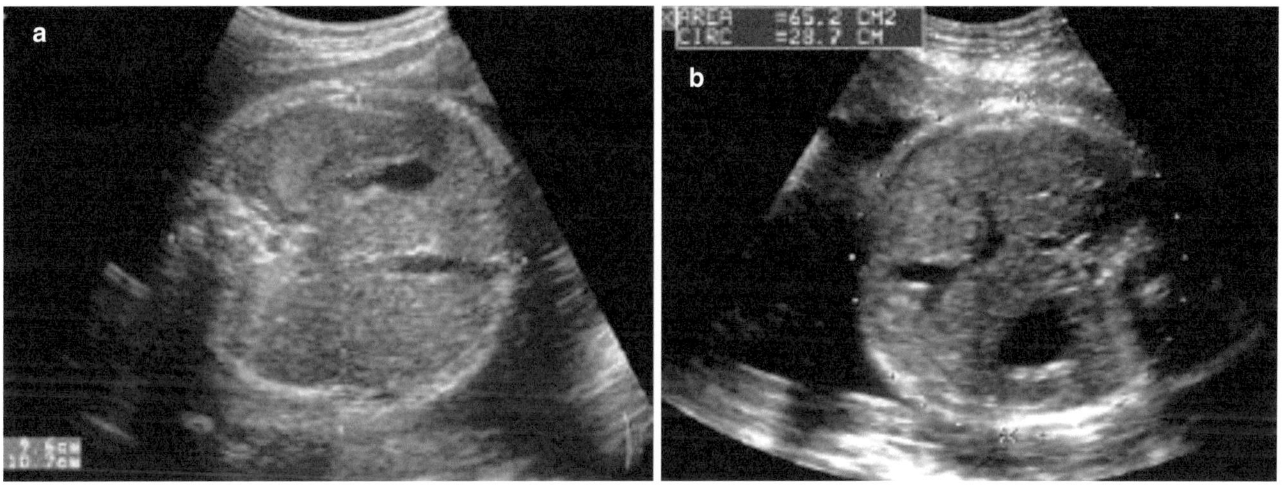

Fig. 2.37 Measurement of fetal AC. (**a**). The first approach for AC measurement: AC = (A + B) × 1.57; (**b**). The second approach: choose the ellipse function button to trace over the outer edge of the abdominal wall

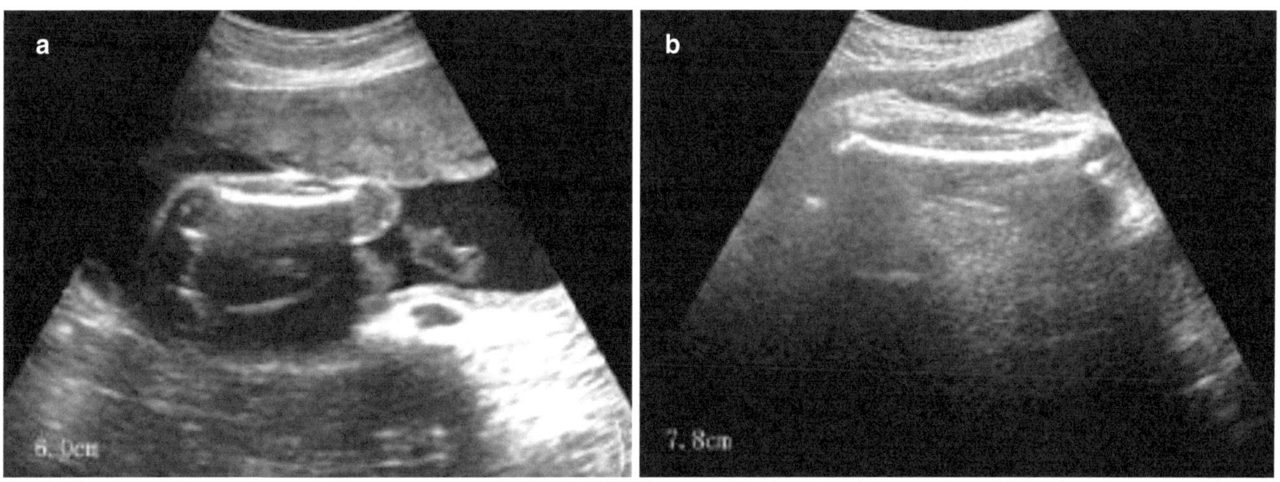

Fig. 2.38 Measurement of FL. (**a, b**). Measure the distance from the top of the proximal arc of the femur to the midpoint of the distal slope

Table 2.3 Predictive parameters of gestational age and fetal development [Unit (cm)]

Item	BPD			TC			AC			FL			
Percentile	10	50	90	10	50	90	10	50	90	10	50	90	FL/AC
19 to 22 weeks	4.25	4.94	5.43	12.09	14.01	15.83	12.72	14.51	16.65	2.76	3.39	4.02	0.23
23 to 26 weeks	5.70	6.29	7.06	16.87	18.54	20.39	15.81	19.29	21.55	3.96	4.68	5.32	0.24
27 to 28 weeks	7.17	7.62	7.84	20.92	22.15	23.69	21.80	23.40	25.00	5.50	5.78	6.12	0.25
29 to 30 weeks	7.72	7.92	8.30	22.18	23.50	25.13	25.53	24.41	25.95	5.78	5.90	6.46	0.25
31 to 32 weeks	7.98	8.29	8.53	23.38	24.66	25.95	24.57	25.86	26.92	5.97	6.36	6.63	0.25
33 to 34 weeks	8.36	8.66	9.00	24.79	25.76	27.11	26.08	26.99	28.34	6.43	6.74	7.09	0.25
35 weeks	8.65	8.91	9.22	26.04	27.11	28.46	27.01	27.99	29.39	6.76	6.98	7.37	0.25
36 weeks	8.81	9.02	9.40	26.86	29.63	28.77	27.83	28.93	30.15	6.88	7.22	7.48	0.25
37 weeks	8.88	9.19	9.41	27.04	28.21	29.34	28.36	29.53	30.59	7.14	7.48	7.85	0.25
38 weeks	9.03	9.33	9.66	27.55	23.71	29.81	28.74	30.09	31.25	7.24	7.65	7.98	0.25
39 weeks	8.99	9.35	9.65	28.24	29.37	30.41	28.80	30.09	31.54	7.36	7.82	8.11	0.25
40 weeks	9.10	9.42	9.65	27.84	29.06	30.35	29.31	30.44	31.73	7.40	7.79	8.16	0.25
41 to 42 weeks	9.15	9.59	9.83	27.65	29.34	30.82	29.63	30.70	32.04	7.68	7.87	8.17	0.25

Note: the data is from the West China Second University Hospital, Sichuan University

Table 2.4 The length of fetal limb bones [Unit: cm, $\overline{x} \pm s$]

Fertilization age	Humerus	Ulna	Radius	Femur	Tibia
12	1.29 ± 0.23	0.96 ± 0.18	0.81 ± 0.23	1.36 ± 0.30	0.93 ± 0.23
13	1.50 ± 0.29	1.32 ± 0.22	1.00 ± 0.27	1.60 ± 0.25	1.22 ± 0.24
14	2.06 ± 0.48	1.78 ± 0.49	1.56 ± 0.46	2.11 ± 0.45	1.61 ± 0.49
15	2.08 ± 0.29	1.86 ± 0.19	1.62 ± 0.17	2.11 ± 0.26	1.74 ± 0.32
16	2.51 ± 0.24	2.23 ± 0.23	2.02 ± 0.20	2.59 ± 0.20	2.14 ± 0.14
17	2.83 ± 0.24	2.59 ± 0.23	2.34 ± 0.19	2.88 ± 0.20	2.52 ± 0.24
18	3.10 ± 0.12	2.91 ± 0.18	2.55 ± 0.21	3.32 ± 0.26	2.88 ± 0.25
19	3.37 ± 0.21	3.10 ± 0.20	2.79 ± 0.19	3.53 ± 0.19	3.06 ± 0.21
20	3.68 ± 0.18	3.34 ± 0.10	2.96 ± 0.14	3.93 ± 0.10	3.33 ± 0.25
21	3.79 ± 0.20	3.58 ± 0.21	3.17 ± 0.20	4.06 ± 0.28	3.48 ± 0.22
22	4.10 ± 0.23	3.85 ± 0.26	3.46 ± 0.34	4.40 ± 0.37	3.76 ± 0.21
23	4.29 ± 0.24	3.94 ± 0.19	3.52 ± 0.15	4.52 ± 0.30	3.95 ± 0.21
24	4.51 ± 0.22	4.06 ± 0.19	3.63 ± 0.20	4.67 ± 0.21	4.29 ± 0.18
25	4.66 ± 0.20	4.34 ± 0.17	3.85 ± 0.18	5.09 ± 0.19	4.45 ± 0.21
26	4.89 ± 0.30	4.43 ± 0.45	3.97 ± 0.41	5.49 ± 0.41	4.69 ± 0.34
27	5.14 ± 0.30	4.60 ± 0.28	4.19 ± 0.30	5.72 ± 0.28	4.98 ± 0.37
28	5.14 ± 0.20	4.73 ± 0.20	4.34 ± 0.17	5.73 ± 0.31	4.96 ± 0.17
29	5.23 ± 0.32	4.86 ± 0.24	4.38 ± 0.26	6.00 ± 0.30	5.22 ± 0.28
30	5.55 ± 0.21	5.15 ± 0.25	4.72 ± 0.24	6.26 ± 0.21	5.52 ± 0.28
31	5.76 ± 0.26	5.28 ± 0.26	4.81 ± 0.36	6.50 ± 0.34	5.66 ± 0.26
32	5.83 ± 0.31	5.31 ± 0.29	4.77 ± 0.28	6.73 ± 0.37	5.79 ± 0.39
33	5.95 ± 0.26	5.45 ± 0.33	4.95 ± 0.36	6.98 ± 0.24	5.93 ± 0.33
34	6.04 ± 0.40	5.52 ± 0.30	5.01 ± 0.37	6.89 ± 0.33	5.92 ± 0.31
35	6.31 ± 0.26	5.89 ± 0.37	5.35 ± 0.37	7.43 ± 0.23	6.22 ± 0.20
36	6.38 ± 024	5.74 ± 0.32	5.31 ± 0.42	7.37 ± 0.17	6.19 ± 0.39
37	6.47 ± 0.19	5.92 ± 0.18	5.36 ± 0.20	7.59 ± 0.13	6.45 ± 0.23
38	6.72 ± 0.40	6.00 ± 0.37	5.56 ± 0.46	7.60 ± 0.43	6.56 ± 0.50

Note: the data is from the West China Second University Hospital, Sichuan University

including BPD, HC, AC, transverse cerebellar diameter, FL, subcutaneous tissue thickness at the middle of the femur, kidney length, and liver length were measured by ultrasound within three days before delivery. Also, the bodyweight of the neonate was measured within 24 hours after delivery. After statistical processing, the linear relationship and relative error of each index were calculated, and transverse cerebellar diameter was best correlated with the fetal weight. No matter which method or formula is used to estimate the fetal weight, the accuracy of ultrasonic measurement affected

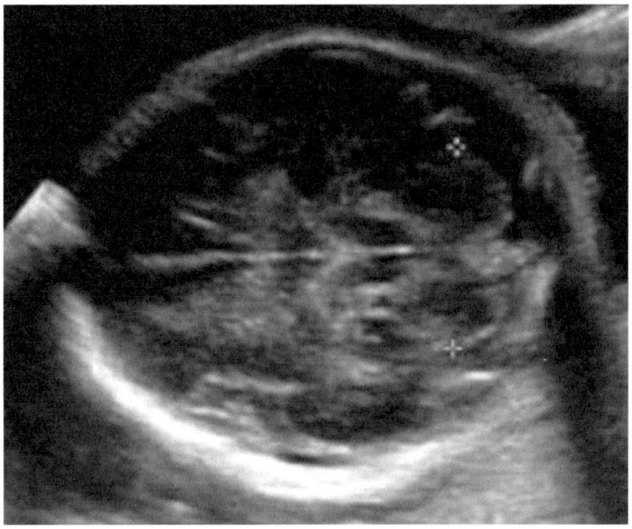

Fig. 2.39 Image of the fetal cerebellum

by many factors must be taken into accounts, such as the verification of menstrual cycle and gestational age, the body shape of pregnant women, complications, drug abuse, and genetic factors (Fig. 2.39).

Special Tips

1. When measuring growth parameters, pay attention to select the standard views, and take the average value after three or more measurements.
2. The measurement methods used must be uniform. There are many parameters and measurement methods introduced at home and abroad. Choose uniform methods and standards, and derive the standard application data of the region.
3. The errors are mostly caused by nonstandard planes, inconsistent measurement methods, and the effects of different fetal positions and head shapes (Fig. 2.40).

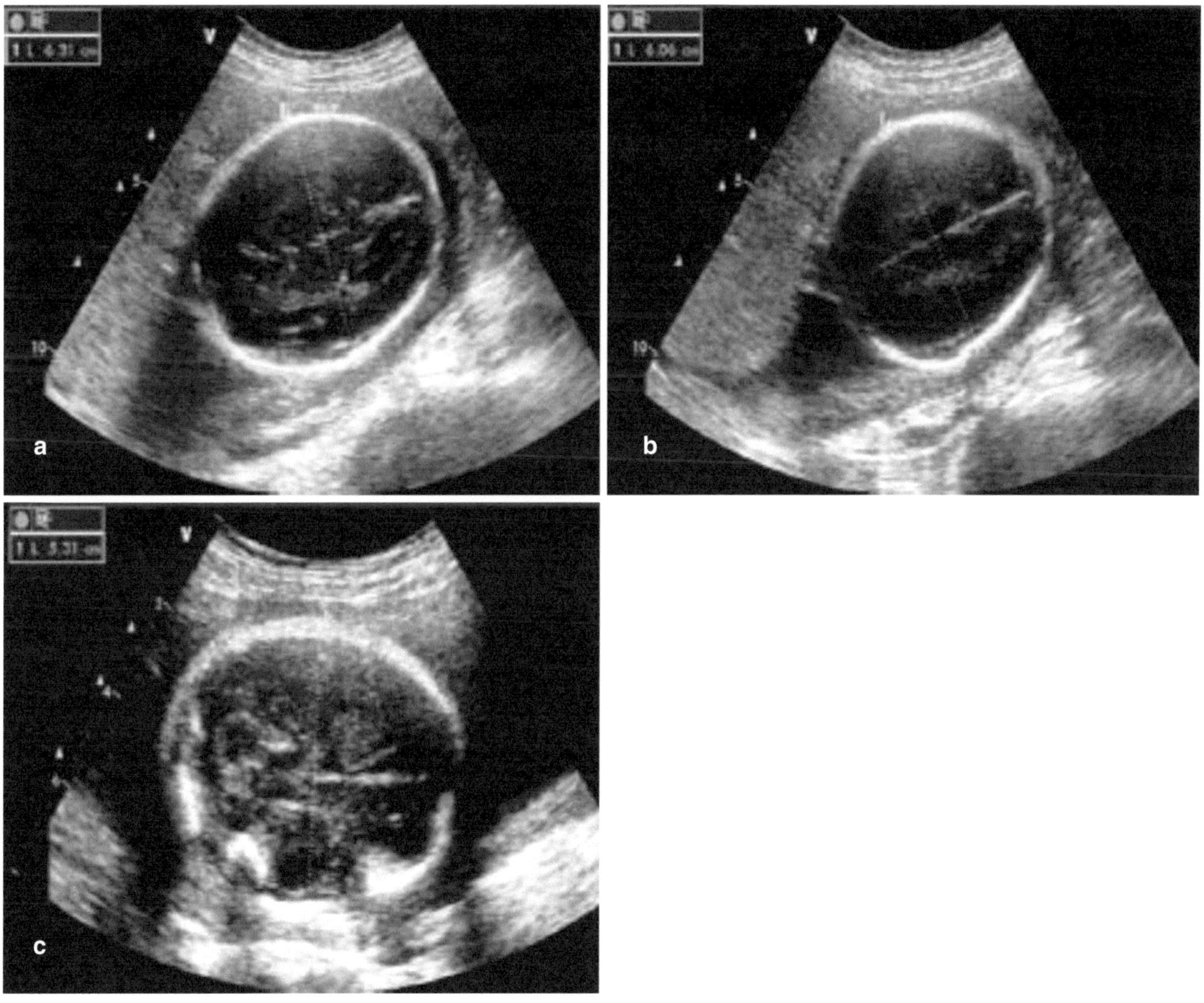

Fig. 2.40 Measurement of BPD in different views. (**a**). Standard view of BPD; (**b**). The brain midline demonstrates a straight line, the intracranial structure is unidentifiable, and the measured value is too small; (**c**). When the bone echo is observed in the head, the measured value of BPD is too small

Table 2.5 S/D ratio value ($\overline{x} \pm s$) of the umbilical artery in normal pregnancy

Gestational age(week)	$20^{+} \sim 24$	$24^{+} \sim 28$	$28^{+} \sim 30$	$30^{+} \sim 34$	$34^{+} \sim 38$	$38^{+} \sim 42$
S/D	3.9 ± 0.8	3.1 ± 0.5	2.8 ± 0.4	2.7 ± 0.4	2.3 ± 0.3	2.1 ± 0.3

Note: The data are from the West China Second Hospital of Sichuan University

2.3.2.6 Clinical Significance of Fetal Umbilical Artery Blood Flow Doppler

Basic Concepts

Fetal placental circulation and maternal placental circulation are respective blood circulation systems during pregnancy. The oxygen and material for fetal growth are exchanged between the mother and the fetus through the placenta barrier. The placenta is a vital organ, which allows for blood and substance exchange, deliver nutrient-rich blood to fetal tissues and organs via blood circulation channels, including umbilical artery, umbilical vein, vein catheter, artery catheter, and patent foramen ovale. Use color Doppler ultrasound to detect the maternal and fetal blood circulations, which indirectly reflects the status of fetal blood supply.

The hemodynamics change of fetal umbilical artery can indicate the function of placenta and the intrauterine state of the fetus indirectly. In normal pregnancy, the hemodynamic characteristics of fetal placenta circulation are represented by the ratio of peak systolic velocity (S)-to-peak end-diastolic velocity (D) of umbilical artery.

Color Doppler ultrasound for fetal umbilical arterial blood flow spectrum is easy to obtain, without any discomfort to pregnant women, and no side effects to the fetus. As a noninvasive prenatal examination, it has been widely used in surveillance of placental function and fetal intrauterine condition.

Detection method of umbilical artery blood flow spectrum: The umbilical artery can be detected at the free-floating portion of umbilical cord in the amniotic fluid, near the beginning of the placenta or the abdominal wall of the fetus. The arteries in the umbilical cord should be located by color Doppler, and the sampling volume was placed at the artery to detect the blood flow spectrum to obtain the S/D ratio.

Normal Spectral Doppler of Fetal Umbilical Artery

Since the application of spectrum Doppler ultrasound in obstetrics, many scholars have studied the fetal umbilical artery hemodynamics and established their own standard umbilical artery S/D value. A large number of studies indicate that the placenta matures during normal pregnancy, with increasing villous capillaries, decreased placental vascular resistance, and increased blood flow. The end-diastolic velocity of umbilical artery increases. Therefore, the S/D ratio value of umbilical artery decreases with gestational age. Most scholars regard the umbilical artery S/D ≤ 3 as normal standard for term pregnancy. The ultrasonic measurement of fetal umbilical blood flow S/D ratio in our hospital is shown in Table 2.5.

Abnormal Spectral Doppler of Fetal Umbilical Artery

With the development of the pregnancy, if the fetal umbilical artery S/D ratio fails to decrease with gestational weeks, or S/D > 3 at term, even with the absent end-diastolic velocity (AEDV) or reversed end-diastolic velocity (REDV), the following abnormalities should be considered: placental insufficiency, intrauterine growth retardation, fetal distress, maternal pregnancy-induced hypertension, fetal malformations, and oligohydramnios. The umbilical artery blood flow of 101 high-risk singleton pregnancy fetuses were detected. According to the ROC curve, the best S/D ratio value for predicting adverse pregnancy outcomes was defined as 2.8, having a sensitivity of 70.6%, a specificity of 97.6%, and an accuracy of 92.0%. Moreover, we compared and analyzed the S/D ratio of the umbilical artery between 59 malformed fetuses and 118 healthy fetuses in our hospital. The umbilical artery S/D ratio of the fetuses with multiple malformations, digestive system malformations, and central nervous system malformations were significantly higher than that in the normal control group, suggesting that increased or abnormal S/D ratio of the umbilical artery should be watched over for fetal malformation.

Typical Cases

When AEDV or REDV appears in the fetal umbilical artery blood flow spectrum, the fetal prognosis is poor (Figs. 2.41 and 2.42).

At 37 weeks and 5 days of gestation, oligohydramnios was observed, and fetal umbilical artery S/D ratio was 4.5. Cesarean section was performed due to markedly decreased fetal movement 2 days later. The neonate exhibited Apgar scores as 6 immediately after delivery, 7 at 1 minute, and 10 at 3 minutes. He was diagnosed with mild neonatal asphyxia clinically.

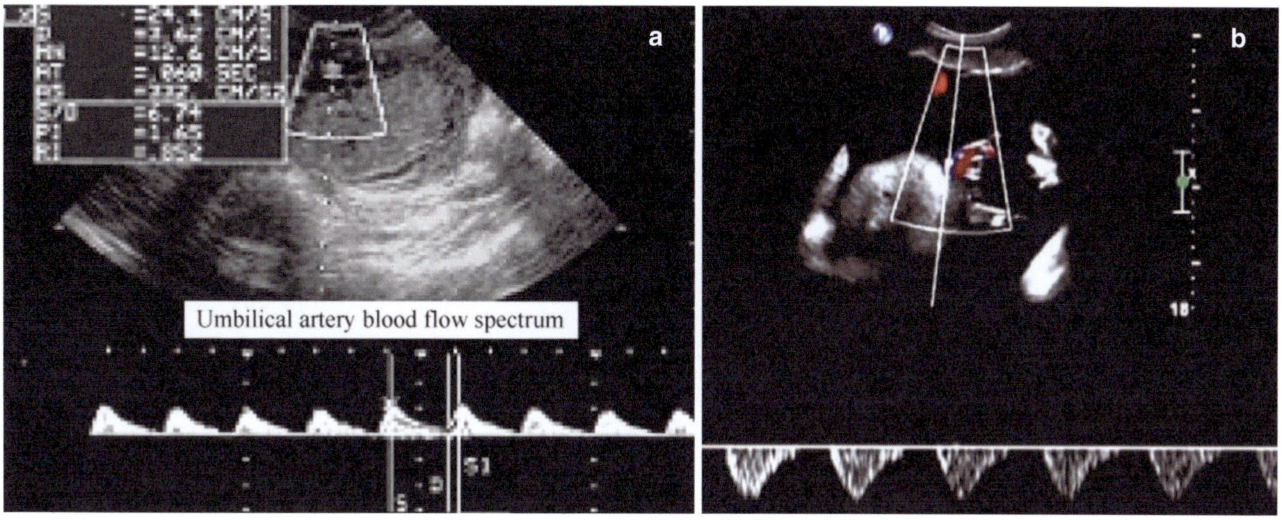

Fig. 2.41 Abnormal fetal umbilical artery blood flow spectrum (1). (**a**, **b**). 33 weeks of pregnancy combined with pregnancy-induced hypertension, oligohydramnios, and IUGR, the first color Doppler ultrasound scan showed the umbilical artery S/D ratio was 6.74. Five days later, the CDFI showed the REDV, with unresponsive NST for many times. Two days later, the intrauterine fetus died. Placental pathological indicated extensive multifocal ischemic infarction with multiple hematomas

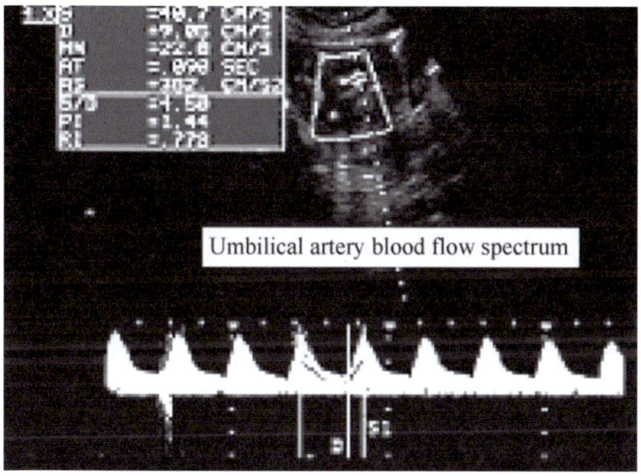

Fig. 2.42 Abnormal fetal umbilical artery blood flow spectrum (2)

2.4 Ultrasonic Diagnosis of Fetal Abnormality

2.4.1 Normal Multiple Pregnancy

2.4.1.1 Basic Concepts

Multiple pregnancy is defined as the presence of two or more fetuses in the uterus during the same pregnancy. The ratio of twins to singleton pregnancy in China is 1: (66 to 104). Family history, multiple parity, and other factors increase the incidence of multiple pregnancy. In recent years, due to the widespread development of assisted reproductive technology, the incidence of twin or more has increased dramatically, even as high as 20%–40%.

In multiple pregnancies, maternal complications are more common, maternal morbidity, perinatal mortality, and the incidence of neonatal disease are higher. Ultrasound is a convenient and practical method to diagnose multiple pregnancy, and the accuracy in early pregnancy is almost 100%. Ultrasound has become an essential method for multiple pregnancy.

There are two types of twins, dizygotic twins and monozygotic twins. Dizygotic twins are formed by the fertilization of two ova respectively, accounting for about two-third of the total number; and monozygotic twins account for one-third. According to the different replication times of oosperm, twins are divided into three types, including dichorionic diamniotic twin, monochorionic diamniotic twin, and monochorionic monoamniotic twin.

Family history of twins, ovulation induction, vitro fertilization and multiple embryos transfer may be found during the process of history taking. Pregnant women have more severe morning sickness and more weight gain than the singleton's. The abdomen distends in the last trimester, accompanied with hydramnios, dyspnea, and walking difficulty. Two or more fetal poles can be detected on obstetric examination, and two fetal hearts can be heard in different parts of the abdomen of pregnant women.

2.4.1.2 Ultrasonic Diagnosis

1. Image of twin or multiple pregnancy in early first trimester shows two or more gestational sacs in the uterus, with the presence of yolk sac, embryo, and fetal heartbeat in each gestational sac (Fig. 2.43).

2. The type of chorionicity and amnionicity in twin pregnancies can be preliminarily determined in the first trimester, according to the intrauterine gestational sac location or the thickness of the membrane. In the first trimester, the two distant gestational sacs or one gestational sac with a thick membrane, or even the lambda sign (λ) can be observed in dichorionic diamniotic twin pregnancy. Monochorionic diamniotic twins represent a single gestational sac, two yolk sacs, and two embryos with fetal hearts. Monochorionic monoamniotic twin pregnancy is rare and susceptible to complications, such as twin-to-twin transfusion syndrome and conjoined twins, and the prenatal mortality is extremely high (Figs. 2.44, 2.45, 2.46, 2.47, and 2.48).

One gestational sac with two yolk sacs and embryos, without intervening membrane.

3. Images of the mid and late period of twin or multiple pregnancy show more than two fetuses in the uterus, one or two placentas, and the intervening membrane in the amniotic cavity (Fig. 2.49).
4. Dichorionic twins and monochorionic twins can be distinguished based on discordant fetal sex, number of the placenta, and the thickness of the intervening membrane (Fig. 2.50).

2.4.1.3 Special Notice

1. When diagnosing twin or multiple pregnancy during early pregnancy, the number of typical gestational sacs

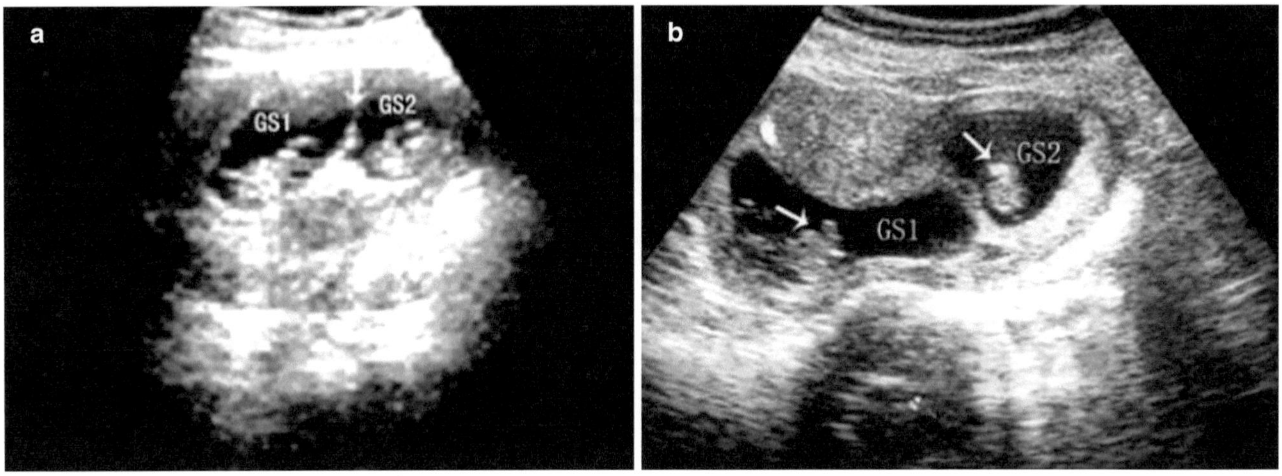

Fig. 2.43 Twins in early pregnancy. (**a**). On the 50th day of gestation, the intervening membrane is observed in the gestational sac, with two visible embryos and fetal hearts; (**b**). On the 57th day of gestation, the intervening membrane is observed in the gestational sac, which contains two embryos with fetal hearts and movement

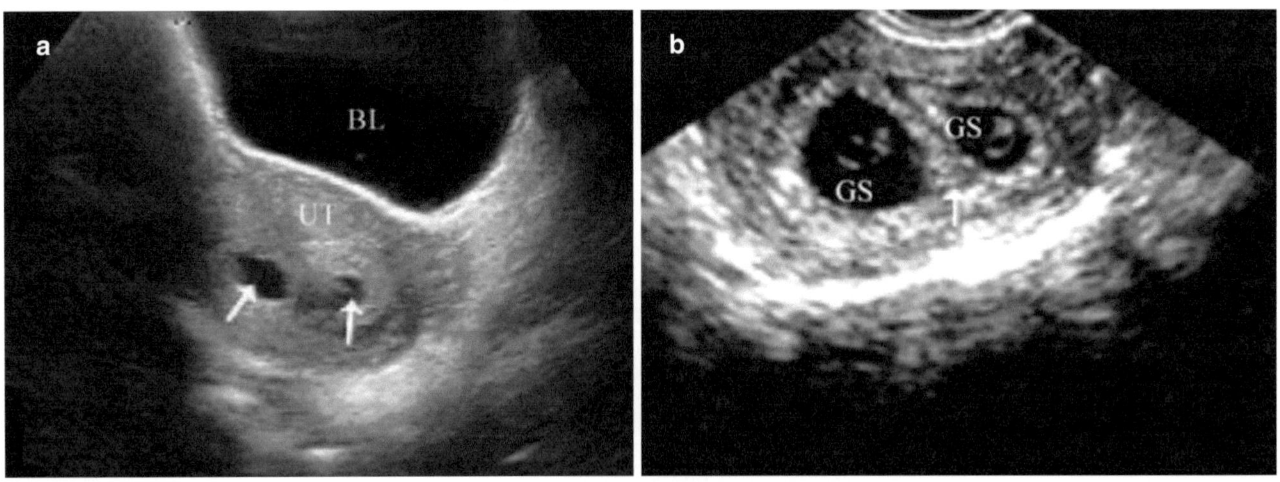

Fig. 2.44 Dizygotic twins. (**a, b**). In early intrauterine pregnancy, the two gestational sacs are relatively far apart, with a thicker intervening membrane

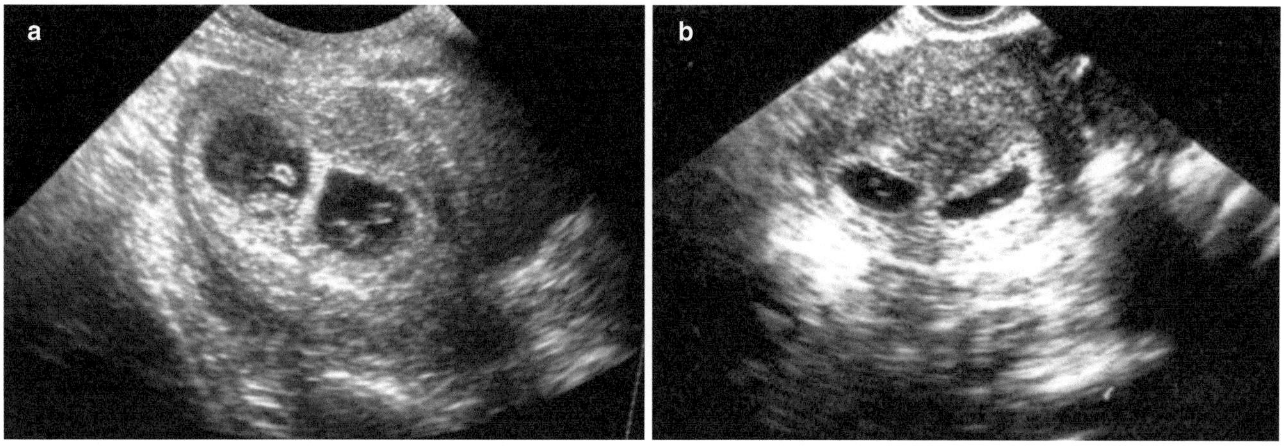

Fig. 2.45 Early twins pregnancy. (**a, b**). Early pregnancy, two intrauterine gestational sacs with a yolk sac, an embryo, and fetal heart, respectively

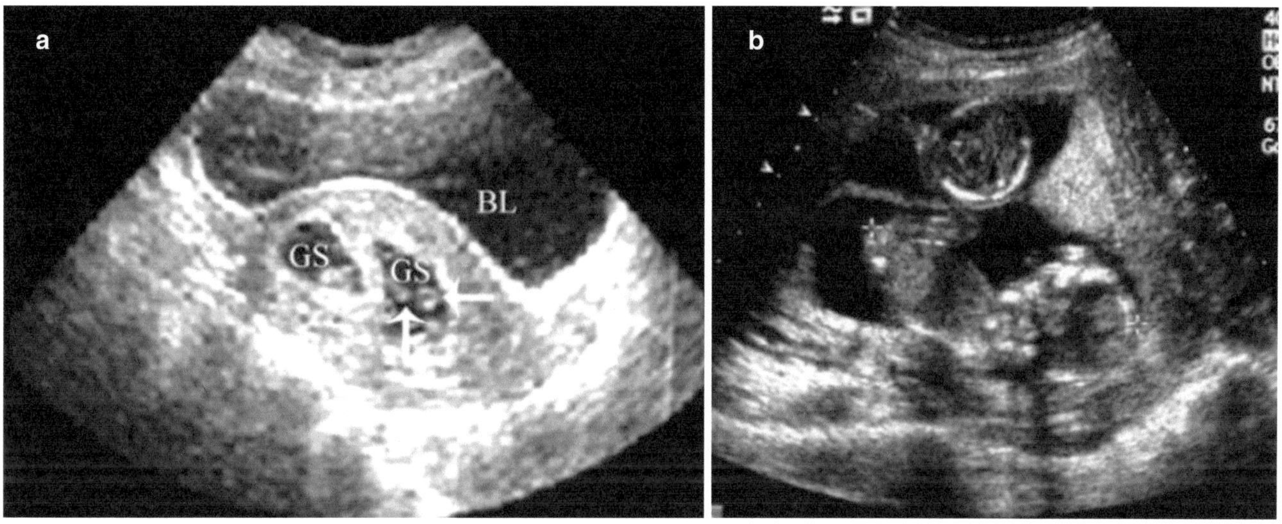

Fig. 2.46 Dichorionic diamniotic twins. (**a**). Three embryos in two gestational sacs, one of which is a monoamniotic twin with two embryos; (**b**). The sign of "λ" between the intervening membrane and the placenta

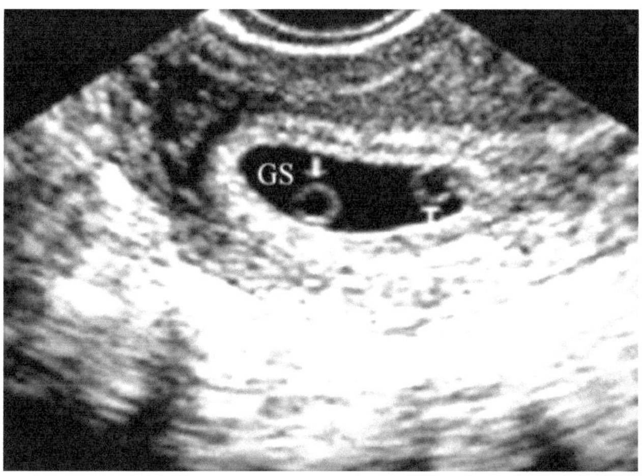

Fig. 2.47 Monoamniotic twin pregnancy. One gestational sac with two yolk sacs and embryos, without intervening membrane

and embryos and fetal heartbeats must be ensured on the sonogram.

2. Since the beginning of the second trimester of pregnancy, dichorionic, or monochorionic twin can be preliminarily judged based on the number of placentas, the thickness of the intervening membrane, and the sex of each fetus. If the intervening membrane is not visible after repeated examinations for monochorionic twins, pay attention to excluding the conjoined twins and umbilical cord entanglement.
3. When meeting potential multiple pregnancy women, pay attention to the scanning direction of the transducer. During the examination, the head, neck, spine, chest, heart, abdomen, and limbs of each fetus should be traced, observed, and measured separately, to avoid false-positive twins or missed diagnoses. The most accurate diagnostic

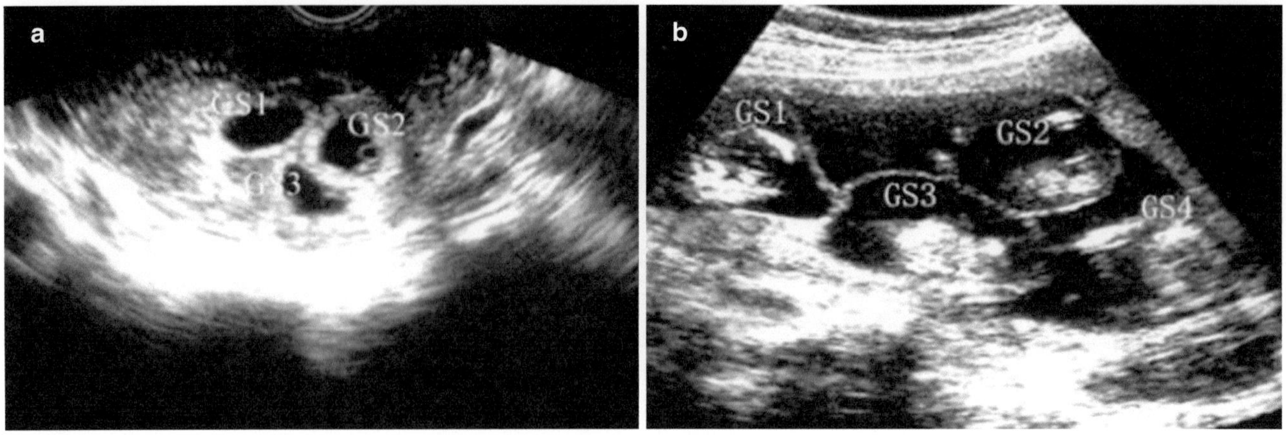

Fig. 2.48 Early multiple pregnancy. (**a**). After successful embryo transferring, three gestational sacs with embryos and fetal heartbeat are observed in the uterus; (**b**). 76 days of natural pregnancy, 5 sacs in the uterus, each with one fetus and fetal heartbeat

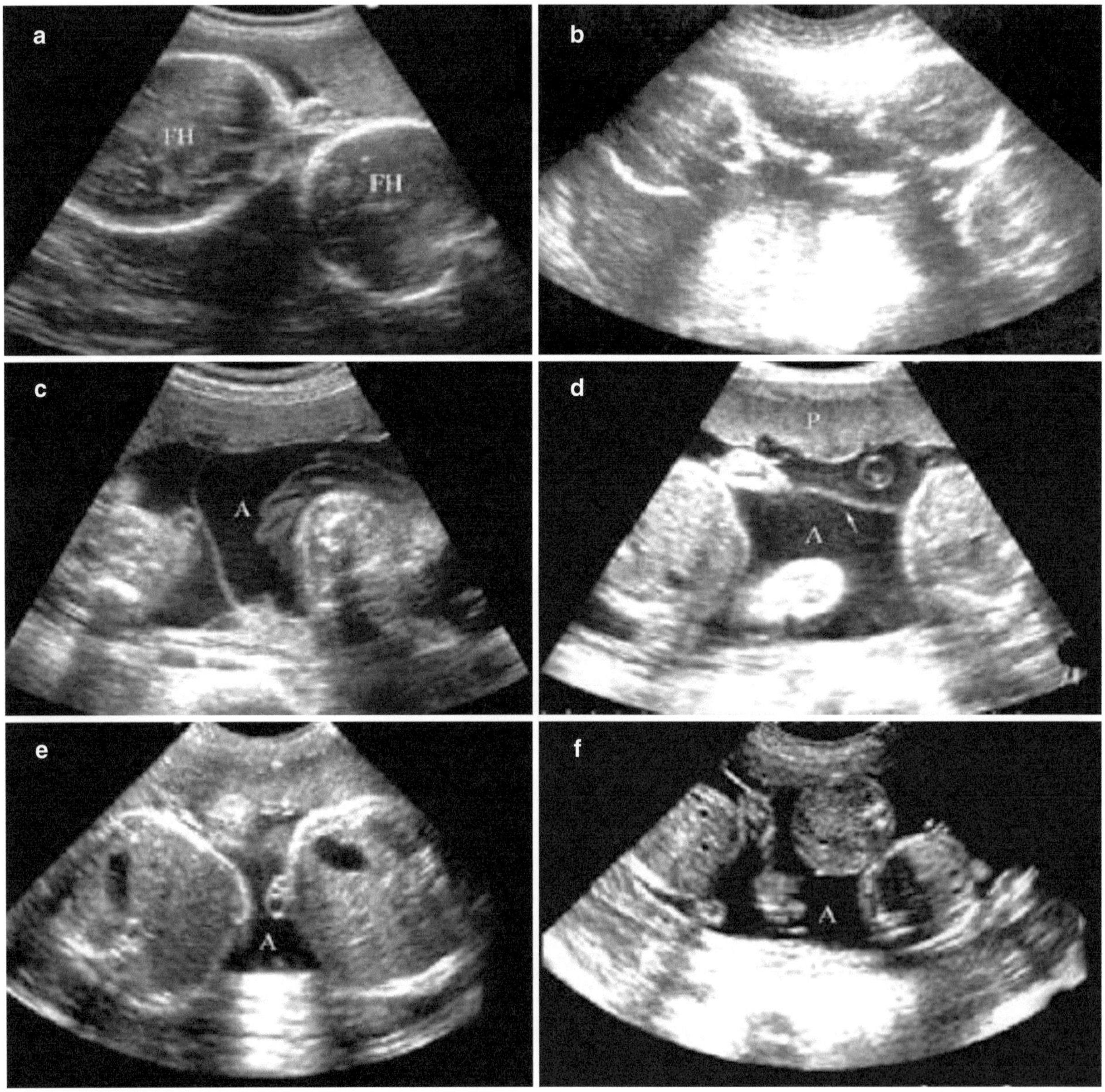

Fig. 2.49 Multiple pregnancy in the second and third trimesters. (**a**). Twin; (**b**). Triplet; (**c, d**). Intervening membrane in the amniotic cavity of twins; (**e**). Transverse view of twin abdomen; (**f**). Transverse view of triplet's abdomen

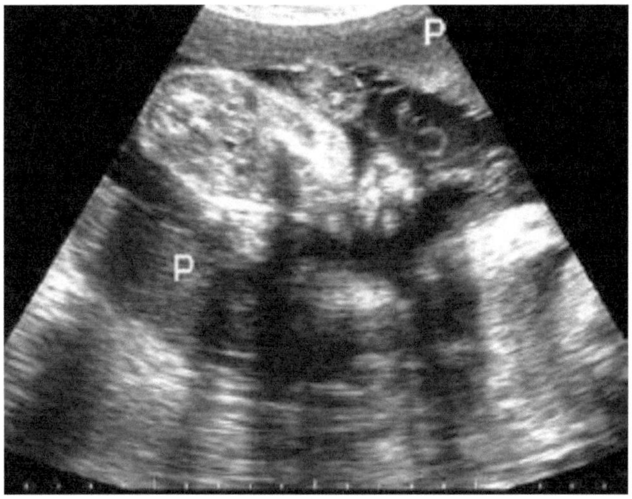

Fig. 2.50 Twin pregnancy, two placentas

image is to show two or more fetal heads on the same view or no less than two fetal trunks on the same transverse section.

2.4.2 Macrosomia

2.4.2.1 Basic Concepts

The fetus with a birth weight above 4000 g is defined as macrosomia. According to data from China, fetal macrosomia accounts for 5.62%–6.49% of all the newborn babies. Because of the increased risk of perinatal morbidity, and the probability of dystocia as a result of cephalopelvic disproportion, the rate of neonatal and maternal complications increases. Therefore, the estimation of fetal weight through ultrasound measurement is helpful for the clinical choice of delivery mode.

Maternal diabetes is the main risk factor for macrosomia. Other related factors include tall parents, multipara with excessive weight gain, post-term pregnancy, more dietary intake with less activity, and hydramnios. Macrosomia can be diagnosed according to the medical history of pregnant women, the symptoms and rapid weight gain in late pregnancy, and larger fundal height and abdominal circumference.

At present, multiple ultrasonic parameters have been proposed for estimating fetal weight. These include several fetal measurements: BPD, HC, FL, AC, as well as body weight predictive values. If these parameters are all above the 90th percentile of normal gestational age, macrosomia should be considered. In addition, other methods, such as measurement of shoulder distance and upper arm soft tissue thickness, are also used.

2.4.2.2 Ultrasonic Diagnosis

1. Fetal parameters are measured by ultrasound, and fetal weight is predicted to be greater than the 90th percentile of corresponding gestational age (Fig. 2.51).
2. The measurement of fetal subcutaneous soft tissue thickness at the middle point of femur and the cheek-to-cheek diameter can be supplemental, and if the shoulder distance of the fetus is larger than BPD, macrosomia should be considered (Fig. 2.52).

Thickened subcutaneous tissue and facial hypertrophy of the fetus.

2.4.3 Fetal Intrauterine Growth Retardation

2.4.3.1 Basic Concepts

Intrauterine growth retardation (IUGR) refers to the birth weight of full-term infant less than 2500 g, or falls below two standard deviations or the tenth percentile of average fetal weight for gestational age. The average incidence in China is 6.39%, which is one of the main complications during the perinatal period.

The causes of IUGR are diverse and complex, and are mainly related to maternal genetic factors, nutrition, pathological pregnancy, pregnancy complications, and other factors. It can also be related to abnormal fetal development, metabolic dysfunction, various growth factors deficiency, intrauterine infections, radiation exposure, as well as abnormal fetal appendages.

IUGR is classified into three types: symmetrical IUGR caused by intrinsic factors, asymmetrical IUGR caused by extrinsic factors, and symmetrical IUGR caused by extrinsic factors. Symmetrical IUGR occurs in the early stage of gestation, all the fetal organs are affected, and the prognosis is poor. Asymmetrical IUGR caused by extrinsic factors often occurs in the middle and late stages of gestation, and the fetal growth is asymmetric. Symmetrical IUGR, caused by extrinsic factors, is mostly the interacted result of various factors, the absence of amino acids and trace elements, or adverse drugs.

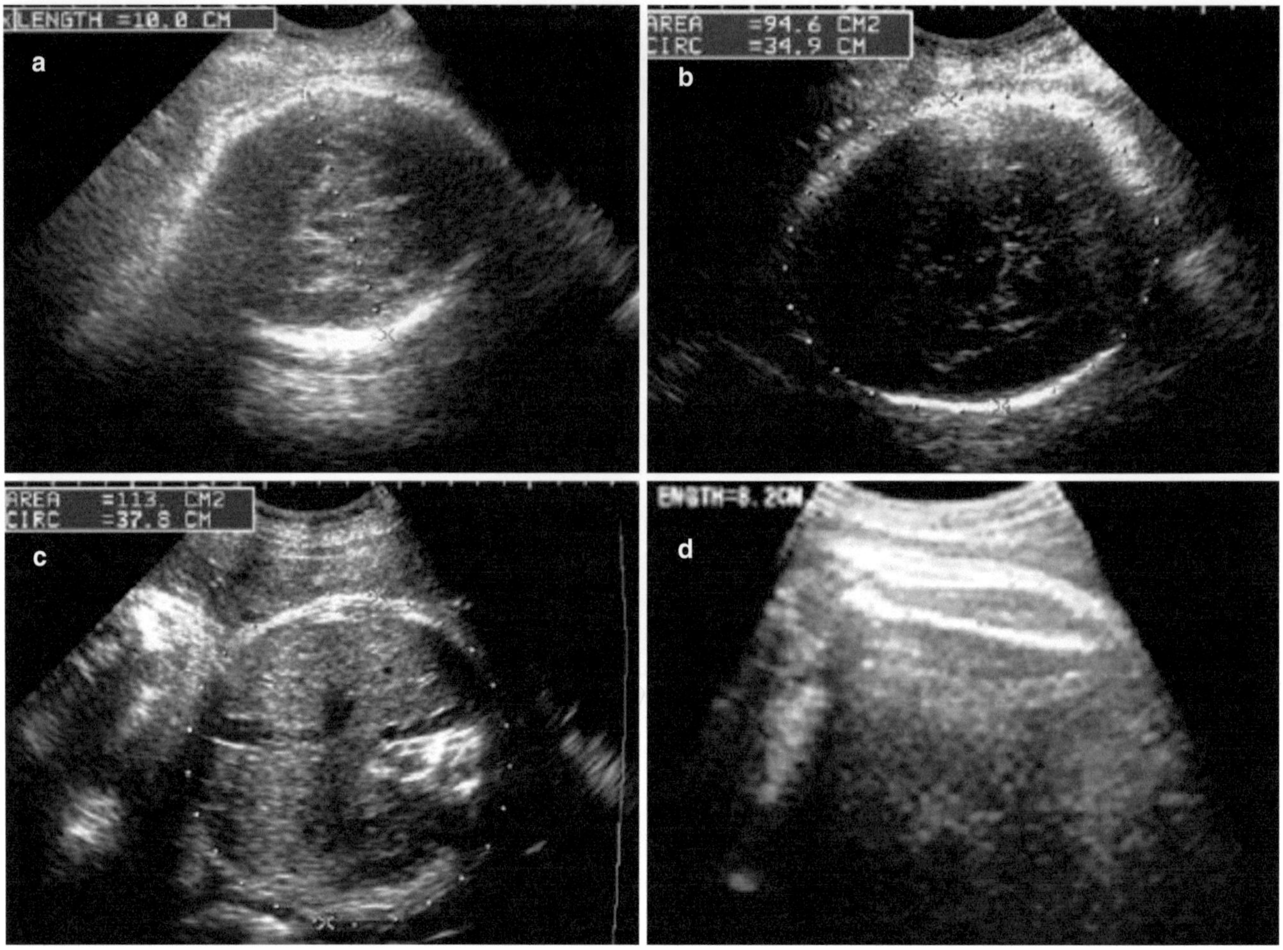

Fig. 2.51 Macrosomia. (**a–d**). At 38 weeks and 6 days of gestation, fetal BPD, HC, AC, and FL are all larger than those of the same gestational age, and the neonatal weight is 4300 g

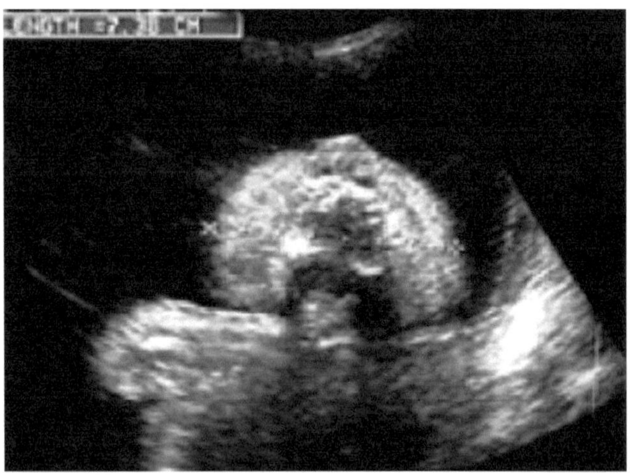

Fig. 2.52 Macrosomia

Dynamically measure the fetal BPD, FL, AC, chest circumference, HC, HC/AC, FL/HG, transverse cerebellum diameter, and umbilical artery S/D ratio, which helps accurately estimate the fetal size for further clinical diagnosis and classification.

2.4.3.2 Ultrasonic Diagnosis

1. After the second trimester of gestation, the values of fetal BPD, FL, and AC are less than two standard deviations below the mean for gestation age. Moreover, the fetal AC is less than the HC after 36 weeks' gestation (Fig. 2.53).
2. The growth rate of the fetus slows down during the whole pregnancy. If the growth rate of BPD and FL is lower than the normal standard after three consecutive weeks of observation, IUGR should be considered.

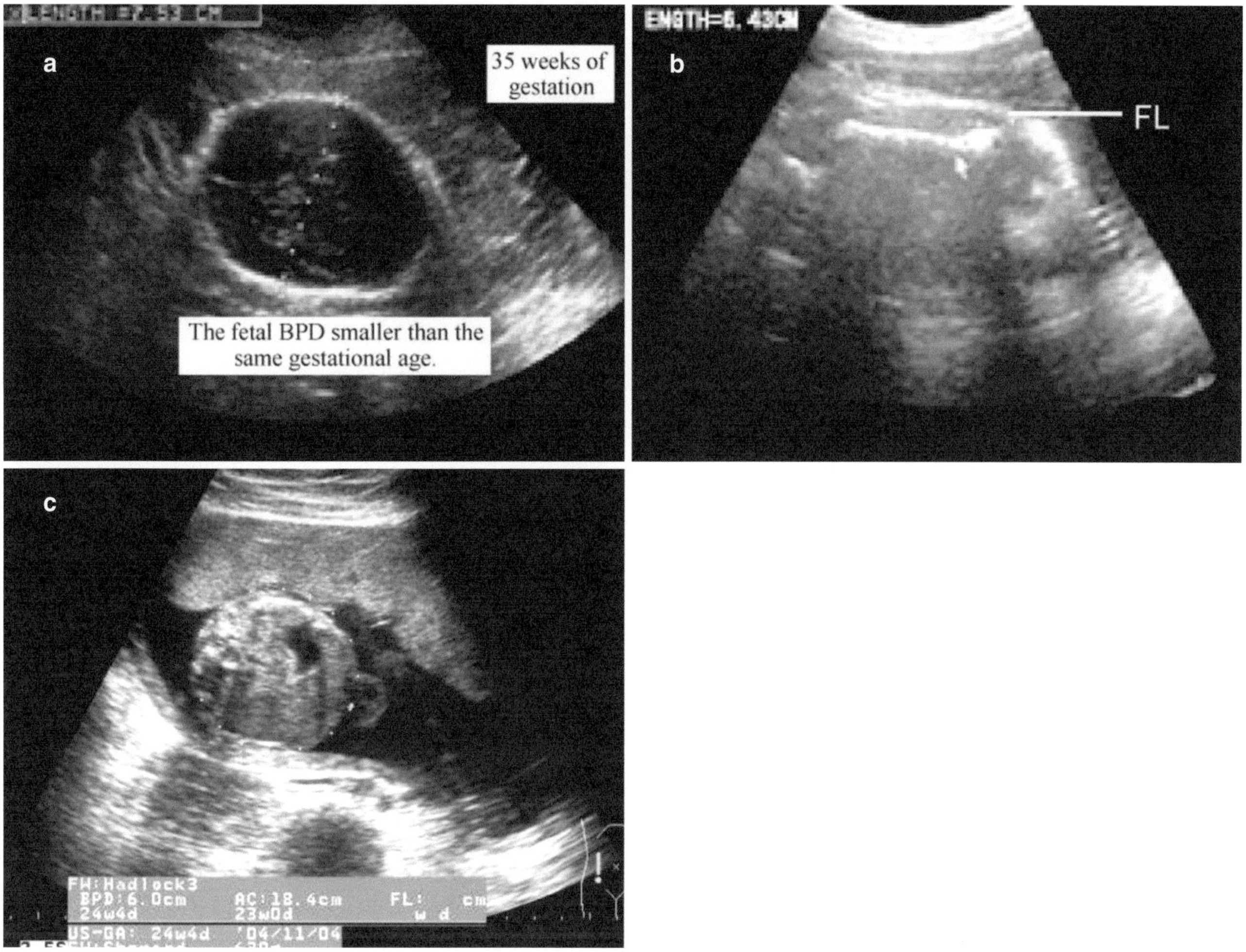

Fig. 2.53 Ultrasonic diagnosis of IUGR. (**a–c**). At 35 weeks of gestation, the fetal BPD, FL, and AC are significantly smaller than those of the same gestational age

2.4.3.3 Special Notice

1. IUGR should not be diagnosed by a single measurement but should be dynamically observed for at least 2 to 3 weeks.
2. When the S/D ratio of the umbilical artery increases during the third trimester, the incidence of IUGR increases significantly.
3. Diagnosis of fetal IUGR should be based on the comprehensive analysis of individual genetic factors and fetal nutritional status.

2.4.4 Intrauterine Fetal Demise

2.4.4.1 Basic Concepts

Intrauterine fetal demise is defined as fetal death that occurs in utero due to maternal or fetal reasons after the 20th week of pregnancy.

Ultrasound can directly observe the fetal heartbeat and movement to identify the fetal demise, and estimate the time of death based on some secondary degenerating signs after stopped growing.

If the dead fetus is retained for more than 3 weeks, degenerative placental tissue will release thromboplastins into the maternal circulation, which may lead to maternal coagulopathy. Once a fetal demise is diagnosed, the pregnancy should be terminated as early as possible.

2.4.4.2 Ultrasonic Diagnosis

1. Fetal heartbeat and fetal movement are not visible. The measurement values of all fetal parts are smaller than that for gestational age (Fig. 2.54).
2. The deformed and overlapping fetal skull bones are caused by the collapse of the fetal brain. The scalp is separated from the skull bones, and the intracranial structure is unclear. If the fetus has been dead for a long time,

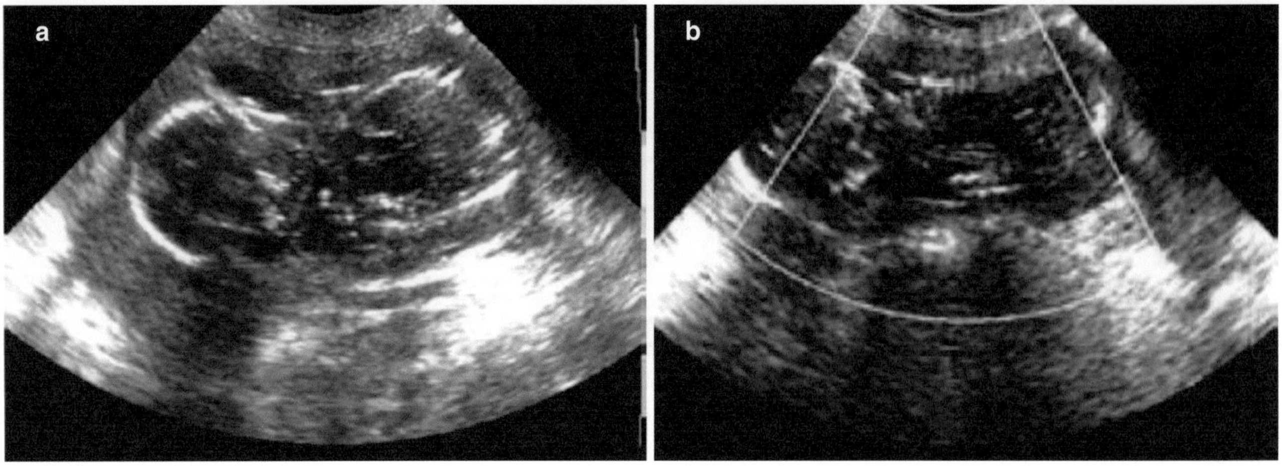

Fig. 2.54 Intrauterine fetal death at 21 weeks of gestation. (**a**). At 21 weeks of gestation, no fetal heartbeat nor fetal movements, and smaller BPD for gestation age; (**b**). No blood flow in the fetal heart is visible

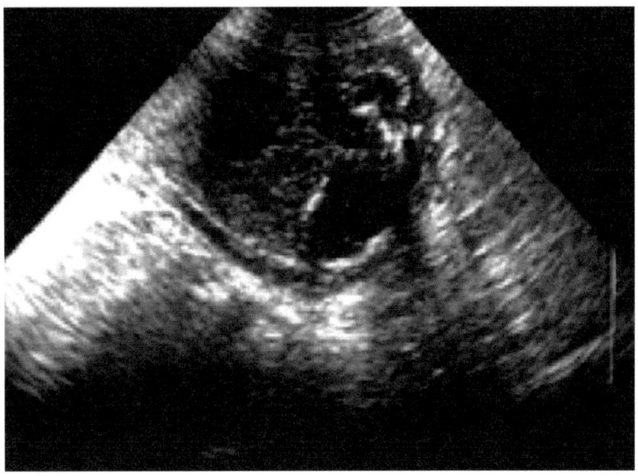

Fig. 2.55 Intrauterine fetal demise at 22 weeks of gestation

the fetal head and gross skin present a double-layer echogenic, the viscera blurs, pleural effusion and ascites appear, and the amniotic fluid reduces or even turns turbid (Figs. 2.55 and 2.56).

At 22 weeks of gestation, rare amniotic fluid and gross distortion of the fetus because of a long time demise.

3. The placenta is indistinct with obscured outlines, and placenta edema presents an inhomogeneous echo (Fig. 2.57).

2.5 Ultrasonographic Images of Common Fetal Congenital Anomalies

Congenital anomalies refer to abnormalities in fetal development whose main features are malformations of morphology and structure. It is a crucial differentiation period of cell tissue, blood vessels, and function of the embryo in the first eight weeks of pregnancy. During the differentiation process, the interference of genetic factors, environmental teratogenic factors, or the combination of genetic and environmental teratogenic factors can lead to fetal abnormalities. Each system of the fetus can be involved with various manifestations, even death. Fetal congenital malformation accounts for a considerable proportion of fetal or infant mortality. According to the statistics, about 30% of stillbirths have deformities, and about 2% of the surviving fetuses have apparent deformities. With the popularization and development of modern ultrasonic technology, the majority of congenital fetal anomalies can be diagnosed by prenatal ultrasonography.

2.5.1 Congenital Abnormalities of the Fetal Neural System

2.5.1.1 Basic Concepts

Neural malformation of fetus refers to anencephaly, exeucephalia, hydrocephalus, encephalocele, meningocele, spina bifida, myelomeningocele, microcephaly, and so on. Internal or external teratogenic factors interfere with the normal development of the central nervous system, from neural tube formation in the early embryo to the formation, growth, development, and transition of various structural primitives of the brain in fetal period. All the above can cause structural, morphological, and even functional abnormalities of the nervous system. The most vulnerable period is between the fifth and 18th week of gestation. 10% of the cases are associated with chromosomal malformations, genetic mutations, maternal diabetes, and ingestion of teratogenic drugs.

The basis of pathological changes is that the neural tube is not developed or closed incompletely. It may cause fetal brain development to be primitive or undeveloped, skull defi-

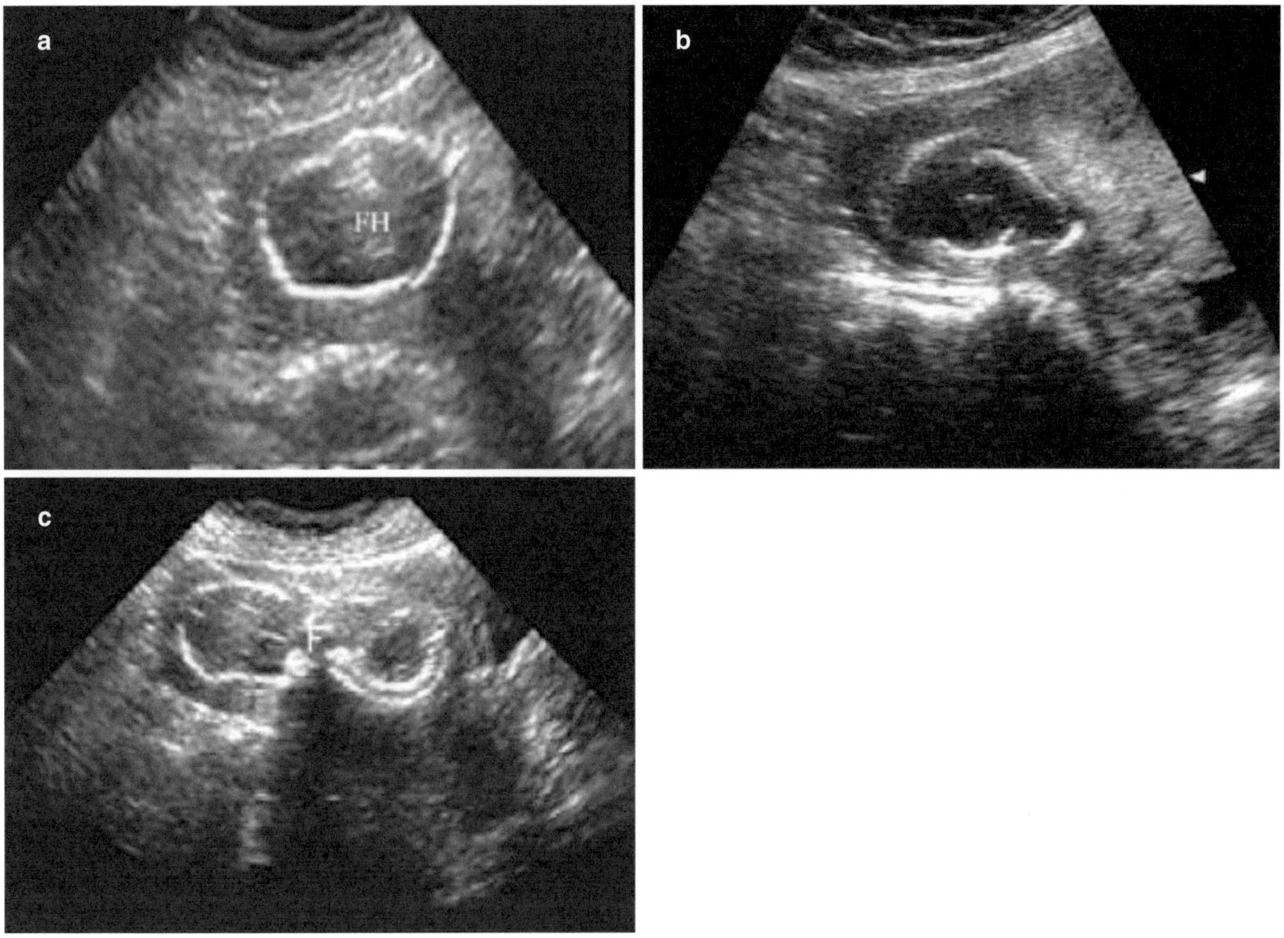

Fig. 2.56 Intrauterine fetal demise. (**a**). Deformed fetal skull bones; (**b**). Deformed fetal skull is imbricate; (**c**). Fetal maceration with unrecognizable head, trunk, and limbs

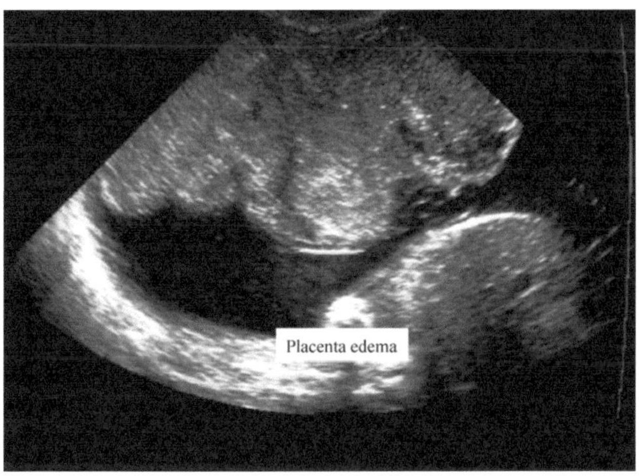

Fig. 2.57 Placenta edema after fetal demise

ciency, abnormal spine, encephalocele, myelomeningocele, and other malformations. Hydrocephalus can occur due to abnormal secretion of fetal cerebrospinal fluid or obstruction of circulatory channels. Chromosomal abnormalities can also lead to abnormal central nervous system development.

Fetal central nervous system malformation is often associated with hydramnios. The clinical manifestations are abdominal distention, distension, discomfort, nausea, and vomiting. Acute hydramnios can cause dyspnea and fail to supine. The obstetric abdominal examination performs to be high uterine tension, high uterine position, an abdominal circumference greater than menopause months, unclear fetus position, and untouchable fetal head. AFP in maternal blood and amniotic fluid increase.

Ultrasound observations of the normal fetal nervous system include cranial morphology and size. Various sections should be taken to show structures like hemicerebrum, lateral ventricle and choroid plexus, third ventricle, brain middle, thalamus, the cavity of septum pellucidum, cerebellar hemisphere and vermis, fossa cranii posterior, fourth ventricle, and the continuity and integrity of spinal echo. The combination of fetal genetics and ultrasound may result in the diagnosis of most fetal nervous system malformations by prenatal ultrasound.

2.5.1.2 Ultrasonic Diagnosis

Anencephaly and Exencephaly

1. Exencephaly: The main features are the absence of skull and skin, and brain tissue disorganized and exposed to amniotic fluid. Because the ears and the hemispheres of the brain are apparently separate, in early period the fetal head ultrasonic image present to be "Mickey sign" (Fig. 2.58).
2. Anencephaly: The full skull and brain echo of the fetus is not visible, with the absent brain midline. With longitudinal scanning along the spine of the posterior neck, there is no echo of the skull ring and brain at the superior apex of the spine. The forehead cannot be shown above the eye socket by facial scan which appears as "frog face" (Figs. 2.59 and 2.60).
3. Most of them combined with hydramnios, spina bifida, or other deformities.

Hydrocephalus

1. Lateral or bilateral ventricles of the fetus are enlarged, or both the third and fourth ventricles are enlarged. The ventricular rate is the ratio of lateral ventricular width to hemispheric width. Lateral ventricles expansion should be suspected if the ventricular rate is more than one-third after 20 weeks of gestation, or the posterior horn of lat-

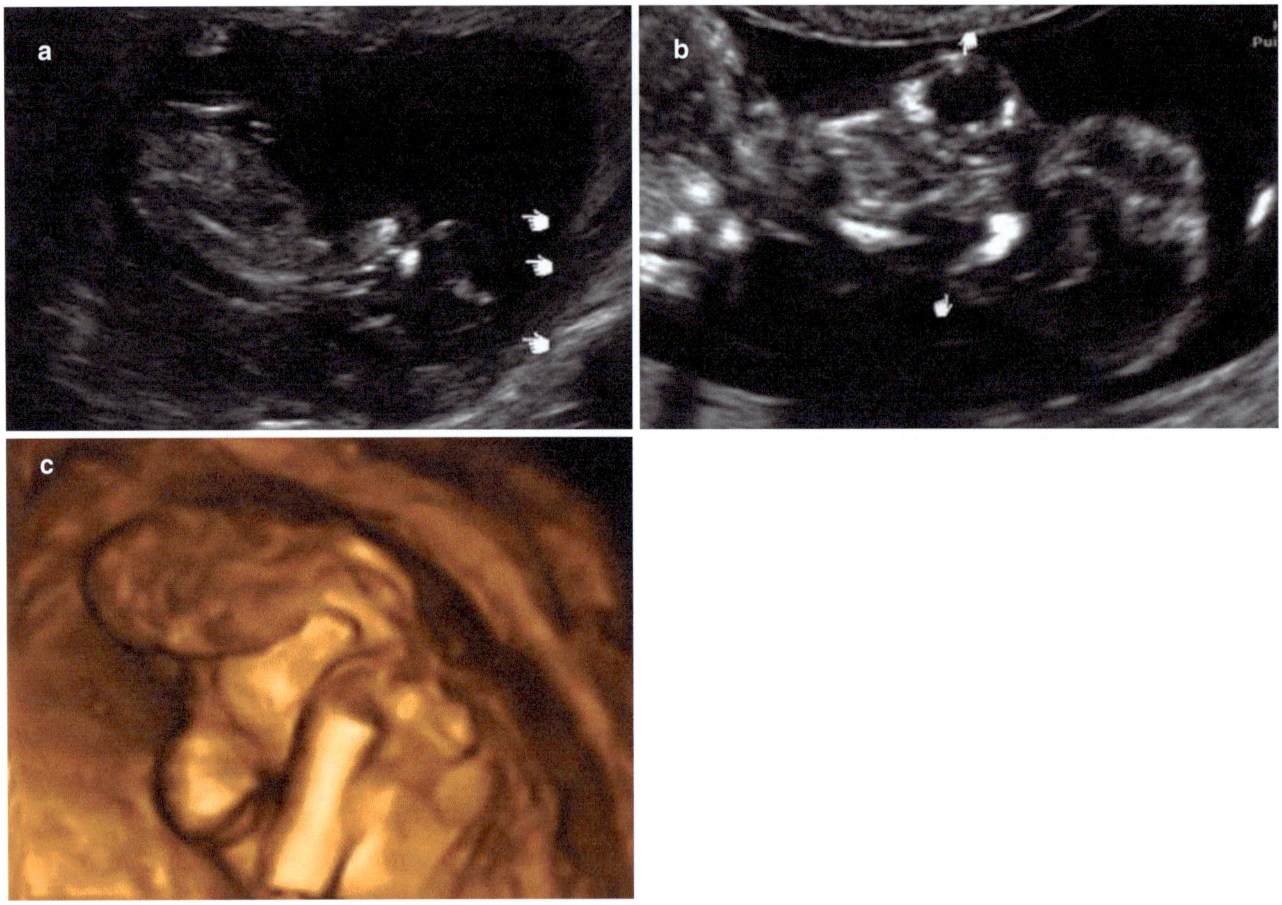

Fig. 2.58 Exeucephalia. (**a**). At 15 weeks of gestation, sagittal view of the fetus shows no skull ring; (**b**). Coronal view presents the "Mickey sign" of the fetal head, only the eye socket is shown. (**c**). 3-D image of visual exeucephalia

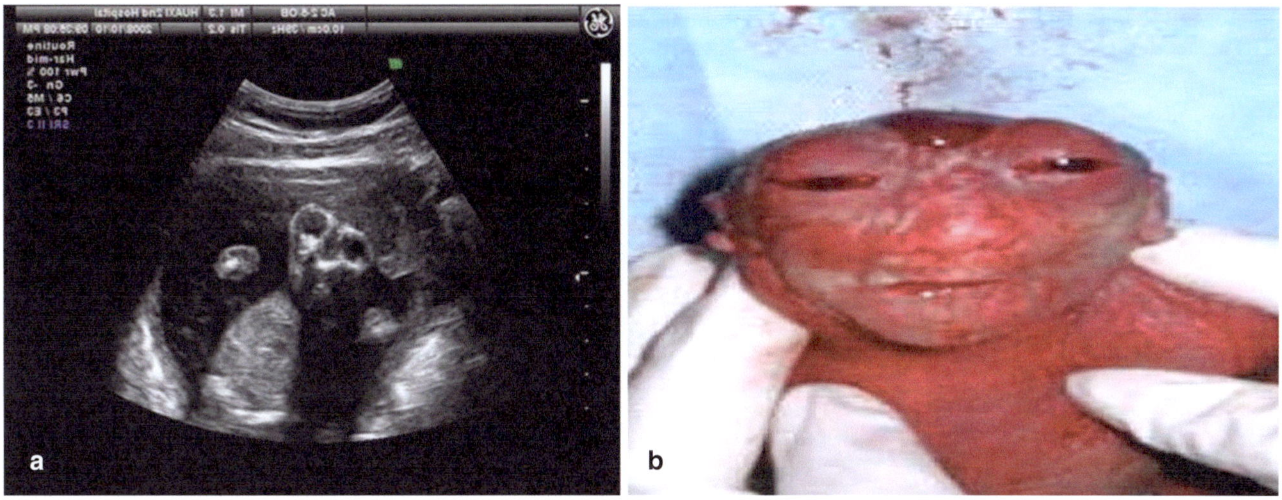

Fig. 2.59 Anencephaly. (**a**). The fetus had no skull or brain, with the eye socket at the highest point and invisible frontal bone, appearing as "frog face." (**b**). The autopsy image

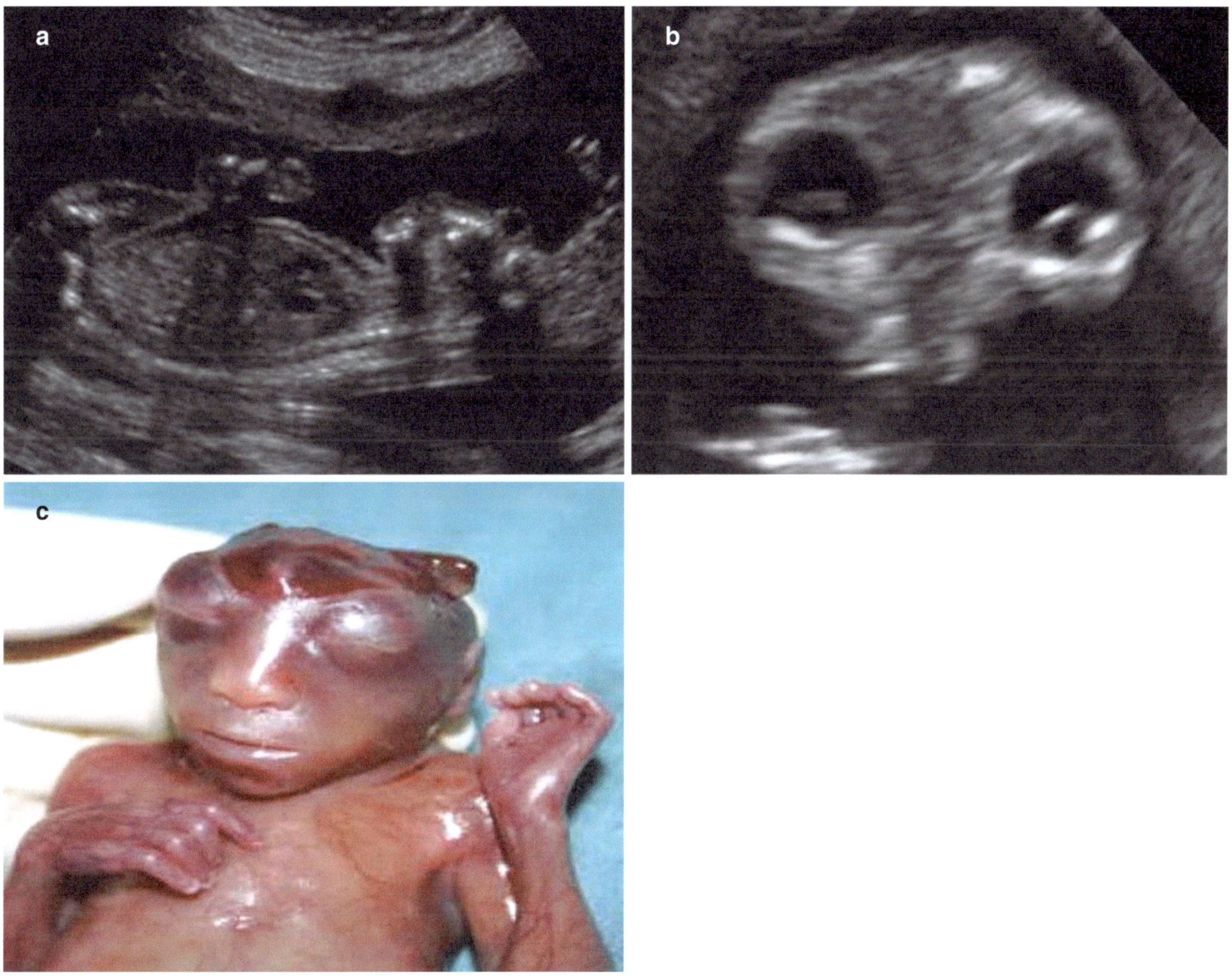

Fig. 2.60 Anencephaly. Prenatal ultrasound performance and images after labor induction. (**a**) Sagittal plane shows the absence of fetal skull and brain. (**b**) Coronal plane shows the "frog face". (**c**) Image after labor induction

eral ventricle is more than 1 cm at any week of gestation. The fetal prognosis is poor when the lateral ventricle expands to ≥1.5 cm (Fig. 2.61).

2. Hydrops of unilateral lateral ventricular is obvious, and the brain midline is shifted to the contralateral side. In the case of severe bilateral hydrops of lateral ventricular, the brain midline can also be shifted (Fig. 2.62).
3. In severe fetal hydrocephalus cases, the brain tissue becomes thinner due to pressure. The BPD and HC are significantly larger than those of the same gestational age (Figs. 2.63 and 2.64).

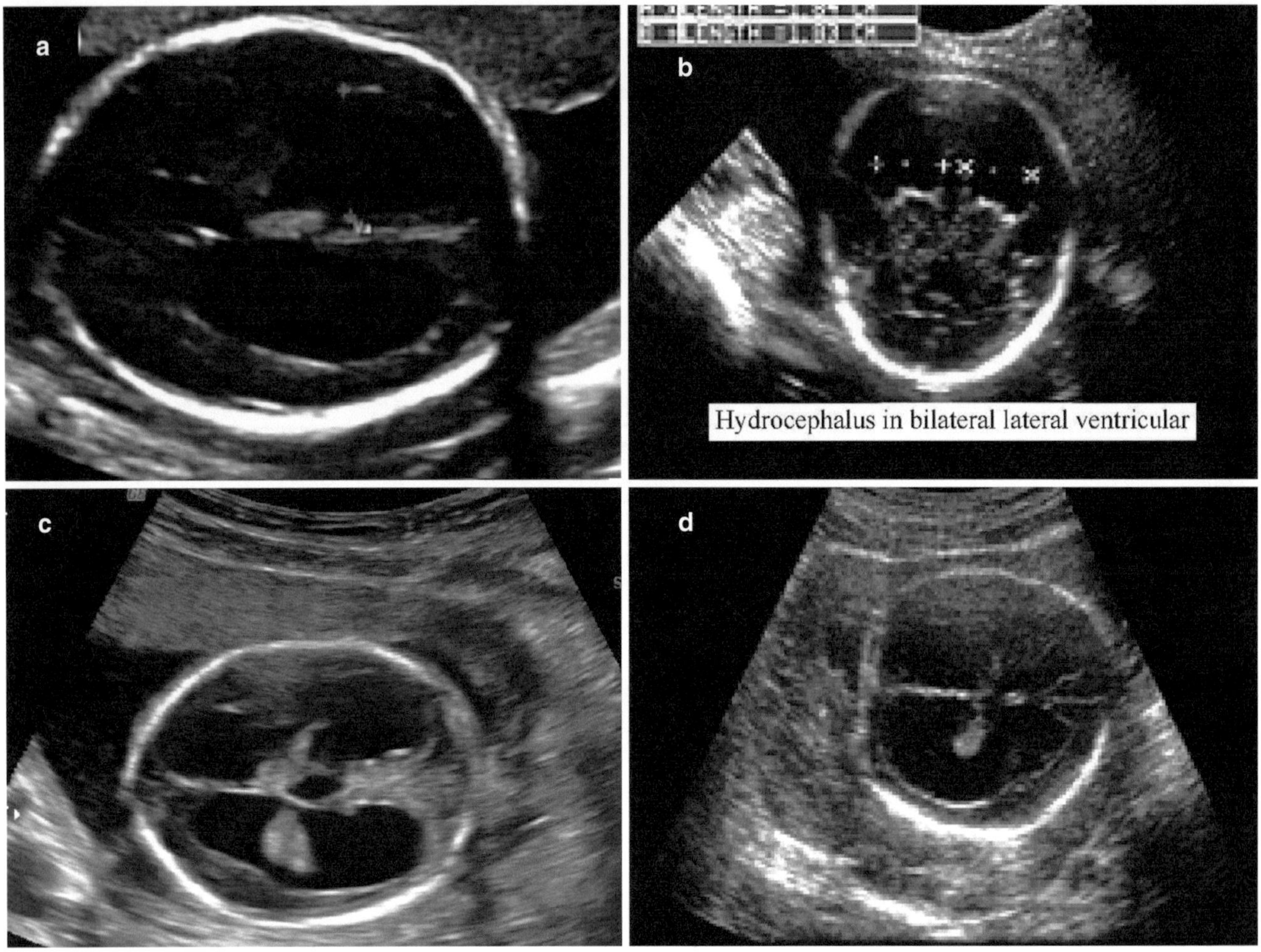

Fig. 2.61 Hydrocephalus. (**a**). The lateral ventricle width and ventricular rate of the fetus increase. (**b**). The bilaterally dilated anterior horn of the lateral ventricle. (**c**). The dilated third ventricle. (**d**). A large accumulation of fluid in the bilateral ventricles of the fetus

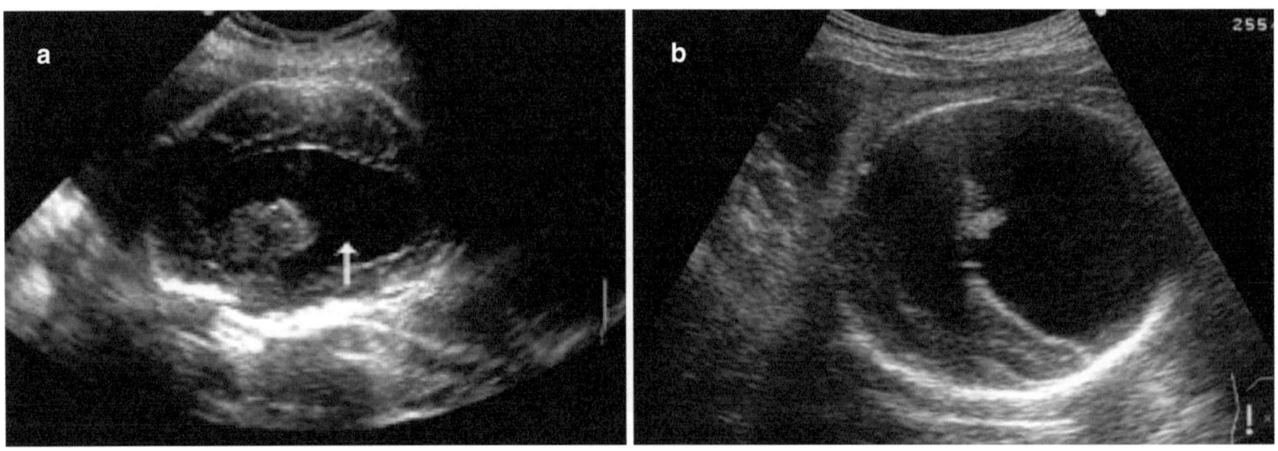

Fig. 2.62 Severe hydrocephalus (I). (**a, b**). Hydrops of unilateral lateral ventricular is obvious, and the brain midline is shifted

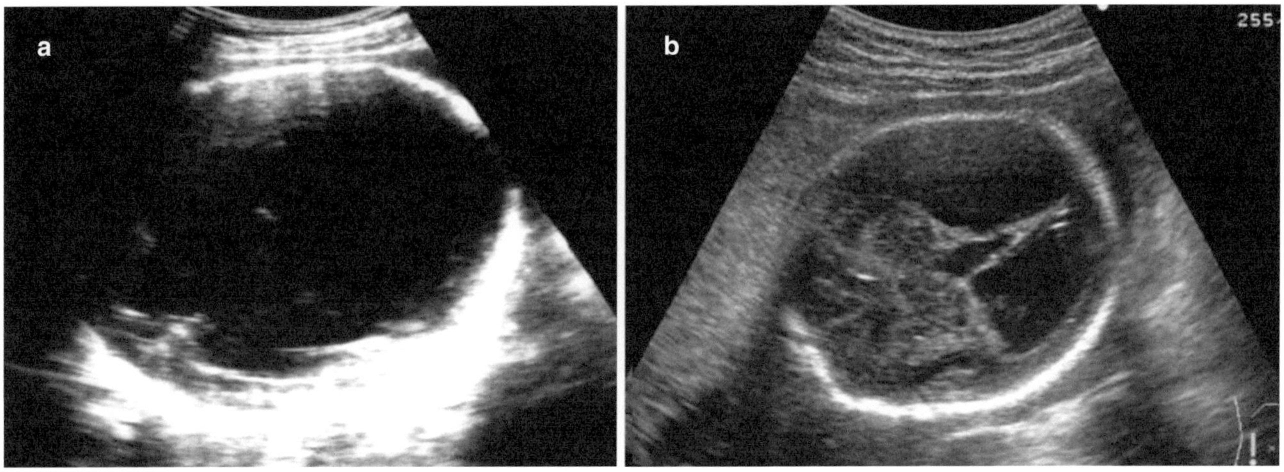

Fig. 2.63 Severe hydrocephalus II. (**a**). There is a large amount of intracranial fluid, leading to the thin cerebral cortex and large HC. The structure of the ventricle is not visible. (**b**). Hydrops in bilateral lateral ventricles and the significantly expanded third ventricle

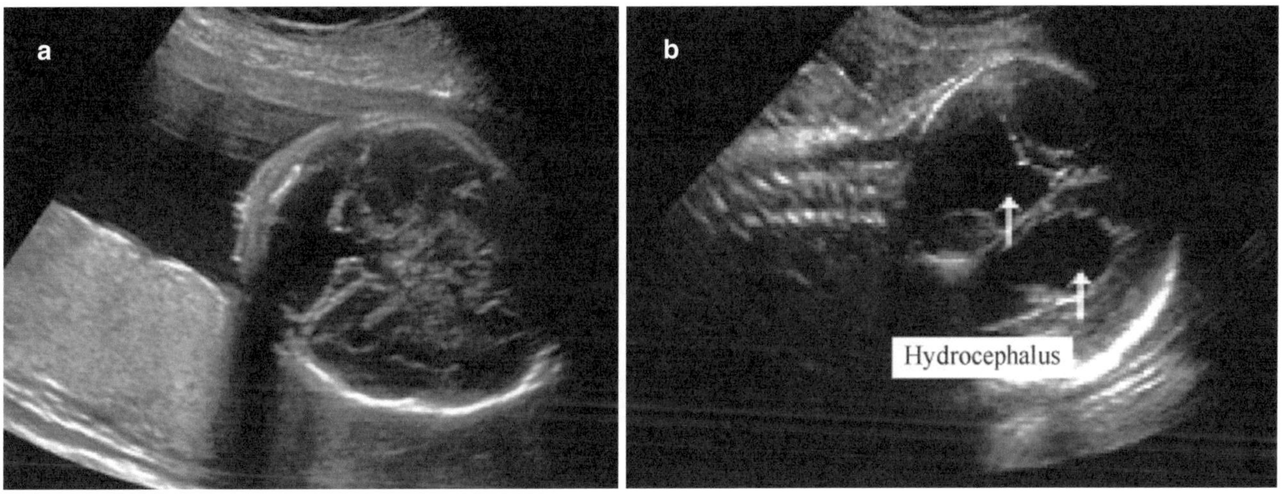

Fig. 2.64 Severe hydrocephalus III. (**a**). Fluid accumulation in the posterior cranial fossa of the fetus. (**b**). Fluid accumulation in the posterior cranial fossa and lateral ventricles of the fetus

Encephalocele and Meningocele

1. Multiple sections show the interrupted and discontinuous echo of fetal skull ring.
2. It appears as an inhomogeneous hypoechoic mass caused by bulging brain tissue and meninges. When a large number of brain tissue is expanded, the fetal head skull ring decreases. Meningocele is primarily considered in cystic mass with thin wall cases (Figs. 2.65 and 2.66).
3. Seventy-five percent of defects are located at the posterior part of the occipital, few in the frontal and apical regions, and fewer in the nasofrontal area (Fig. 2.67).

Spine Bifida and Meningomyelocele

1. On the longitudinal section of the spine from the fetal dorsal direction, defects of the skin, and soft tissue at the site of spina bifida show interrupted echo (Fig. 2.68a).
2. On the transverse view, the triangular ossification centra of the spine is abnormal, which represents a typical "V" or "U" shape (Fig. 2.68b).
3. An expanded mass at the cleft of the spine is visible. Spinal meningocele is the case that only the meninge and hydrops inside the mass. Meningomyelocele is the case that both the meninge and the nervous tissue inside the

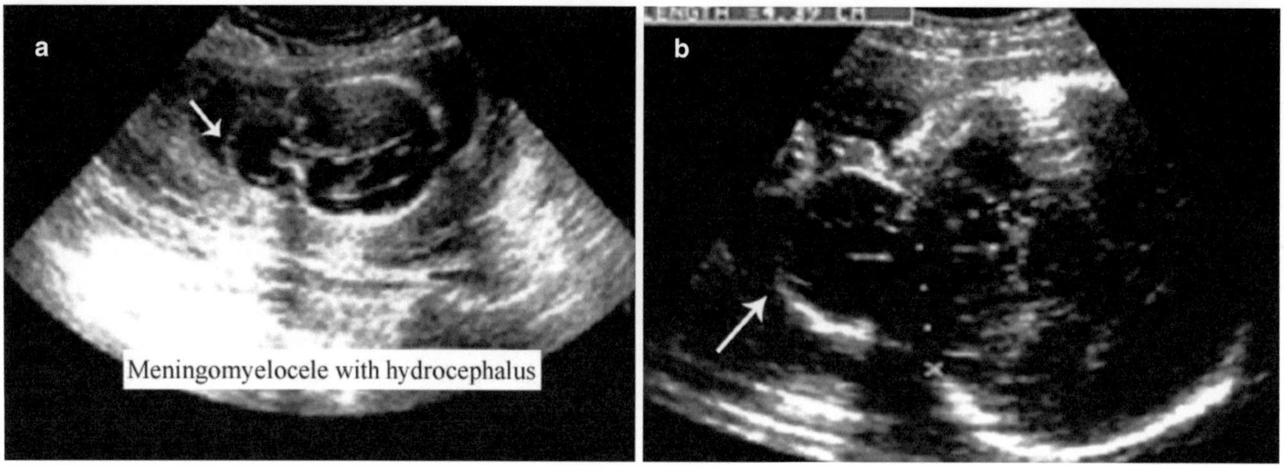

Fig. 2.65 Skull defect with encephalocele. (**a, b**). Partial defect of fetal skulls, shows interrupted skull echo and meninges bulging sacculate

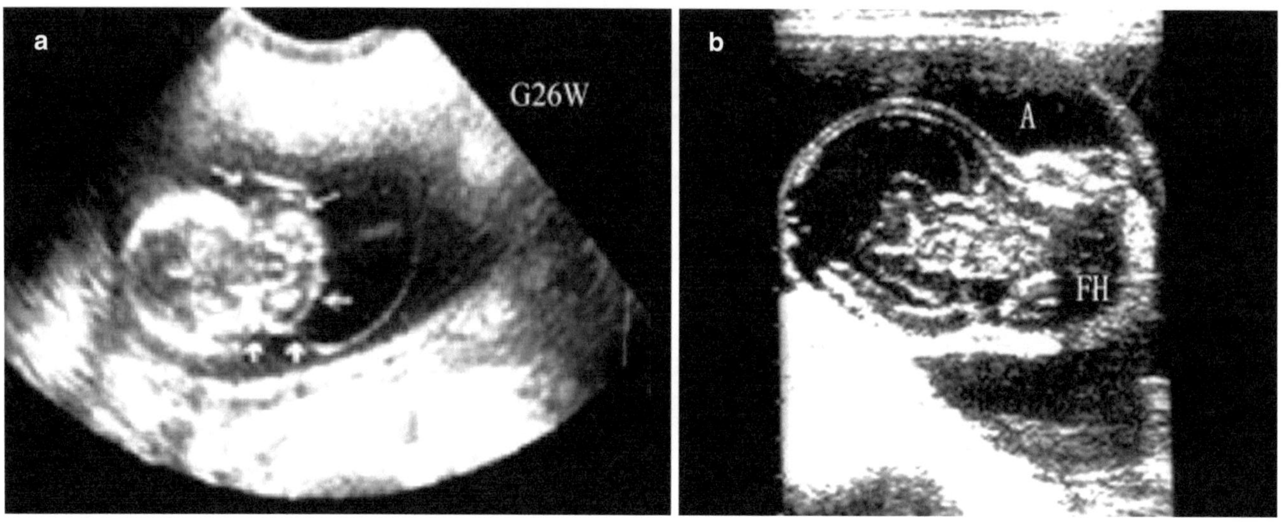

Fig. 2.66 Meningocele. (**a, b**). Obviously defected fetal skull. The bulging meninges and brain tissue appear as a mixed echo

mass. The echo of most protrusions is cystic anechoic (Fig. 2.69).

4. Spina bifida can be accompanied by a series of brain abnormalities, including cerebellar abnormality, effacement of cisterna magna (the banana sign), the lemon sign, and ventriculomegaly. If any of the above suspicious signs are found during the examination, the fetal spine should be scanned carefully. (Figs. 2.69 and 2.70).

Microcephaly

1. The microcephaly is diagnosed by ultrasonic biological measurements, without obvious abnormality in skull morphology. It is one of the indicators to diagnose microcephaly that the measurement of fetal BPD and HC are less than three standard deviation away from mean of the same gestational age (Fig. 2.71).
2. Ultrasound measurements of other fetal growth parameters are within the normal range.

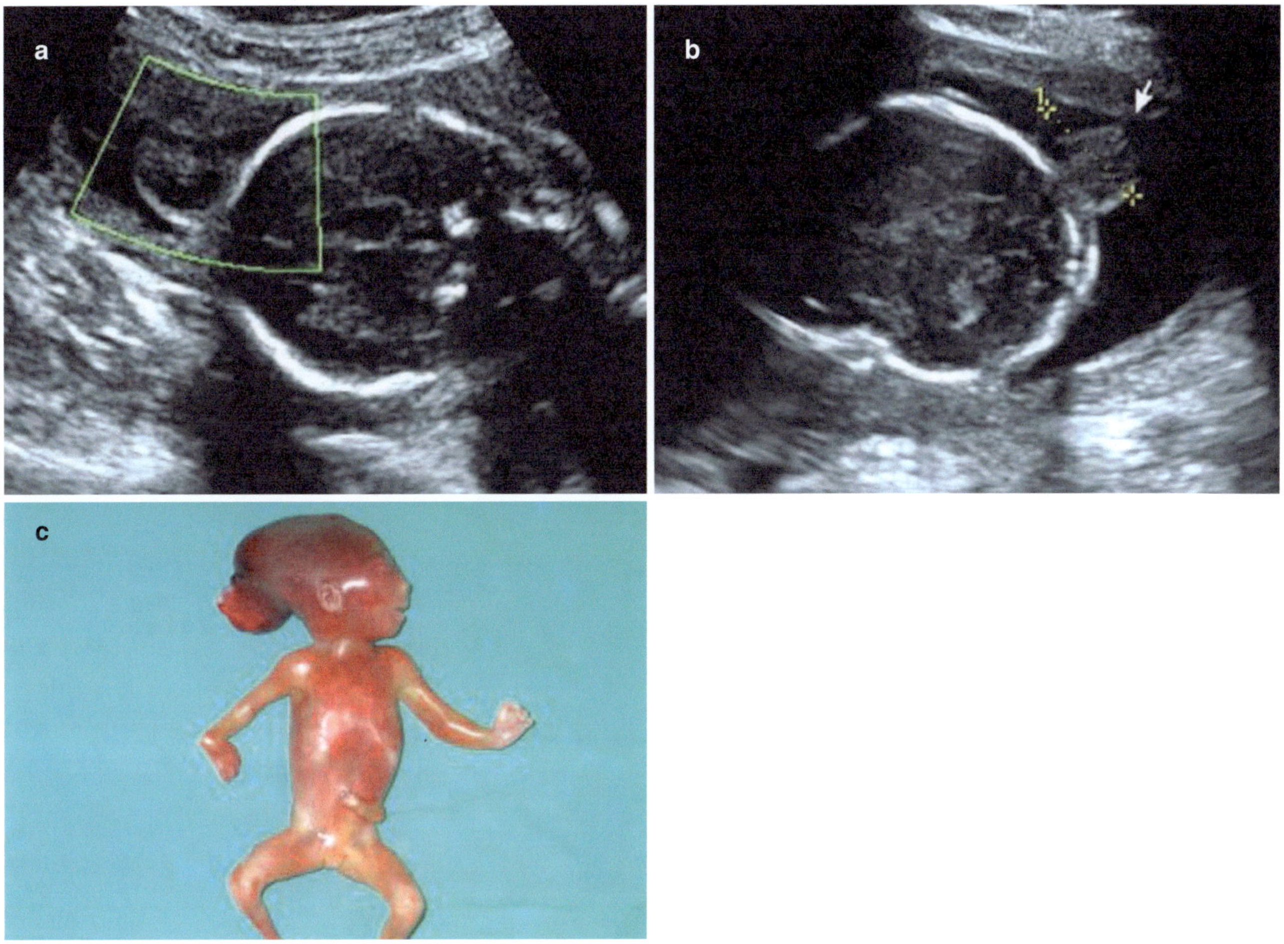

Fig. 2.67 Occiput posterior encephalocele. (**a–c**). Prenatal ultrasound performance and images of the autopsy

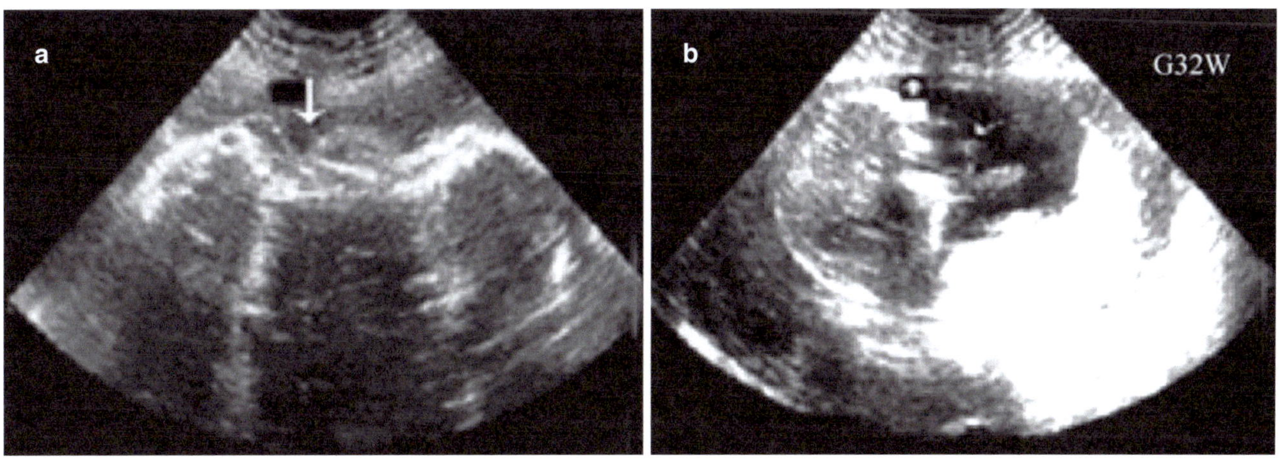

Fig. 2.68 Spine bifida. (**a**) Sagittal view shows interrupted echo of skin and missing vertebra at the thoracic and cervical segments of the fetal spine. (**b**). The transverse view shows a cystic protrusion at the skull defect

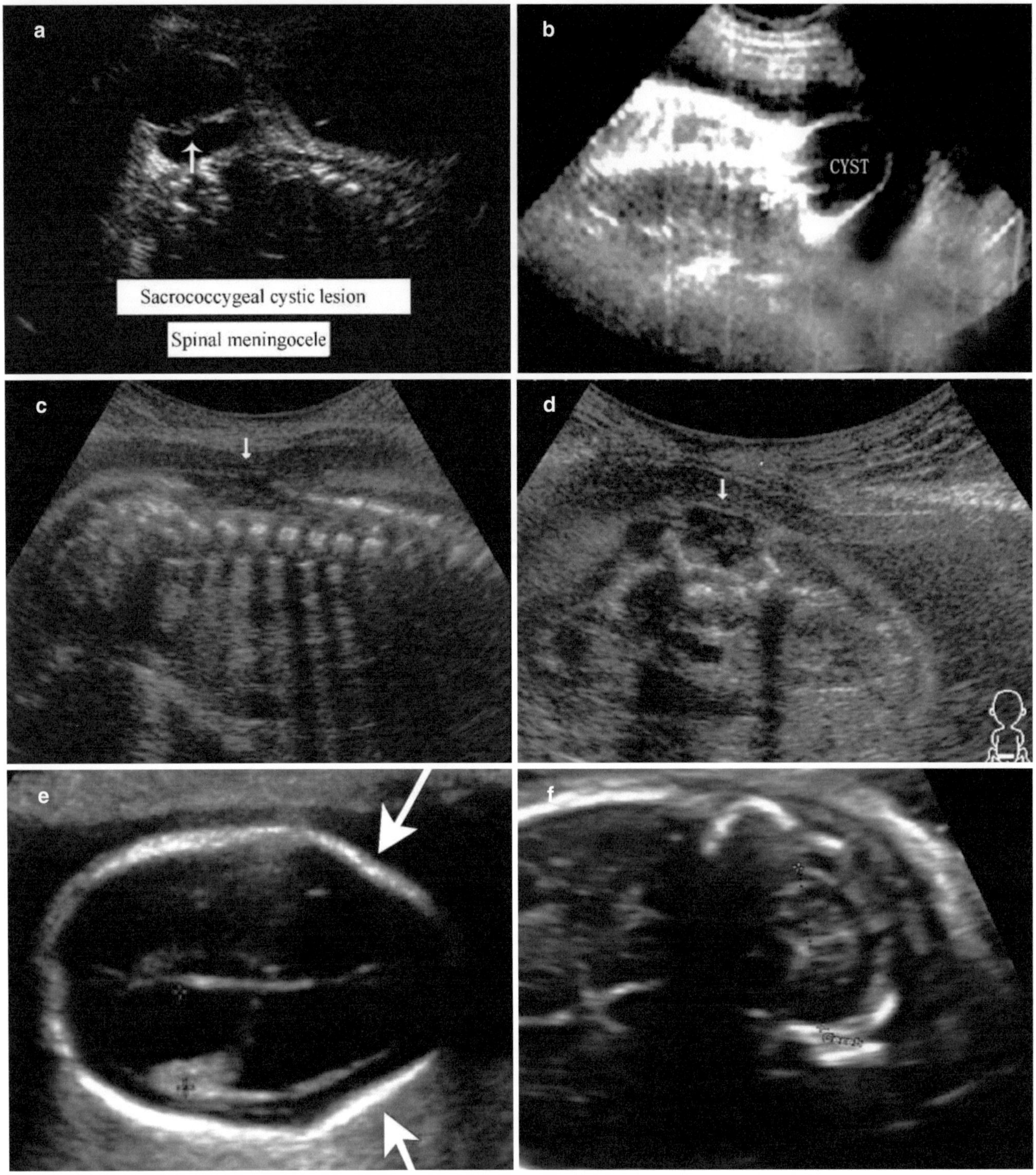

Fig. 2.69 Spine bifida with meningomyelocele I. (**a, b**). The fetal sacrococcygeal cystic mass is meningomyelocele. (**c, d**). Sagittal and transverse view shows the interrupted skin echo and widened spinal canal. (**e, f**). Ultrasonographic images of the banana sign and the lemon sign

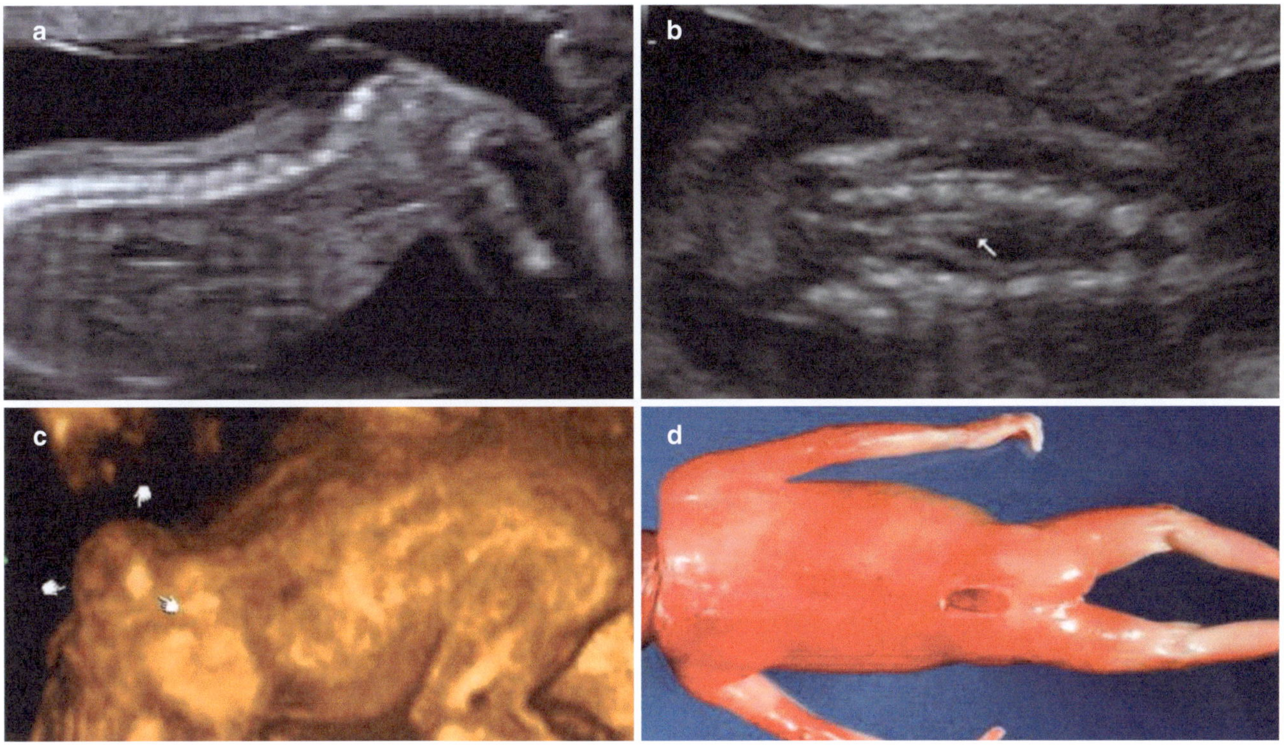

Fig. 2.70 Spine bifida with meningomyelocele II. (**a–d**). Prenatal ultrasound performance and images after labor

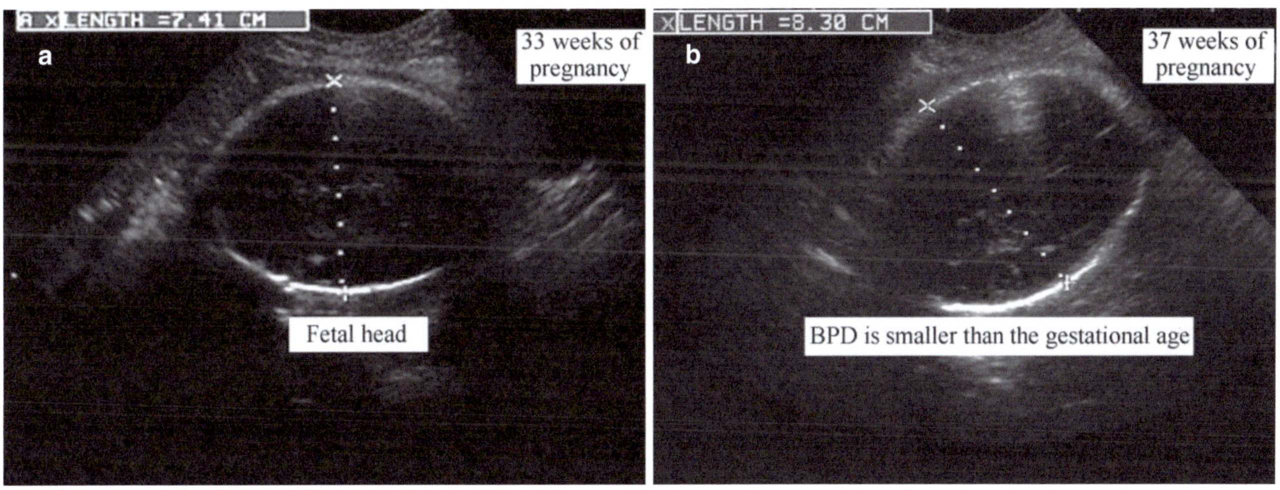

Fig. 2.71 Microcephaly. (**a**). At 33 weeks of gestation, BPD: 7.4 cm, FL: 5.6 cm. (**b**). At 37 weeks of gestation, BPD: 8.3 cm, FL: 7.0 cm, with cleft lip confirmed after induced labor

3. The ratios of fetal HC/AC, BPD/AC, BPD/FL are significantly lower than normal. Moreover, the smaller the HC, the more severe the dysnoesia.
4. Other accompanied deformities.

Other Rare Malformations of the Nervous System

1. Holoprosencephaly: Holoprosencephaly represents as an intracranial structural disorder. There is only a sizeable primitive ventricle without brain midline, septum pellucidum, the third ventricle, bilateral lateral ventricles, and bilateral thalamus. The facial structure is severely abnormal. What is more, the fourth ventricle and posterior cranial fossa present enlarged cystic masses (Fig. 2.72).
2. Choroid plexus cyst: Round and smooth anechoic cyst in the hyperechoic choroid plexus is visible in choroid plexus cyst cases after ten weeks of gestation. It can be unilateral or bilateral, single, or multiple. Most of them can disappear after 26 weeks of gestation. If the cysts are

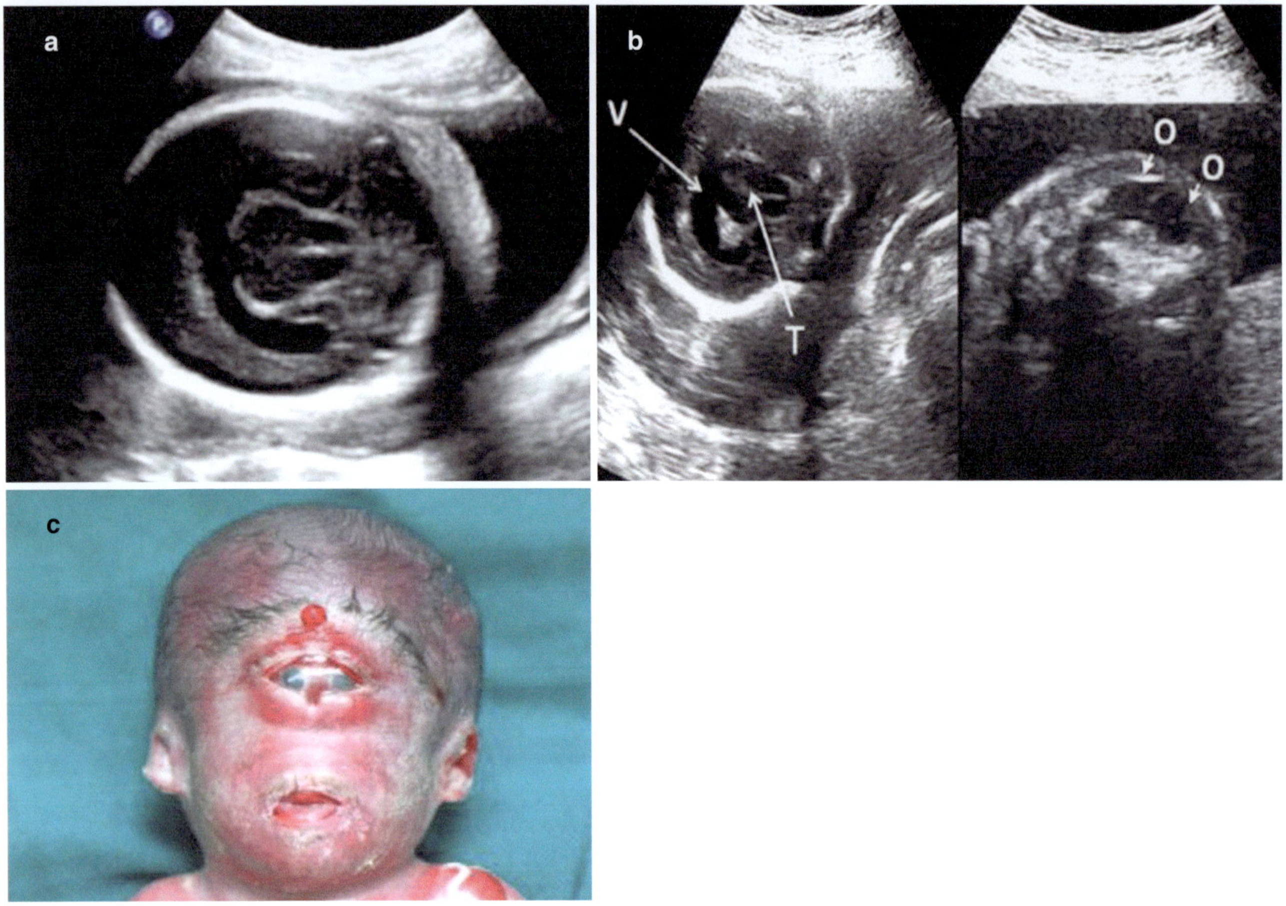

Fig. 2.72 Holoprosencephaly. (**a**). Typical ultrasonic imaging. (**b, c**). Combined hypotelorism

bilateral and keep existing or growing, further chromosome examination should be performed (Fig. 2.73).

3. Arachnoid cyst and congenital porencephaly: Arachnoid cysts represent round or irregular anechoic cystic areas in the brain with thin and smooth cystic walls. The cyst is not connected to the lateral ventricle. The prognosis is poor if the cyst keeps growing or is associated with other malformations, and further chromosomal examination should be performed. Congenital porencephaly is characterized by one or more irregular cystic anechoic areas in the fetal brain. The cyst is connected to the lateral ventricle and may accompany with hydrocephalus. It is extremely rare (Fig. 2.74).
4. Dandy-Walker syndrome: Sonography shows the completely absent cerebellar vermis and the two separated cerebellar hemispheres. The posterior cranial fossa and the fourth ventricle are enlarged and communicated with the posterior cranial fossa. Dilated lateral ventricles can be found in some cases (Fig. 2.75).
5. Intracranial tumor: Intracranial tumor is extremely rare. Teratoma is the most common intracranial tumor. It often occurs in the tentorium. The tumor may result in compression and displacement of normal intracranial structures like brain middle or hydrocephalus. Most of them are discovered until the middle or third trimester. Intracranial tumors can be lethal.

2.5.1.3 Special Tips

1. The majority of the fetal central nervous system malformations have a poor prognosis, such as anencephaly, severe hydrocephalus, encephalocele, meningocele, spina bifida, and myelomeningocele. The neonates usually die a few hours after birth. Pregnancy should be terminated immediately after a confirmed diagnosis.
2. Fetal neurological abnormalities have the risk of recurrence. Those who had already given birth to a fetus with neural tube defects have a risk of recurrence at about 5%. Moreover, the recurrence risk of those who had two children with neural tube defects is 10%. The recurrence risk is 15% to 20% for those who have had three such children. Pregnant women with high-risk factors should be examined multiple times at different gestational weeks.
3. Half of the patients who suffer from anencephaly, exencephaly, or hydrocephalus are often associated with spina bifida or other malformations. Be careful and patient when scanning the spine and other areas of the fetus.

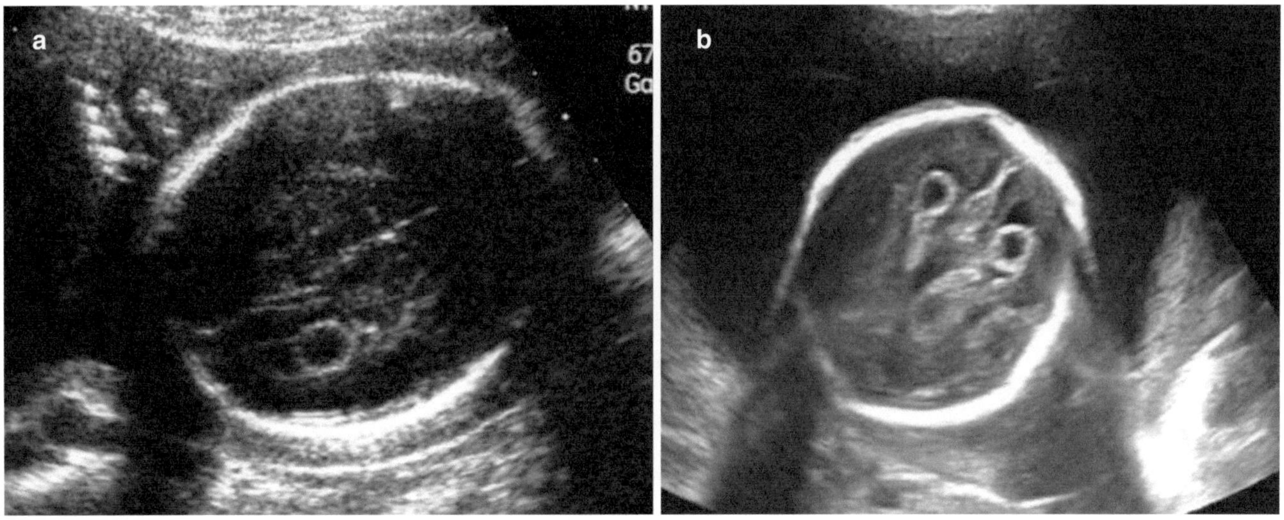

Fig. 2.73 (**a**). The unilateral fetal choroid plexus cyst usually disappears spontaneously after 26 weeks of gestation. (**b**). Bilateral choroid plexus cysts should be observed regularly. If it does not vanish after 26 weeks of gestation, a chromosome examination should be performed

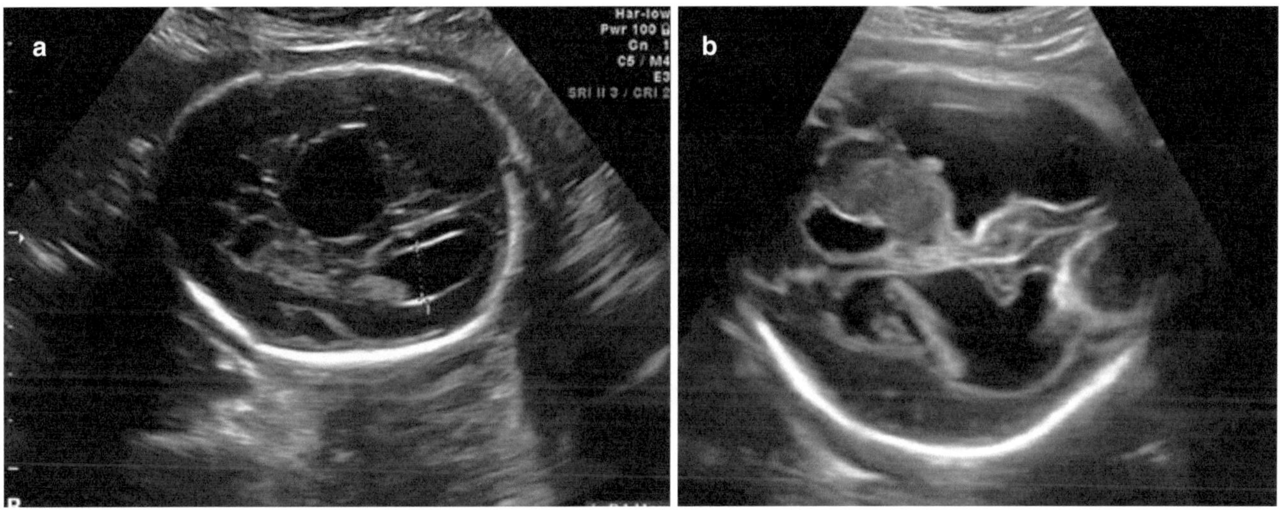

Fig. 2.74 Arachnoid cyst and congenital porencephaly. (**a**). Arachnoid cysts appear as sharply defined cystic lesions with thin and smooth cystic walls. The surface of the cyst is often attached to the endocranium directly. (**b**). Congenital porencephaly appears as an asymmetric cerebral hemispheric cavity

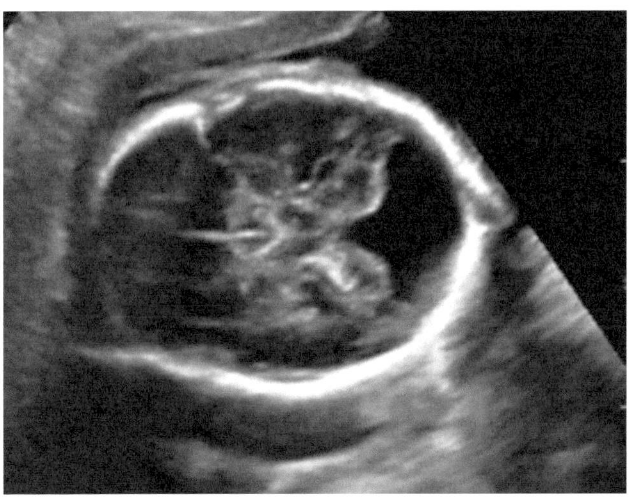

Fig. 2.75 Dandy-Walker syndrome. The posterior fossa cyst is communicated with the fourth ventricle. And the third ventricle is enlarged

4. When the fetal posterior fossa effusion is larger than 1.2 cm, regular surveillance, and follow-up by sonography are suggested. Be cautious about diagnosing microcephaly, only cases that the fetal growth values such as BPD and HC below more than three standard deviations from the normal values of the same gestational age should be highly suspected after regular dynamic measurement. Attention should be paid to the small measurement value of fetal head due to the particular head shape and parental genetic factors (Fig. 2.76).
5. It is essential to improve the ultrasonic accuracy of fetal malformation in the early diagnosis. The doctor who is engaged in ultrasonic diagnosis should remember all kinds of anatomical and sonogram features in different developing stages of the fetus. The technique of scanning should be programmed and standardized to avoid missed diagnosis and misdiagnosis. Choose further relevant

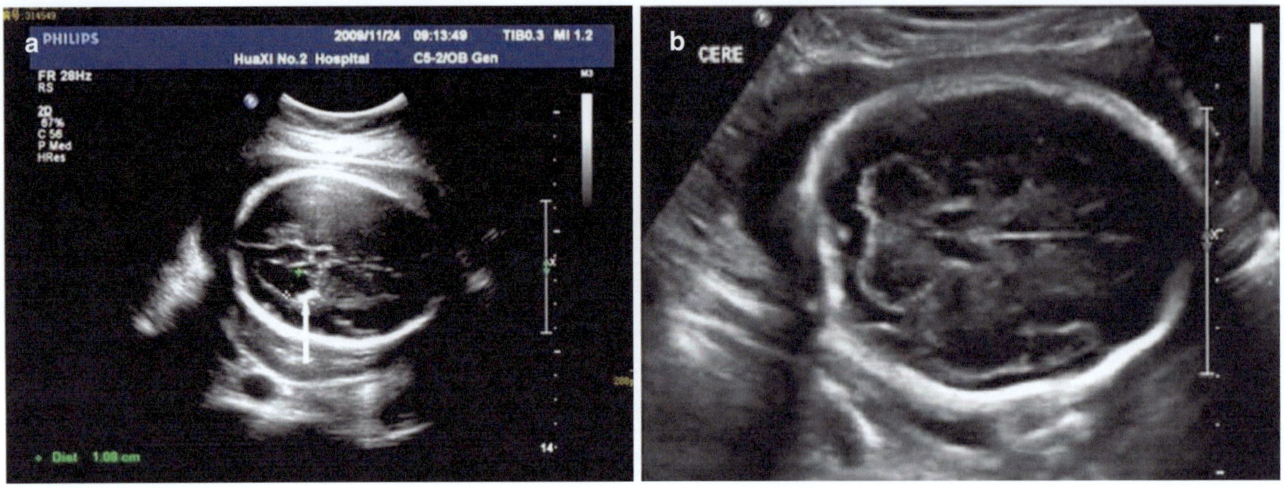

Fig. 2.76 It must be cautious to make the diagnosis of hydrocephalus when fetal lateral ventricle is less than 1.0 cm and fetal posterior fossa effusion below 1.5 cm. (**a**) The width of the lateral ventricle is 1.08 cm. (**b**) This image shows the mild enlarged cisterna magna

laboratory tests according to the actual situation, such as karyotype analysis and percutaneous umbilical blood sampling.

6. Ultrasonic result is affected by fetal position or maternal factors. Undertake the examination after the fetus or the pregnant women is properly promoted. Be patient and careful during the examination. Pregnant women are suggested to review regularly when suspicious lesions in a system or part of the fetus cannot be confirmed immediately. The decision should be taken after consultation by two or more physicians or transfer to the superior hospital for confirmation.
7. Pay attention to multi-section scanning of the fetal head and spine and avoid missing small encephalocele or meningocele.

2.5.2 Gastrointestinal Abnormalities of the Fetus

2.5.2.1 Basic Concepts

Fetal gastrointestinal malformation, a common congenital malformation, includes esophageal atresia and stenosis, duodenum stenosis and atresia, intestinal atresia and stenosis, and colon atresia and stenosis. The formation of such deformities may be related to the following reasons: the esophagus forming different types of blind ends during the development of laryngopharyngeal tracheal fold in embryo; the blocked or incomplete vacuolization of esophagus and intestine; embryonic mesenteric blood supply or the disordered vacuolization of the midgut.

In cases of esophageal atresia, duodenal stenosis, or atresia, some are accompanied by other congenital malformations. Among them, cardiac defect is the most common one, followed by gastrointestinal malformation, urinary malformation, and skeletal deformity. Some fetuses may be associated with chromosomal abnormalities, and the risk of developing trisomy 21 syndrome (Down's syndrome) is significantly increased. A few abnormalities are related to genetic factors, such as congenital megacolon.

As a result of fetal deglutition and functional disorders of digestion, absorption, and so on, digestive tract malformations are often associated with polyhydramnios. Pregnant women present with abdominal distension, chest tightness, and inability to lie on the back. Congenital esophageal atresia often coexists with tracheoesophageal fistula, which is changeling to diagnose prenatally. The neonate may have a cough and cannot eat. The diagnosis is confirmed after further examination.

Ultrasound has a certain value in the diagnosis of digestive tract malformations. The prognosis of simple gastrointestinal stenosis or obstruction relates to the associated deformities. Some of these simple deformities can be corrected by surgical treatment. Gastrointestinal dysplasia with other abnormalities or chromosomal abnormalities has a poor prognosis.

2.5.2.2 Ultrasonic Diagnosis

Esophageal Atresia

1. Esophageal atresia is highly suspected if no stomach bubble in the abdominal cavity is found, or the stomach bubble is very small with polyhydramnios after 18–20 weeks of gestation (Figs. 2.77 and 2.78).
2. In the case of partial esophageal atresia, the upper esophagus represents the anechoic cystic area. After 26 weeks, the fetal swallowing motion is visible under ultrasound, and the anechoic cyst is evident in the coronal section of the fetal neck, whose size changes with the swallowing.
3. Esophageal atresia often accompanies congenital heart malformation and chromosome abnormality.

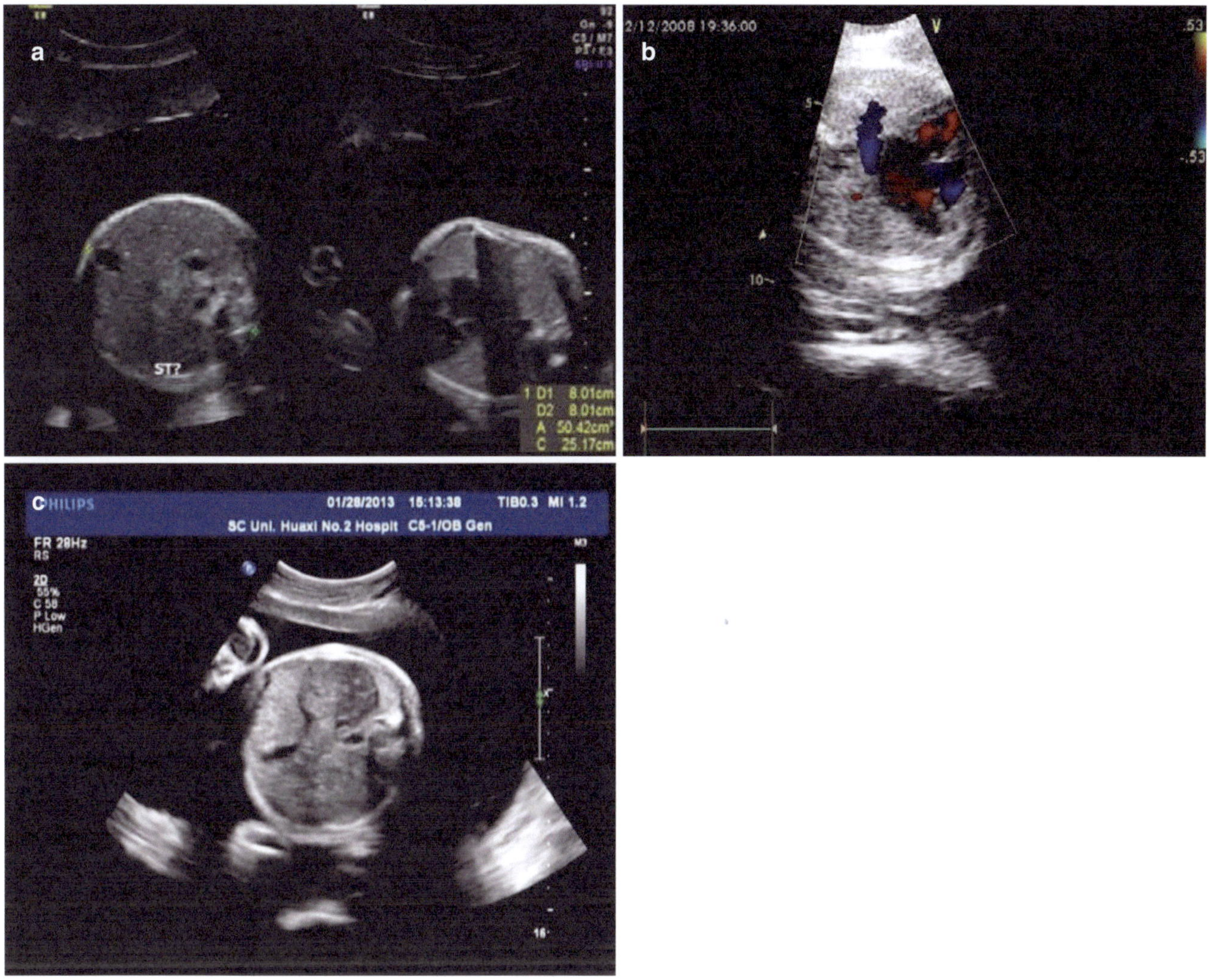

Fig. 2.77 Esophageal atresia. (**a, b**). The image shows no stomach bubble in the abdominal cavity with polyhydramnios at 28 weeks of gestation. Fetal echocardiography shows an atrial septal defect. (**c**). An absent stomach bubble with polyhydramnios at 35 weeks of gestation. The fetus died from digestive tract atresia after birth

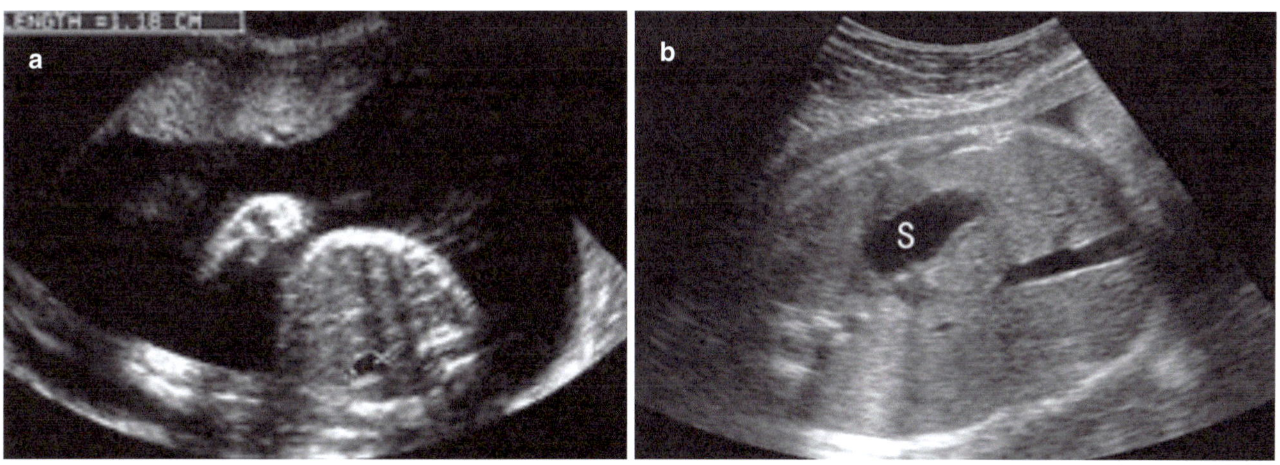

Fig. 2.78 Small fetal stomach bubble. (**a**). The image shows the diameter of gastric bubble is only 1.18 cm with polyhydramnios at 26 weeks of gestation. (**b**). The same patient was reviewed 3 weeks later, the diameter of gastric bubble is 2.0 cm and the digestive tract is normal after birth

Duodenal Stenosis or Atresia

1. The classic "double bubble" sign appears as two similar anechoic masses in the transverse view of the fetal abdomen, representing the expended stomach and duodenum. The bubble at the left upper abdomen and inferior to the heart is gastric bubble, and the bubble at the right lower side of liver is the expended duodenum (Fig. 2.79).
2. Adjust the direction of the probe and the connection between the two bubbles can be found (Fig. 2.80).
3. It is often accompanied by hydramnion. The degree of hydramnion and the occurrence time are related to the severity of duodenal obstruction.

Jejunoileal Stenosis or Atresia

1. The section of the middle and lower abdomen of the fetus demonstrates multiple anechoic areas in the abdominal cavity, which are persistent with peristalsis. The lower the atresia, the more dilated the jejunoileal (Fig. 2.81).
2. The small intestinal diameter is dilated more than 7 mm, and the diameter gradually increases during multiple examinations, indicating the small intestinal obstruction (Fig. 2.82).
3. Ultrasonography shows significantly enhanced intestinal peristalsis, with fetal ascites. Most of the cases are accompanied by hydramnion (Fig. 2.83).

Colon Stenosis or Atresia

1. The expended colon in the middle and lower fetal abdomen, which is more than 1.8 to 2.0 cm in diameter, increases with the gestational age. The expended colon appears like a multilocular cyst, with an irregular shape. Duplicature is visible on the inner wall of the dilated bowel (Fig. 2.84).
2. The fetal lower bowel in pelvic dilates is in a "V" or "U" shape in anal atresia cases. Fetal anal atresia should be highly suspected if there is an apparent half-septum in liquid area of the expended bowel (double leaf sign).
3. It often combines with hydramnion.

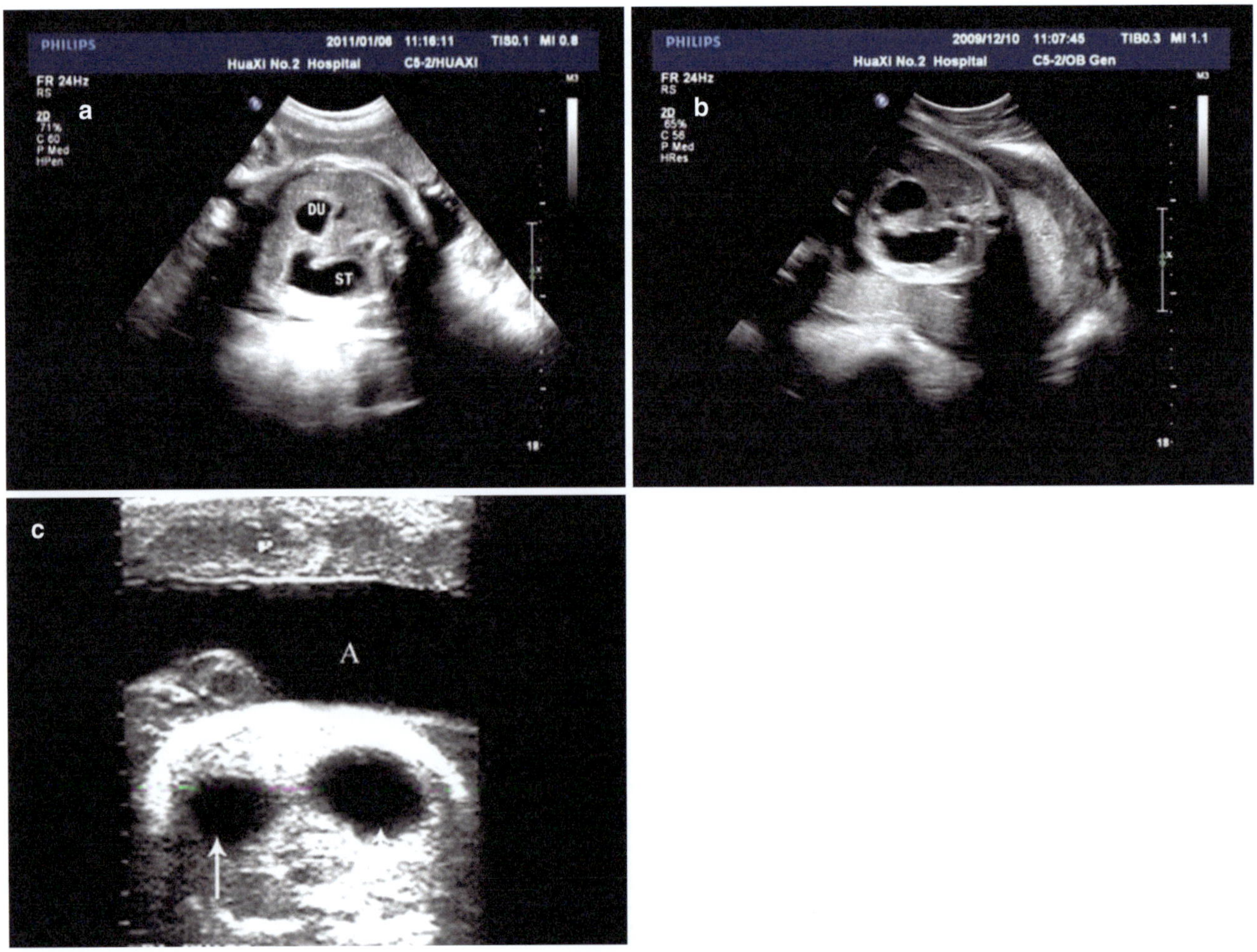

Fig. 2.79 Duodenal stenosis or atresia I. (**a–c**). The transverse section of the fetal abdomen shows two sonolucent bubbly anechoic areas, combined with hydramnion

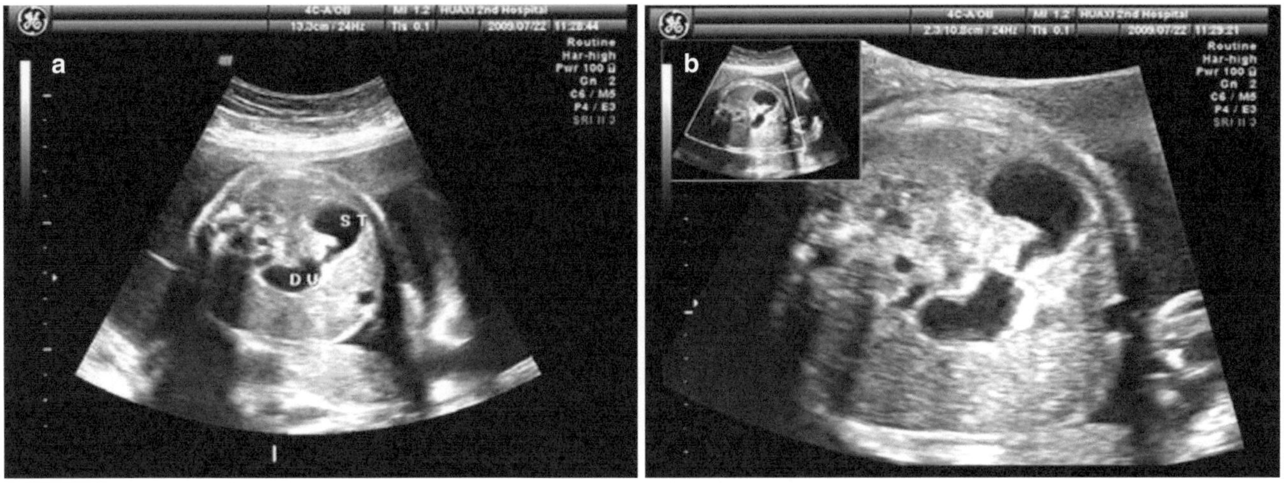

Fig. 2.80 Duodenal stenosis or atresia II. (**a, b**). After adjusting the probe, the connection between the stomach bubble and dilated duodenum is visible

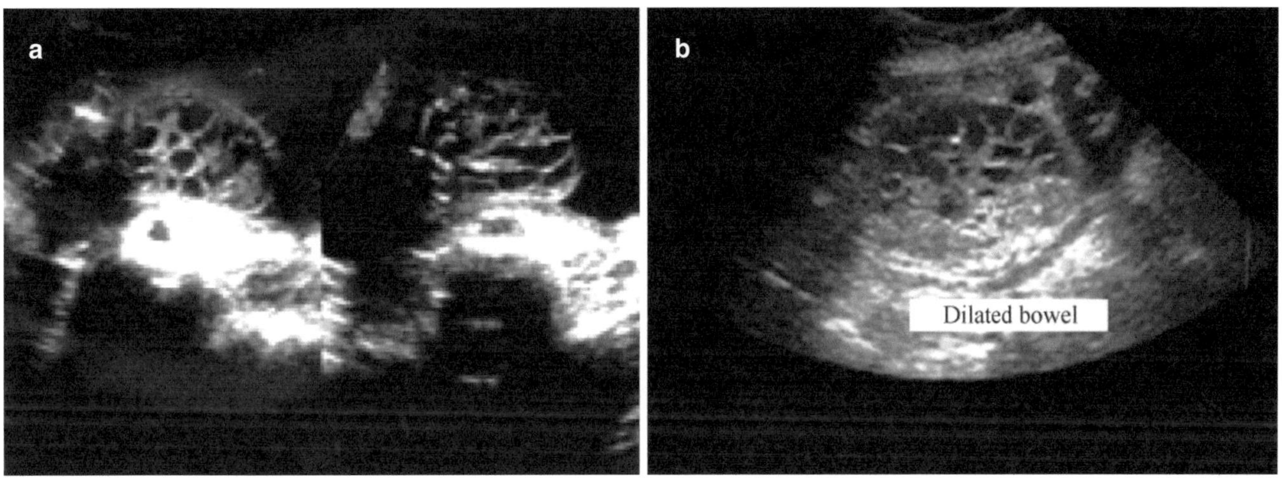

Fig. 2.81 Jejunoileal stenosis or atresia I. (**a, b**). The images show the fetal dilated small intestine, like a "honeycomb" appearance

Other Rare Fetal Intestinal Abnormalities

1. Megacolon: The bowel expands obviously in ultrasound. It is difficult to diagnose by ultrasound if there is no significant expansion of the bowel. Take it seriously if there is positive family history.
2. Meconium ileus: It is rare. The echo of intestine is significantly enhanced, similar to the echo of bone. The bowel above the obstruction dilates (Fig. 2.85).

Space Occupying Lesions of Liver

1. Intrahepatic calcification: Antenatal ultrasound shows a strong echo in the liver, and the big ones are accompanied by posterior shadow. Most of them will disappear after birth (Fig. 2.86).
2. Liver tumor: Liver tumors of the fetus are rare. The most common liver tumors in literature are hepatic cyst, hepatic hemangioma, hepatoblastoma, hepatic hamartoma, and so on. The echo of the hepatic tumor can be cystic, solid, or mixed. The boundary of the mass is generally clear with regular and orderly margins. Hepatic hemangioma and hepatoblastoma can lead to the enlargement of the liver. The echo of the tumor is chaotic, with abundant blood flow under CDFI (Figs. 2.87 and 2.88).

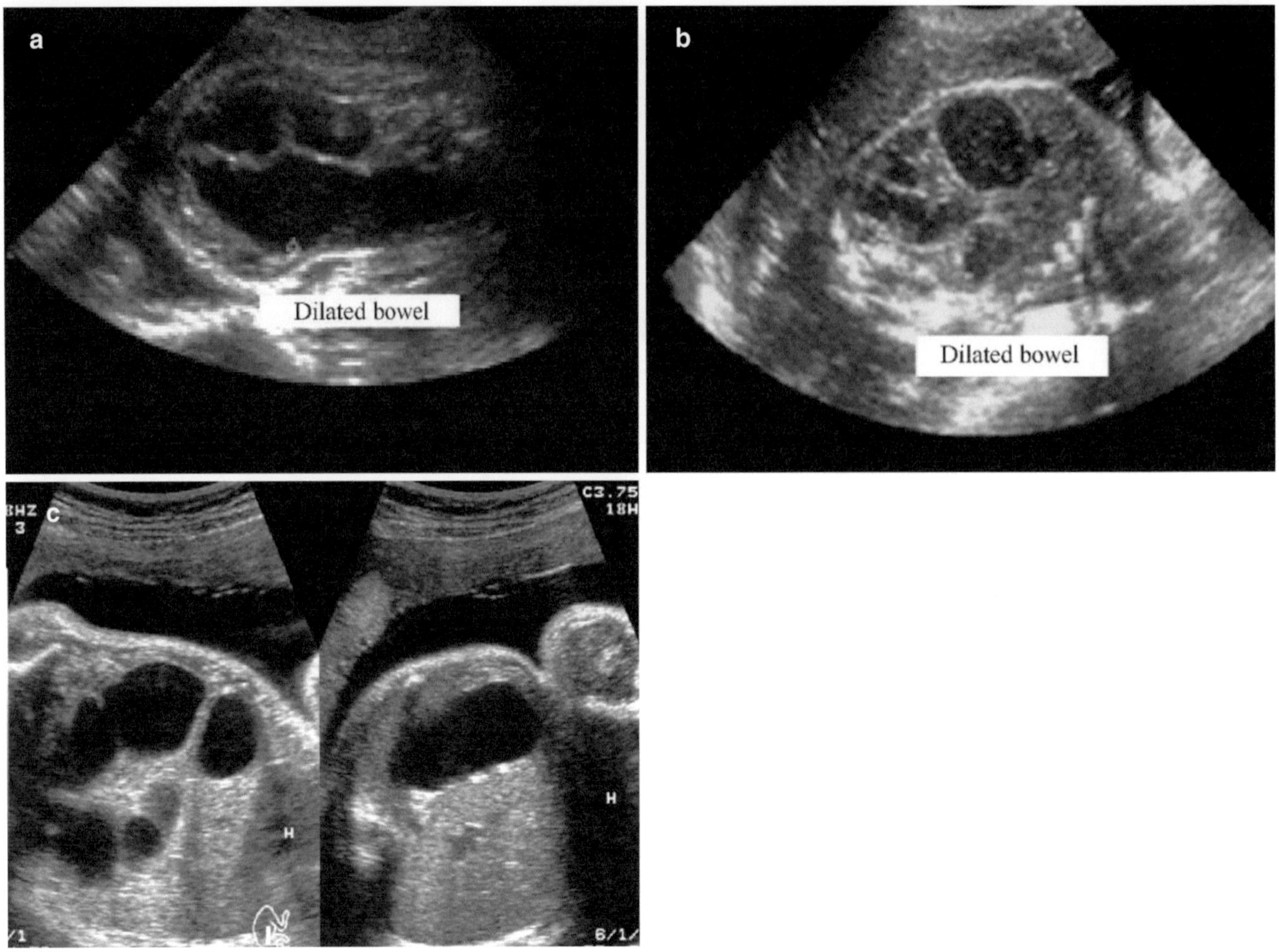

Fig. 2.82 Jejunoileal stenosis or atresia II. (**a–c**). The fetal bowel is dilated, with more than 2.0 cm in diameter, and septum is visible in the cavity

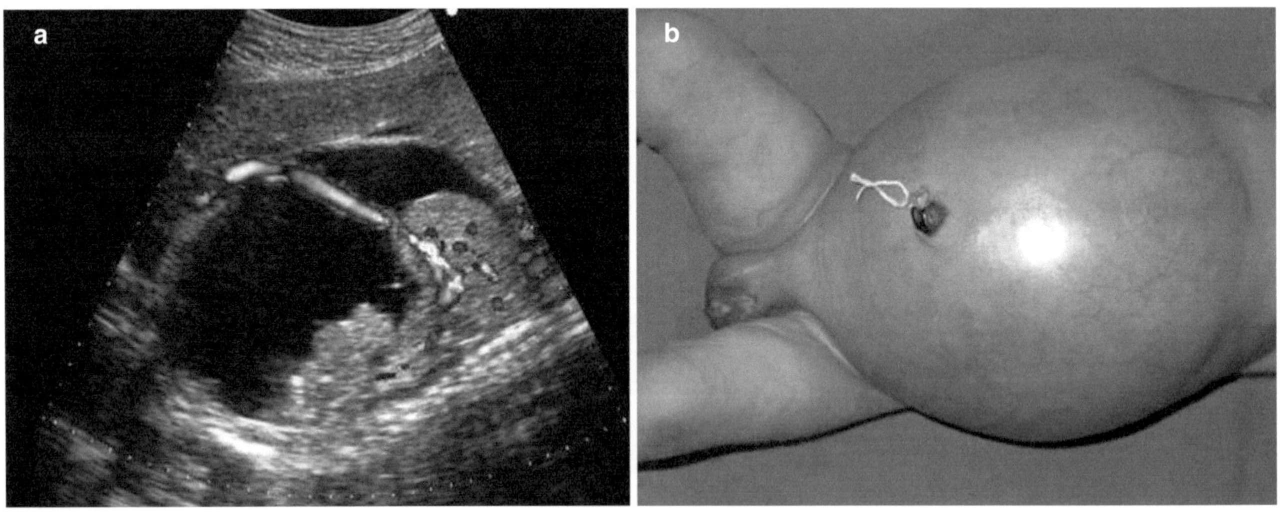

Fig. 2.83 Fetal ascites. (**a**). A large amount of ascites in abdominal cavity on the sagittal section. (**b**). The extremely distended abdomen

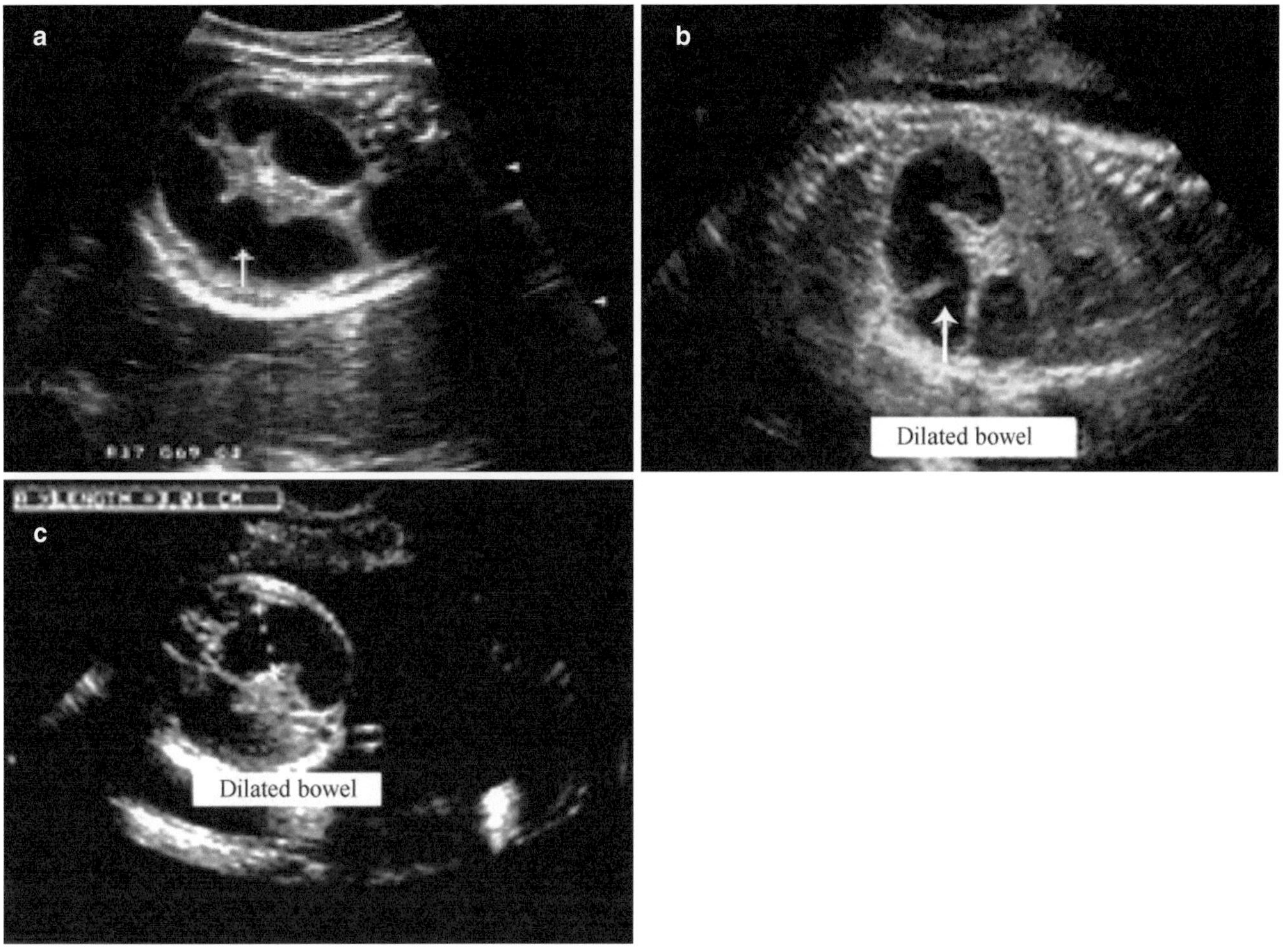

Fig. 2.84 Colon stenosis or atresia. (**a–c**). Septal or lobulate cystic masses in the lower fetal abdomen, most of which are colonic atresia or stricture and anal atresia

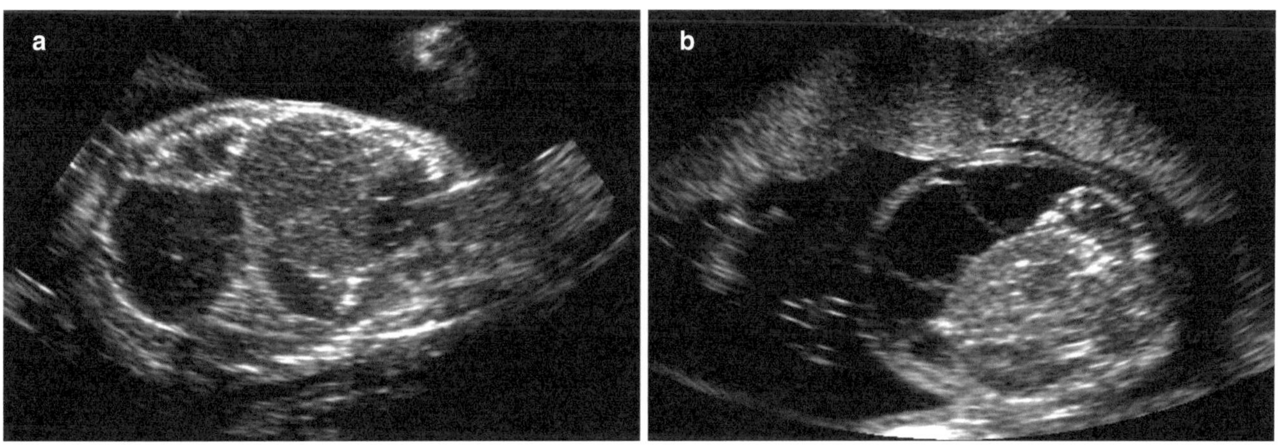

Fig. 2.85 Meconium ileus. (**a, b**). The involved bowel is dilated, and the bowels below are hyperechoic

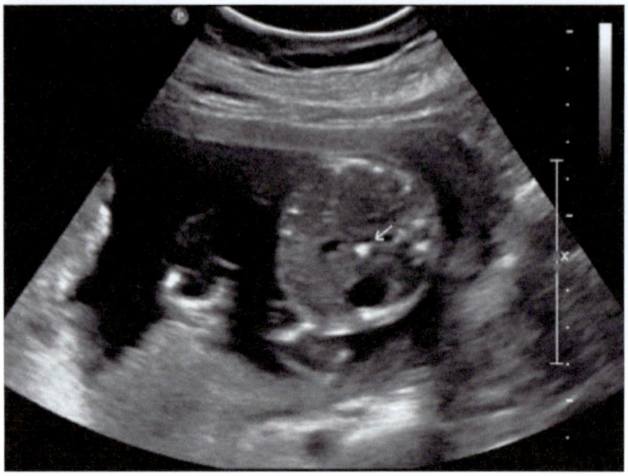

Fig. 2.86 Intrahepatic calcification of fetus

2.5.2.3 Special Tips

1. Note that the fetal bowel can be segmental hyperechoic in the third trimester of pregnancy, 1.8–2 cm in diameter, or hyperechoic clumps in the intestine with different sizes and no echo attenuation. It can disappear after birth and is easy to be misdiagnosed as intestinal abnormalities (Fig. 2.89).
2. Intestinal dilatation should be distinguished from dilated ureteral and intraperitoneal cysts. Colon dilatation often occurs in the third trimester, which should be distinguished from the fetal bladder, renal cyst, and abdominal cyst. Change the scanning angle of the probe for further diagnosis (Fig. 2.90).
3. Irregular transverse section of the abdomen should be avoided. When the stomach and bladder, or the stomach

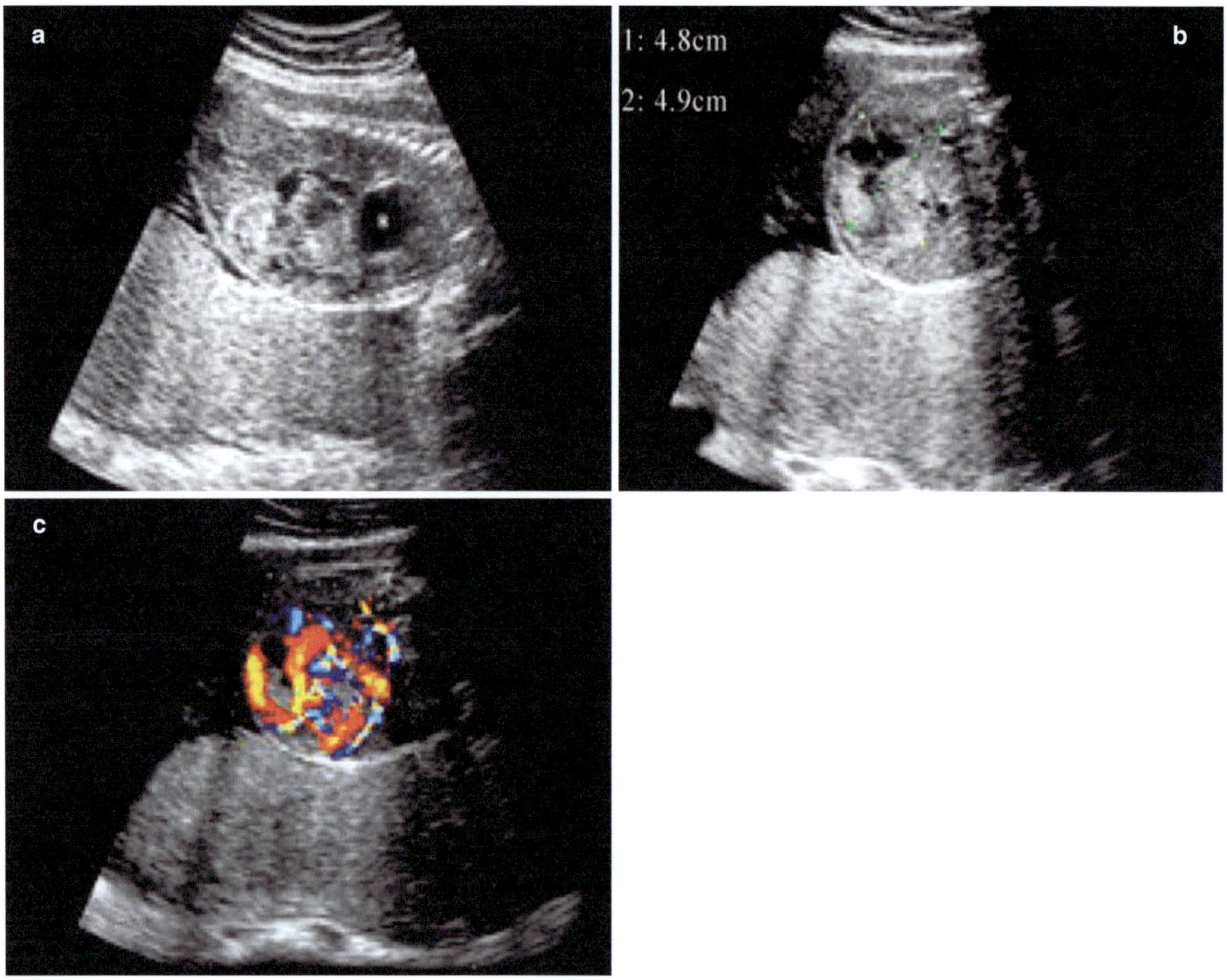

Fig. 2.87 Liver tumor. At 26 weeks of gestation, the ultrasound revealed a solid lesion in the liver with a diameter of about 5.0 cm. (**a**). The sagittal view of the liver tumor. (**b**). The transverse view of the liver tumor. (**c**). CDFI shows the blood flow in the mass

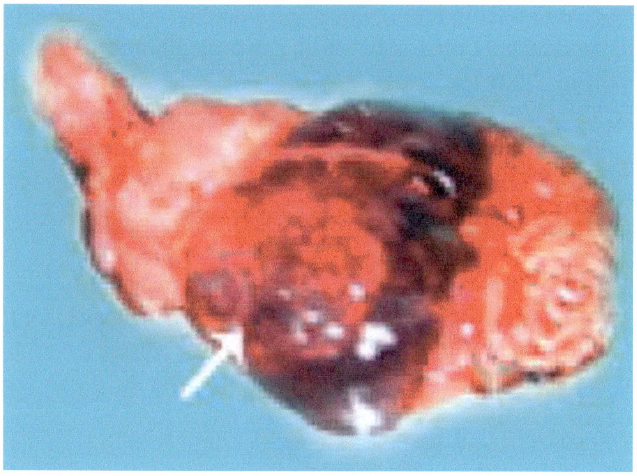

Fig. 2.88 The image shows a solid liver tumor, which is the postoperative specimen of the same fetus in Fig. 2.87

and fluid-containing intestines are showed in the same section, it is similar to the "double bubble" sign (Figs. 2.90 and 2.91).

4. Anal atresia and megacolon are lack of specificity. The anal atresia cannot be completely excluded when there is no significant intestine dilatation in ultrasound.
5. Even if there is a standard size stomach bubble in the fetal abdominal cavity, esophageal atresia with tracheoesophageal fistula cannot be wholly excluded.

2.5.3 Fetal Gastroschisis (Anterior Abdominal Wall Defect)

2.5.3.1 Basic Concept

1. At 6–10 weeks of the pregnancy, the digestive tract grows faster than the abdominal cavity and abdominal wall,

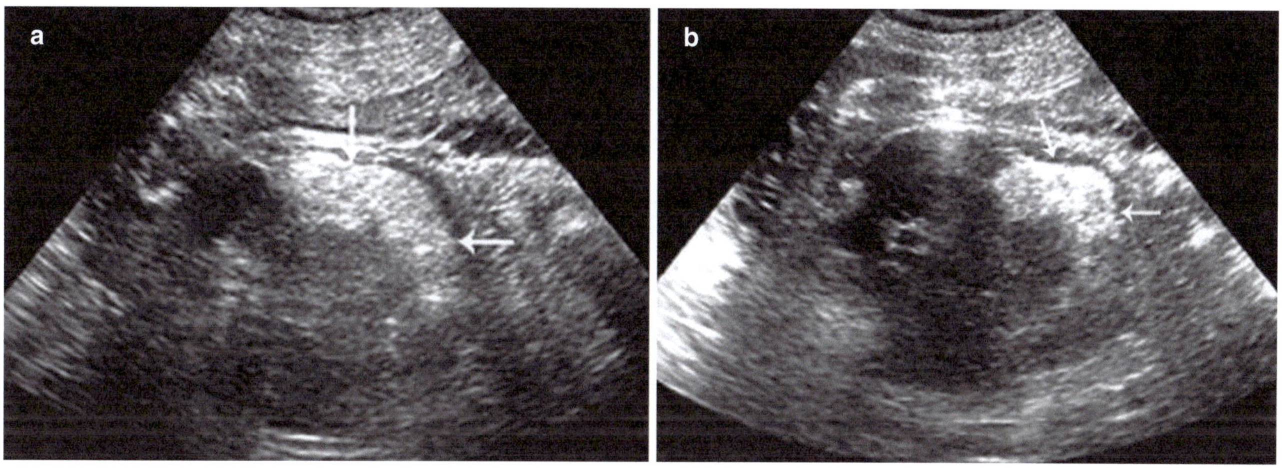

Fig. 2.89 Bowel of fetus. (**a, b**). The images show a strong echogenic mass in the fetal bowel at 38 weeks of gestation. There is no digestive tract abnormality after birth

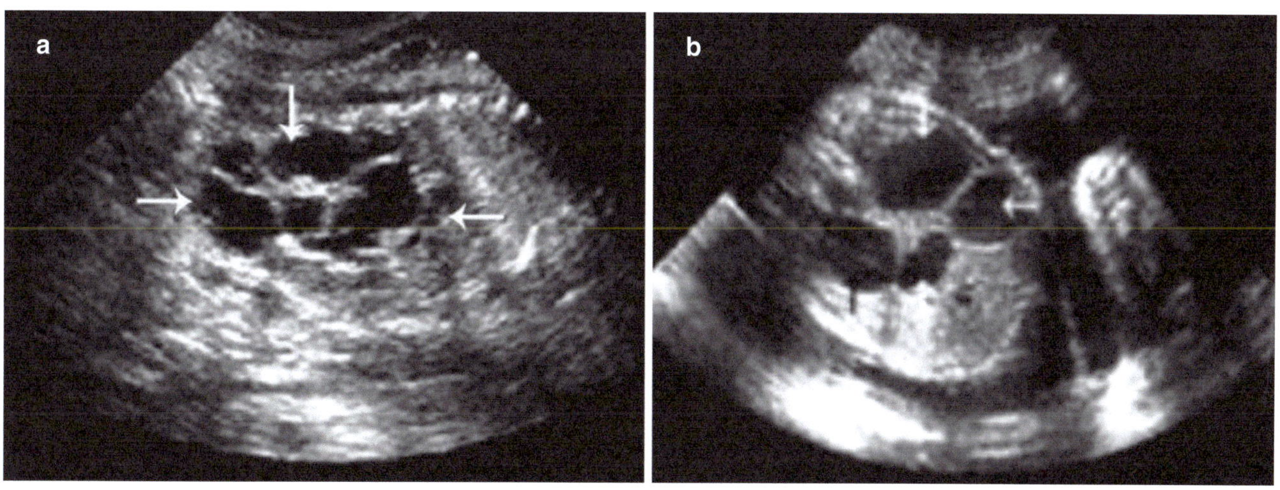

Fig. 2.90 Cystic lesions in abdominal cavity. (**a**). Fetal renal cysts. (**b**). The dilated bowel. We should pay attention to the distinction between the two diseases

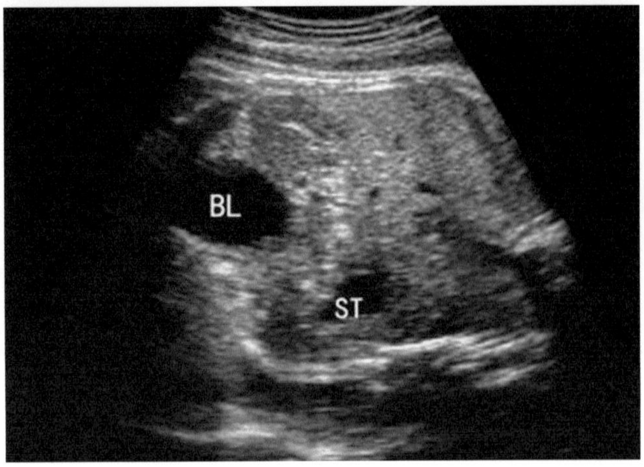

Fig. 2.91 False "double bubble" sign. Bladder and stomach bubble are displayed in the same section, because of the unstandardized view, which is easy to be misdiagnosed as "double bubble" sign

resulting in the midgut being pushed to the bottom of the umbilical cord and formed a physiologic midgut hernia. After 10 weeks of gestation, the abdominal cavity grew faster with expanded volume. The head fold and tail fold of anterior abdominal wall along with skin and muscles on both sides close and fold rapidly from the lateral dorsal midline. The midgut which protrudes outside the body cavity recedes into the abdominal cavity gradually. The midgut rotates and merges with the abdominal wall to form the umbilical ring in the center.

During the formation of the fetal abdominal wall, the formation of the abdominal wall is inhibited or delayed, affected by some factors, leading to the defects of the abdominal wall and the umbilical region. All the above may result in prolapse and abdominal cavity content bulging.

Fetal omphalocele is caused by the failed fusion of the ectoderm and mesoderm along the midline, resulting in hypoplasia of the anterior abdominal wall. Defects in the muscles and skin around the midline umbilical cord lead to the bulging of partial the peritoneum or abdominal organs. The expanded contents are covered with an amniotic membrane and peritoneum.

Fetal gastroschisis, also known as visceral valgus, is characterized by a defect of the entire anterior abdominal wall, where valgus abdominal organs floating in the amniotic cavity. Fetal gastroschisis is caused by some teratogenic factors during the formation of the abdominal wall.

2.5.3.2 Ultrasonic Diagnosis

Omphalocele

1. The interruption of hyperechoic fetal skin continuity of the anterior abdominal wall is visible. There is an extruding mass with unequal size in the fetal umbilical cord, covered with a strong linear echo on the surface. There is an anechoic area between the two membranous echoes (Fig. 2.92).
2. The umbilical cord entrance is usually located on the surface of the mass, attached to the center of the mass or one side. CDFI shows the mass is attached to the entrance of the umbilical cord. This disease is often combined with other abnormalities.
3. The content of small puffed mass is mostly bowels, and that of larger masses can be stomach, liver, pancreas, and spleen. Ultrasound is utilized to identify the inside contents.

Gastroschisis

1. The echo of the fetal abdominal wall is discontinuous. The transverse section of the abdomen reveals the width of the abdominal wall defect. The abdominal cavity is empty, and the measured value of AC is less than that of the corresponding gestational week.
2. The viscera in the abdominal cavity, such as liver, stomach, intestines, and bladder, emerge from the defect and protrude into the amniotic cavity.
3. The umbilical cord entrance is in normal position or on the left inferior abdominal wall aside protrusions. Color Doppler blood flow shows the relationship of blood flow between the umbilical cord and viscera. Confirm the structure of the organ according to the presence of blood flow inside (Fig. 2.93).
4. Fetal gastroschisis is often combined with polyhydramnios.

2.5.3.3 Special Tips

1. The surface of omphalocele is covered with peritoneum and amniotic membrane. There is an anechoic strip between the two membranes, which is the differential point from gastroschisis. Pay attention to the difference between the abdominal skin mass, umbilical cord mass, fatal omphalocele, and gastroschisis.
2. Gastroschisis often occurs after the second trimester and even in the third trimester. Therefore, we should notice the integrity of the fetal abdominal wall in late pregnancy.
3. When there is only a small amount of intestine in the protrusion, it is easy to be mistaken for fetal external genitalia (Fig. 2.94).
4. Physiological bowel herniation usually appears in the 6th–tenth week of pregnancy, so omphalocele should not be diagnosed before 12 weeks of pregnancy. If the diameter of the umbilical cord mass is >7 mm, or the diameter of the umbilical cord mass is bigger than the diameter of AC, it should be alert to the omphalocele and reviewed regularly.
5. The image of pseudo bulged out viscera is caused by the lack of amniotic fluid, the nonstandard scanning, or

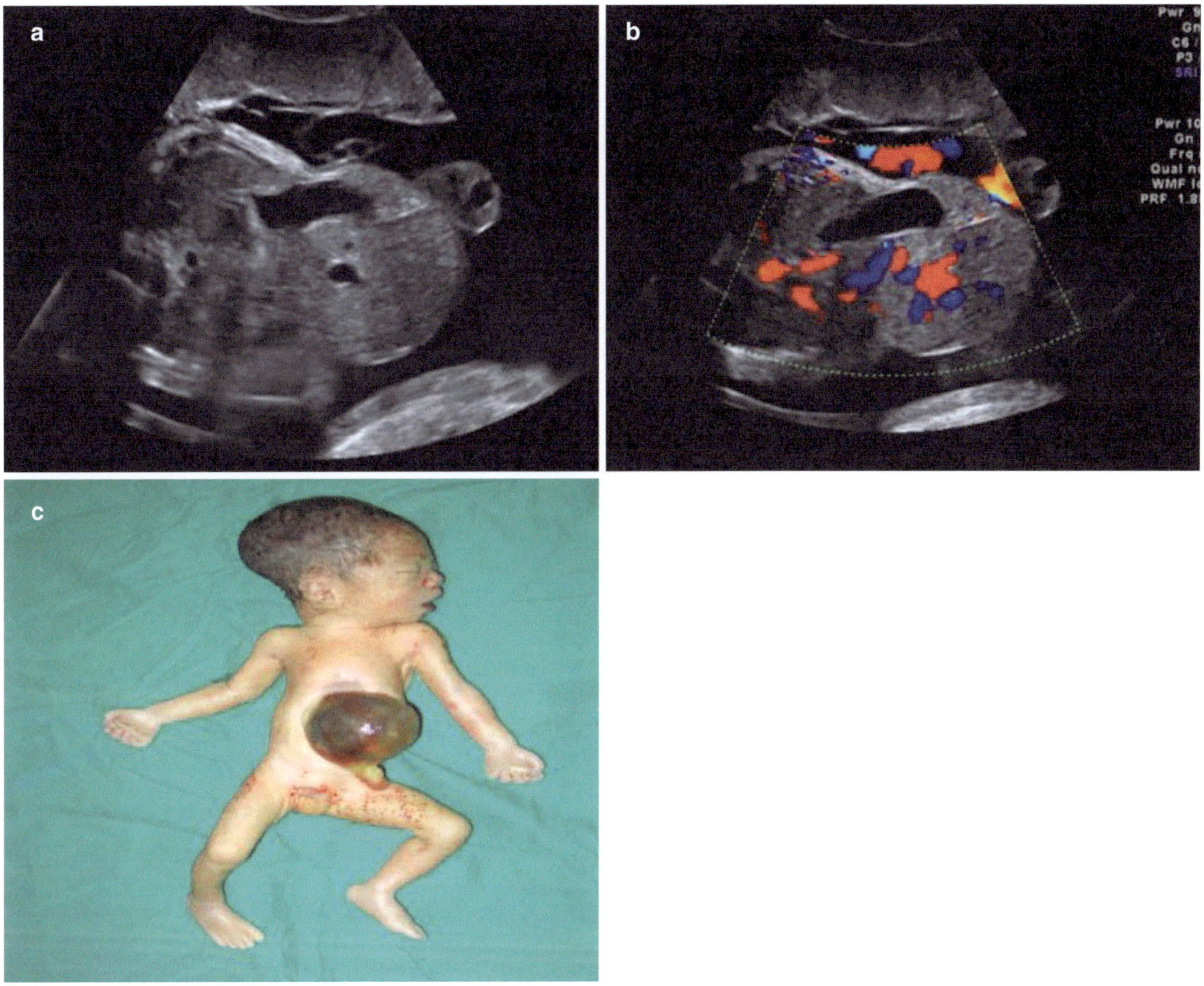

Fig. 2.92 Omphalocele. (**a, b**). Omphalocele in transection of the abdomen. The umbilical cord is attached to the expanded mass. (**c**). Omphalocele is confirmed after labor induction

overexertion of the probe. It can be distinguished by changing the angle of the probe and changing the position of the pregnant woman and fetus (Fig. 2.95).

2.5.4 Urogenital System Abnormalities of Fetus

2.5.4.1 Basic Concepts

The urogenital system of the fetus develops at the end of the third week in the human embryo. It is developed from the intermediate mesoderm. During the embryo, the nephrotome forms and differentiates into the pronephros, then the mesonephros, and finally evolves into the metanephros. The metanephros develops into a permanent kidney of the adult. The mesonephros duct develops into the ureter, renal pelvis, calyces, and collecting tubules.

Various factors affect the process of urinary tract development process, resulting in urethremphraxis and congenital kidney malformations—polycystic kidney, ectopic kidney, renal absence, and duplex kidney.

After 13 weeks of gestation, the fetal bladder is visible. After 16 weeks of gestation, the structures of the fetal kidney can be shown clearly. The prenatal ultrasonic detection rate of urinary system malformation is varied. The main cause of false-positive diagnosis is the slight dilatation of the renal collecting system. Different authors have different criteria for diagnosing fetal hydronephrosis, which is not easy to unify at present. Most domestic and foreign scholars believe that follow-up is necessary if the dilated renal pelvis ranges from 0.5 to 1.0 cm and is associated with ureter or bladder expansion.

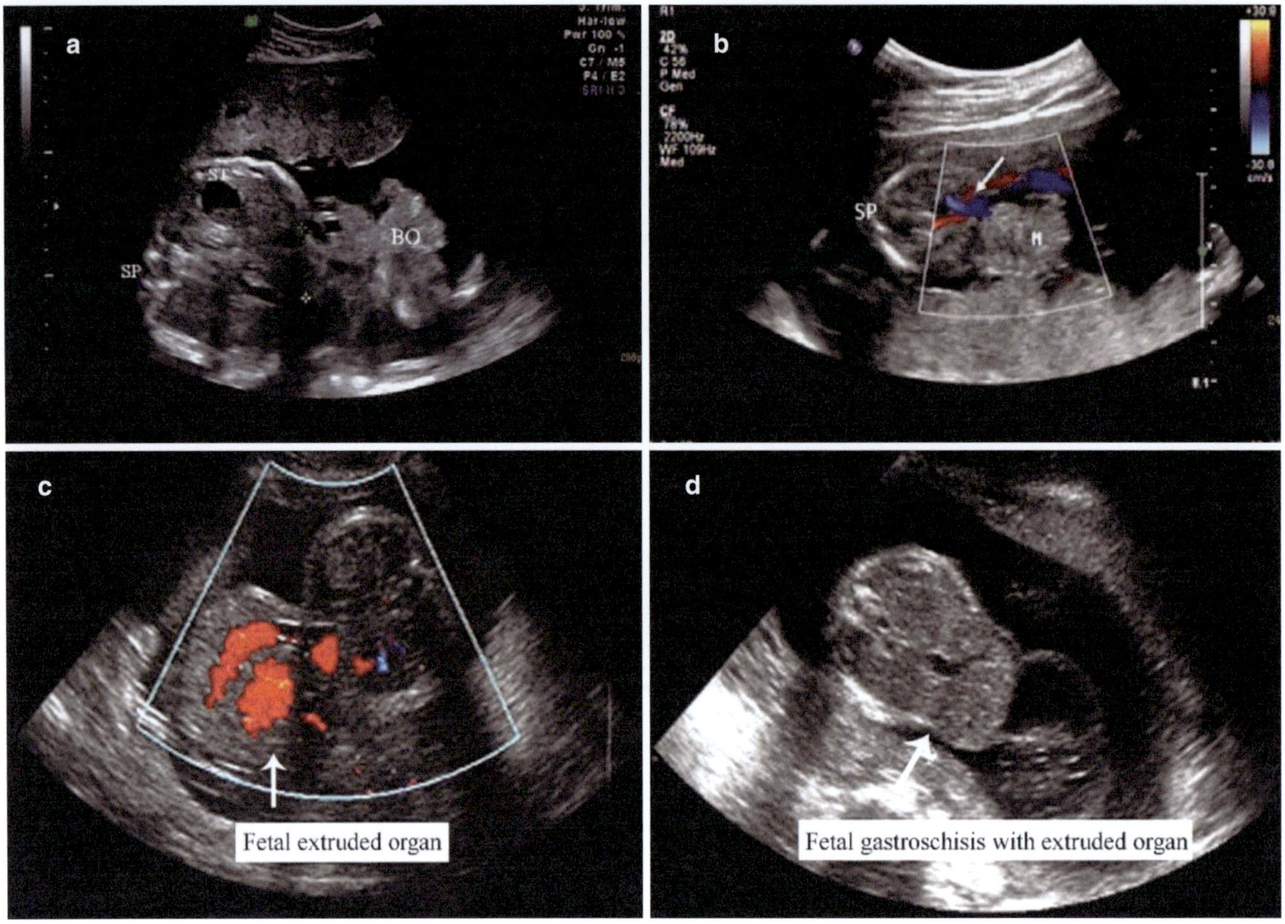

Fig. 2.93 Fetal gastroschisis with extruded organ. (**a**). Fetal gastroschisis with extruded liver. (**b**). Fetal gastroschisis with extruded bowel. (**c**). CDFI shows the blood flow of extruded liver. (**d**). Fetal gastroschisis with extruded bowel and liver

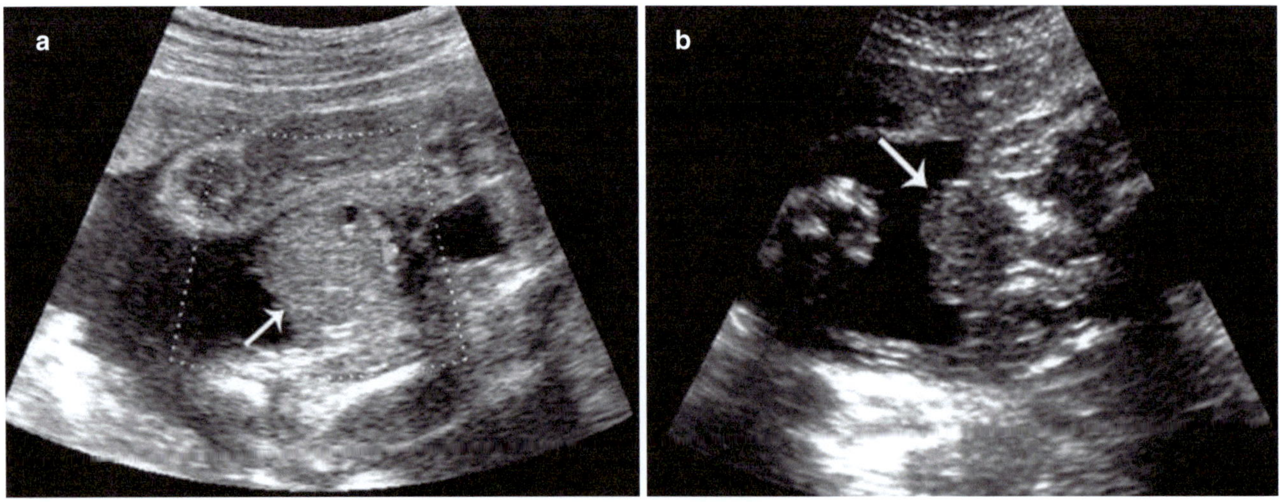

Fig. 2.94 The difference between the intestine and fetal external genitalia. (**a**). The image shows a small amount of intestine in the protrusion, which is easy to be mistaken for fetal external genitalia. (**b**). The external genitalia of the fetus

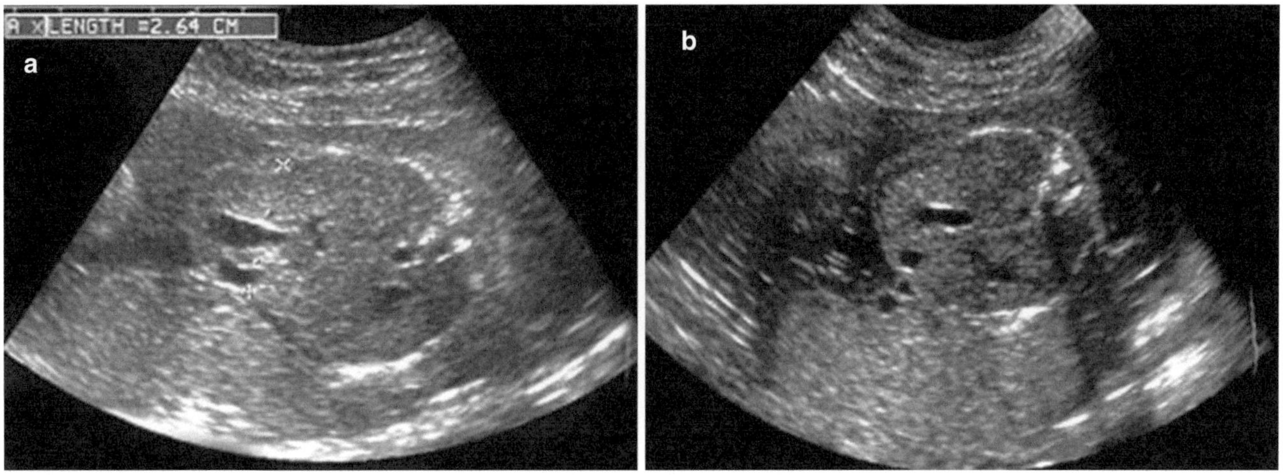

Fig. 2.95 Pseudo bulged out viscera caused by the nonstandard tranesection scanning. (**a**). Pseudo bulged out viscera caused by overexertion. (**b**). The image shows a normal abdominal transverse view of the same fetus after adjusting the probe

2.5.4.2 Ultrasonic Diagnosis

Renal Absence

1. The renal structure is not visible in the kidney area on both sides of the fetal spine nor in the abdomen or pelvis. Renal absence may be unilateral or bilateral.
2. After 16 weeks of gestation, sonography shows no kidneys and bladder, with oligohydramnios. If unilateral renal deficiency does not affect the bladder, the amniotic fluid may be in the normal range, and the contralateral kidney is compensatorily enlarged.
3. In cases of unilateral or bilateral renal absence, color Doppler flow imaging fails to show the unilateral or bilateral renal artery (Fig. 2.96).

Polycystic Kidney

1. Infantile polycystic kidney (autosomal recessive inheritance)
   (a) Both kidneys are enlarged uniformly with an intact capsule and normal shape.
   (b) The echo of the kidney is diffusely enhanced. The boundary between the renal cortex and the collecting system is not clear. The cut surface appears to be spongy.
   (c) 3)Abnormality in kidney size and echo is obvious after 24 weeks of gestation, with a poor prognosis. The recurrence rate is 25% (Figs. 2.97 and 2.98).
2. Adult polycystic kidney
   (a) Adult polycystic kidney is characterized by a unilateral or bilateral renal lesion represents as a multilocular cystic mass, without normal kidney morphology. The abnormal kidney is enlarged.
   (b) There are many vesicular echoes in different sizes, without communication between the sacs, representing a grape, or honeycomb shape.
   (c) No renal cortex beneath the renal capsule and collecting system in the center is visible in severe renal cyst cases. Some renal cysts appear as a large cysts in the center with small ones in peripheral, resembling hydronephrosis. Communication between the sacs is vital to identify the cysts or hydronephrosis (Fig. 2.99).
   (d) In unilateral polycystic kidney cases, the other kidney is healthy. The prognosis is good. Regular follow-up is suggested after birth.

3. Other kidney dysplasias
   (a) Duplex kidney.
      (I) The enlarged kidney has upper and lower renal pelvises, which are not connected. Most of the upper renal pelvises are dilated, and the lower ones are normal in size (Fig. 2.100).
      (II) The ureter is dilated. The expanding and circuitous ureter in the fetal pelvis is visible.

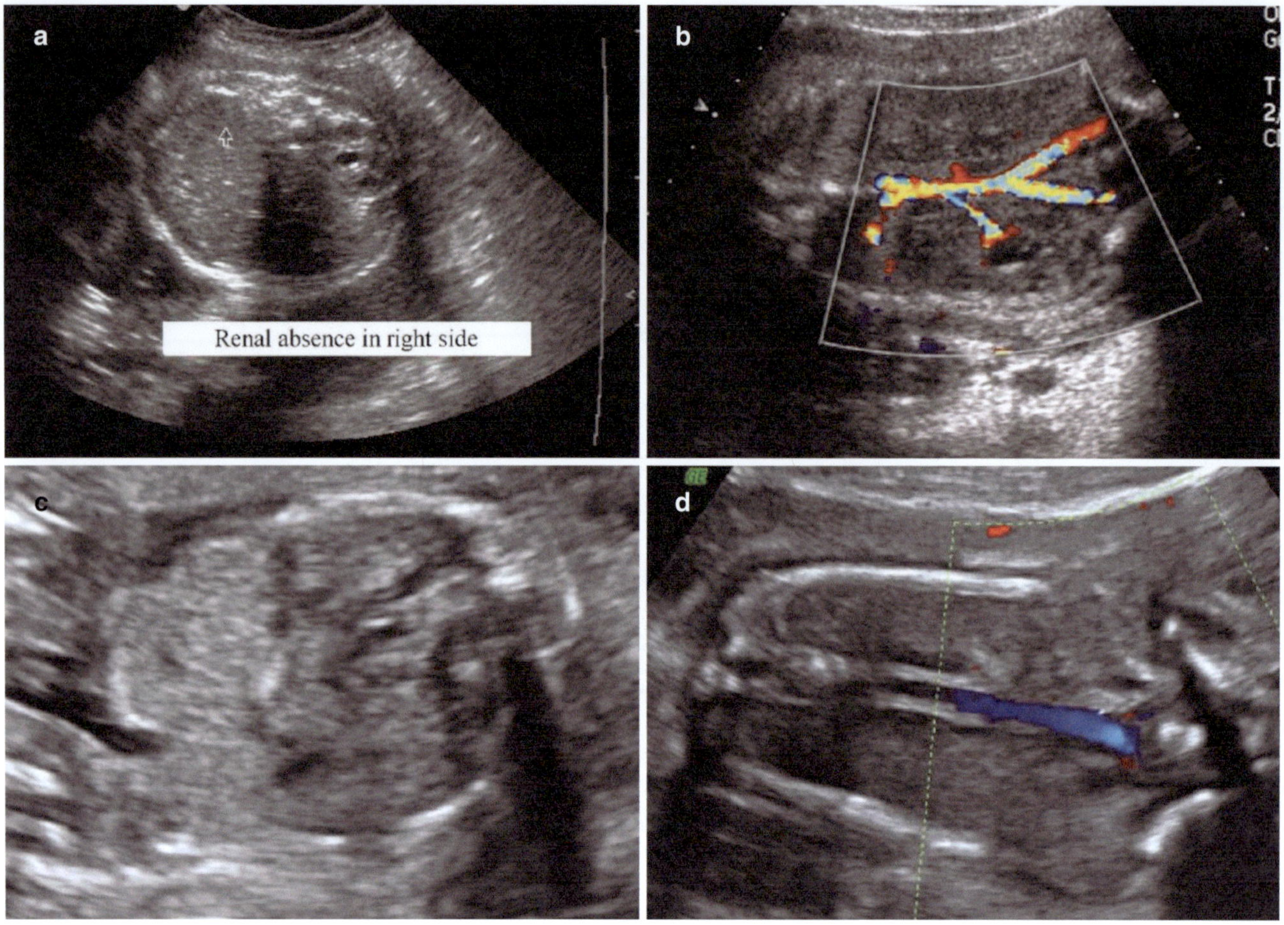

Fig. 2.96 Renal absence (**a, b**). The transverse images show no right kidney and the enlarged left kidney. Only one renal artery is shown. (**c, d**). The bilateral kidneys and renal arteries are absent

(III) The ureteral hernia is a bulbous vesicle located behind the bladder and extending toward the bladder.

(b) Ectopic kidney.
   (I) No renal is found in the renal region on one or both sides. The kidney could be found in other parts of the abdominal cavity or pelvic cavity by careful scanning (Fig. 2.101).
   (II) Pay attention to the differentiation from unilateral kidney absence and horseshoe kidney.

4. Urethremphraxis
   (a) Hydronephrosis: The most common type of urethremphraxis is hydronephrosis, most of which is unilateral. Hydronephrosis can also be bilateral. If the hydronephrosis is less than 1.5 cm, it usually disappears spontaneously after birth. If the measured value is more than 1.5 cm and accompanied by ureteral dilatation, we should exclude the urethremphraxis or bladder regurgitation. It should be regarded as abnormal when the renal pelvis is cystic dilated with septum around the cyst, and thinner renal column and cortex (Figs. 2.102 and 2.103).
   (b) Megabladder and megaloureter: The megabladder should be considered when a giant bladder increases gradually, which is more than 5 cm in diameter, without shrink during dynamic surveillance. Most of the megaloureter are functional obstruction,

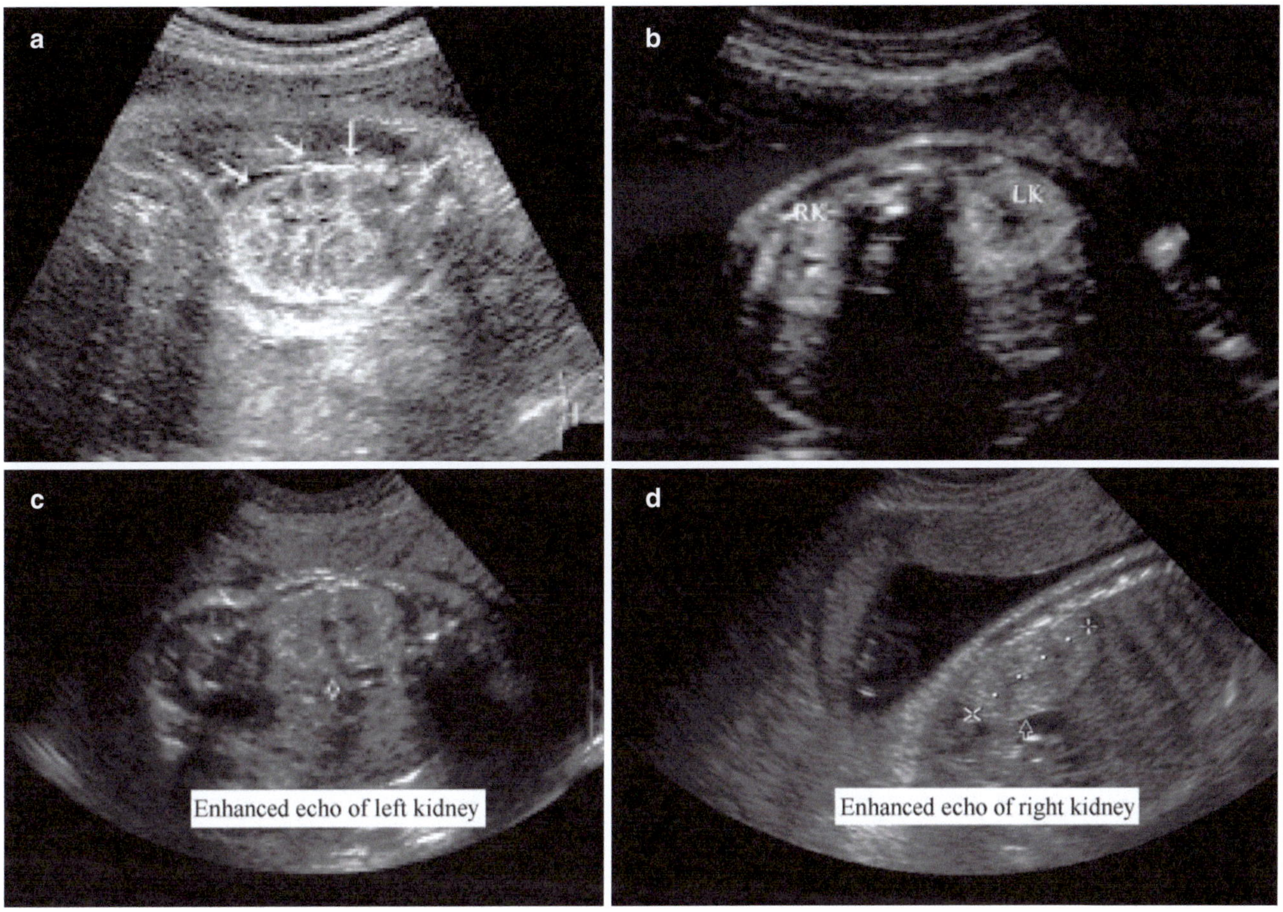

Fig. 2.97 Polycystic kidney. (**a, b**). The echo of both kidneys is enhanced, and the boundary between the renal cortex and the collecting system is unclear at 21 weeks of gestation. This sagittal section demonstrated the increased fetal renal volume. (**c, d**). At 32 weeks gestation, the longitudinal and transverse sections of the fetus show increased renal volume and enhanced renal parenchymal echo with normal amniotic flow. The pregnant woman had two previous pregnancy histories with infantile polycystic kidney. One infant died at four months, and the other died one year after birth. Infantile polycystic kidney is confirmed after induction of the present fetus

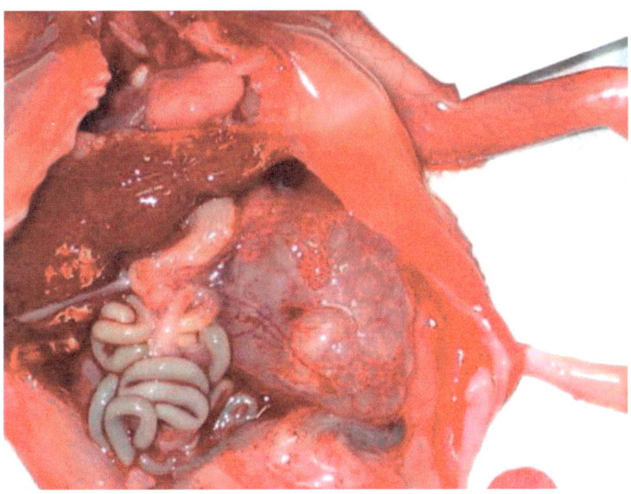

Fig. 2.98 Infantile polycystic kidney after labor induction

resulting in dilatation of the ureter and renal pelvis. Ultrasound shows obvious hydronephrosis and tortuous dilated ureter, which can disappear spontaneously after birth or after surgery (Fig. 2.104).

5. Other rare abnormalities of the fetal urinary system
   (a) Posterior urethral valve: It only happens in males. The bladder is extremely dilated with a thickened wall. The posterior urethra and double ureters are dilatated, with renal pelvis effusion (Fig. 2.105).
   (b) Exstrophy of the bladder: When the kidneys and amniotic fluid volume are normal with the absence of a full bladder, we should scan the lower abdomen of the fetus to find the lower umbilicus and inferior abdominal wall defects (Fig. 2.106).

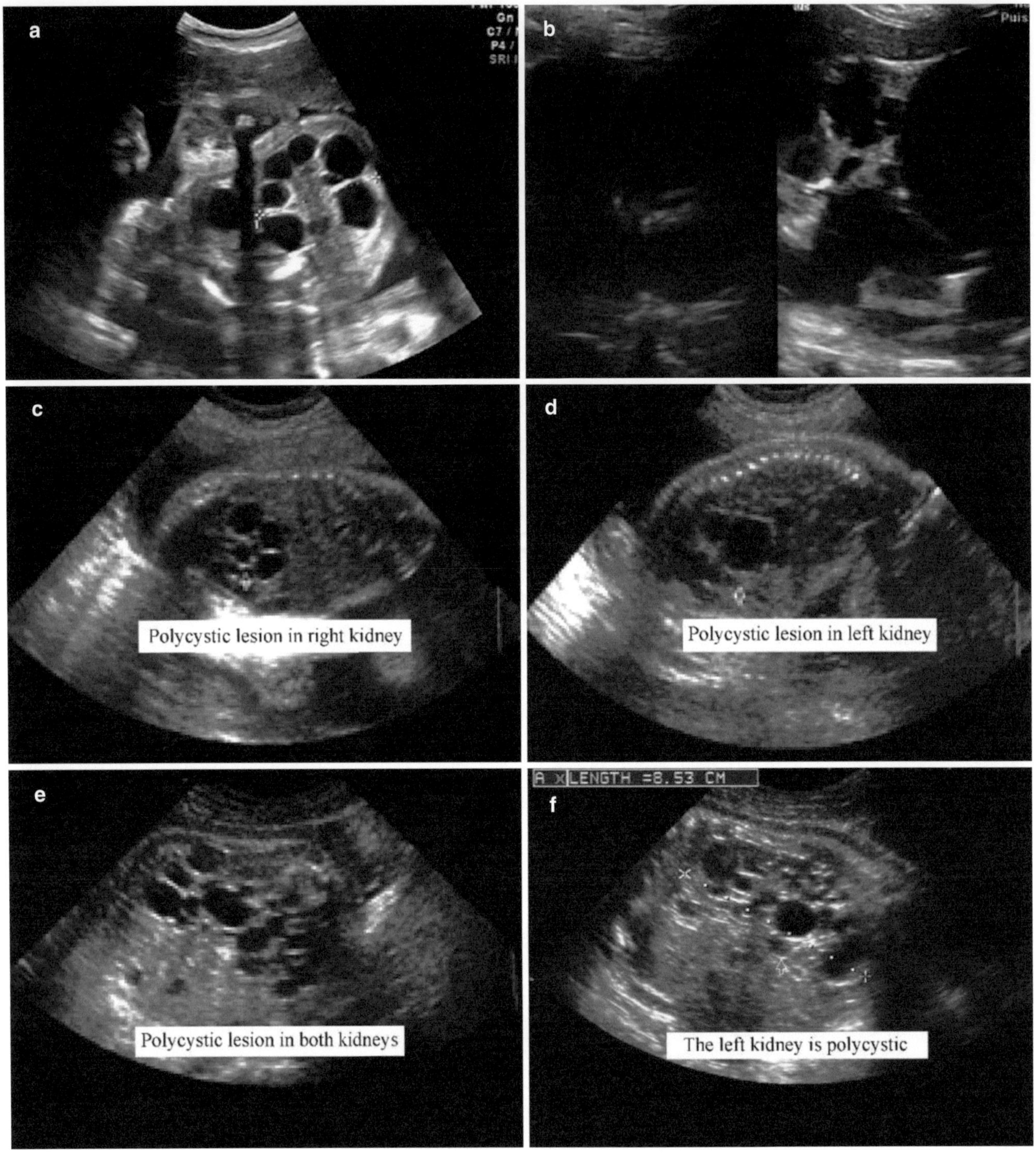

Fig. 2.99 Adult polycystic kidney. (**a**). Unilateral solitary renal cyst; (**b**). Single cyst in bilateral kidney; (**c**). Polycystic lesion in right v; (**d**). Polycystic lesion in left kidney; (**e, f**). For the same fetus, bilateral renal volume increased with abnormal shape, and several cysts in the kidneys

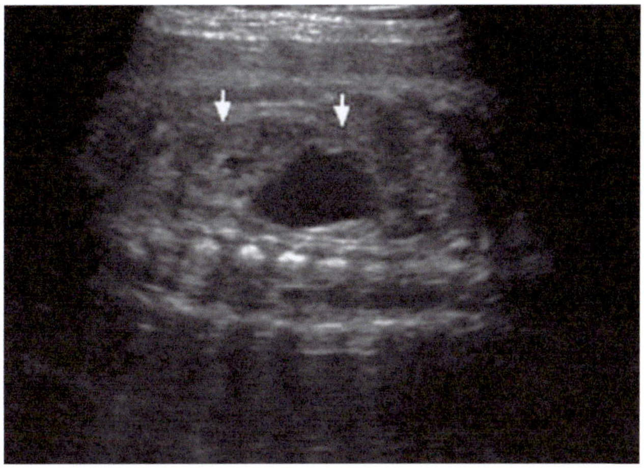

Fig. 2.100 Duplex kidney. There are two renal pelvises in left fetal kidney, and the upper one is dilated

(c) Renal tumors: A heterogeneous solid mass in renal region with an irregular shape. Hamartoma is the most common (Fig. 2.107).

(d) Congenital bladder diverticulum: The bladder shows "double capsule" sign and the filling degree and morphology of the "double capsule" may change during dynamic surveillance.

2.5.4.3 Special Tips

1. It is conducive to display the kidney in occiput anterior position and sacroanterior position. If unilateral or bilateral renal absence is suspected, scan the pelvic and abdominal cavity for a possible ectopic kidney. Renal cysts should be distinguished from abdominal mass and intestinal dilatation.

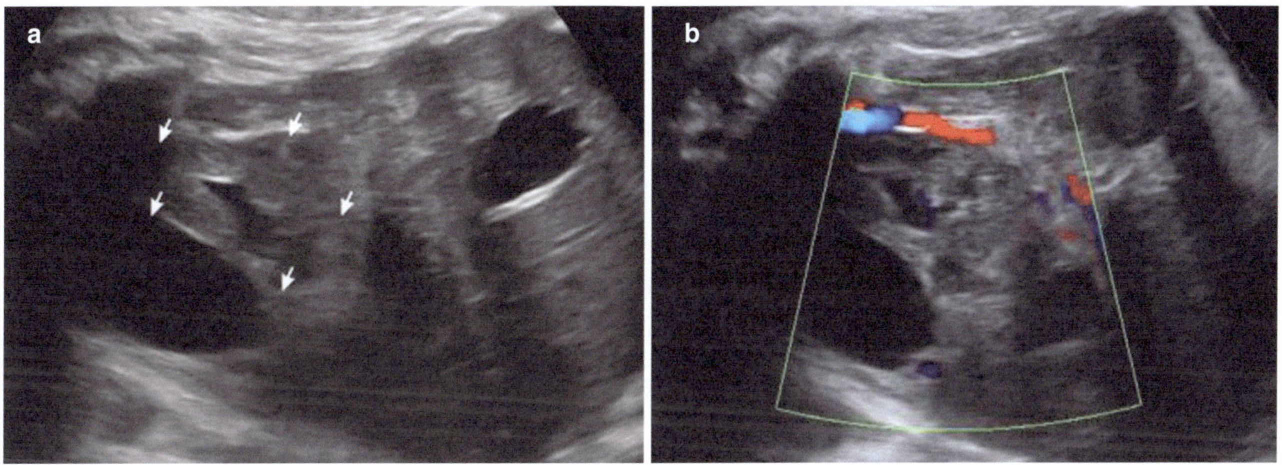

Fig. 2.101 Pelvic ectopic kidney. (**a, b**). No renal is found in the left renal region of the fetus. Renal-like echo is detected in the left side of the pelvic cavity

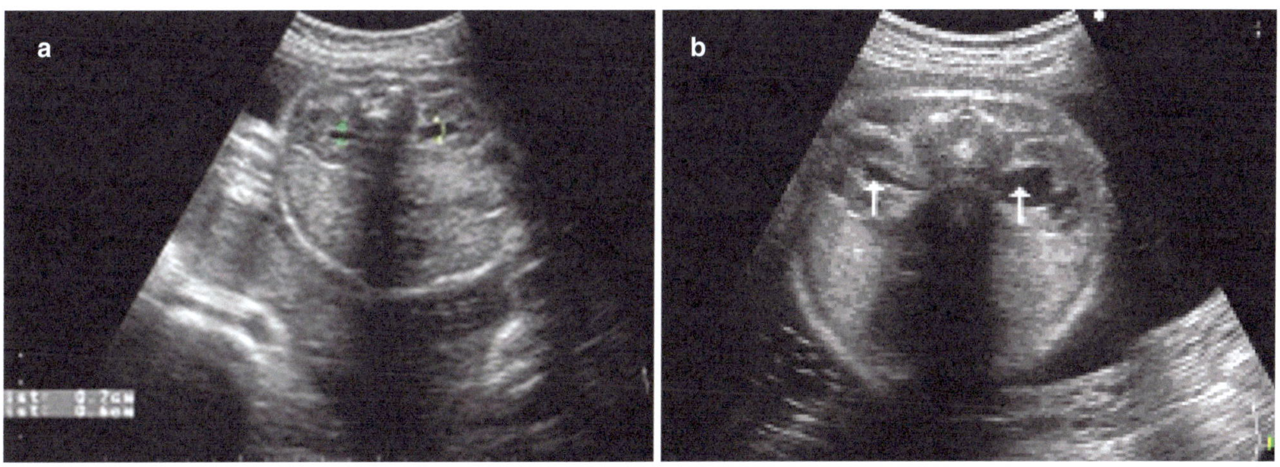

Fig. 2.102 Fetal hydronephrosis I. (**a**). At 34+ weeks of gestation, fetal bilateral renal pelvis is separated about 0.6–0.7 cm, and the anechoic area of renal pelvis separation disappears after birth. (**b**). At 34+ weeks of gestation, left fetal renal pelvis is separated about 1.7 cm, and the separation disappears after birth

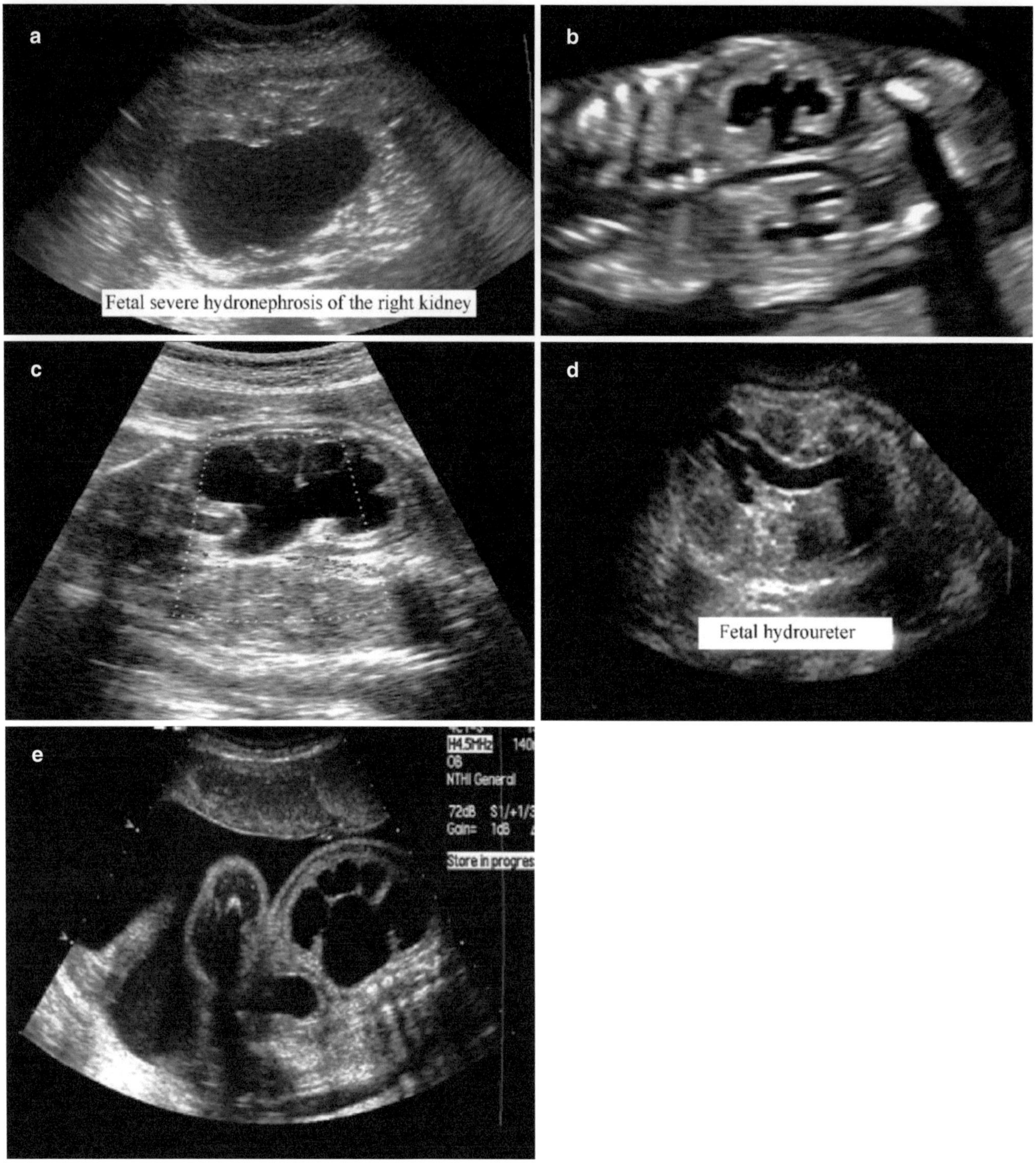

Fig. 2.103 Fetal hydronephrosis II. (**a**). At 22+ weeks gestation, there is a huge effusion in renal pelvis. (**b**). The renal pelvis and calyces are obviously dilated in the form of a "color palette". (**c, d**). The renal pelvis is obviously dilated with ureteral dilatation, and the ureter appears as strip-shaped anechoic. (**e**). The renal pelvis is dilated and the renal cortex is thinner

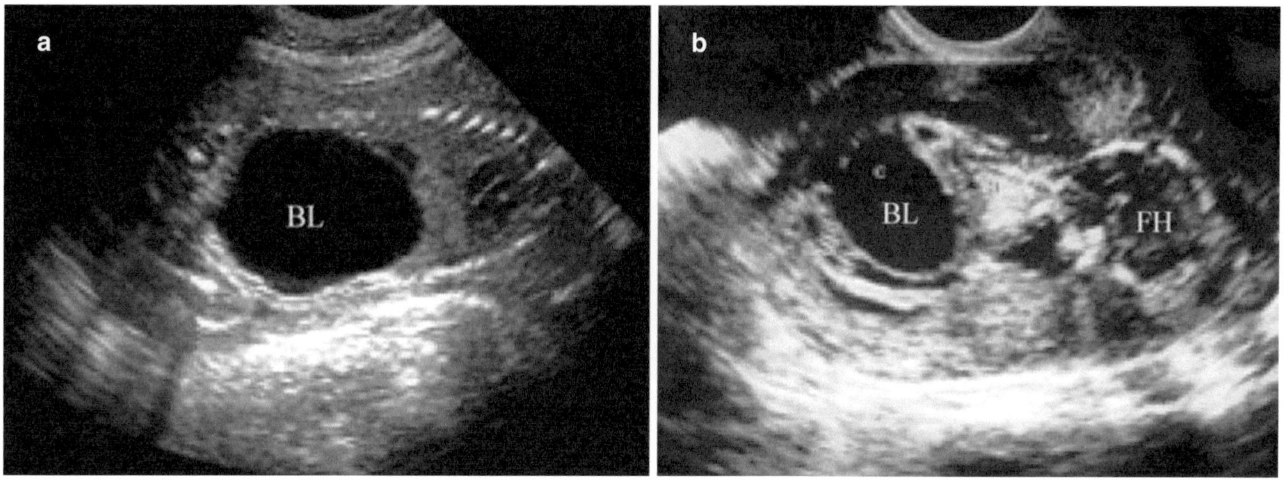

Fig. 2.104 Megabladder. (**a, b**). The diameter of the fetal bladder is greater than 5 cm, without significant reduction half an hour later

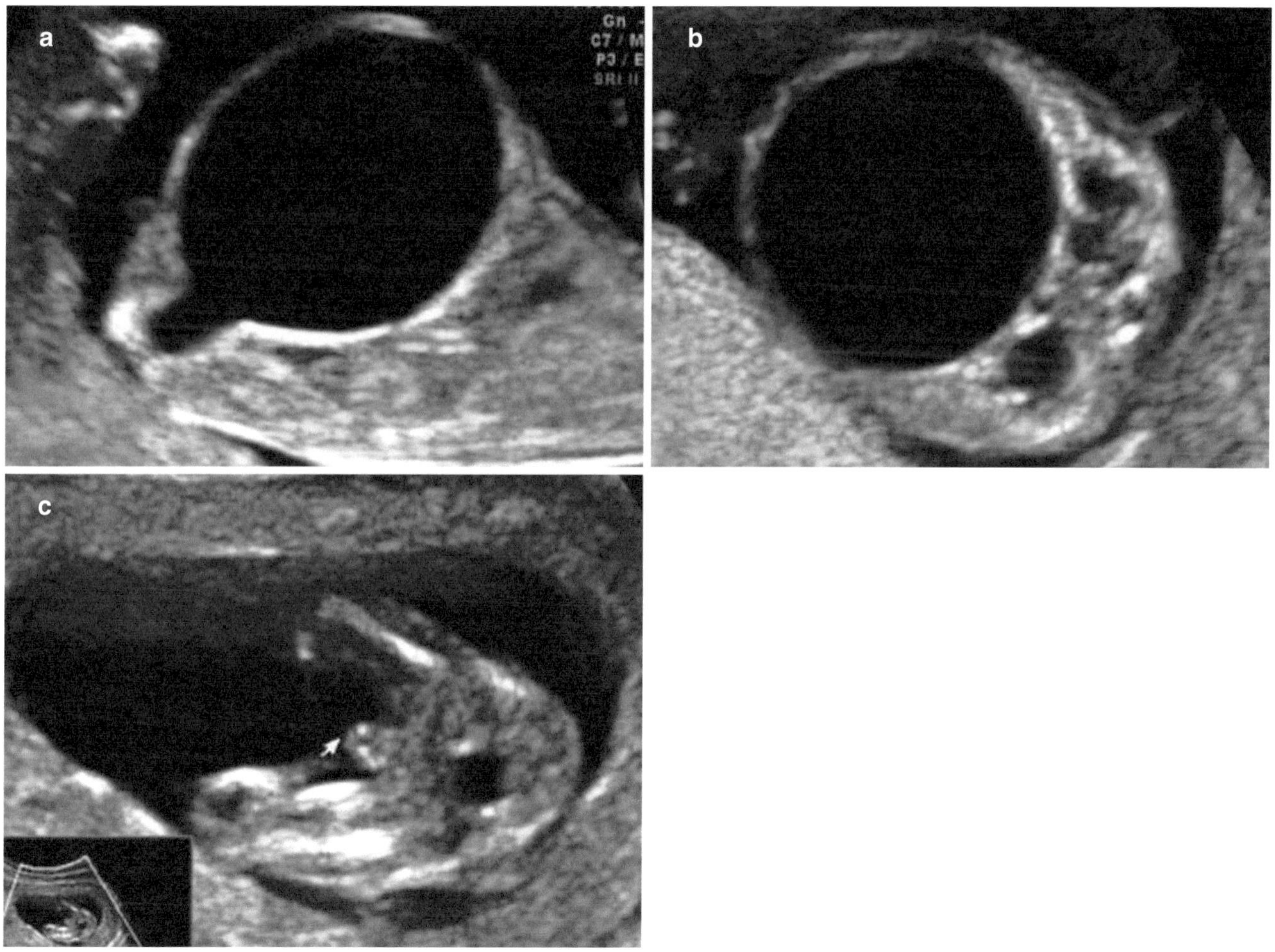

Fig. 2.105 Posterior urethral valve. (**a**). The posterior urethra is obviously dilated, like a "keyhole" that communicates with the bladder. (**b**). The bladder is obviously enlarged with bilateral hydronephrosis. (**c**). Image shows male genitalia

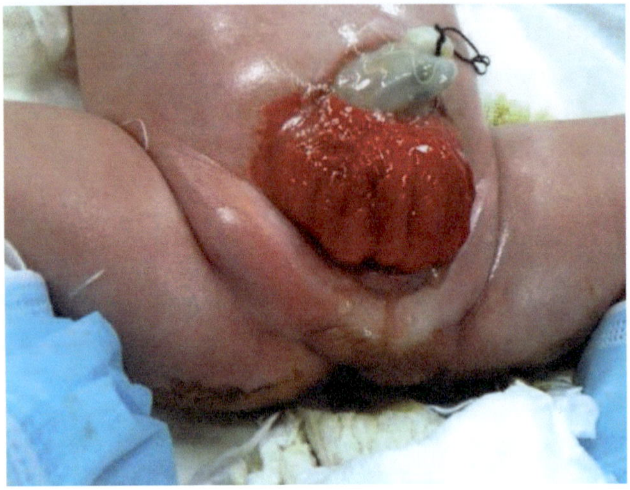

Fig. 2.106 The postnatal image shows exstrophy of bladder

2. Focus on scanning the fetal urinary system in oligohydramnios cases. However, oligohydramnios is not the only sign of urinary system malformation.
3. The majority of urinary system malformations are nonfatal and can be corrected by surgery after birth. Ultrasound diagnosis should be cautious and serial prenatal ultrasound surveillance and long-term postpartum follow-up are essential. Some malformations are of high occurrence rate or a positive family history. Detailed clinical history and family history are important.

2.5.5 Fetal Skeletal and Limb Abnormalities

2.5.5.1 Basic Concepts

By the end of the fourth week after fertilization, the skeleton and skeletal muscles develop in the embryonic meso-

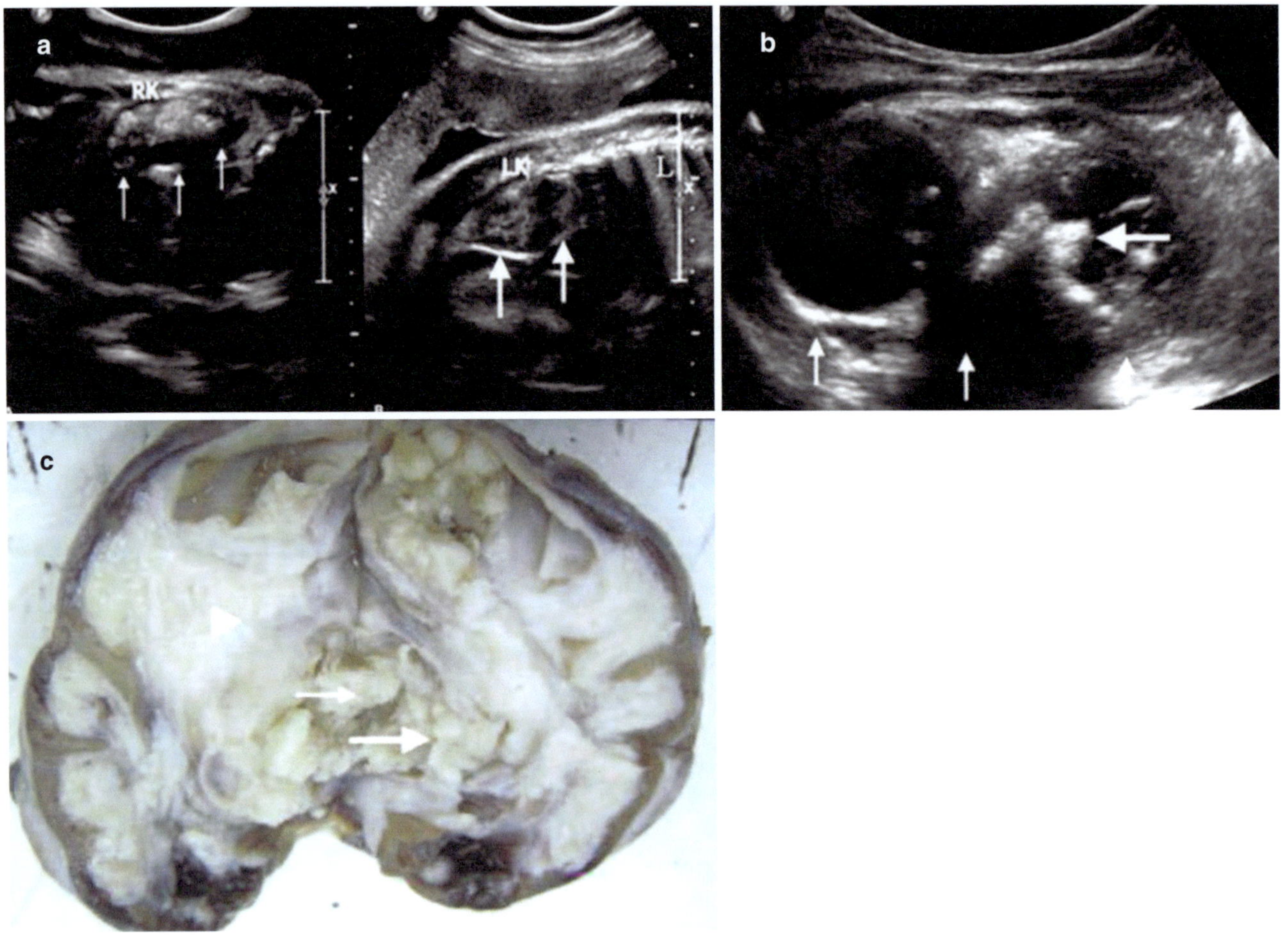

Fig. 2.107 Right renal teratoma. (a–c). The images are prenatal sonogram, postpartum sonogram, and postoperative pathological image

derm and the following somites. Each somite is divided into myotome, sclerotome, and dermatome, and then differentiated into cartilage. By the end of the eighth week, the limbs of the fetus are basically formed, and the bones of the fetus are not ossified yet. They are all cartilages. In this process, the fetal limbs are easy to damage, resulting in limb malformation.

After the fetal cartilage reaches a specific volume, the central part of the cartilage forms the primary ossification center. This center grows in both directions of the forming bone. The ossification center of epiphyseal cartilage is the secondary ossification center, which appears gradually after birth. Malformations in the ossification process of cartilage in embryo, and the osteogenesis of bone hypoplasia can lead to the abnormal development of fetal bones and limbs. It is mostly related to autosomal dominant or recessive inheritance.

There are many kinds of fetal skeletal system malformations, involving a wide range, including skull, spine, limbs, hands, and feet.

Fetal skeletal ossification echoes appear earlier than other organs on ultrasound images. Therefore, most skeletal system malformations can be detected early by prenatal ultrasound through the observation of the characteristics of ossification, morphology, and the echo of fetal bones in various parts, and through the measurement of the length of long bones, which should combine with the intrauterine posture and movement of the fetus.

2.5.5.2 Ultrasonic Diagnosis

Osteogenesis Imperfecta

1. Fetal limb skeletons are short, and the long bone is short and thick. It can fracture into an angle and bending.
2. Multiple fractures can be seen in the ribs, leading to the deformed chest.
3. The fetal skull bone is thin, and the echo is lower than the normal one. The skull ring deforms when the head is slightly pressurized by the probe (Figs. 2.108, 2.109, and 2.110).
4. It may be accompanied by polyhydramnios.

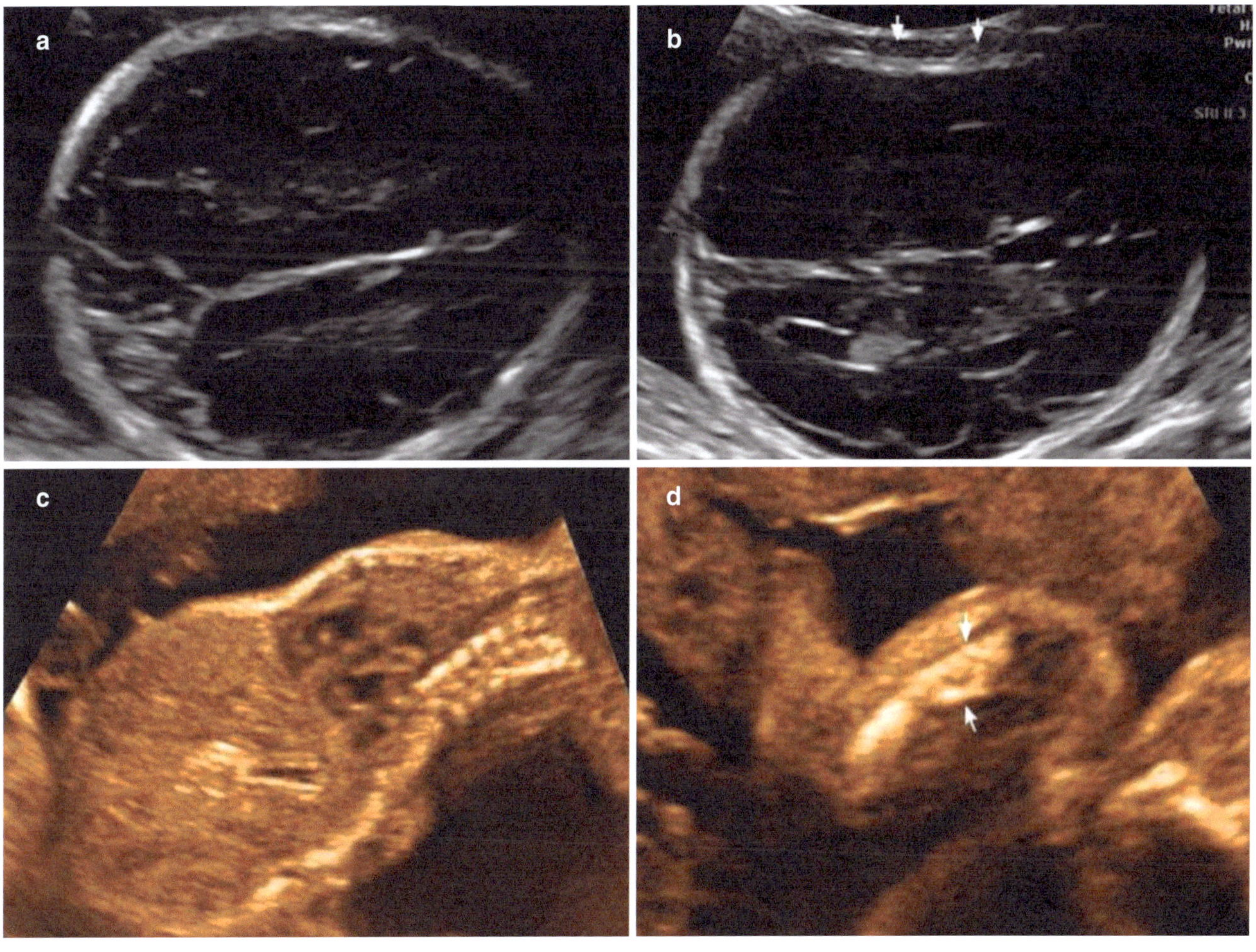

Fig. 2.108 Osteogenesis imperfecta I. (**a, b**). Images show poor cranial calcification. The skull echo is almost equal to the echo of the cerebral midline. The skull ring is deformed by the pressurized probe. (**c**). Narrow chest. (**d**). Enlarged femur which is fractured into an angle

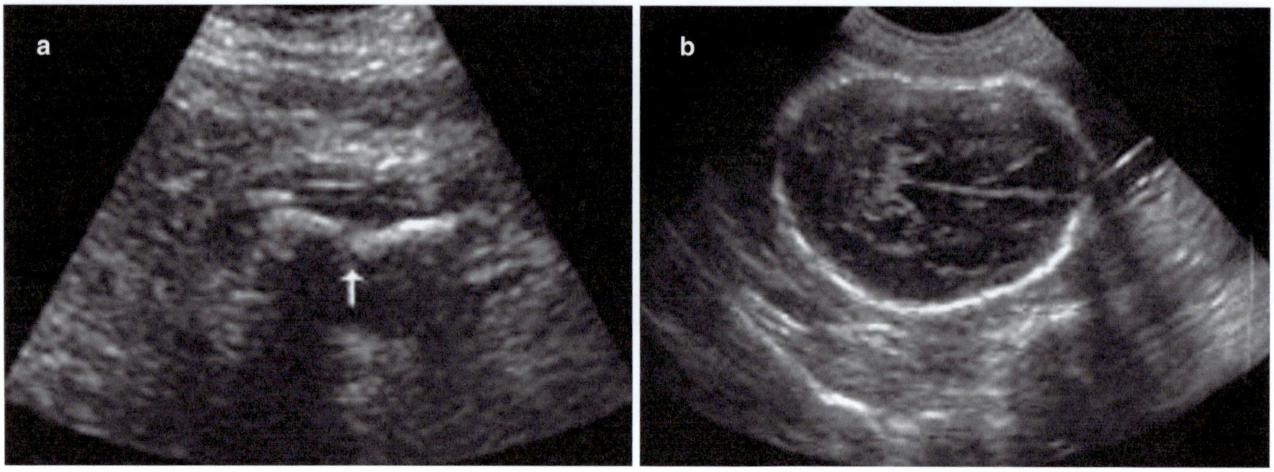

Fig. 2.109 Osteogenesis imperfecta II. (**a**). A pregnant woman's first fetus was diagnosed with osteogenic dysplasia after birth and died 42 days later. At 35 + 3 weeks of gestation in present pregnancy, ultrasound shows callus formation on one femur and fracture on the other. (**b**). In the same fetus, the head echo is weakened, and the head ring is deformed after the probe pressurized

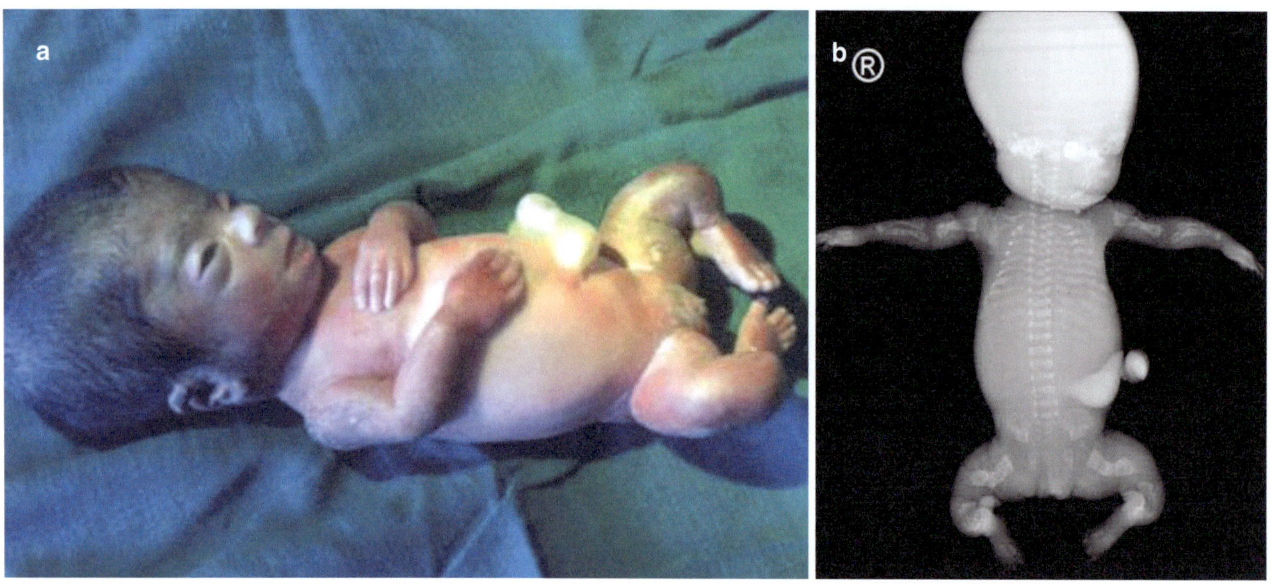

Fig. 2.110 The same fetus as Fig. 2.109. Osteogenesis imperfecta is confirmed after induced labor. (**a**). Image of the fetus after induced labor. (**b**). X-ray of the same fetus

Achondroplasia

1. The size of the fetal BPD is consistent with or more significant than that of the gestational age, and the shape of the head ring is normal. Long limb bones are short and thick with enhanced echo. The acoustic shadow behind the bone is not obvious.
2. Some fetuses can be accompanied by anasarca, serous effusion, and hygroma colli (Figs. 2.111 and 2.112).
3. More than half of them combined hydramnios and other malformations.

Thanatophoric Dysplasia

1. Limbs are very short and shaped like a seal.
2. The skeleton of the limbs is not clear, even unable to distinguish the shape of the fetal hands and feet.
3. Fetal limbs are excessively short, and the soft tissue increased relatively (Figs. 2.113 and 2.114).
4. Thanatophoric dysplasia can combine with hydramnion. Some cases represent decreased fetal movement.

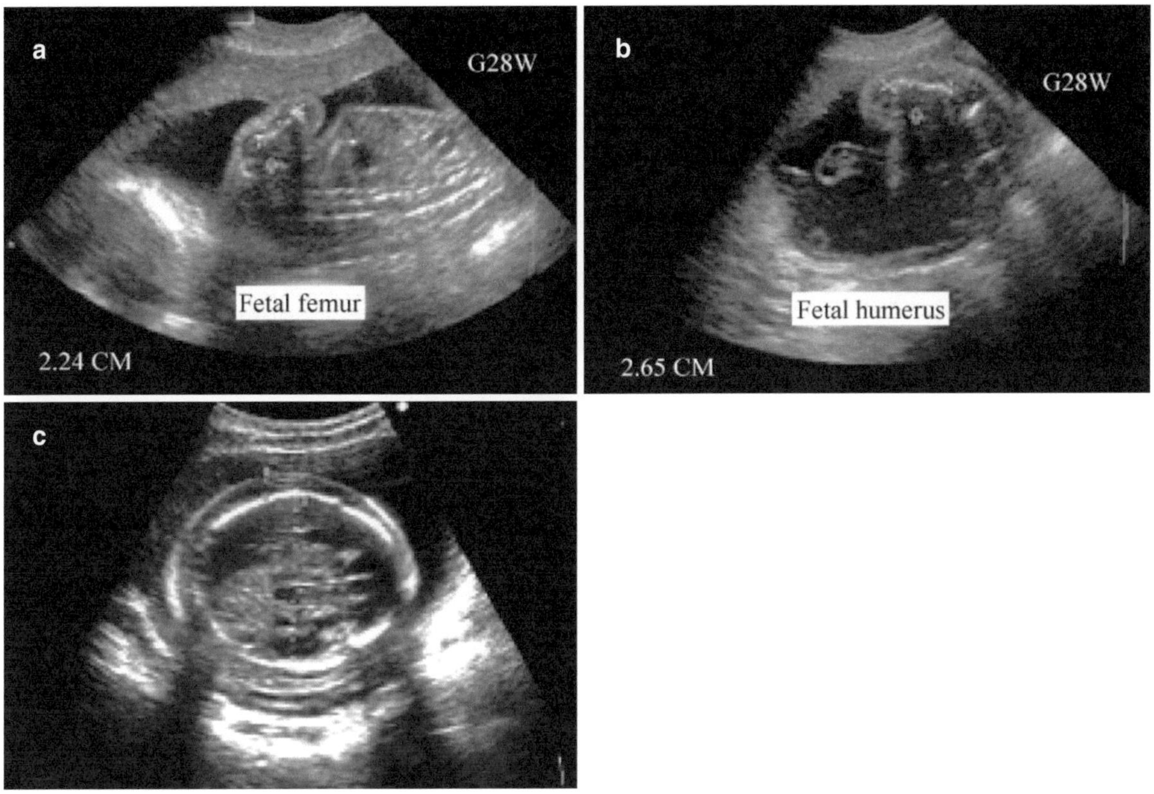

Fig. 2.111 Achondroplasia I. (**a**). At 28 weeks gestation, the length of the fetal femur is 2.24 cm. (**b**). The length of the fetal femur at the same gestational week is 2.65 cm. (**c**). The same fetus with head and body edema

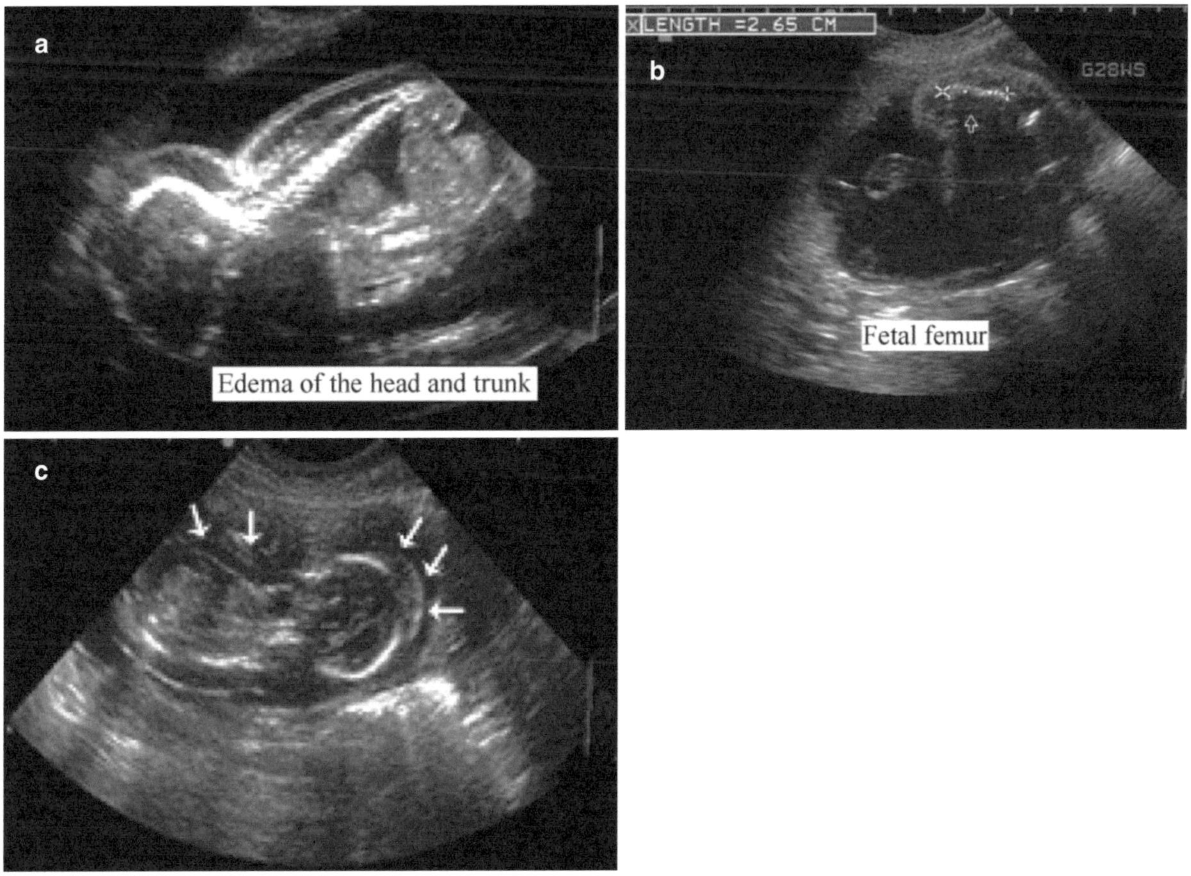

Fig. 2.112 Achondroplasia II. (**a**). Edema from fetal scalp to the whole body. (**b**). Short limb bone. (**c**). Fetal body edema, like "cocoon"

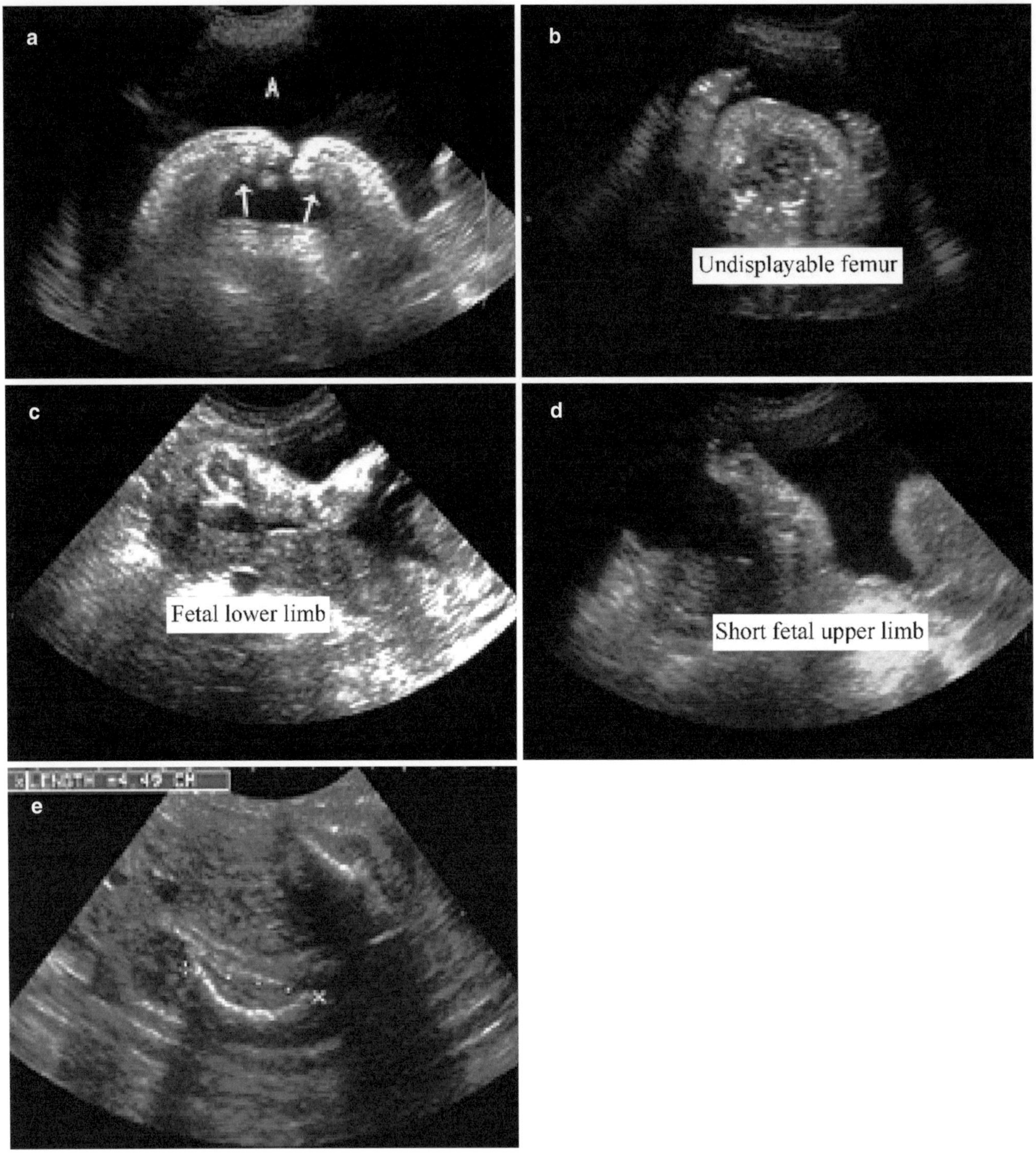

Fig. 2.113 Thanatophoric dysplasia I. (**a, b**). Images show the extremely short fetal limbs with narrow chest. (**c, d**). Pictures without obvious limbs echo but mainly with soft tissue echo. The echo is dominated by soft tissue. e. Long bones are short and curved like a telephone

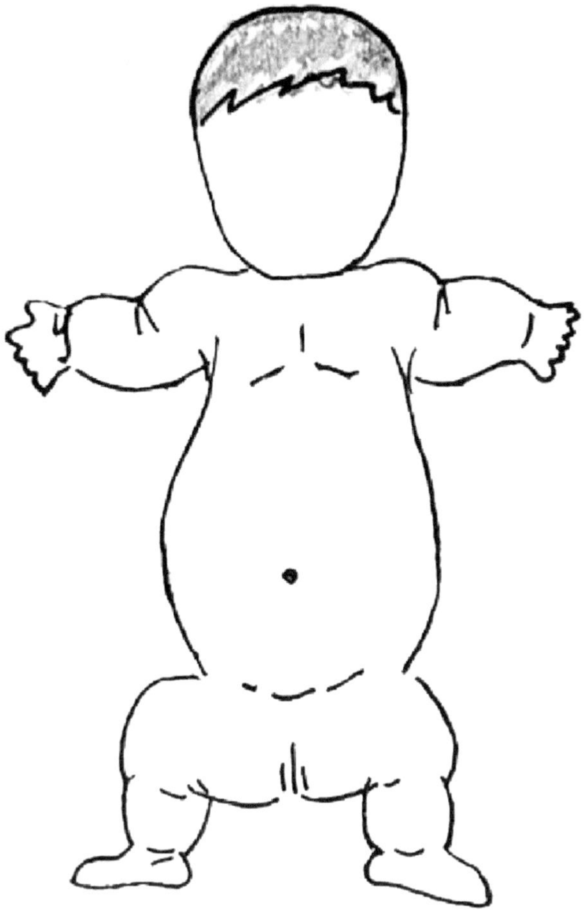

Fig. 2.114 Thanatophoric dysplasia II

Partial Deformity of Fetal Limbs, Hands, and Feet

1. Absent forearm bone: Only one bone is visible in the longitudinal and transverse sections. The normal distal ulna and radius are on the same level. The distal radius is shorter than the ulna when it is hypoplastic or absent. The ulna can be identified according to the relationship between the hand and the hypothenar muscle (Figs. 2.115 and 2.116).
2. Congenital hand malformation.

The absent or hypoplasia ulna and radius can cause hand malformation and dysfunction. Common hand malformations include hands agenesis, ectrodactyly, polydactyly, syndactyl, and split hands. The display of fetal hand and finger are affected by the amniotic fluid, fetal position, and fetal movement. The club hand is characterized by the display of the angular metacarpal bones in the section of the ulna and radius. The diagnosis should be confirmed after the fetal movement or the change of position (Figs. 2.117 and 2.118).

3. Congenital malformation of the foot: Congenital talipes equinovarus is a common deformity in malformations of the fetal foot. Typically, the calves and the vola cannot be shown in the same view. If the tibia, fibula, and vola are found simultaneously in the same section, congenital talipes equinovarus should be considered (Fig. 2.119).

Fetal Limb Tumors

1. Limb tumors are rare. Ultrasound images show the swelling, thickening, and hypoechoic limb with tumor lesion.
2. The benign and malignant nature of the tumor can be preliminarily judged according to the richness of blood supply in the tumor. However, ultrasound could not confirm the pathological result (Fig. 2.120).

2.5.5.3 Special Tips

1. The best time to detect fetal skeletal dysplasia is 16–26 weeks of gestation. The bone structure is easy to show at this time. Most abnormalities can be detected by prenatal ultrasound examination.
2. The ultrasonic measurement and observation of the bone are reliable clues to find the fetal bone malformation. Fetal bones should be thoroughly examined.
3. Ultrasound examination of fetal limbs should be continuously traced from the proximal end of the limb to its distal end, combining the longitudinal section and the transverse section.
4. Affected by amniotic fluid, fetal movement, and fetal position, it is challenging to show fetal hands, feet, and the number, shape, and structure of fingers and toes. Sonographers should observe for enough time for every fetus and be patient and careful.

2.5.6 Complex Twin Pregnancy

2.5.6.1 Basic Concept

The incidence of miscarriage and malformation in twin pregnancy is high. The common abnormalities are one of the twins' malformations, death or disappearance; twins intrauterine growth retardation; conjoined twins; twin–twin transfusion syndrome, etc. All kinds of malformations that can occur in a single pregnancy can occur in a twin pregnancy.

The rate of congenital malformations is higher in multiple pregnancies than in a single pregnancy. There is a higher rate of malformation of monozygotic twins, represented by conjoined twins.

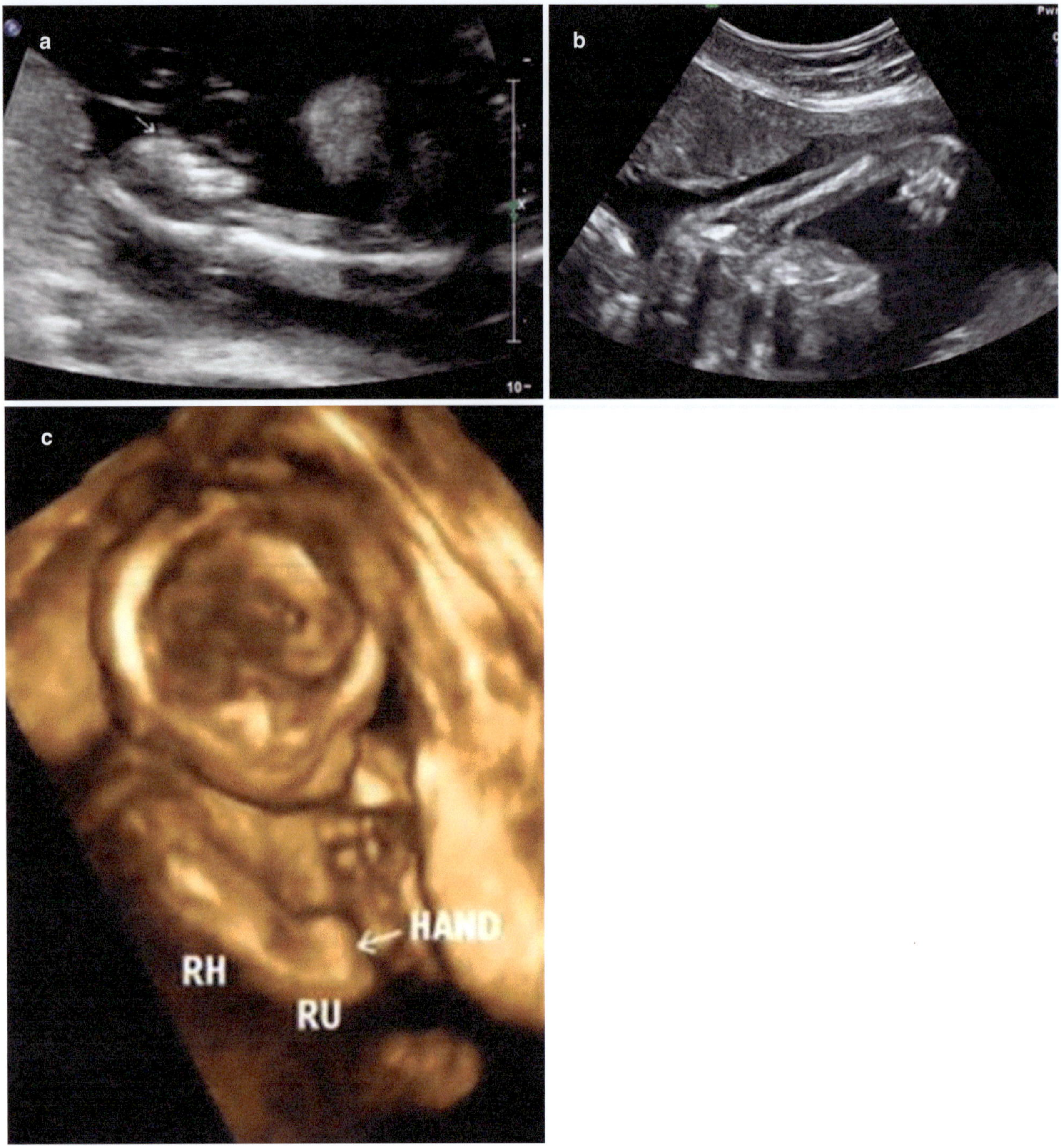

Fig. 2.115 Absent bilateral fetal radius

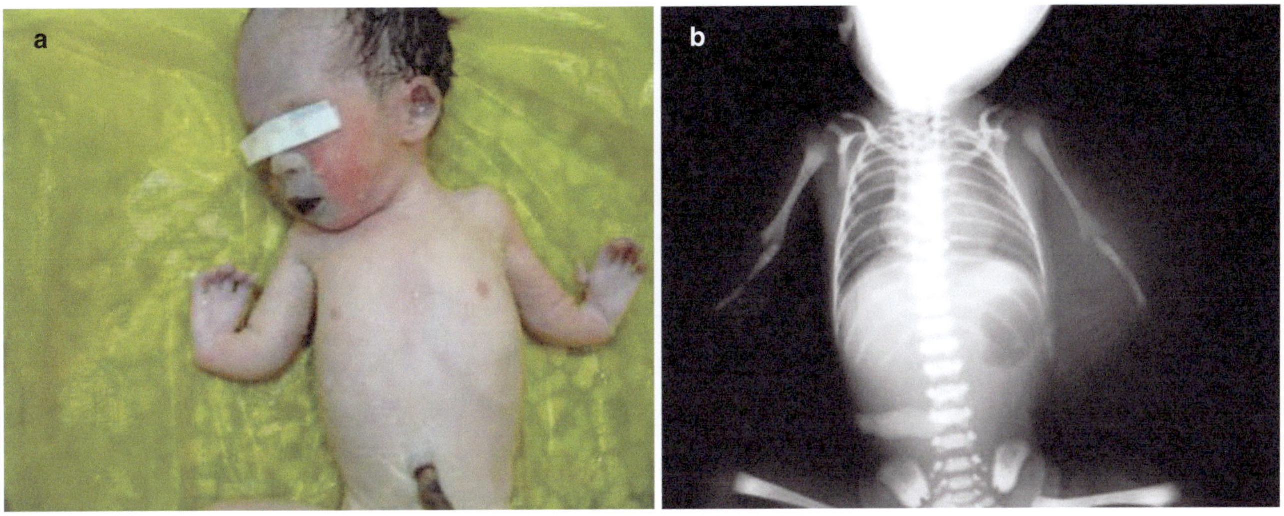

Fig. 2.116 Absent radius in the forearm after induction labor. (**a**). Picture after labor induction (**b**). X-rays of the same induced fetus

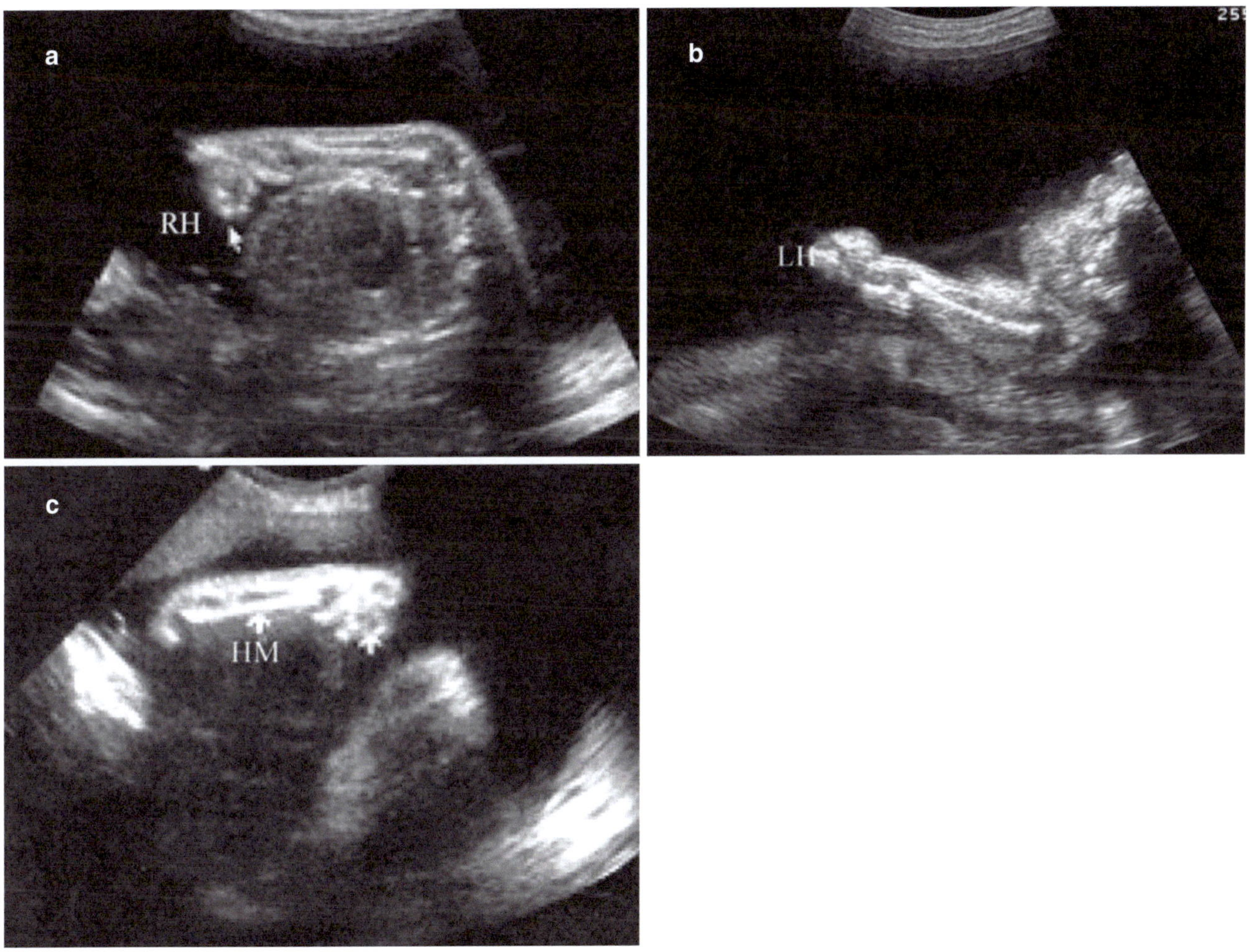

Fig. 2.117 Deformity of fetal limb bone. (**a–c**). Fetal forearm absence with hand deformity

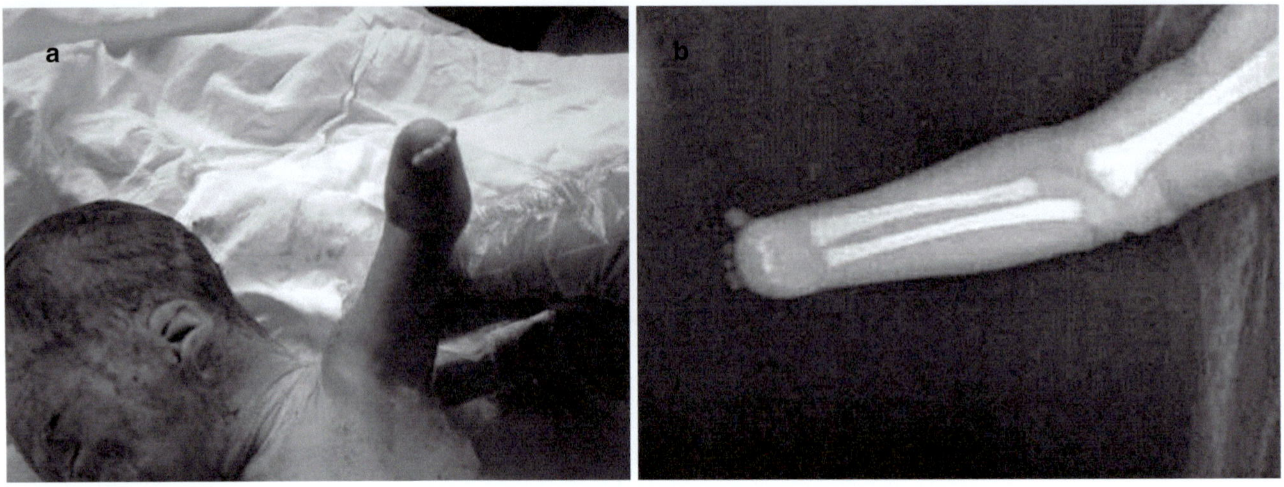

Fig. 2.118 Fetal forearm absence with hand deformity after induction labor. (**a**). Picture after induction labor. (**b**). X-rays of the same induced fetus

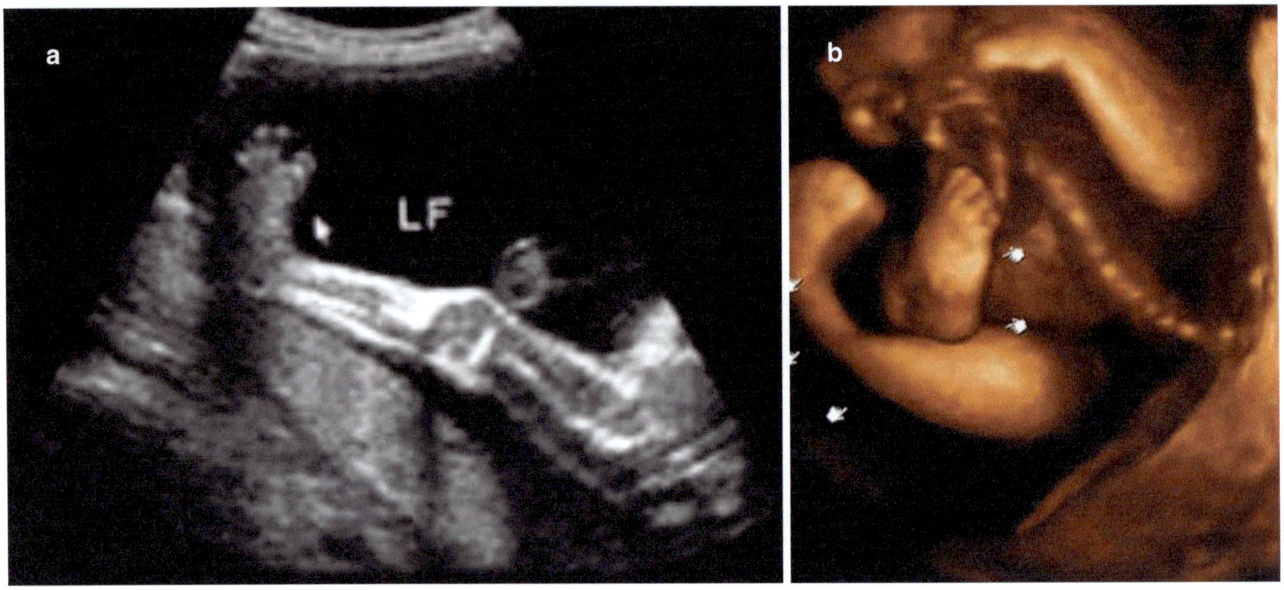

Fig. 2.119 Fetal congenital talipes equinovarus. (**a**, **b**) The calves and the vola are shown in the same section

In recent years, due to various reasons, the number of twin pregnancy increases, and the incidence of deformity is also significantly increased.

2.5.6.2 Ultrasonic Diagnosis

Conjoined Twins

1. Craniopagus twins: One type is a partial connection, that is, the head of one fetus is joined to the other's scalp or bone. The image shows the heads of the two fetuses stick close to each other. The other type is complete craniopagus twins, sharing the brain and facial features (Fig. 2.121).
2. Most cases of thoraco-omphalopagus twins share the hearts and livers, always combined with congenital cardiac abnormalities, kidney abnormalities, and omphalocele (Fig. 2.122).
3. Some parts of the body of two fetuses are connected, which may occur in the upper abdomen, the lower abdomen, even the entire abdomen. The skin of the conjoined area is continuous (Fig. 2.123).
4. The heads of the two fetuses are separated, the two bodies fused, and only a trunk and one set of limbs can be seen (Figs. 2.124 and 2.125).
5. Hydramnios, without septum in the amniotic cavity.

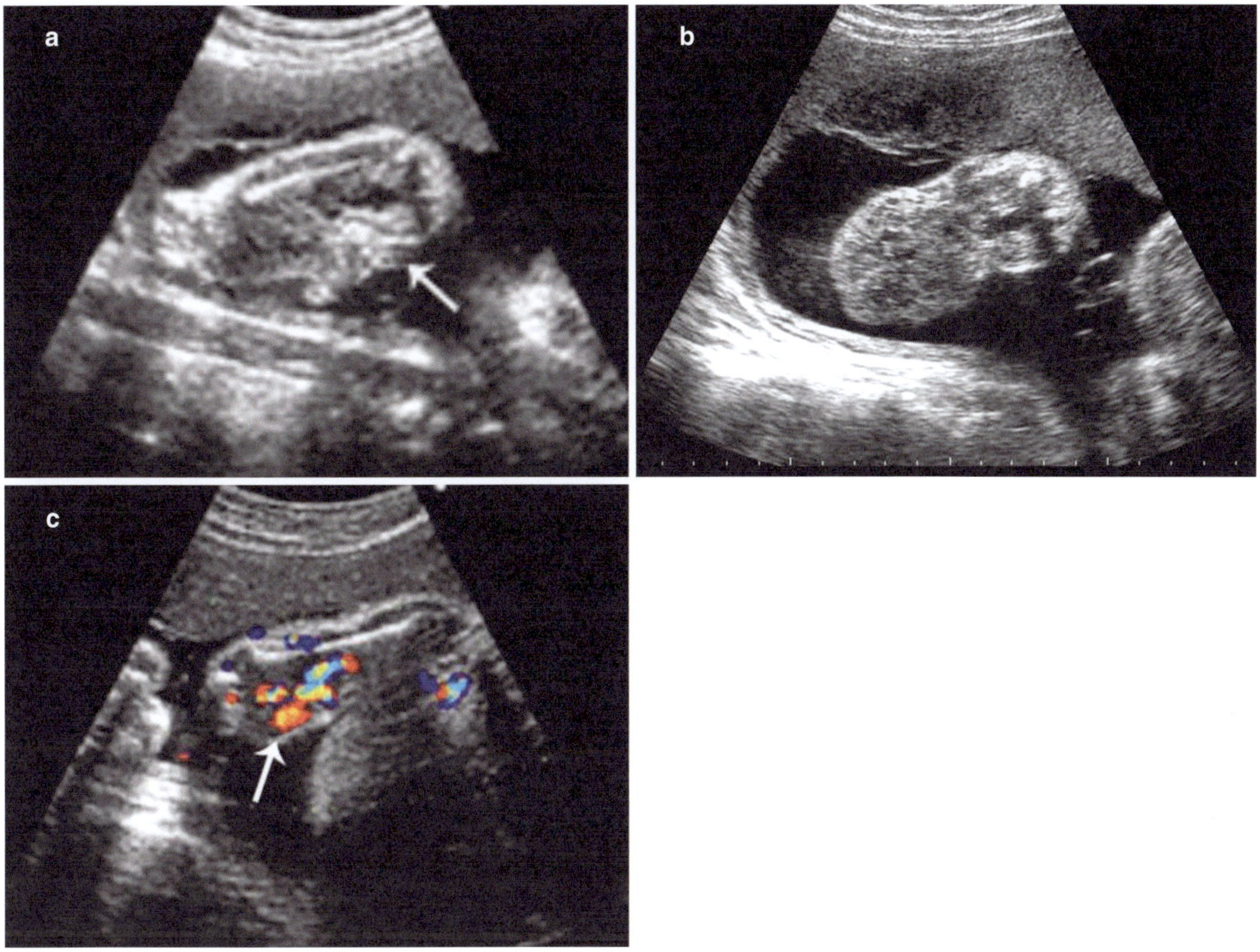

Fig. 2.120 Fetal limb tumor. (**a–c**). At 33+ weeks of gestation, the right upper limb is swollen and thickened with abundant blood flow in the swollen tissue. The humerus is normal. The fetus is diagnosed as rhabdomyosarcoma after labor induction

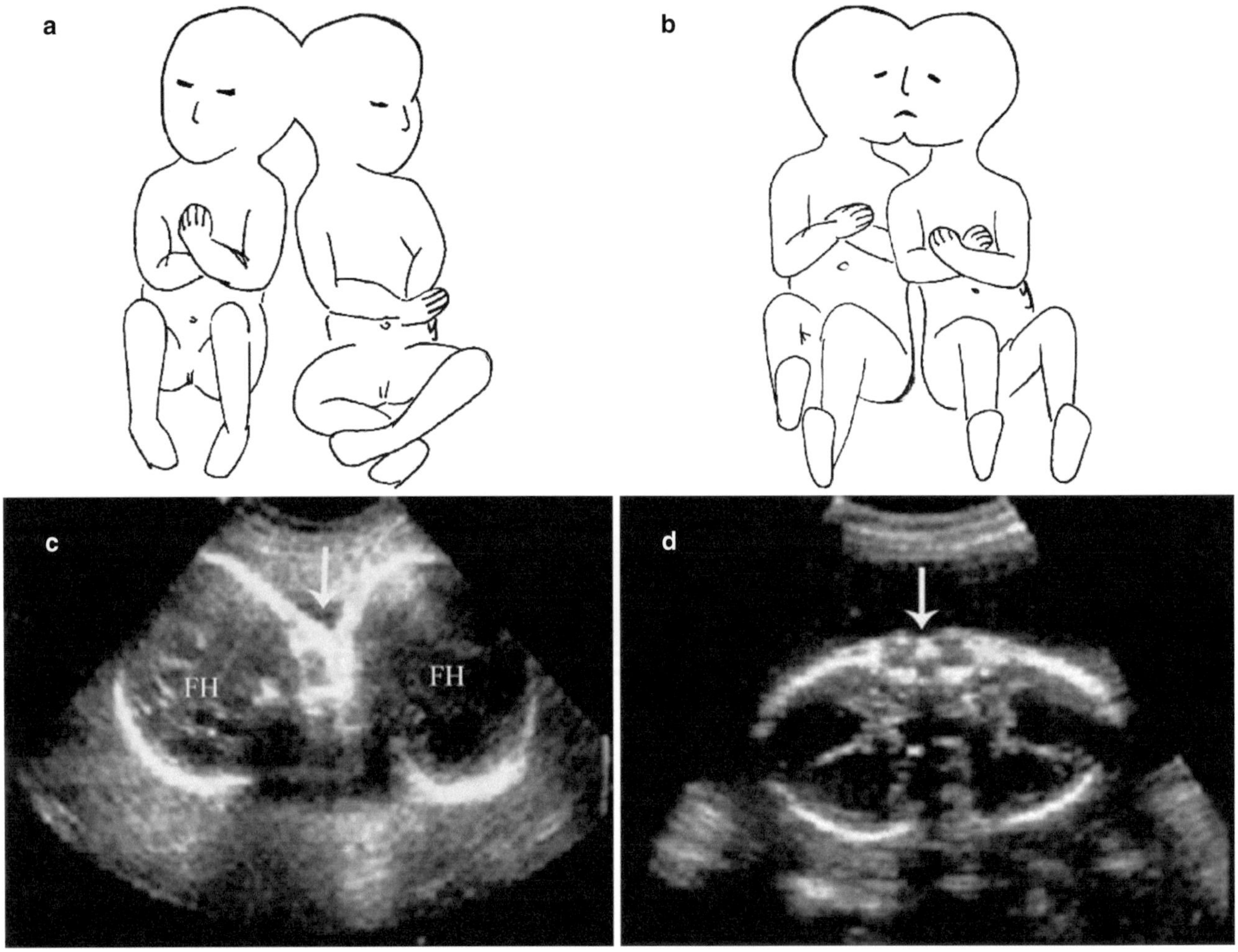

Fig. 2.121 Conjoined twins I. (**a, b**). Diagrams of joined twins. (**c**). The partially joined two skulls. (**d**). The completely joined skull

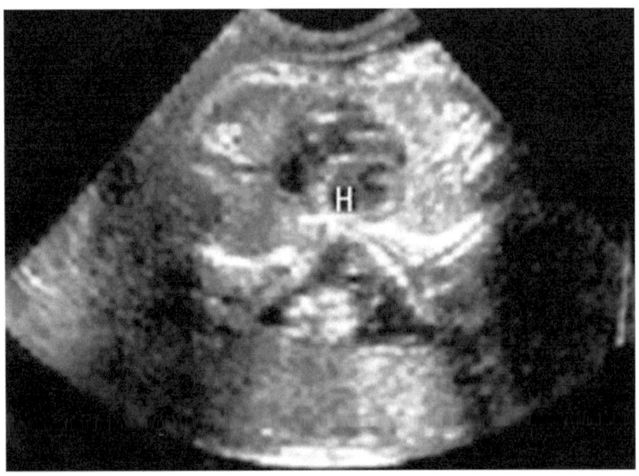

Fig. 2.122 Conjoined twins II. The image shows the twins' thorax is connected and the twin share one heart

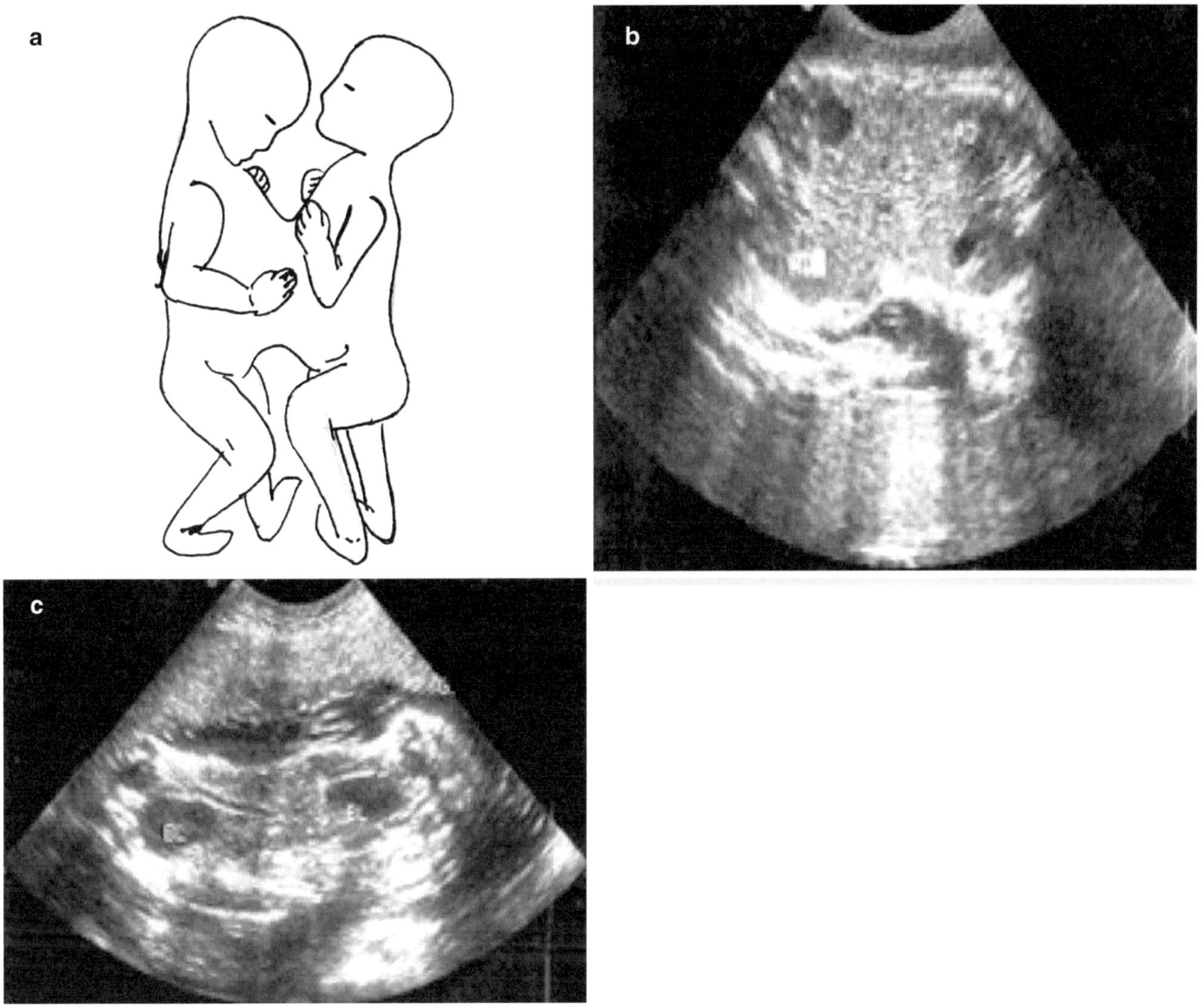

Fig. 2.123 Conjoined twins III. (**a**). Diagrams of conjoined twins. (**b**). The picture shows the twins share a common liver in the upper abdomen and there are two stomach bubbles. (**c**). The image shows the twins are attached to the lower abdomen with two bladders

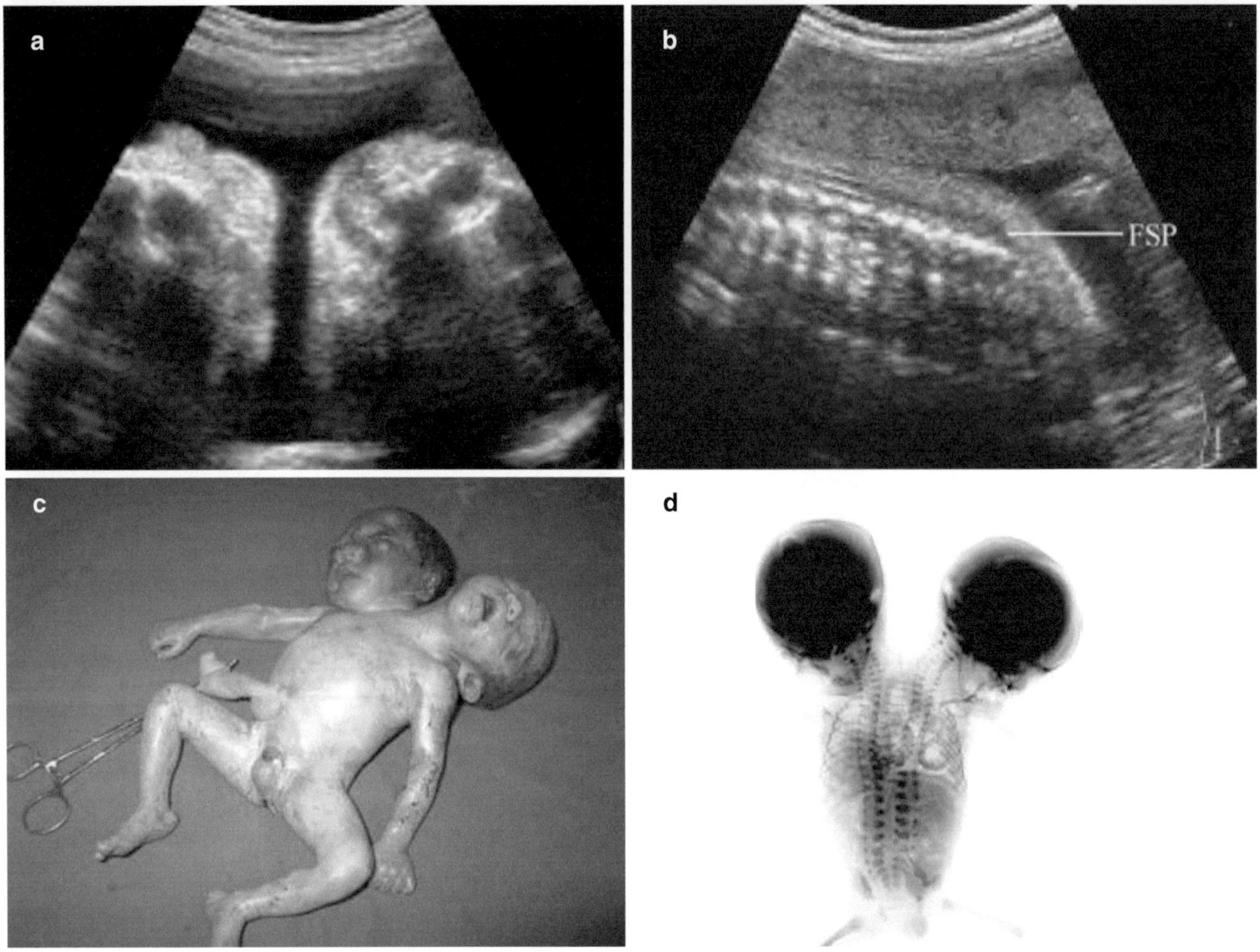

Fig. 2.124 Conjoined twins IV. (**a**). Two separate fetal heads echo; (**b**). Two widened spines echo; (**c**). There are two heads and one body after induction of labor. (**d**). X-ray images of conjoined twins after labor induction

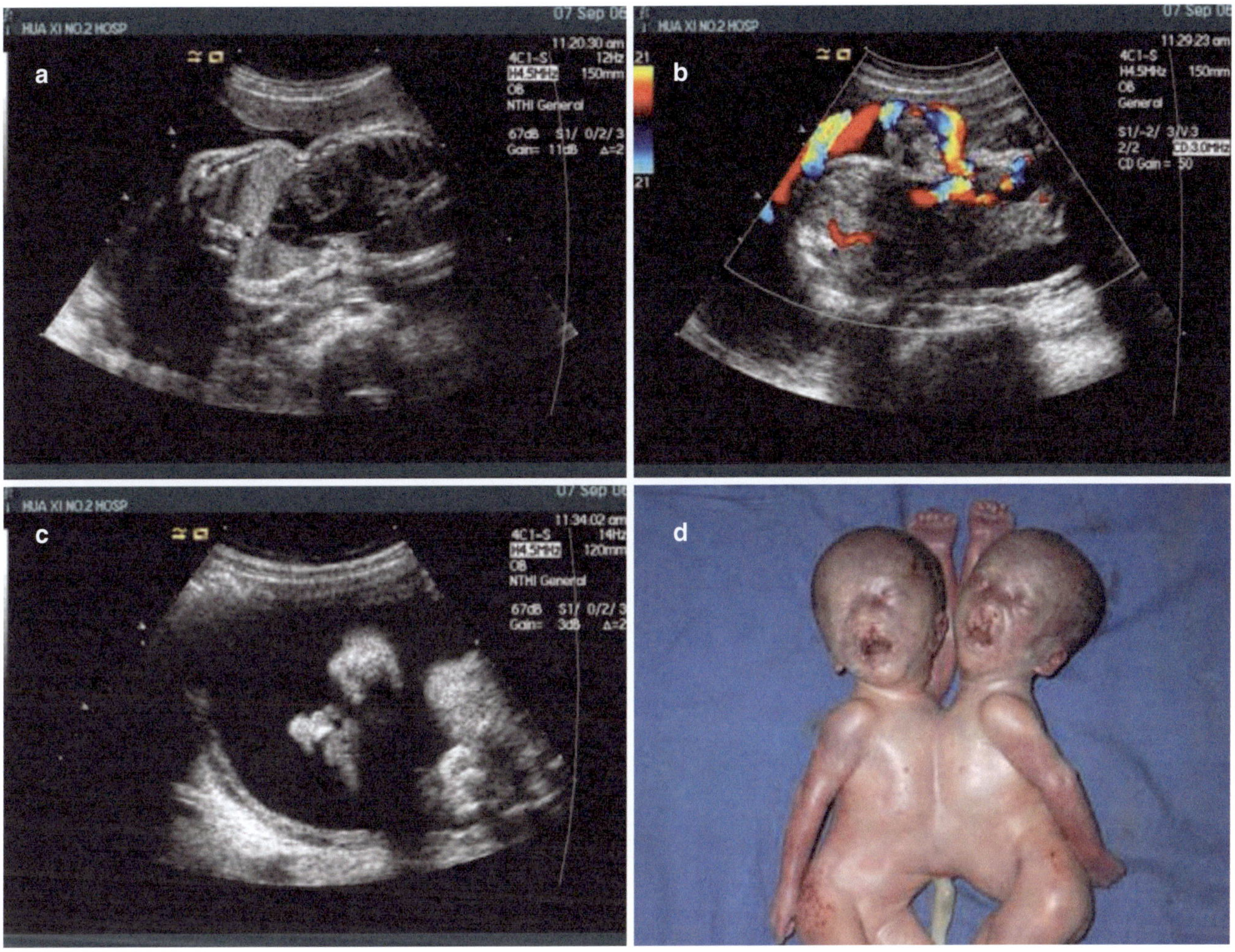

Fig. 2.125 Conjoined twins V. (**a, b**). The images show the twins are connected throughout the abdominal cavity. (**c**). Image shows both twins have cleft lip. (**d**). Picture of conjoined twins after labor induction

6. Asymmetric conjoined twins are called fetus in fetu. Two fetuses are in different sizes. One is developing normally, while the other is undeveloped and connected to the regularly developing fetus. It can also attach to a part of the normal fetal body (Fig. 2.126).

Deformity in One of the Twins

1. Acephalocardius in one of the twins.
   (a) There is one normally developing fetus in the uterus and the other with a severe deformity. The malformed fetus may have no heart and head, and hypoplasia limbs, in the same amniotic cavity as the normal fetus (Fig. 2.127).
   (b) Color Doppler ultrasound shows the umbilical cord is inserted into the malformed fetus, and the other end of the umbilical cord is connected to the placenta.
   (c) Most cases are accompanied by hydramnios.
2. Other deformities in one of the twins.
   (a) Most of the deformities in one of the twins are anencephaly and hydrocephalus, while the other fetus is normal (Fig. 2.128).
   (b) One of the twins died, and the other normal fetus has heart beating and fetal movement (Fig. 2.129).

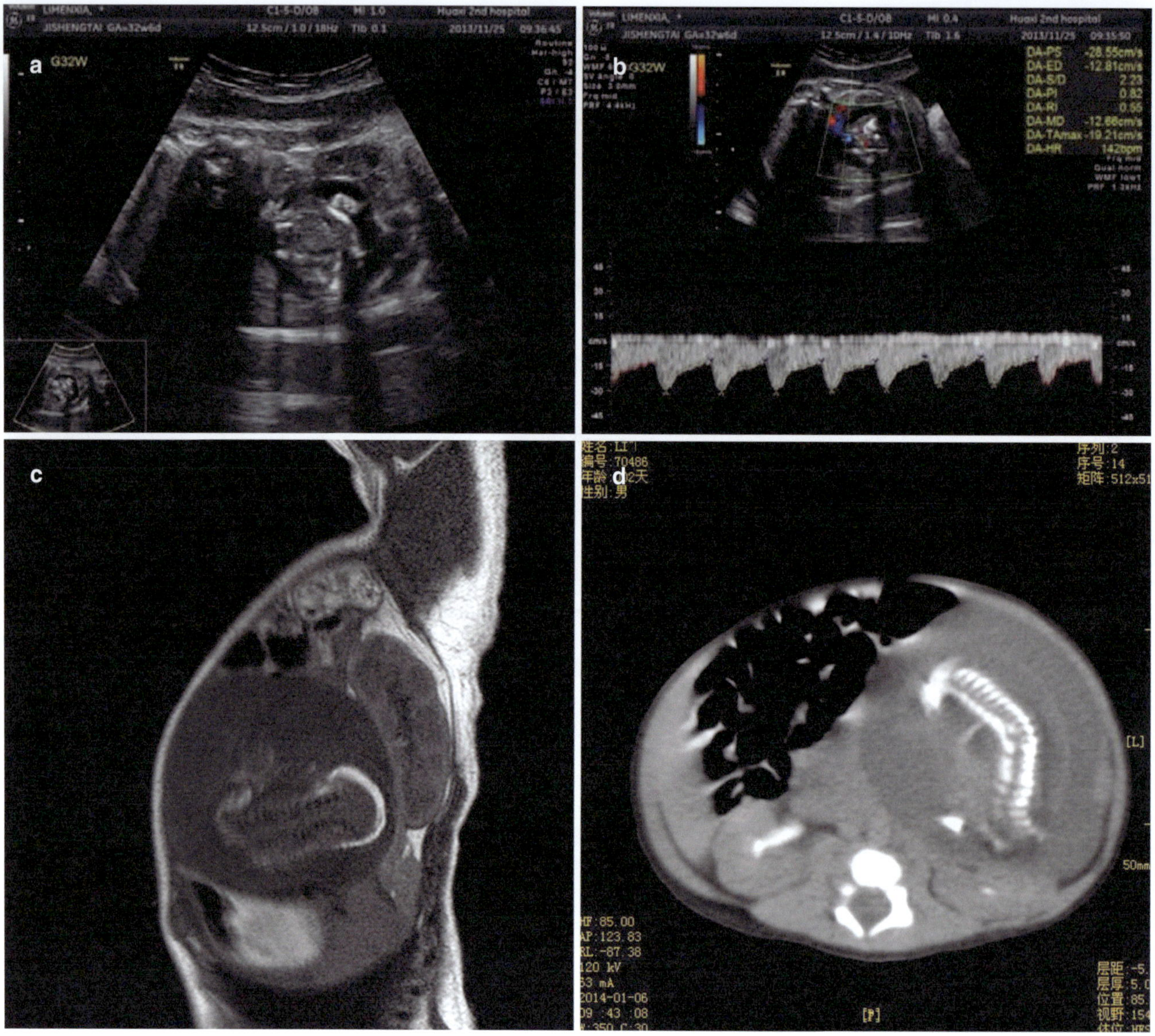

Fig. 2.126 Fetus in fetu. (**a, b**). Prenatal ultrasound images; (**c**). Prenatal MRI image; (**d**). Postpartum CT image

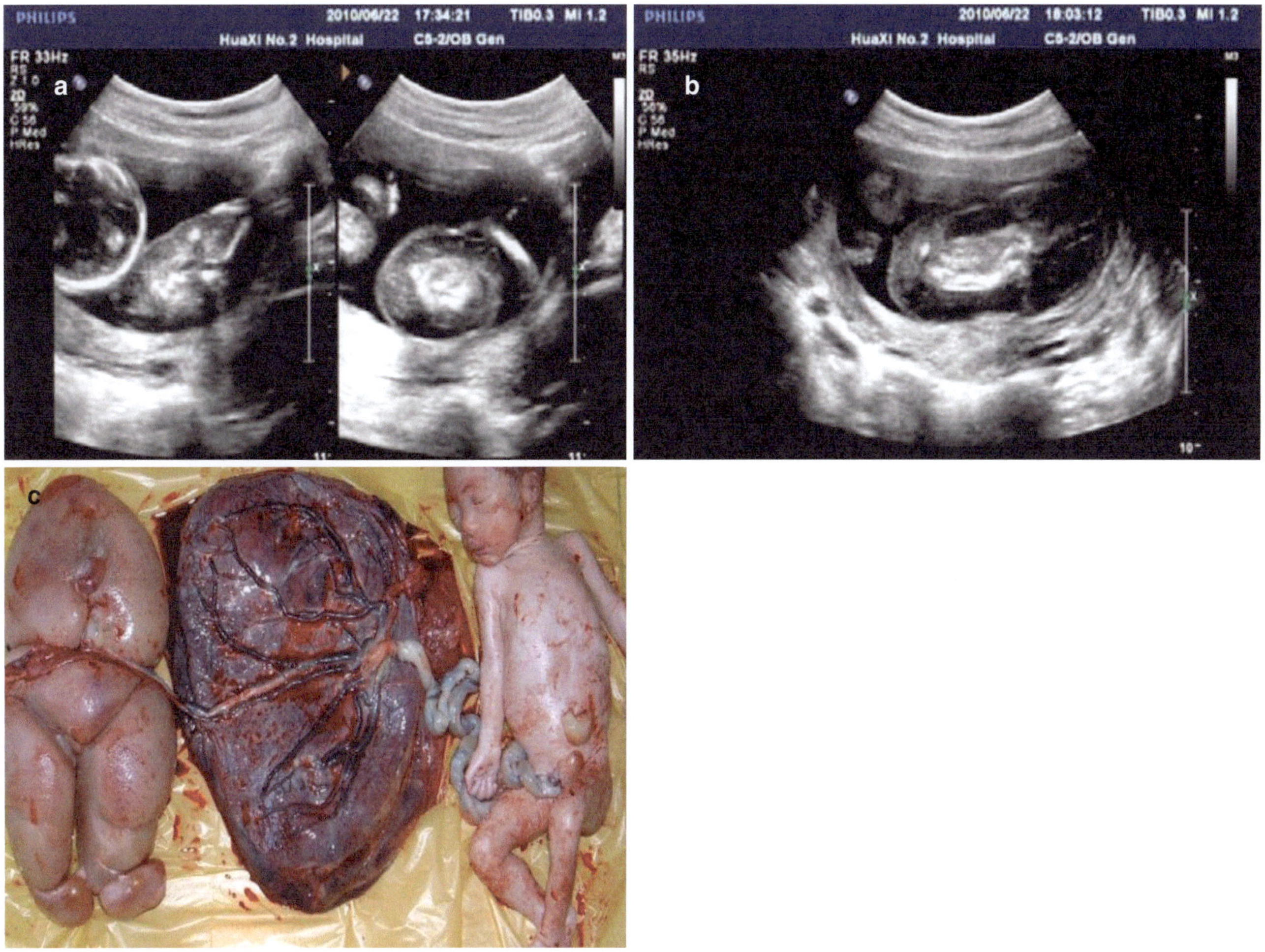

Fig. 2.127 Acephalocardius in one of the twins. (**a, b**). At 25 weeks of gestation, one of the twins is normal. The other fetus was headless and heartless, with the visible spinal column and hypoplastic lower limbs. It has fetal movements. (**c**). Pathology after labor induction confirms the mass is an acephalocardius

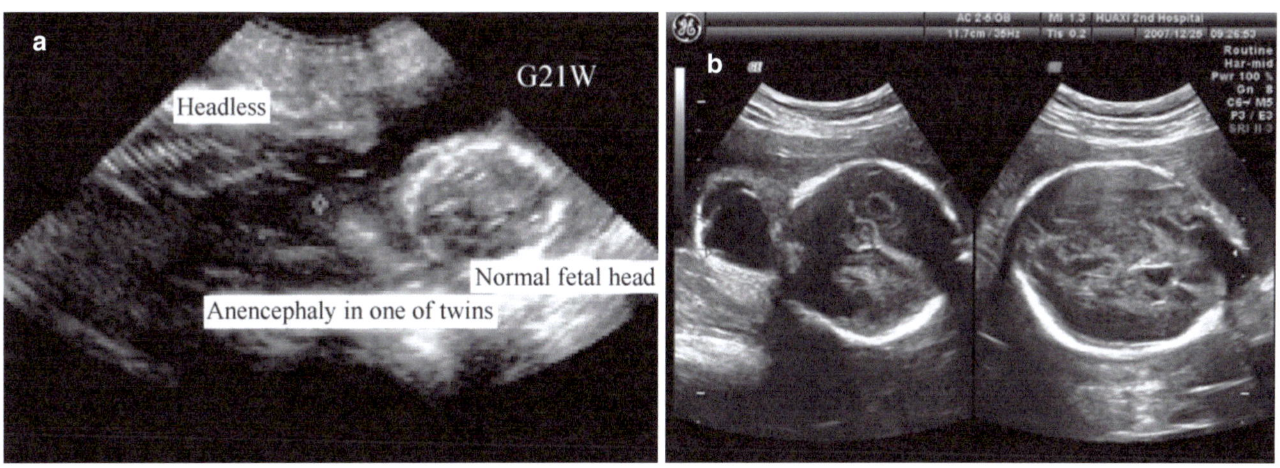

Fig. 2.128 Deformities in one of the twins. (**a**). At 21 weeks gestation, one of the twins is anencephaly. (**b**). At 30 weeks gestation, one of the twins is meningoceles

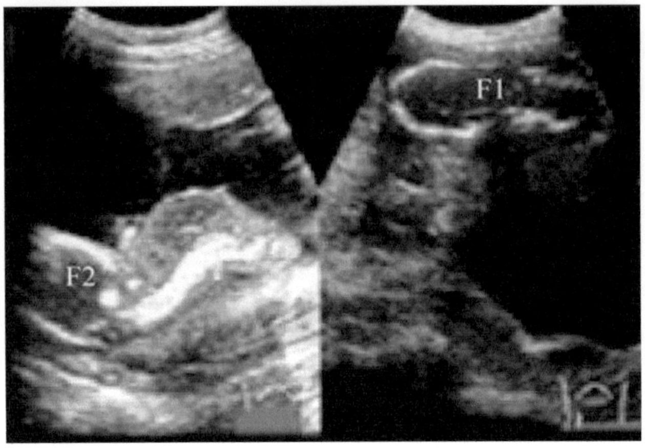

Fig. 2.129 Stillborn in one of the twins

2.5.7 Twin–Twin Transfusion Syndromes

2.5.7.1 Basic Concept

Twin–twin transfusion syndrome (TTTS) occurs in monochorionic twins with artery–artery, venous–venous, and artery–venous anastomosis between placentas. It is now believed that TTTS may occur whenever there is vascular anastomosis with different pressures between the placentas. The donor fetus supplies blood to the recipient fetus, which leads to two unbalanced fetal blood and produces a series of pathological changes.

TTTS may occur early in pregnancy, causing one of the twins to disappear. If it occurs in the second trimester of pregnancy, the donor fetus may have anemia, IUGR, and even death. The recipient fetus is hypervolemic with anasarca, weight gain, and even death.

Clinical diagnostic criteria: ① The difference in birth weight between the two fetuses is more than 20%. ② The difference in hemoglobin between the two newborns is ≥50 g/L. ③ The amniotic septum is thin with two layers of the amniotic membrane or no amniotic septum. The twins share one placenta. ④ Placental pathology shows anastomotic branches formation.

2.5.7.2 Ultrasonic Diagnosis

1. Ultrasound image shows only one placenta with a thin septum between the twins, and two fetuses have the same sex.
2. Polyhydramnios/oligohydramnios sequence: Amniotic fluid depth of the recipient is >8.0 cm, and the depth of the donor is <2.0 cm. The donor one even appears stuck in some severe cases (Fig. 2.130).
3. There is a significant difference in fetal growth measured by ultrasound. The difference between the BPD and FL between the donor and the recipient is ≥5 mm. The expected difference in fetal weight is higher than 25%. The AC of recipient increases significantly, with a difference of 20%.
4. The bladder of the recipient is enlarged, and the bladder of the donor is small or unfilled.
5. One of the twins shows edema, combined with pleural effusion, ascites, or the death of one of the fetuses.
6. The S/D and PI of the umbilical artery are abnormal in one of the twins. Even, the end-diastolic blood flow inversion is detected (Fig. 2.131).

2.5.7.3 Special Tips

1. Identify the type of twins from the following aspects: the diaphragm in the amniotic sac, the thickness of the membrane, the number of placentas, the twin peak sign, and the sex of the fetus.
2. Distinguish the relationship between the head, trunk, and limbs of each fetus to judge the fetal position correctly.
3. When twin pregnancy is diagnosed in early pregnancy, note the morphology, size, and spacing of the two typical sacs. Moreover, confirm the number of embryos in the sacs and fetal heartbeats.
4. If there is an intrauterine neoplasm, pay attention to the relationship between the tumor-like echo in the amniotic cavity and the fetus. CDFI is used to show the blood supply of the mass, and the relationship between the mass, umbilical cord, and placenta.

2.5.8 Facial Anomalies

2.5.8.1 Basic Concept

The embryonic development of the face is a very complicated process. The development of the eye begins at the fifth week of the embryo, and its basic structure forms at the end of the eighth week. Moreover, nasal primordium is initially located above the eye level, gradually migrates to the middle and lower direction, and merges in the midline below eye level and forms the nose.

The lips and palates of the fetus are formed between 7 and 12 weeks of the embryo. Affected by teratogenic factors in the process of formation, some organs which should be fused do not fuse completely, resulting in the cleft, that is, the cleft lip. Cleft palate occurs when the palate fusion is abnormal. Cleft lip and palate can be simultaneous or single.

Facial anomaly is not simply a problem of deformity, but an important issue that deeply affects a person's psychology and spirit. Therefore, the prenatal diagnosis should be as accurate as possible, which is of great significance.

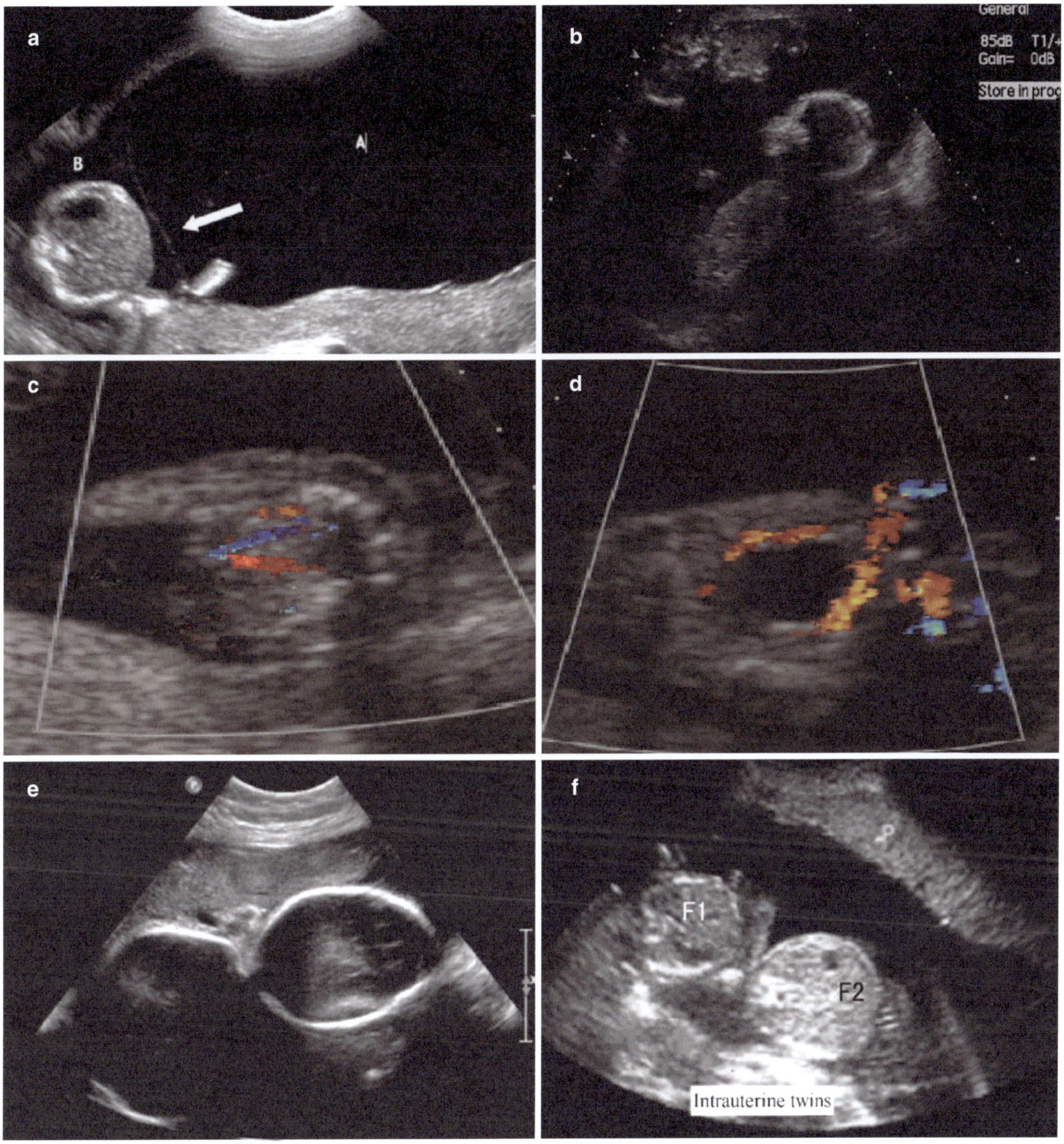

Fig. 2.130 Twin–twin transfusion syndrome I. (**a, b**). Polyhydramnios/oligohydramnios sequence. b The donor is a stuck twin with oligohydramnios. (**c, d**). The bladder of the recipient is enlarged and the bladder of the donor is filled poorly. (**e, f**). The growth and development of twin fetuses are inconsistent

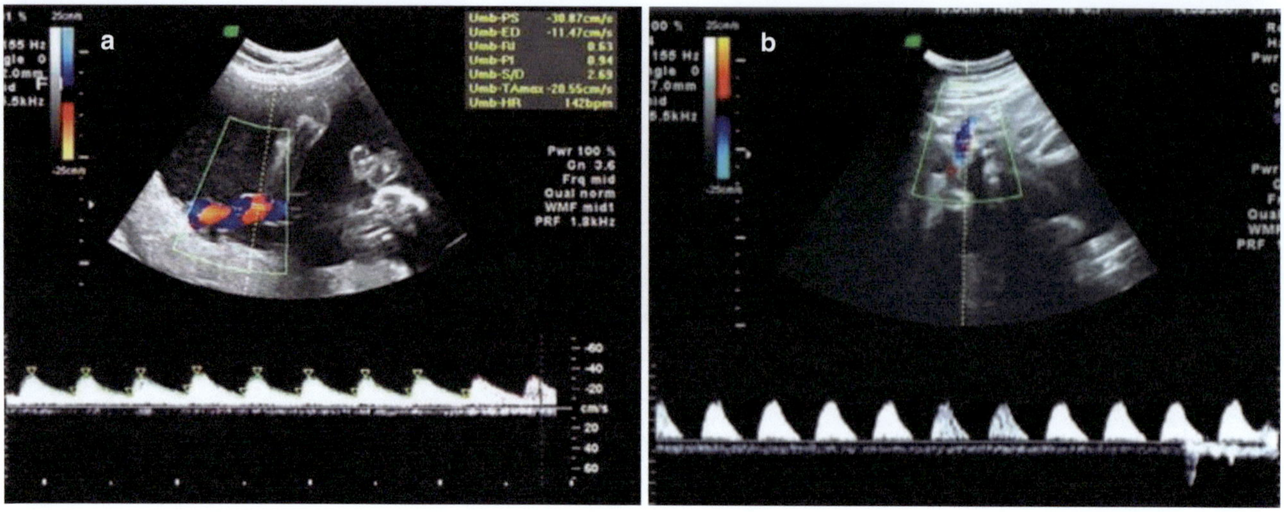

Fig. 2.131 Twin–twin transfusion syndrome II. (**a**). The recipient fetus. (**b**). Abnormal unimodal spectrum of umbilical artery in the donor fetus

2.5.8.2 Ultrasonic Diagnosis

Cleft Lip and Palate

1. On the coronal and transverse views, the upper and lower lips of the fetus can be clearly displayed. The cleft lip is characterized by an interrupted echo in one side or both sides of the upper lip.
2. When the interrupted echo reaches the nostril, it can cause a deformed and flat nostril on the same side, often with cleft palate.
3. When the cleft lip is accompanied by alveolar cleft or complete cleft palate, the alveolar continuity is interrupted simultaneously with the continuous interruption of the upper lip, showing an extremely protruded hyperechoic mass below the nose (Figs. 2.132 and 2.133).

External Nasal Abnormalities

1. Arhiny is caused by the absent or hypoplastic embryonic frontonasal process. It mainly occurs in the holoprosencephaly and combined with facial deformities, such as hypotelorism and hypertelorism.
2. Proboscis and beak nose deformity: Except for facial and intracranial structural changes of the arhiny, the external nose is like a proboscis or elephant trunk above the eye or between the orbits. It represents a columnar soft tissue echo and protrudes forward, often without nostrils in the middle of the proboscis. The proboscis is common in holoprosencephaly cases.
3. Flat nose or single nostril deformity: It is characterized by the flat nose, single nostril deformity, and hypotelorism (Fig. 2.134).

Ear Anomalies

1. Anotia: Anotia is characterized by the absence of unilateral or bilateral auricles, often accompanied by atresia of the external auditory canal.
2. Microtia: The normal ear morphology disappears. Instead, there is a clump, dot, or distinctly abnormal soft tissue, which often accompanies the absence of external auditory canal.
3. Low-set ears: Compared with the temporal bone level, the external ear moved down significantly, and the distance from the shoulder is significantly shortened (Fig. 2.135).

Eye Abnormality

1. Hypotelorism: It mainly exists in the holoprosencephaly cases, rare in other syndromes (Fig. 2.136a, b).
2. Hypertelorism: It can be a major independent defect or a secondary manifestation of multiple syndromes. These syndromes are mostly related to chromosome abnormality or maternal exposure history of teratogenic factors (Fig. 2.136c).

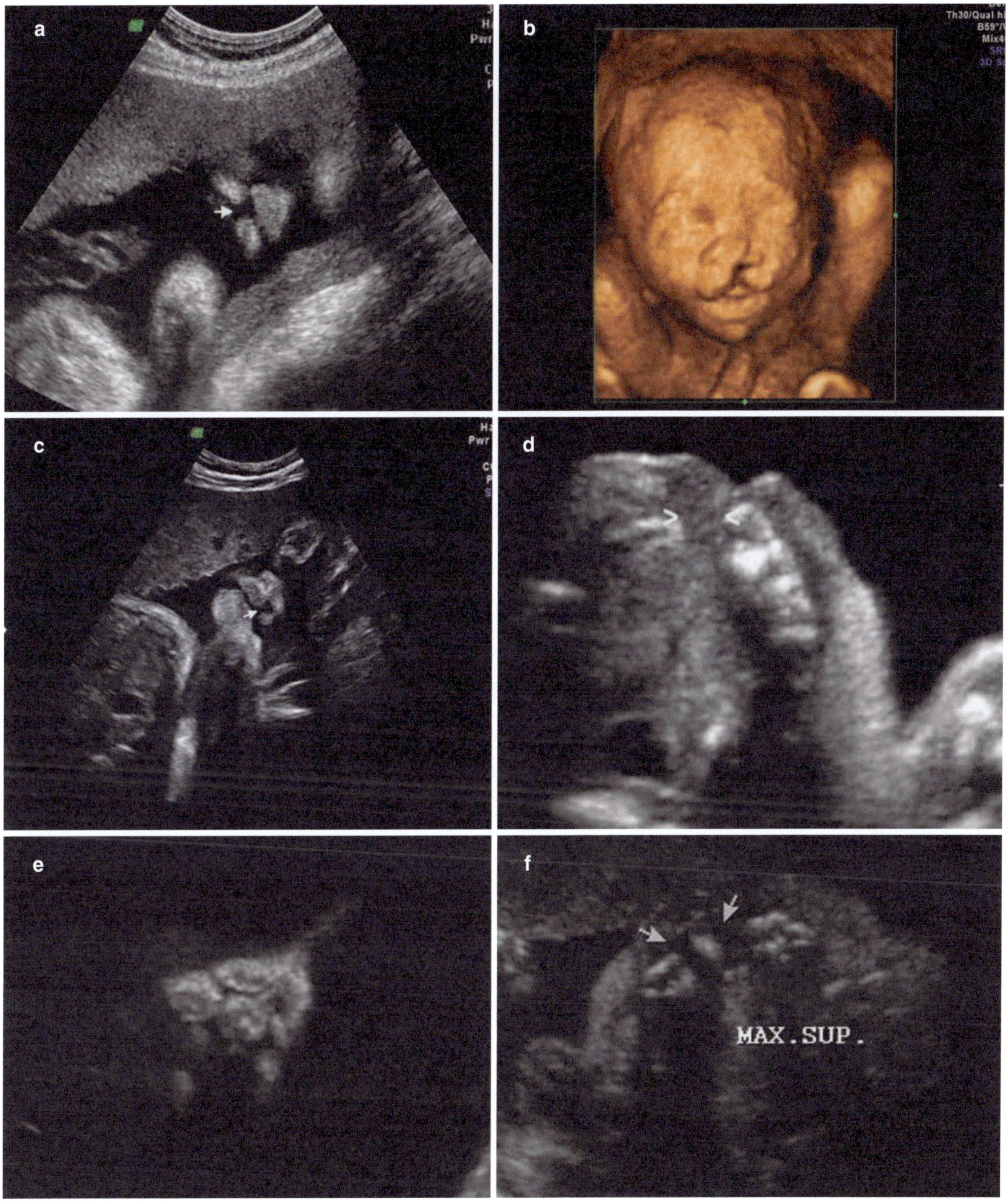

Fig. 2.132 Fetal cleft lip and palate I. (**a, b**). Cleft lip, (**c, d**). Unilateral cleft lip with cleft palate (**e, f**). Bilateral cleft lip with cleft palate

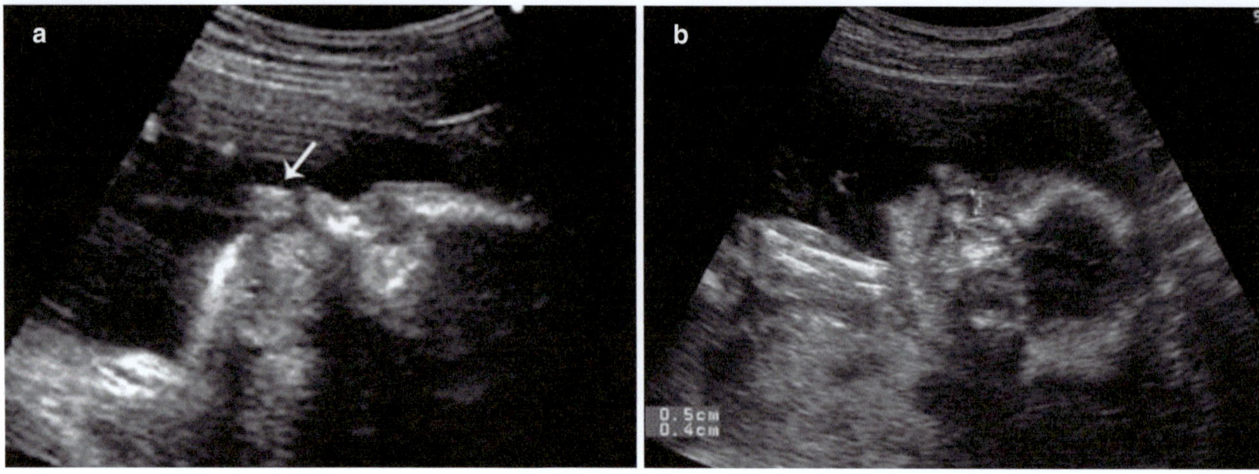

Fig. 2.133 Fetal cleft lip and palate II. (**a, b**). Fetal alveolar bone protrudes forward with abnormal upper lip morphology. There is a solid hyperechoic protuberance in front of the nose

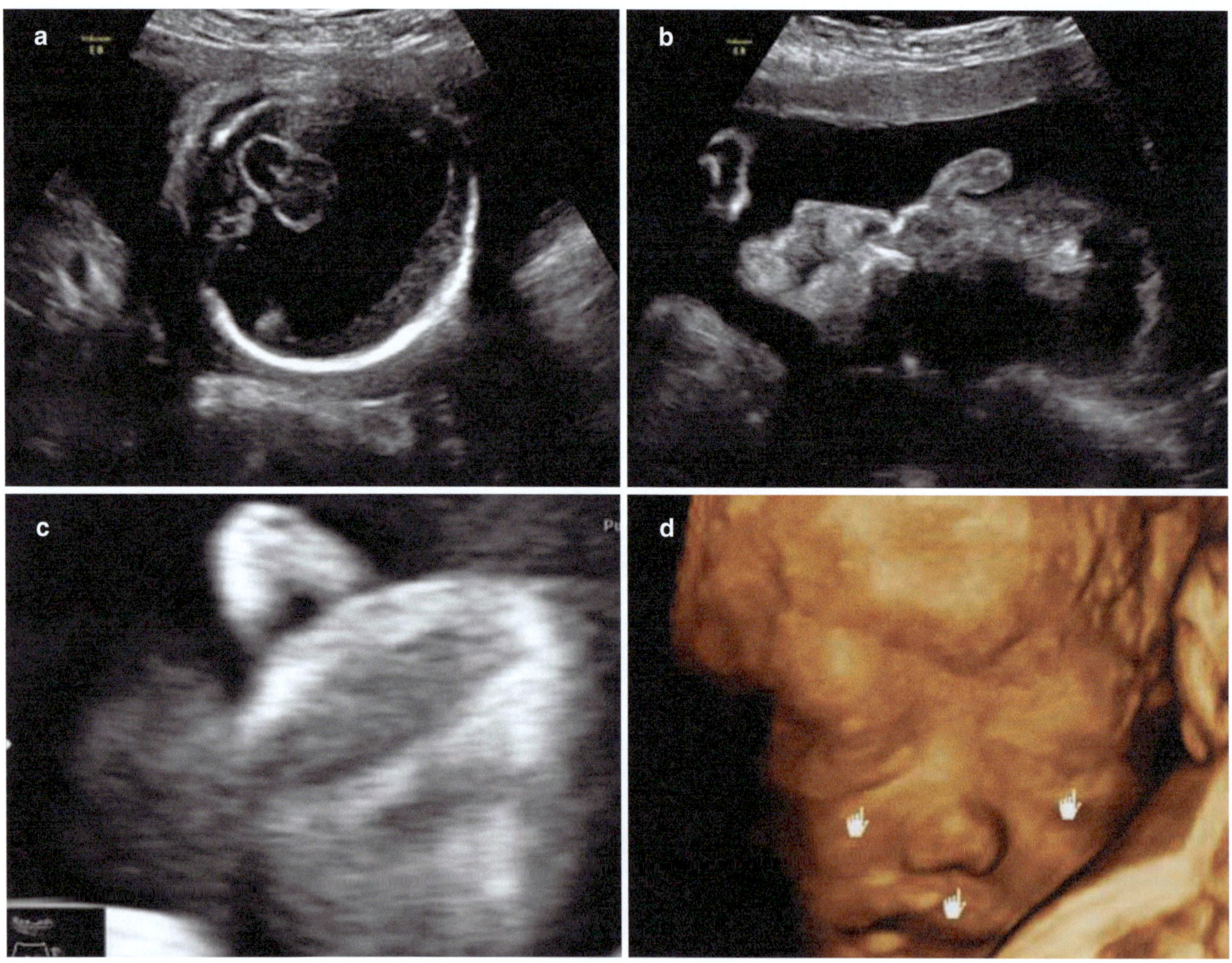

Fig. 2.134 Congenital nasal deformity. (**a, b**). Holoprosencephaly associated with beak nose deformity (**c, d**). Single nostril deformity

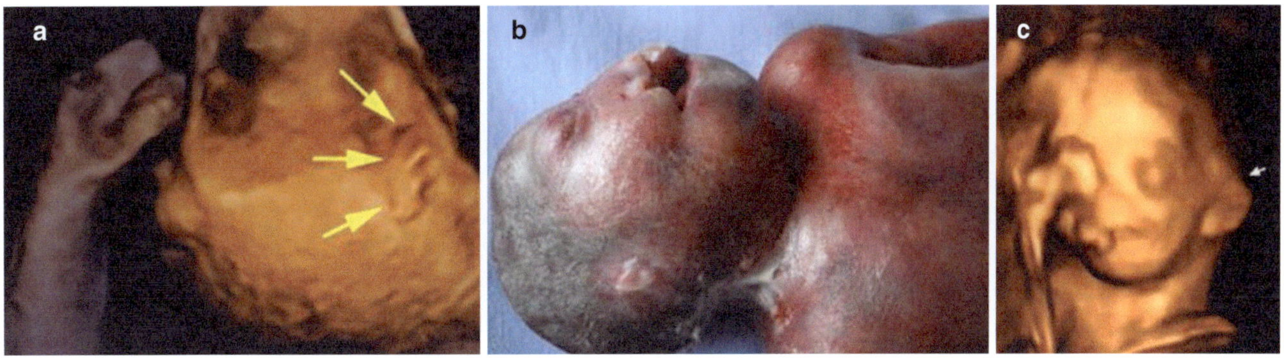

Fig. 2.135 Congenital ear anomalies. (**a, b**). Microtia. (**c**). Low-set ear

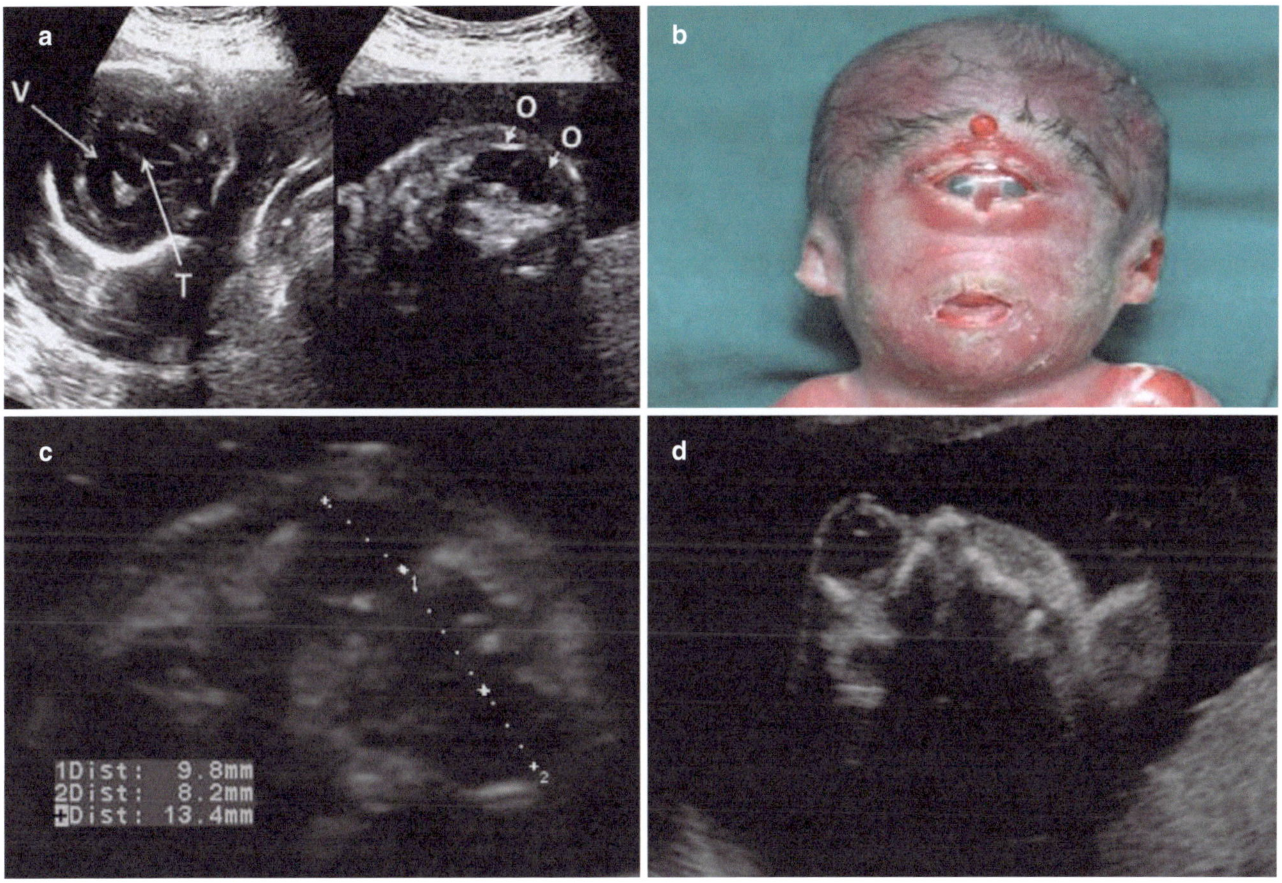

Fig. 2.136 Congenital eye anomaly. (**a, b**). Holoprosencephaly associated with hypotelorism. (**c**). Hypertelorism (Trisomy 18). (**d**). Right anophthalmia

3. Anophthalmia: The sonography shows the absence of one or both sides of the orbits and eyeballs on the horizontal transection of the eyes. An arcuate hyperechoic is visible at the area of the orbit (Fig. 2.136c).

Micrognathia

1. A standard midsagittal view of the fetus shows a forward protruded forehead, nasal tip, upper lip, lower lip, and chin. The lower lip forms an "S" or reverses "S" shape with the chin. The chin retracts and the lower lip moves back, which make the curve into a small circular arc. The more severe the deformity, the smaller the chin and the straighter the curve are (Fig. 2.137).

2. The length of the normal fetal mandible is about half of the BPD, which is significantly shorter in micrognathia cases.

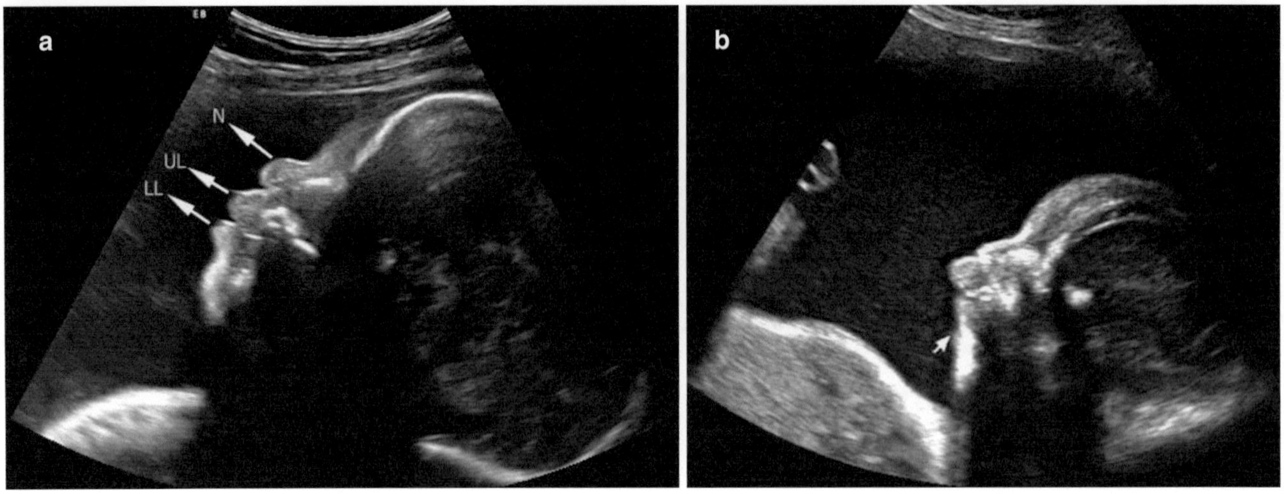

Fig. 2.137 Micrognathia. (**a**). Normal fetal face in midsagittal view. (**b**). Micrognathia

2.5.8.3 Special Tips

1. Common reasons for misdiagnosis of cleft lip and palate are as follows: A. Lack of experience in diagnosis. B. The section is not standardized, and anomalies are not shown through two orthogonal sections at the same time. C. A deep philtrum can be mistaken for the cleft lip. D. It also can be mistaken for a cleft lip when the umbilical cord is pressed vertically against the lip. Color blood flow, fetal mouth movement, and fetal movement are helpful in this situation. E. The squeezed fetal upper lip is mistaken for cleft lip, where dynamic observation is suggested.
2. It is challenging to scan the fetal maxillofacial and external ear malformation. We should pay attention to acquire the standard view and try to change the fetal position.

2.5.9 Chest Abnormality

2.5.9.1 Basic Concepts

There are five distinct stages of the human lung development, including the embryo stage, pseudoglandular stage, canalicular stage, saccular stage, and alveolar stage. At the fourth week of embryonic development, the laryngotracheal sulcus is formed and gradually differentiated. By the end of the sixth week, the bronchus form and bifurcate irregularly and small vesicles differentiate into respiratory bronchioles, alveolar tubes, blastocysts, and alveoli. By the end of the 16th week, the bronchial tree has formed. At 16–20 weeks, the number and complexity of airways, great vessels and capillaries in the lung increase significantly. After 24 weeks, the cubed epithelial cells lining the airway gradually become flattened (Alveolar type I epithelial cell). Alveolar type II epithelial cells secrete alveolar surface-active substances at the same time. It is fully prepared for an effective arterial gas exchange after birth. In the development process of the fetal lung, the fastest growth happens in the three months before delivery. Its weight is about 1/70 of fetal body weight, and its volume is about 1/2 of fetal chest cavity.

The diaphragm of the fetus gradually forms between 6 and 14 weeks, and the posterolateral part of the diaphragm is formed by the chest wall and closed in the end. The defect of the diaphragm may result from weak or failed fusion of the related structures before the formation of the diaphragm. The stomach, intestine, liver, and spleen in the abdominal cavity enter the chest cavity through the diaphragm defect, which compresses the lungs and causes pulmonary dysplasia. The fetus often dies of respiratory failure after birth.

2.5.9.2 Ultrasonic Diagnosis

Pulmonary Hypoplasia

1. The diagnosis of pulmonary hypoplasia by 2-D ultrasound is mainly according to the area and the length of the lung, chest circumference, thoracic area measurement, and other relevant ratios, such as increased cardiothoracic ratio, decreased chest circumference/AC ratio, and decreased chest circumference/FL ratio (Fig. 2.138).
2. 3-D ultrasound is a hot topic in current research, which mainly focuses on the measurement of lung volume and a series of parameters derived from it, such as the ratio of lung weight-to-fetal weight, and the ratio of actual lung volume to the expected value. However, it is not thorough enough to put forward a specific evaluation standard, which needs further study. We measured the lung volume of 402 fetuses between 20 and 32 weeks of normal pregnancies and established the normal values (Fig. 2.139, Table 2.6).

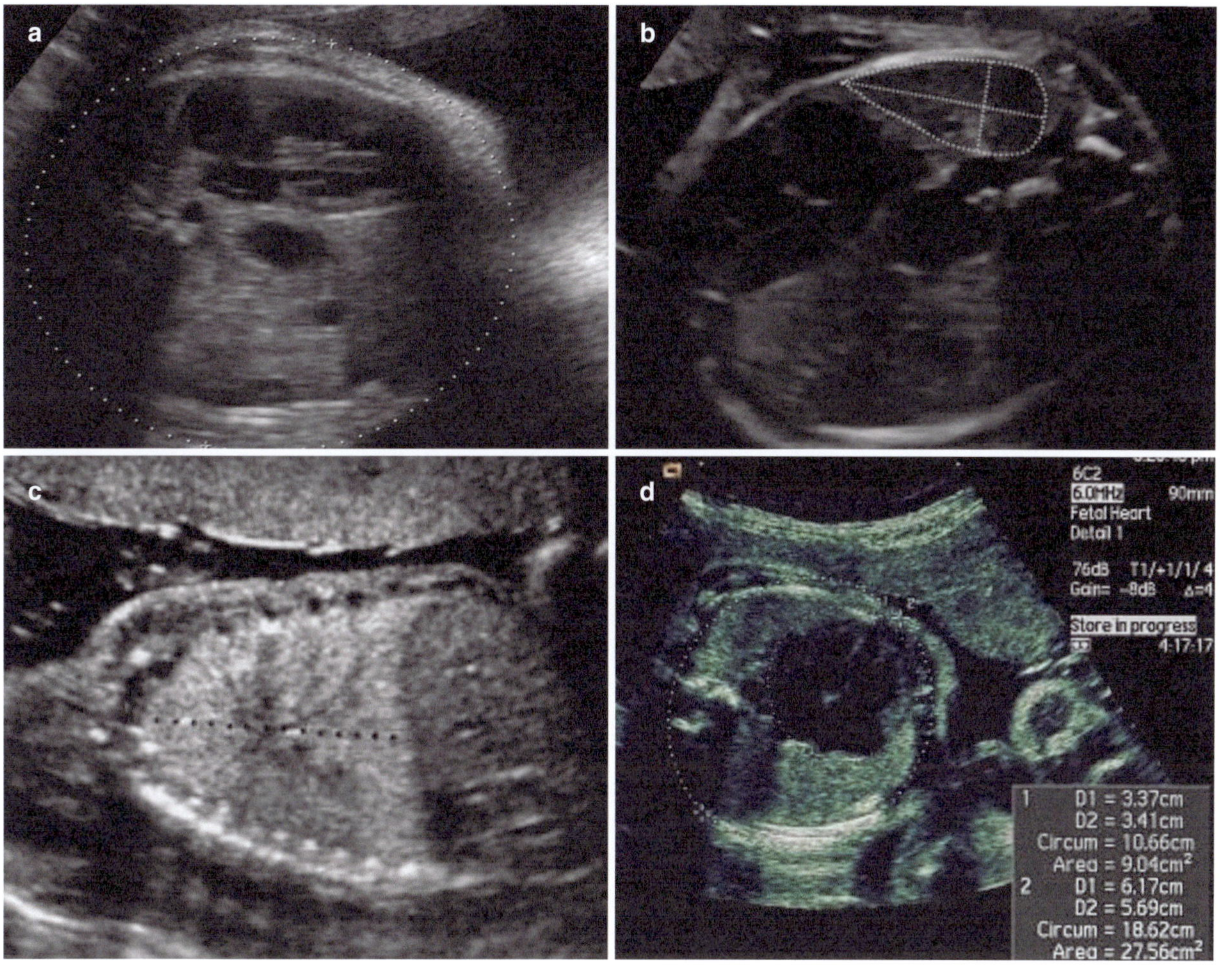

Fig. 2.138 Common 2-D ultrasonic parameters of pulmonary dysplasia. (**a**). Chest circumference. (**b**). Pulmonary area. (**c**). Pulmonary length. (**d**). Cardiothoracic ratio

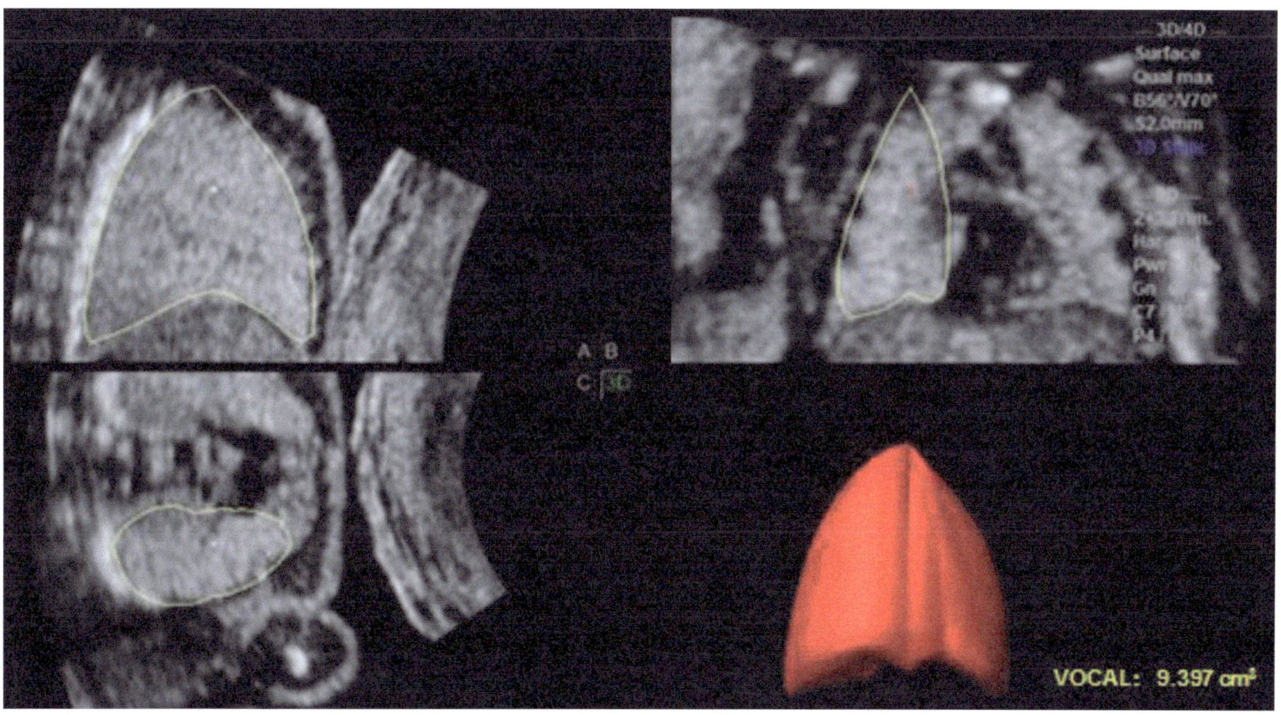

Fig. 2.139 The measurement of lung volume by 3-D ultrasound

Table 2.6 Normal fetal lung volume at 20–32 weeks of gestation ($\overline{x} \pm s$, 95% *CI*)

Gestation (week)	Number	Lung volume (ml) Left lung volume	Right lung volume	Total lung volume
20	23	4.38 ± 1.09(2.24–6.52)	6.09 ± 1.49(3.17–9.01)	10.5 ± 2.54(5.47–15.5)
21	25	5.65 ± 1.20(3.30–8.00)	7.80 ± 1.66(4.55–11.1)	13.5 ± 2.93(7.70–19.2)
22	25	6.71 ± 1.64(3.50–9.93)	9.23 ± 2.05(5.22–13.2)	15.9 ± 3.68(8.74–23.1)
23	27	8.17 ± 2.07(4.10–12.2)	11.5 ± 2.47(6.65–16.3)	19.7 ± 4.52(10.8–28.5)
24	35	9.54 ± 2.04(5.54–13.5)	13.1 ± 2.90(7.45–18.8)	22.7 ± 4.91(13.1–32.3)
25	40	11.1 ± 2.54(6.07–16.0)	14.9 ± 3.31(8.40–21.4)	26.0 ± 5.80(14.6–37.3)
26	40	12.8 ± 3.08(6.76–18.8)	16.9 ± 3.43(10.2–23.6)	29.7 ± 6.44(17.1–42.3)
27	39	14.0 ± 3.05(7.98–19.9)	18.6 ± 4.29(10.2–27.0)	32.5 ± 7.27(18.3–46.8)
28	38	15.4 ± 3.53(8.43–22.3)	21.5 ± 5.11(11.5–31.5)	36.8 ± 8.57(22.0–53.6)
29	35	17.3 ± 3.65(10.1–24.4)	23.3 ± 5.14(13.2–33.4)	40.6 ± 8.75(23.4–57.8)
30	35	18.6 ± 3.77(11.2–26.0)	25.8 ± 6.35(13.4–38.3)	44.4 ± 10.0(24.7–64.1)
31	22	21.1 ± 4.50(11.3–30.9)	29.7 ± 6.56(16.9–42.6)	50.8 ± 11.5(28.2–73.4)
32	18	21.8 ± 5.29(11.4–32.1)	31.7 ± 7.37(17.3–46.2)	53.5 ± 12.5(28.9–78.1)

Extralobar Sequestration (ELS)

1. The performance of 2-D ultrasound: A triangular or leaf-like hyperechoic mass in the thorax or abdomen. The internal echo is homogeneous with a clear boundary.
2. The color Doppler examination shows that the nourishing blood vessels originate from the systemic circulation artery or its branches (Fig. 2.140).
3. 3-D power ultrasound is more sensitive to detect abnormal blood supply vessels.
4. Prognosis and clinical management depend on whether the fetus is combined with pleural effusion and edema. It also depends on whether the size of the mass can gradually recede.

Congenital Cystic Adenomatoid Malformation (CCAM)

Ultrasound images of congenital cystic adenomatoid malformation can be simply divided into the macrocytic type and microcystic type (mainly the solid portion). The macrocytic type presents as a solid, strong echogenic mass or mixed echogenic mass in the chest cavity with cysts of different sizes. In contrast, the microcystic type tends to be a solid hyperechoic tissue (Fig. 2.141).

Diaphragmatic Hernia

1. Abdominal viscera-like echo is seen in the fetal chest, with the cardiac mediastinum pushed to the opposite side.
2. The fetal stomach and heart are at the same level in transverse chest section, and the heart moves to the right side.
3. If the intestines herniate into the chest cavity the peristalsis can be observed and if stomach herniates the size of it will change. AC is smaller than normal (Figs. 2.142 and 2.143).
4. A diaphragmatic hernia is more common on the left than on the right.

Pleural Effusion and Ascites

1. Irregular fluid anechoic area is observed in the fetal chest cavity and even around the heart. The fetal lungs are evident in large amounts of fluid (Fig. 2.144).
2. Free liquid anechoic areas are found in the abdominal cavity, between the intestines, and in perihepatic area (Fig. 2.145).

2.5.9.3 Special Tips

1. Fetus with severe bilateral lung dysplasia cannot survive after birth. Fetus with unilateral lung dysplasia may survive after birth, but neonatal mortality can reach 50%. The prognosis is worse when combined with other severe malformations. Besides, the prognosis also depends on the cause of pulmonary dysplasia.
2. The diagnosis of ELS is influenced by instrument resolution, pregnant women's abdominal wall thickness, fetal movement, operator's professional level, and other factors. The abnormal blood supply is detected only in 40% to 65% of cases. Therefore, MRI is recommended for pregnant women in controversial cases. 50%–70% of the ELS cases can decrease or even completely disappear with the progression of pregnancy, and the mechanism is unknown. Therefore, if there are no other severe malformations, it is recommended to continue pregnancy surveillance with the comprehension of the family. The interval time of follow-up should be as short as possible, so that the complications such as pleural effusion and pulmonary dysplasia can be detected and treated timely.
3. About 70% of CCAMs have a stable mass size in literature, about 20% of cases get atrophic or disappeared before birth, and only 10% of the cases are gradually increased. So the patients without fetal edema and polyhydramnios can be dynamically observed in 2 to 3 weeks.

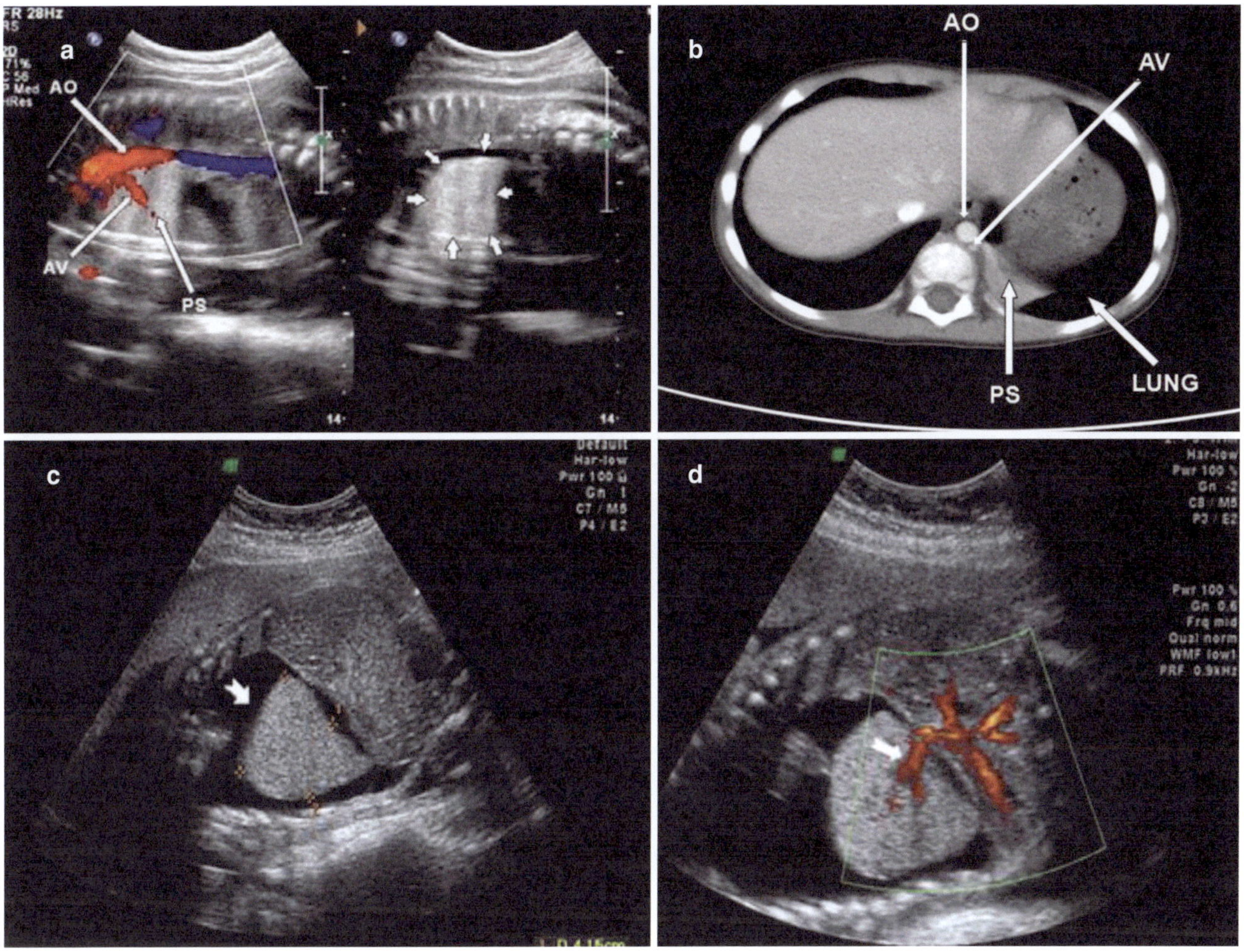

Fig. 2.140 Extralobar sequestration. (**a**). At 25 weeks of gestation, the 2-D ultrasound shows a lobulated or triangular hyperechoic mass with clear boundaries at the base of the left lung. The supply vessel is originated from the aorta. (**b**). Postpartum CT proves the ELS. The patient underwent mass resection, with good prognosis. (**c, d**). ELS with pleural effusion

4. For communicating diaphragmatic hernia, the abdominal content herniated into the chest cavity changes with the abdominal pressure. The abdominal contents herniate into the chest cavity when the abdominal pressure increases, and return to the abdominal cavity when the abdominal pressure decreases. The sonogram shows that the size of hernial mass varies at different times.

2.5.10 Other Congenital Malformations (Cystic Hygroma, Sacrococcygeal Teratoma, Amniotic Band Syndrome, Pelvic Cysts)

2.5.10.1 Basic Concepts

The abnormal development of the fetal lymphatic system may be caused by the failure of the normal connection between cervical lymphatic vessels and internal jugular vein during the development of the lymphatic system. Lymphatic circumfluence obstacle causes the edema of fetal neck, partial upper limb, and even whole body.

1. Cystic hygroma: Most of the cases are associated with chromosomal abnormalities (Turner syndrome, Trisomy 21 syndrome) and cardiovascular abnormalities. The common cystic hygromas are mostly located on the dorsal side of the fetal head and neck. Capillary lymphangioma is another kind of lymphangioma. It often occurs in the fetal neck, chest, upper arm, and other parts of the subcutaneous tissue.
2. Sacrococcygeal teratoma: It is a congenital germ cell tumor and composed of three germ layers. Most are located near the sacrococcyx of the fetus. It can be classified as benign, malignant, and immature teratoma.
3. Amniotic band syndrome: During the early and second trimester of pregnancy, the mesodermal fibrous bands on the surface of the amnion chorionic membrane leak out,

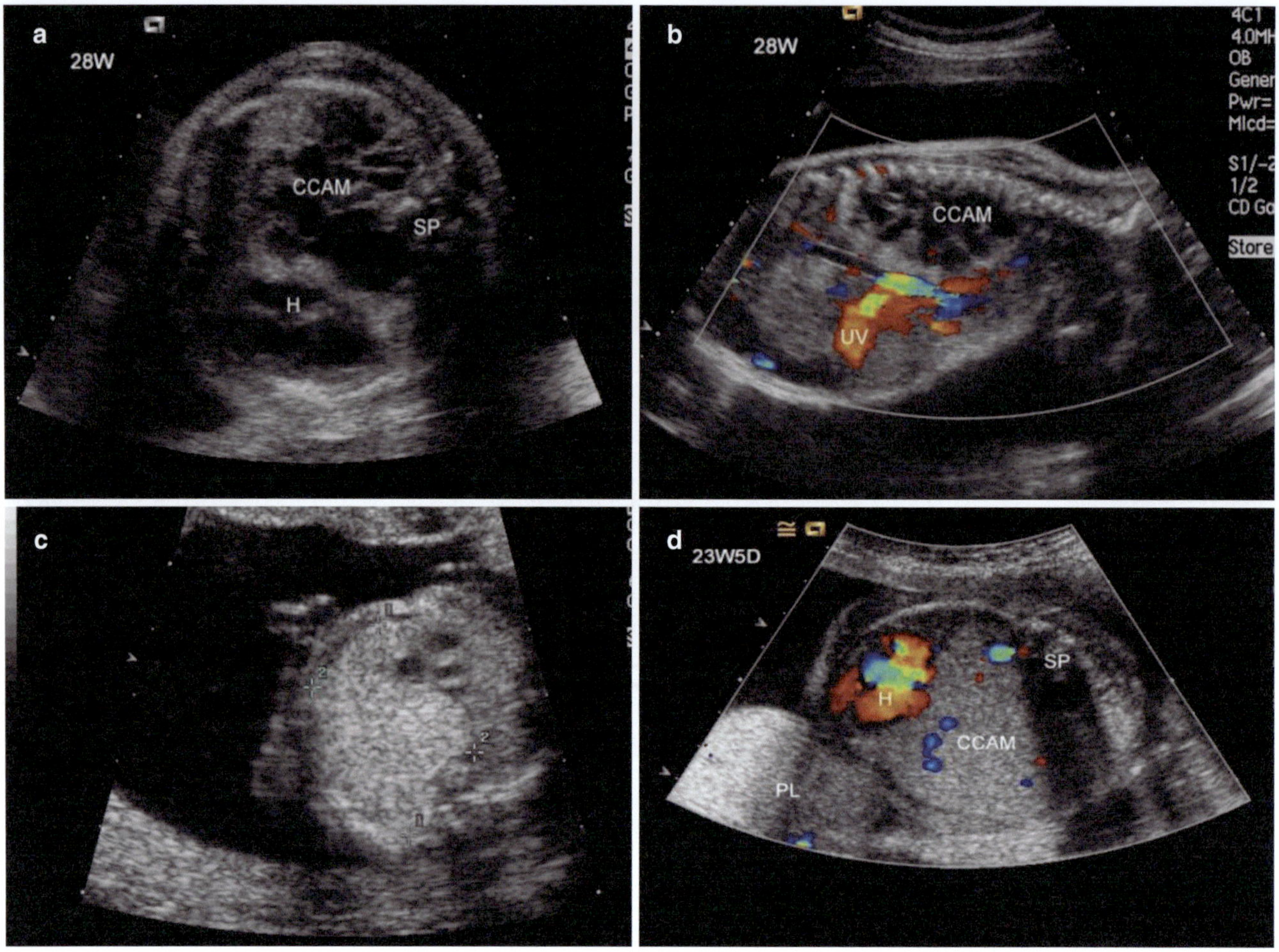

Fig. 2.141 Congenital cystic adenomatoid malformation. (**a, b**). The macrocytic type is characterized by one or more circular anechoic area in the lung parenchyma with distinct boundary and the size of cysts vary. (**c, d**). The microcystic type is characterized by homogeneous strong echo without cyst

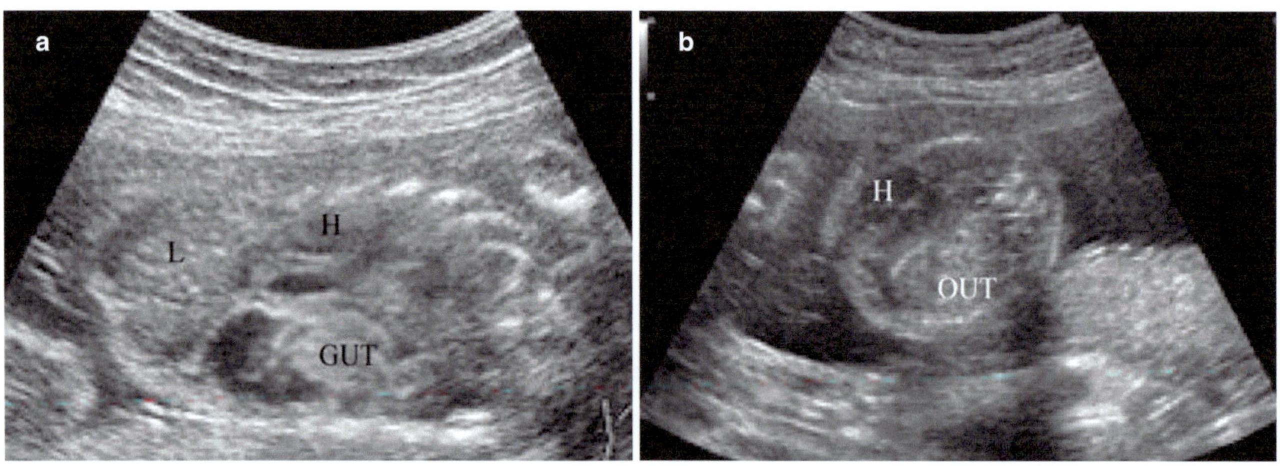

Fig. 2.142 Diaphragmatic hernia I. (**a**). At 32 weeks of gestation, the sagittal section of the fetus shows the heart and the gastric bubble are at the same level with the bowel moving above the diaphragm. (**b**). The transverse section of the abdomen of the same fetus shows the fetal heart moving to the right with intestinal peristalsis next to the heart

infiltrating and wrapping around the body of the fetus. All the above may result in fetal malformation. Once it is attached to the fetus, amniotic banding can easily lead to amputation, narrow ring around limbs, and immobilization of the fetus in a certain position. The earlier the amniotic membrane is damaged, the more serious the abnormalities are.

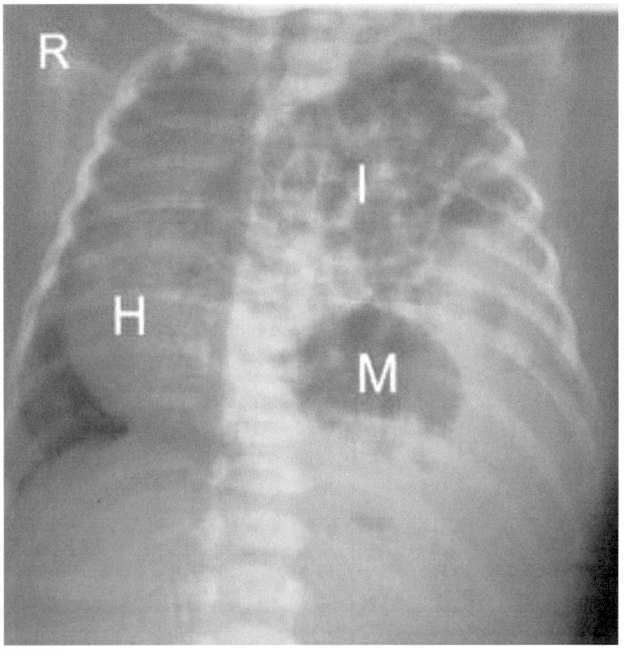

Fig. 2.143 Diaphragmatic hernia II. Postpartum X-ray confirms gastric and bowl punching above the diaphragm

4. Pelvic cysts: Fetal pelvic cysts have a wide range of sources, in which the most common are female fetuses' ovarian cysts. Ovarian cysts are often found in the third trimester of pregnancy. No definite cause has been found, and most studies believe it is related to maternal hormone overstimulation.

2.5.10.2 Ultrasonic Diagnosis

Cystic Hygroma

1. It appears as an irregular anechoic cystic mass on the back of the fetal head and neck, clinging to the back of the neck tightly.
2. Septum is visible in the cystic mass in the neck. The cystic area extends upward to the head and surrounds the fetal head (Fig. 2.146).
3. The fetal scalp is edema with low echo. It can also appear as "cocoon" like anasarca, and be accompanied by skeletal variations and malformations (Figs. 2.147 and 2.148).

Sacrococcygeal Teratoma

1. A cystic, mixed, or solid mass that are attached to the fetus is visible at the sacrococcygeal or perineal regions of the spine on the longitudinal view of the fetal back.
2. The sacrococcygeal mass protrudes into the amniotic cavity and oscillates with fetal movement. Complete cystic teratoma is indistinguishable from spinal meningocele in the sacrococcygeal region.
3. Color Doppler flow image shows abundant blood flow in the heterogeneous echogenic mass, suggesting that the tumor is most likely malignant (Fig. 2.149).

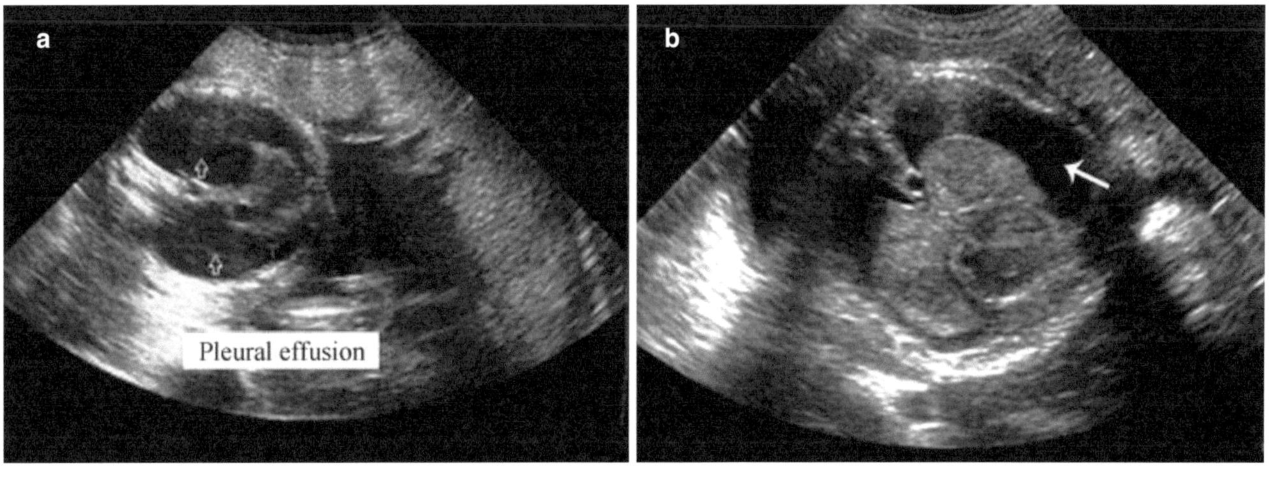

Fig. 2.144 Pleural effusion. (**a, b**). The transverse view of the fetal chest shows bilateral pleural effusion and visible echo-enhanced lungs

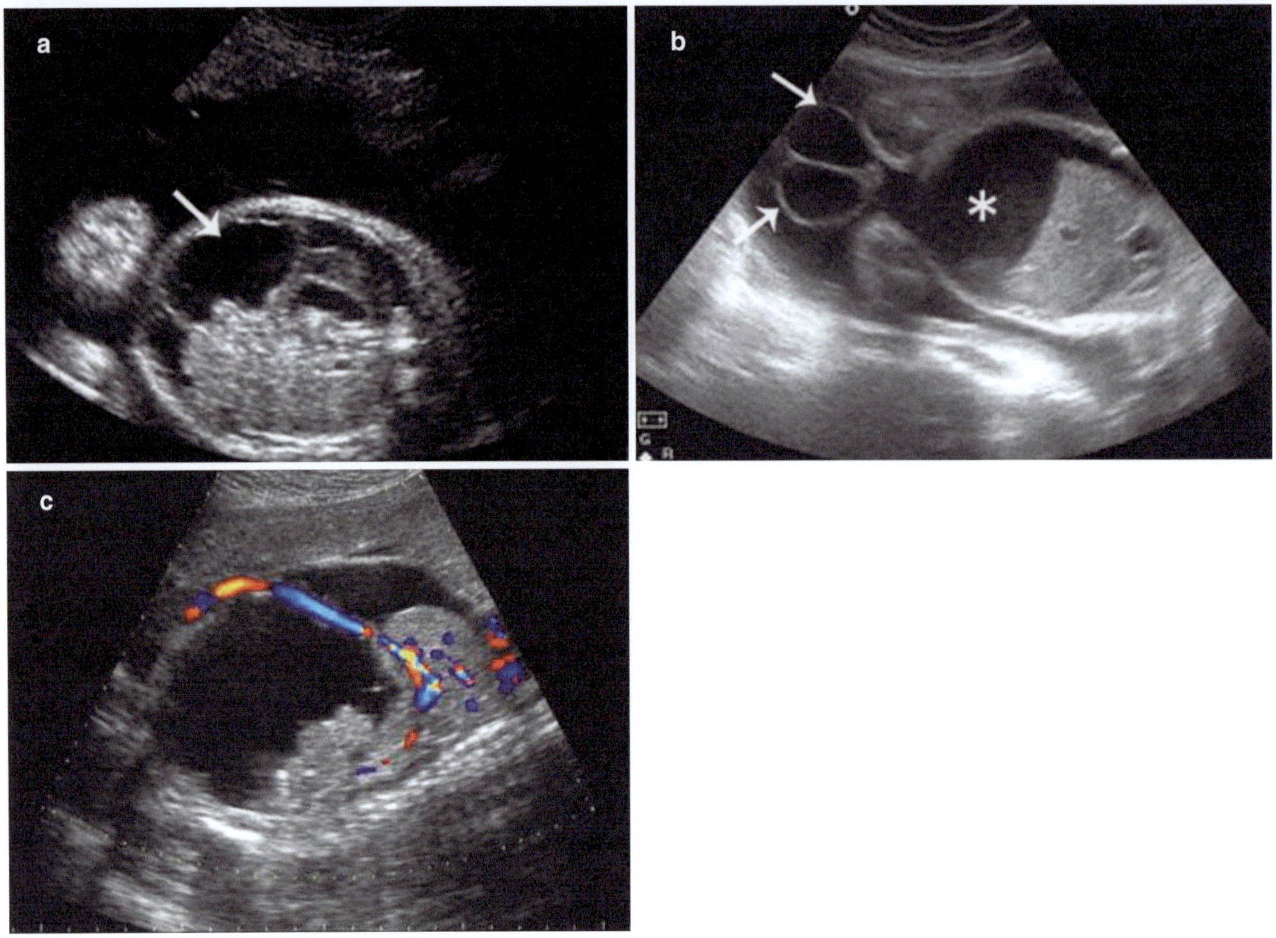

Fig. 2.145 Ascites. (**a**). Transverse view of the abdomen shows fluid between intestines and floating bowl. (**b**). A large amount of ascites with scrotal effusion. (**c**). A large amount of ascites

Amniotic Band Syndrome

1. In the amniotic cavity, the strip-like enhanced echo is observed and attached to a part of the body.
2. In malformation cases, it is necessary to search for the amniotic band at the malformation part (Fig. 2.150).
3. Fetal movement is limited and may combine with oligohydramnios.

Pelvic Cysts

1. The majority of pelvic cysts are from the ovary and are prevalent in female fetuses.
2. Ultrasound shows a cystic mass on one side of the bladder or above it, which is in a round or oval shape with a clear boundary and capsule. Its shape does not change with the change of planes and fetal movement (Fig. 2.151).
3. The position and shape of double kidneys, bladder, and stomach bubble are normal.

2.5.10.3 Special Tips

1. In any period of pregnancy, if we find cystic hygroma, chromosome examination should be taken. In cases with chromosome abnormality, the fetus should be terminated in time.
2. Fetal cystic hygroma in early or middle pregnancy is prone to abort. If the tumor is small and located on the body surface, the abortion may occur in the third trimester.

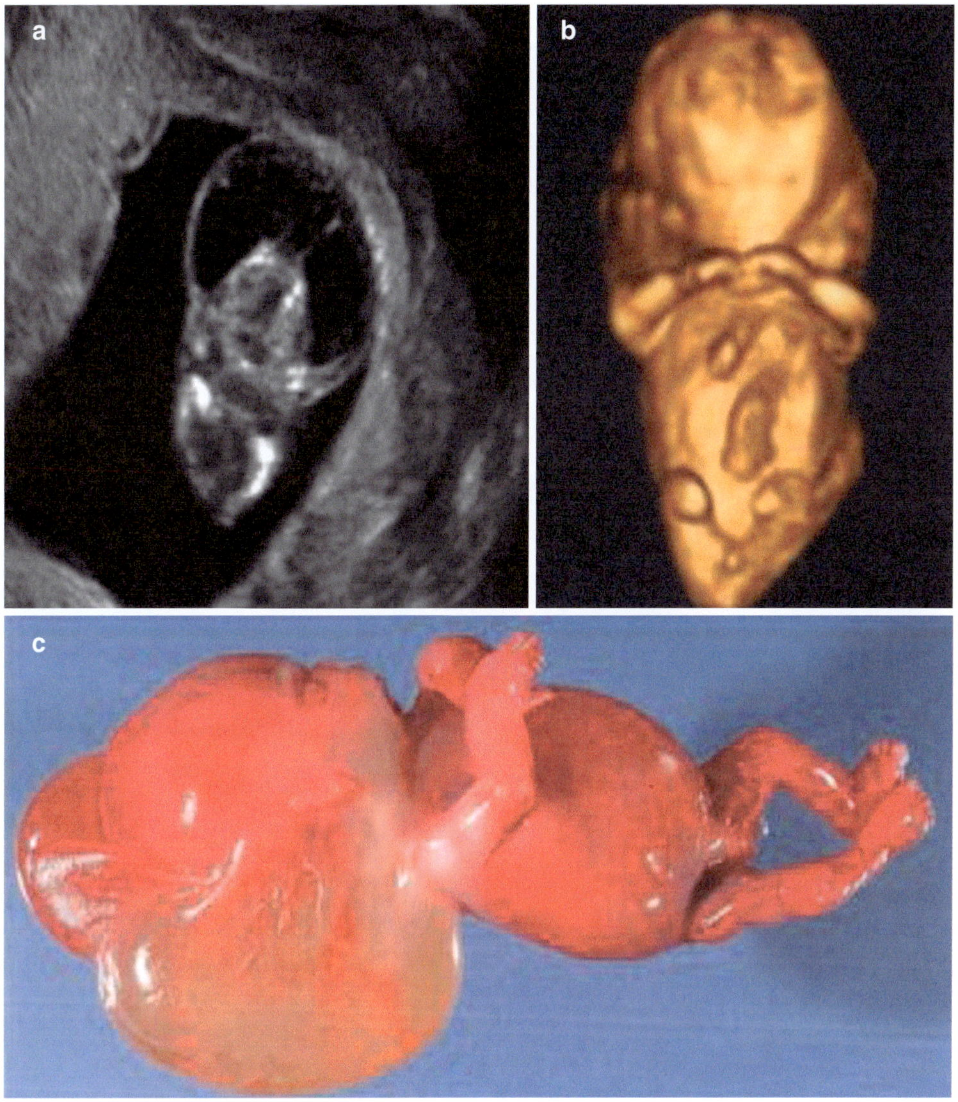

Fig. 2.146 Cystic hygroma I. (**a**). There is cystic echo in the back of the head and neck, with septum inside. (**b**). 3-D ultrasound shows "cocoon" like edema. (**c**). Induced labor confirms the cystic hygroma

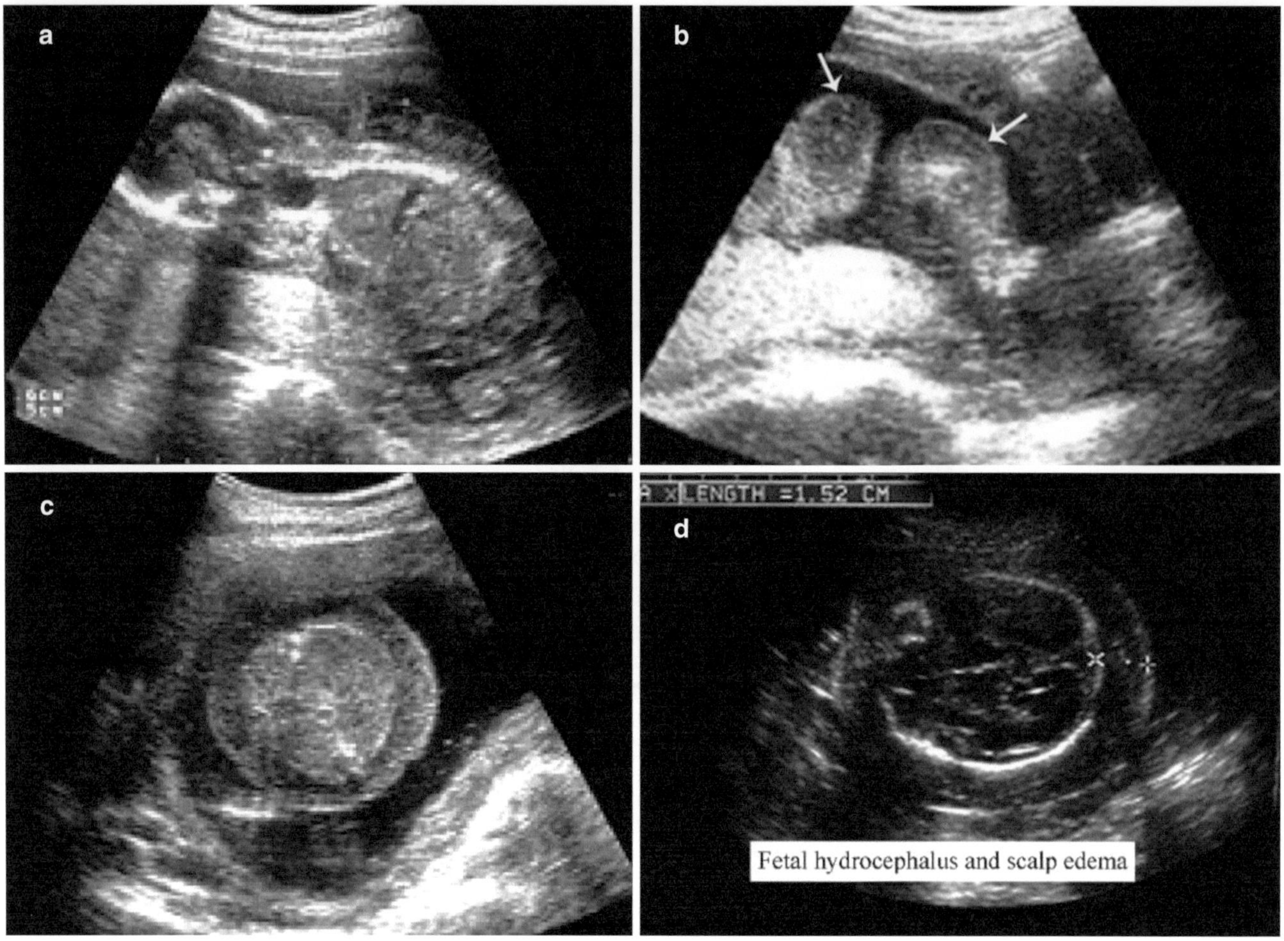

Fig. 2.147 Cystic hygroma II. (**a**). At 24 weeks of gestation, an enlarged mass around the neck. (**b**). "Cocoon" like edema of fetal limbs and trunk. c. Separated skull and scalp of the same fetus

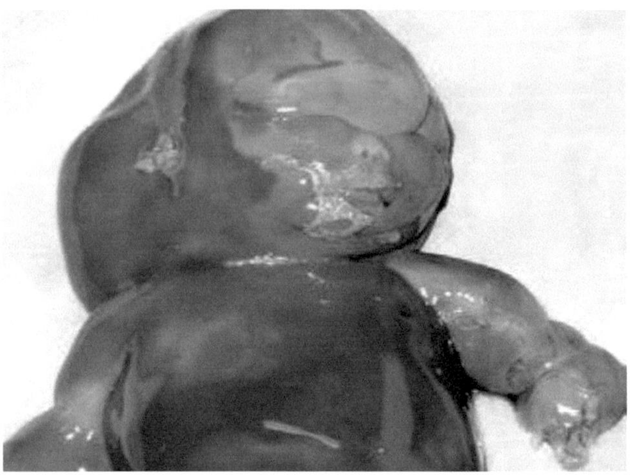

Fig. 2.148 Anasarca in fetus

Fetuses without chromosomal abnormalities have a better prognosis. Due to the compression of the respiratory tract, fetal separated cystic hygroma accompanied by edema, and cystic hygroma located in the front of the neck have an extremely poor prognosis.

3. When the cord or lamellar enhanced echo is found in the amniotic cavity, pay attention to whether there is adhesion with the fetus. It should be differentiated from unfused amnion and chorion, intrauterine adhesion, intrauterine adhesion, and amniotic membrane separation of twins.
4. Note the difference between sacrococcygeal cystic teratoma and spinal meningocele.
5. Avoid the missed diagnosis of small swelling in the skull and spine.

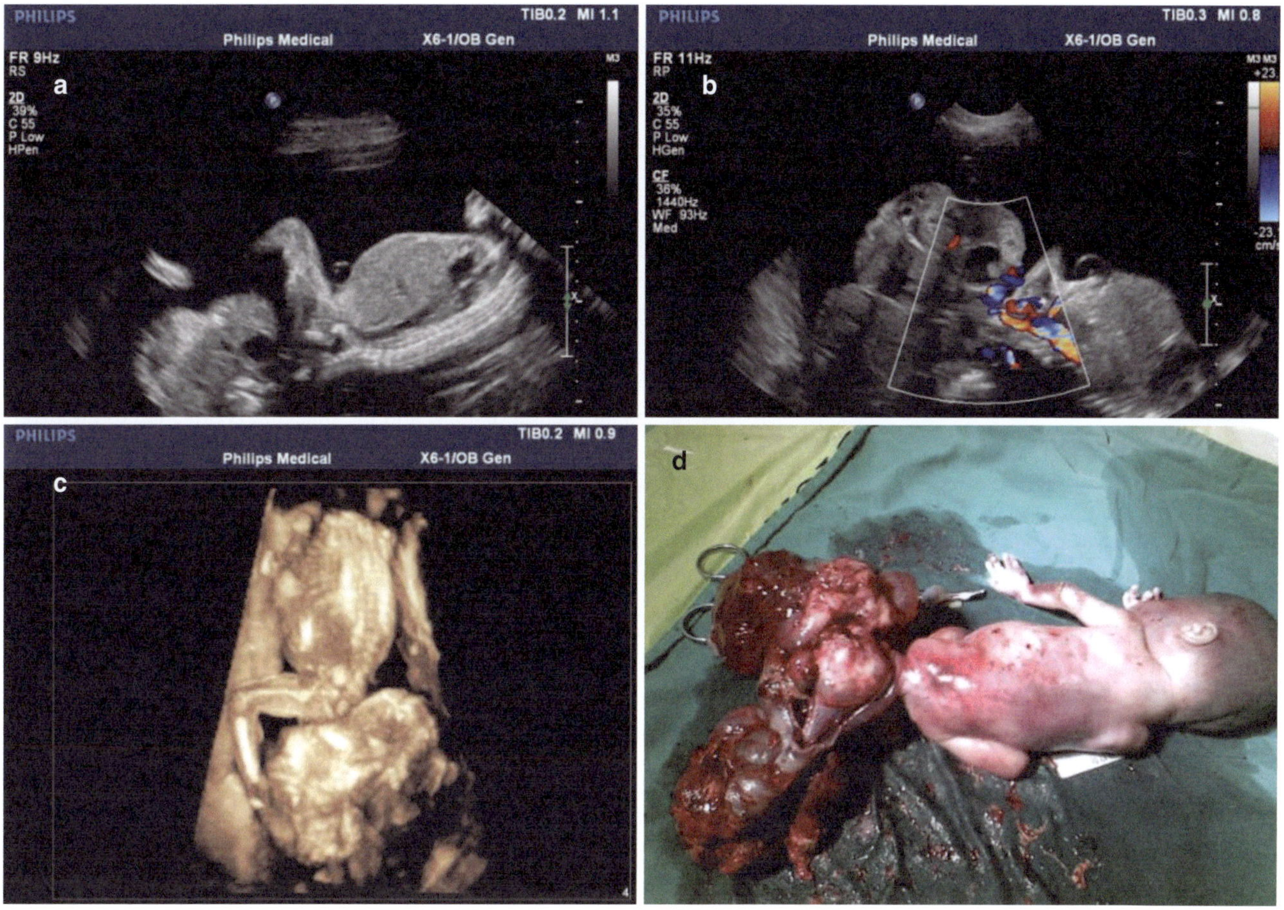

Fig. 2.149 Sacrococcygeal teratoma. (**a**). 2-D ultrasound shows a large heterogeneous mass in the sacrococcygeal region with the fluid area. (**b**). CDFI shows abundant blood flow in the mass. (**c**). 3-D ultrasound image. (**d**). Induced labor confirms sacrococcygeal teratoma

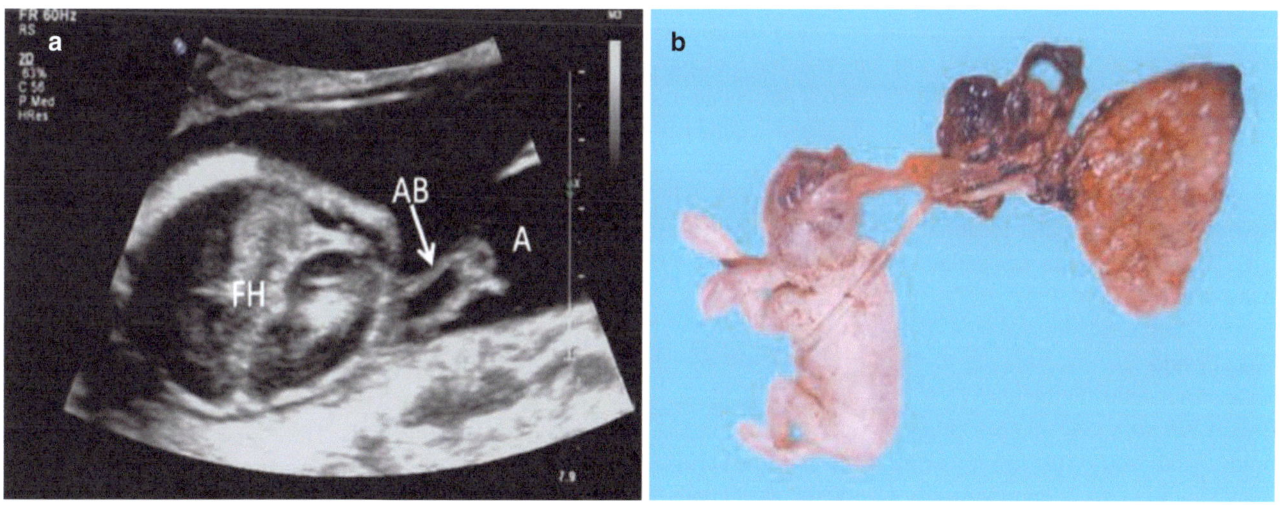

Fig. 2.150 Amniotic band syndrome. (**a**). Image shows that the amniotic tape attaches to the fetal skull and causes exeucephalia. (**b**). The specimen after labor induction shows amniotic band attached to the fetal head

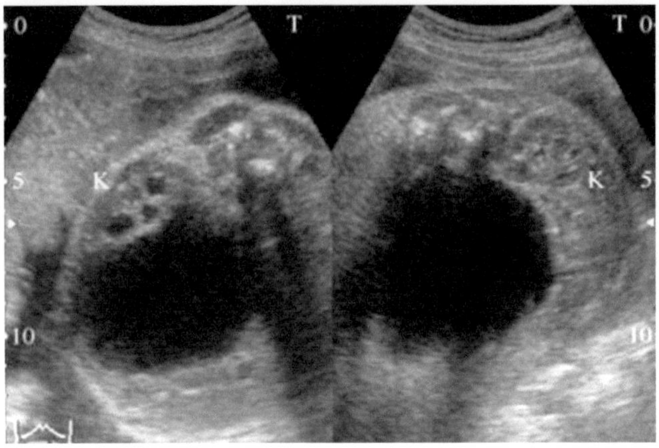

Fig. 2.151 Pelvic cyst. It is proved to be ovarian cyst after birth

2.6 Ultrasonic Diagnosis of Abnormal Fetal Appendages

2.6.1 Placenta Previa

2.6.1.1 Basic Concepts

Placenta Previa

Placenta previa is defined as the condition that the placenta wholly or partly covers the internal cervical os after 28 weeks of gestation, which happens when the placenta attaches to the lower segment of the uterus with its inferior edge below the fetal presentation. Risk factors include endometrial disease, large placenta, succenturiate lobe, developmental retardation of the trophoblast, smoking, and drug abuse.

The most common clinical manifestation is painless bleeding from the vagina during the second and third trimesters, leading to anemia and even shock. The fetal position is abnormal in one-third of the cases, mainly the breech presentation.

The placenta is relatively large in the first and second trimesters. Part of women observed with temporary condition of placenta previa or low-lying placenta before 30 weeks will have a normal placental location in advancing gestational age. This phenomenon was called "Placental Migration" by King (Fig. 2.152).

Vasa Previa

Vasa previa refers to the fetal vessel, which lacks the protection of Wharton jelly and placenta, crosses within the membranes, and overlies the lower uterine segment or the cervix. Vasa previa occurs in approximately 1/2500 to 1/6000 deliveries, which is relatively rare. High-risk factors of vasa previa include placenta previa or low-lying placenta, velamentous placenta, succenturiate lobe, placenta duplex, multiple pregnancy, and IVF. According to its cause and the shape of the placenta, vasa previa can be classified into two types: type I, unilobar placenta with vasa previa (89.5%) (Fig. 2.153); type II, multilobate with vasa previa (10.5%) (Fig. 2.154).

Pernicious Placenta Previa

Pernicious placenta previa was first proposed by Saudi scholar Chattopadhyay in 1993. Pernicious placenta previa is characterized by the placenta previa with the previous cesarean section history, and the placenta is attached to the original uterine scar, often accompanied by placenta implantation. 30% ~ 50% cases of the pernicious placenta previa combine with placenta implantation. The mortality rate of pregnant women in these cases is up to 10%. The etiology is not detailed, which might be related to the erosion ability of placental villi and the imbalance between decidual tissues. High-risk factors could be maternal age, multiparous history, multiple cesarean sections, placenta previa, submucous myoma, uterine infection, and so on.

The main clinical manifestation is painless vaginal bleeding in mid and late pregnancy. Ultrasound is the most commonly used diagnostic method. The characteristics of 2-D ultrasound are as follows: ① Vortex formation in placenta (also known as "Swiss cheese"); ② A locally exophytic mass encroaches on the bladder; ③ Thinning or interruption of the vesical peritoneum; ④ Irregular retroplacental clear space. The characteristics of color Doppler ultrasound are as follows: ① Abnormal diffusion or concentration of blood flow in the lacunae;② Pasty dark areas with chaotic blood flow; ③ Highly vascularized vesical peritoneum; ④ The vessels in the sub-vesical and adjacent regions are dilated significantly. When failing to diagnose by using the abdominal ultrasound, the transvaginal ultrasound should be recommended, which is safe and more accurate (Fig. 2.155).

2.6.1.2 Ultrasonic Diagnosis

According to the relationship between the inferior placental edge and the internal cervical os, placenta previa is divided into four types:

1. Low-lying placenta: The inferior placental edge is less than 2 cm away from the internal cervical os (Fig. 2.156).
2. Marginal placenta previa: The edge of placenta is attached to the lower part of the uterus, even to the internal cervical os, but does not completely cover the internal cervical os (Fig. 2.157).

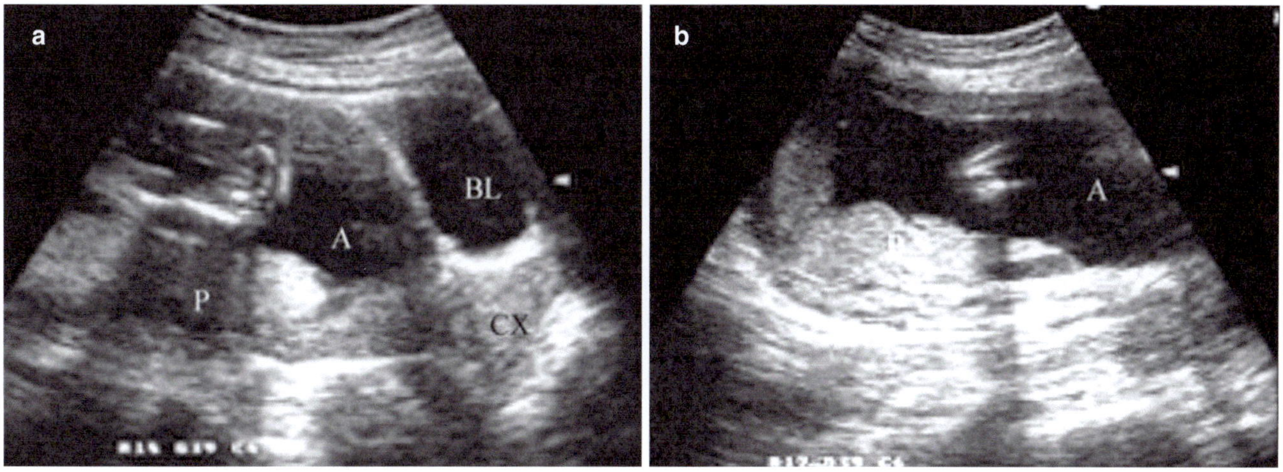

Fig. 2.152 Placental migration. (**a**). The inferior placental edge is 2.3 cm away from the cervix. (**b**). In the same case, the placental position is normal

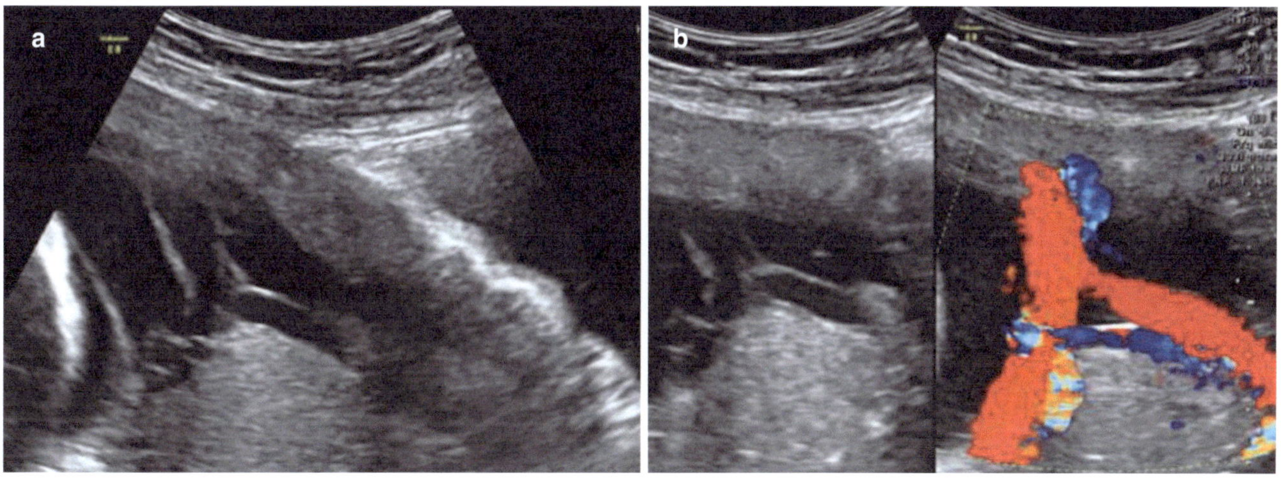

Fig. 2.153 Placenta previa combined with vasa previa and marginal cord insertion, type I

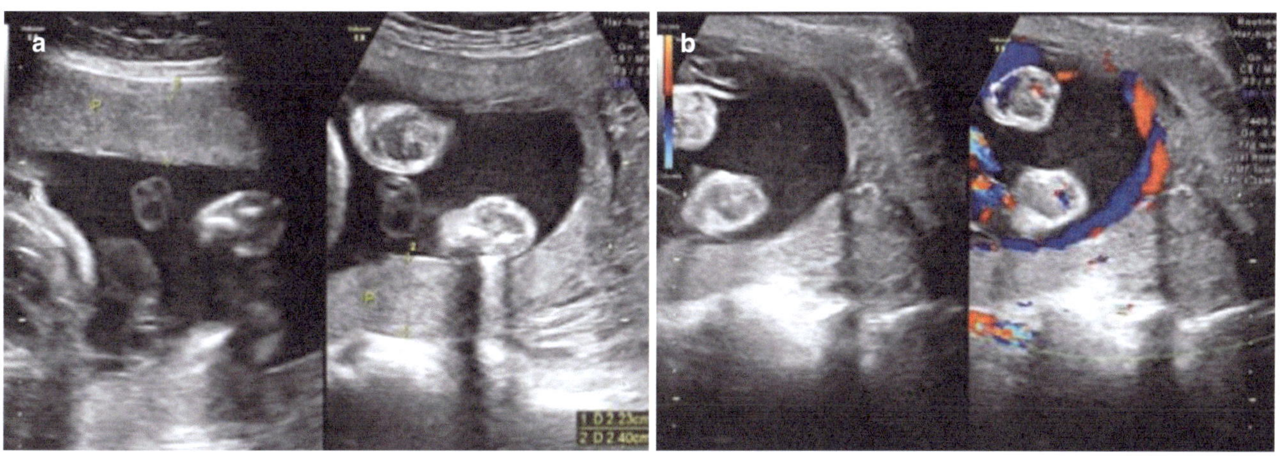

Fig. 2.154 multilobate with vasa previa, type II

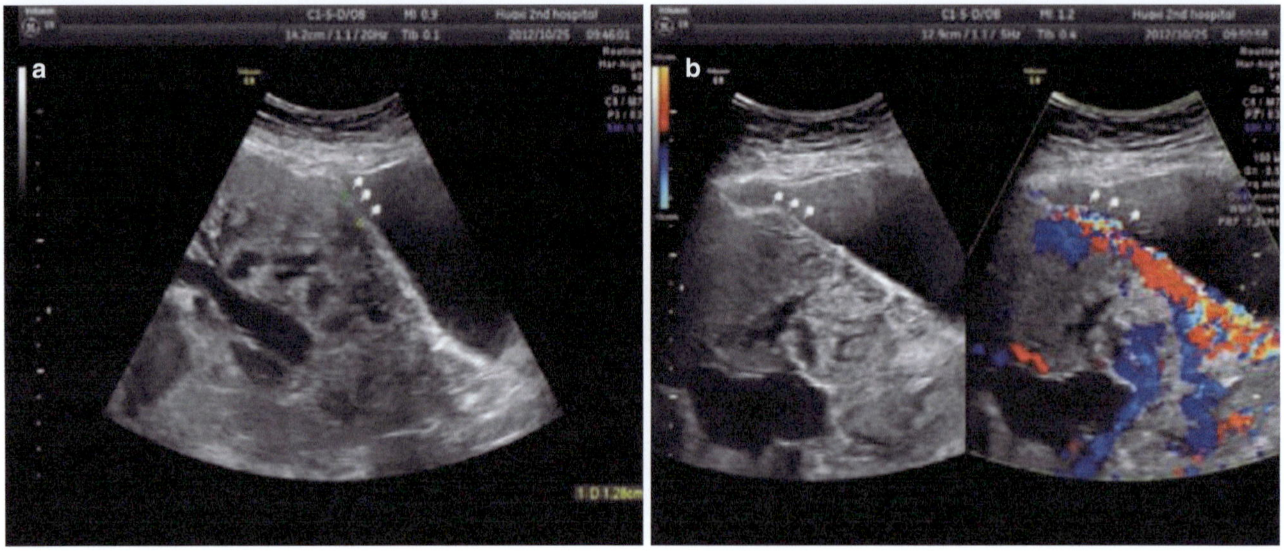

Fig. 2.155 Pernicious placenta previa. (**a**). 2-D Sonogram shows the vortex formation in placenta and the thinned vesica peritoneal extension. (**b**). Color Doppler flow imaging shows abundant blood vessels in the vesical peritoneum

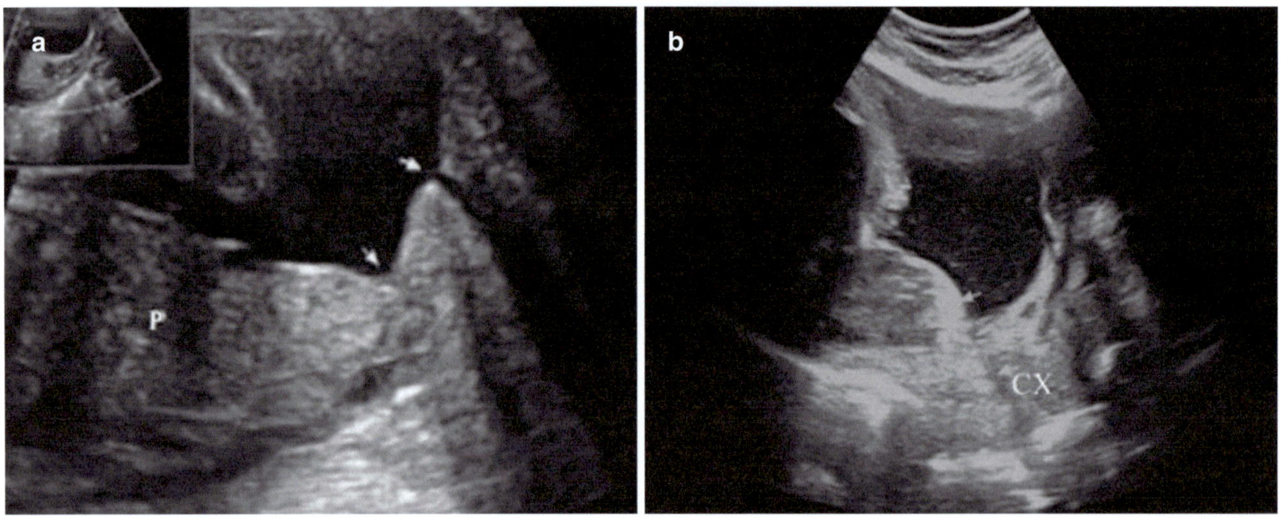

Fig. 2.156 Low-lying placenta. 33 years old and 33+ 4 weeks of gestation, the inferior placental edge is 1.56 cm away from the internal cervical os

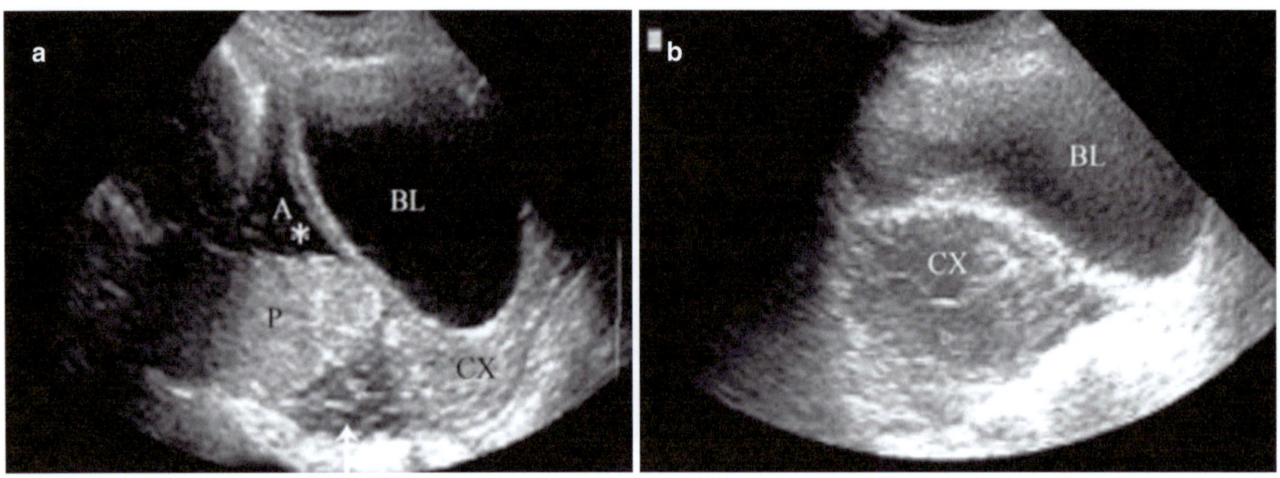

Fig. 2.157 Marginal placenta previa. 30 years old and 36 weeks of gestation, the inferior edge of the posterior placenta reaches the margin of the internal cervical os, but not cover the internal cervical os

33 years old and 33^{+4} weeks of gestation, the inferior placental edge is 1.56 cm away from the internal cervical os.

30 years old and 36 weeks of gestation, the inferior edge of the posterior placenta reaches the margin of the internal cervical os, but not cover the internal cervical os.

3. Partial placenta previa: The placenta partially covers the cervical os (Fig. 2.158).
4. Complete placenta previa: The placenta completely covers the internal cervical os (Fig. 2.159).

34 weeks of gestation, irregular vaginal bleeding for 2 weeks. a. Longitudinal section; b. Transverse section, the placenta completely covers the internal cervical os.

2.6.1.3 Special Tip

1. During transabdominal ultrasound scanning, the inferior edge of the placenta can be stretched by the overfilled bladder, resulting in the false appearance of placenta previa (Fig. 2.160).

30 years old, 28 weeks of gestation. The image shows an overfilled bladder and stretched lower uterine segment, which needs to recheck to exclude false placenta previa.

2. Due to the phenomenon of "placenta migration," it is not suitable to make a definitive diagnosis of placenta previa until followed up to about 34 weeks of gestation.
3. The median longitudinal view is utilized to distinguish the type of placenta previa by ultrasonography.

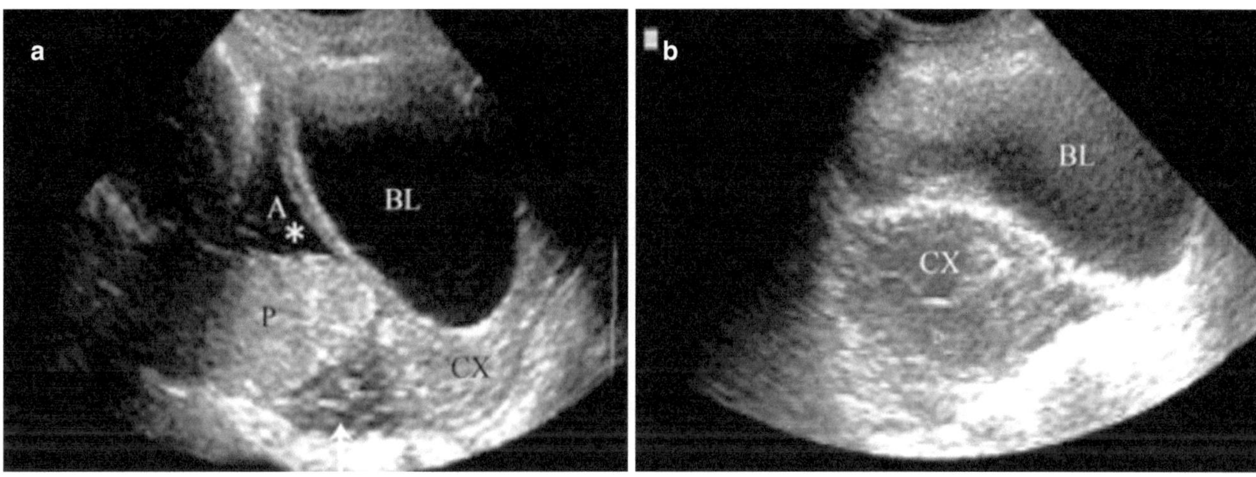

Fig. 2.158 Partial placenta previa. (**a**). At 30^{+2} weeks of gestation, the inferior edge of the posterior placenta covers the internal cervical os, with a fluid echolucent area between the internal cervical os and the region behind the placenta. (**b**). In the same case, the transverse section shows that part of the placenta covers the internal cervical os. The asterisk presents the Crucial triangle, and the arrow shows the post placental hemorrhage

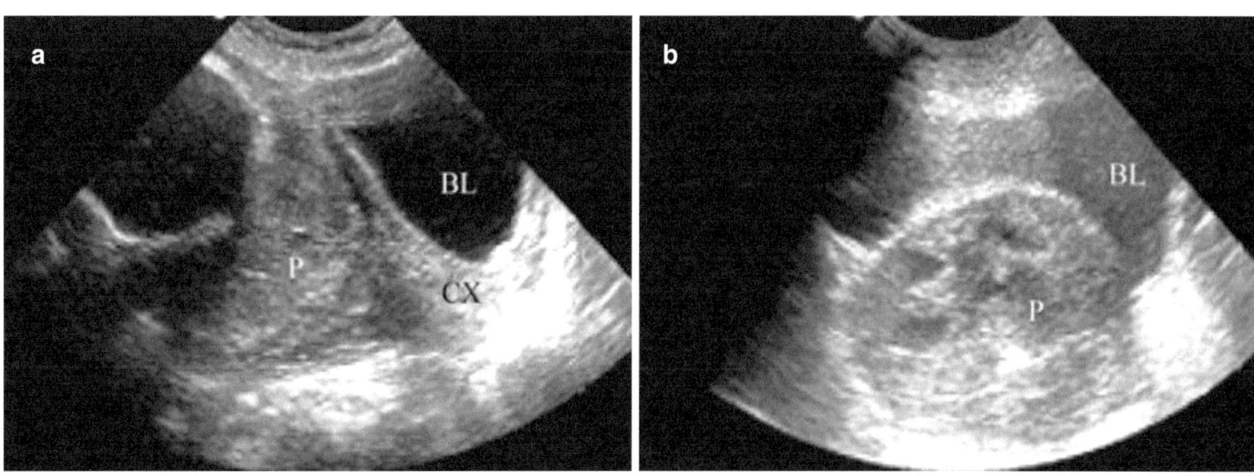

Fig. 2.159 Complete placenta previa

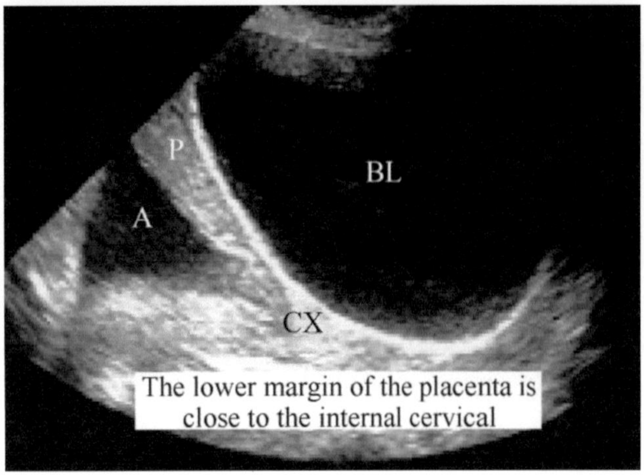

Fig. 2.160 False low-lying placenta

4. The placenta previa attached to the posterior wall is easily blocked by the fetal presentation, and is not easy to show the relationship between the inferior placental edge and the internal cervical os, which might lead to miss diagnosis. The Crucial triangle is helpful in determining the type of placenta previa. The three sides of the Crucial triangle (Fig. 2.158) are composed of the bladder wall, part of the fetal cranial ring, and part of the chorionic plate. Through the amniotic fluid in the Crucial triangle, the relationship between the inferior edge of the posterior placenta and the internal cervical os can be shown on the sonographic image.
5. Transvaginal ultrasound can accurately distinguish the relationship between the inferior placental edge and the internal cervical os. Please be gentle in examining.
6. Vasa previa have no obvious clinical manifestation before delivery, which is challenging to be detected by 2-D ultrasound features, resulting in a low prenatal diagnosis rate. Vasa previa is an obstetric emergency and the absolute indication of cesarean section. If the vasa previa is not diagnosed promptly in prenatal period, the perinatal mortality is very high. The sagittal view of the cervix and the placental umbilical cord insertion view can facilitate to improve the detection rate of vasa previa during middle pregnancy.

2.6.2 Placenta Accreta

2.6.2.1 Basic Concepts

Placenta accreta refers to the implantation of placental villi into the myometrium due to decidual dysplasia. The villi will invade the myometrium when the decidua is of defect or the decidual layer is damaged. Placenta accreta is a severe obstetric complication, which can lead to postpartum hemorrhage.

The prenatal detection rate of placenta accreta is low, which is only 2.6% reported by Gielchinsky et al.

Common risk factors include endometrial injury, placental attachment abnormalities, and cicatricial uterus.

1. Endometrial damage: Multiple abortion, intrauterine infection, intrauterine surgery, and multi-pregnancies are causes of endometrial damage.
2. Abnormal placental attachment: The placenta is attached to the lower uterine segment, cervix, and uterine horn, where the endometrium is thin and vulnerable to the invasion of villi into the uterine muscularis.
3. Cicatricial uterus: Placenta accreta happens when the placenta attaches to the scar of the uterine incision.

2.6.2.2 Ultrasonic Diagnosis

1. The placenta is slightly thickened than that of normal, the implanted placenta invades the myometrium, with an unclear boundary between the placenta and uterine wall. Some even penetrate the myometrium, forming a local protrusion. The placenta that invades the myometrium is usually hyperechoic, a few times isoechoic.
2. There are many fluid echolucent areas in the placenta, which are irregular in shape and different in size.
3. Color Doppler ultrasound shows the formation of placental vascular lacunae, which is more than 1 cm wide. There is abnormal blood flow in the retroplacental space, which is jet like.

2.6.2.3 Special Tips

1. It is challenging to diagnose placenta accreta prenatally.
2. Carefully observe the boundary between the placenta and uterine muscle wall in complete placenta previa or cesarean scar pregnancy cases, and pay attention to whether there is placenta accreta.

2.6.2.4 Typical Cases

Pregnant woman, 38 years old, G3P1 + 2. At 32 + 3 weeks of pregnancy, she is hospitalized because of vaginal bleeding for half an hour. Sonogram shows that the fetal position is normal, and the placenta is attached to the posterior uterine wall—completely covers the internal cervical os. There are multiple dilated blood sinuses in the placenta, with a maximum diameter of 4.3 cm. The retroplacental space at the lower part of the posterior uterine wall is not apparent, with

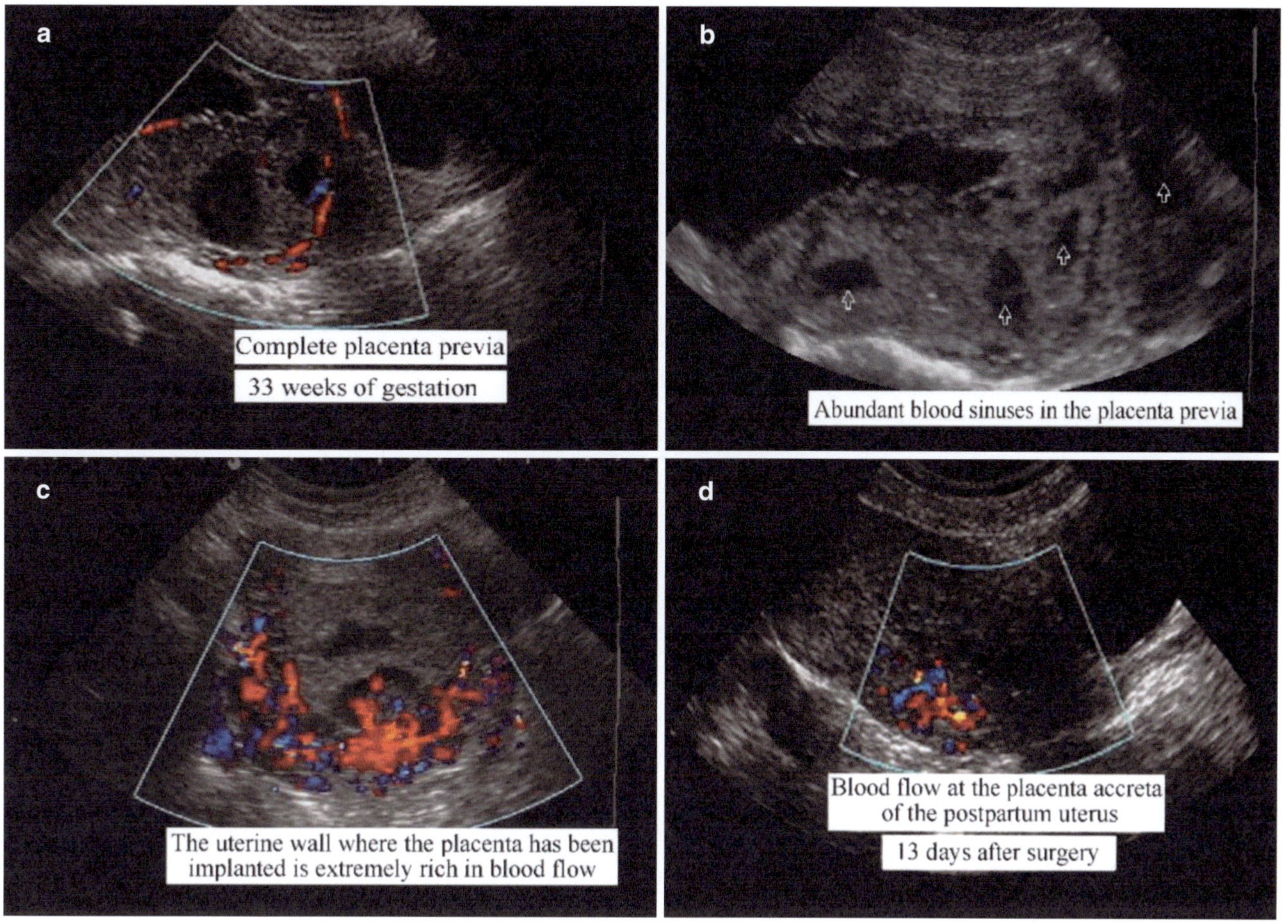

Fig. 2.161 Complete placenta previa with placenta accreta. (**a**). Complete placenta previa. (**b**). Abundant blood sinuses in the placenta. (**c**). Normal retroplacental space disappeared but with abnormal blood flow. (**d**). Blood flow at the placenta accreta of the postpartum uterus

rich blood flow. The diagnosis opinions: intrauterine live fetus; complete placenta previa; suspected partial placenta accreta. Cesarean section is performed at 34 + 4 weeks. Intraoperatively, the placenta is attached to the posterior wall and the right anterior wall of the uterus, completely covering the internal cervical os, and partially adhered or implanted to the uterus (Fig. 2.161).

2.6.3 Placental Abruption

2.6.3.1 Basic Concepts

Placental abruption is defined as a normally implanted placenta partially or completely separating from the uterine wall after 20 weeks of gestation or during the delivery period, before the delivery of the fetus. Placental abruption can be divided into the dominant abruption, recessive abruption, and mixed abruption. The incidence rate is 0.46%–2.10% in China and 1% abroad.

The placental abruption is related to severe pregnancy-induced hypertension syndrome, hypertension, placental vascular abnormality, twins, premature rupture of membranes, trauma, correction of fetal position by external transfer, excessively short umbilical cord, and other factors.

Placental abruption is divided into mild placental abruption and severe placental abruption, and vaginal bleeding is divided into dominant bleeding and recessive bleeding. The patient may have mild abdominal pain in mild placental abruption cases, and persistent abdominal pain, back pain, board-like rigidity, and even shock in severe placental abruption cases.

2.6.3.2 Ultrasonic Diagnosis

1. There are liquid echolucent areas with an unclear boundary between the placenta and uterine wall, without visible blood flow. Depending on the course of bleeding, the irregular masses may appear in enhanced or sonolucent echo (Figs. 2.162 and 2.163).

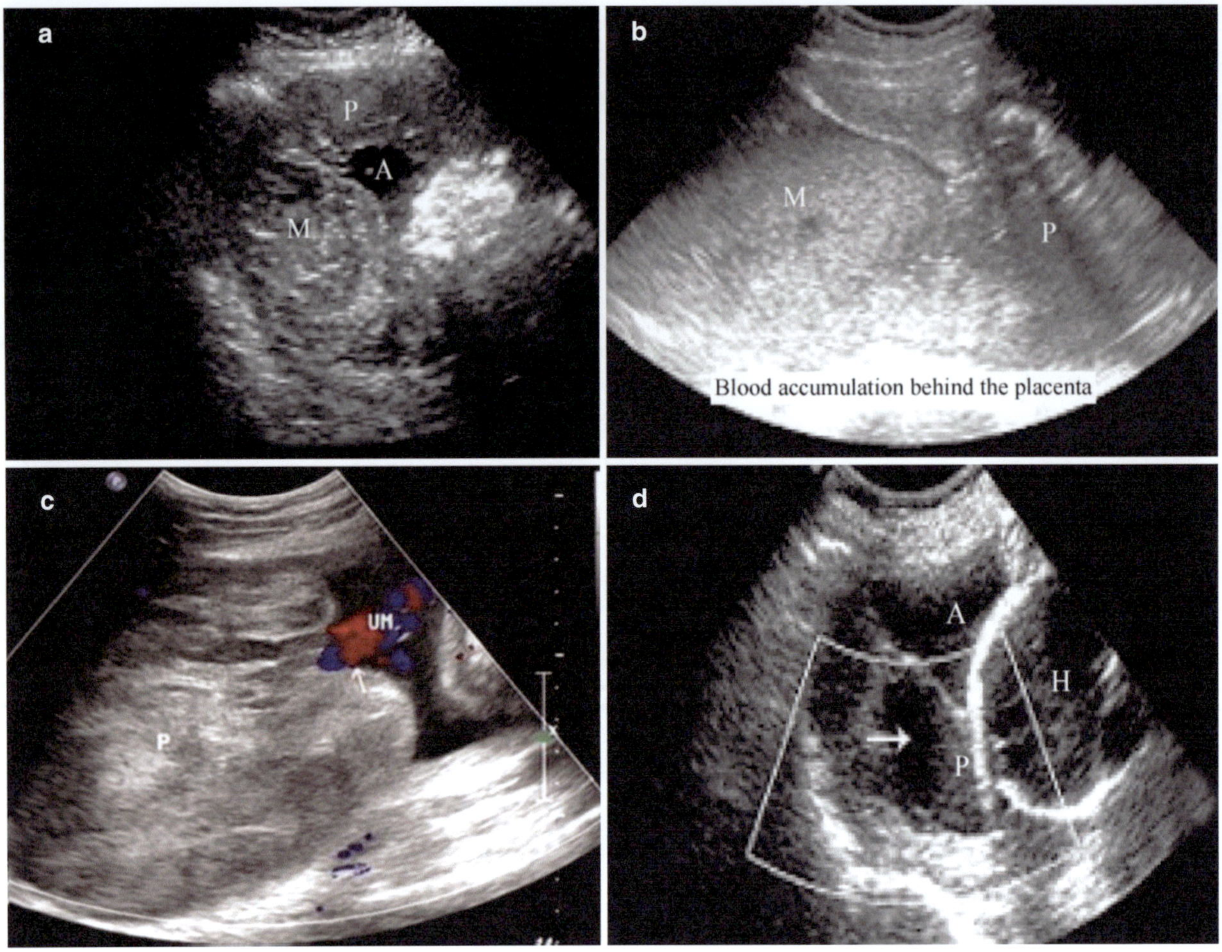

Fig. 2.162 Placental abruption (I) (**a**). The patient is 31 years old and at 31 weeks of gestation. The placenta is located in the right anterior wall, and there is a heterogeneous hyperechoic mass, 9.6 cm × 7.4 cm × 10.7 cm, in the maternal surface of the right posterior placenta, protruding into the amniotic cavity; (**b**). The patient is 27 years old and at 23 weeks of gestation. The placenta is located in the posterior uterine wall. A homogeneous hypoechoic mass, 5.1 cm × 5.4 cm × 10 cm, is observed between the maternal surface of the placenta and the muscle wall; (**c**, **d**). The patient, 25 years old and at 27 weeks of gestation, is suffering from abdominal pain and vaginal bleeding. The placenta is located at the right anterior wall, 7.1 cm in thickness, and protrudes into the amniotic cavity

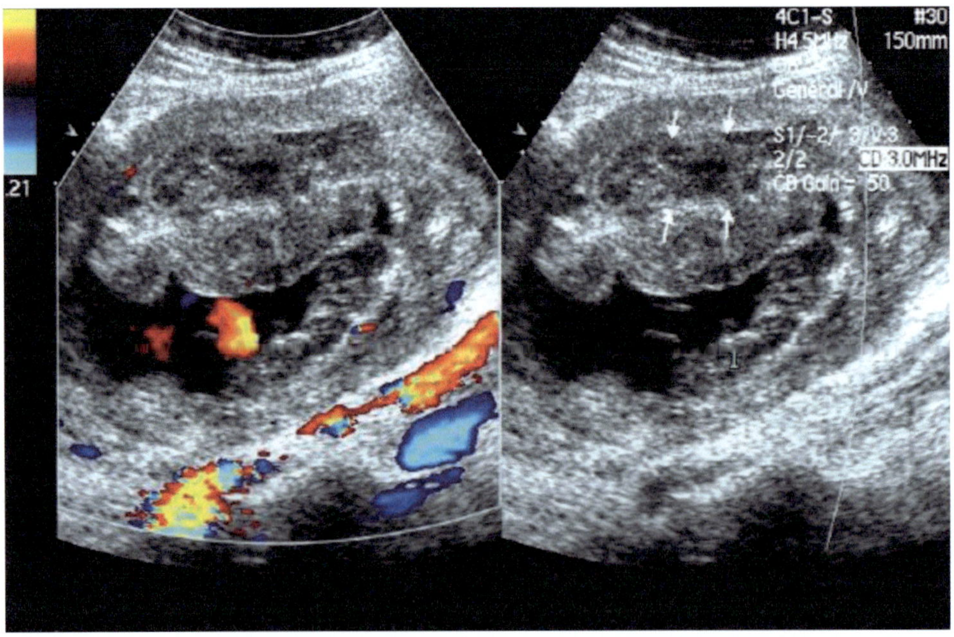

Fig. 2.163 Placental abruption (II). The fluid echolucent area is visible between the fetal membrane and the posterior uterine wall

A subchorionic fluid echolucent area with an unclear boundary is visible under the fetal surface of the placenta.

2. The placenta protrudes into the amniotic cavity.
3. If blood breaks into the amniotic cavity, floating hyperechoic dots or mass—representing the clot, can be observed in the amniotic fluid.
4. Extremely large abruption area may lead to decreased fetal heart rate, even the disappearance of fetal heartbeat and fetal movement.
5. When detecting the blood or blood clot posterior to the placenta and the sign that fetal membrane peeling from the uterine wall, Michael considered that the diagnosis of placental abruption is valid.

2.6.3.3 Special Tips

1. The sonographic appearance of placental abruption is extremely variable depending on the location, type, amount of bleeding, and the bleeding course in different placental abruption cases.
2. Ultrasound has some limitations in the diagnosis of mild placental abruption because of its untypical clinical symptoms and physical signs.
3. In the case of posterior placenta abruption, ultrasonography diagnosis may be influenced by the thickness of the abdominal wall and the placental position.
4. The placental abruption should be distinguished from the retroplacental venous plexus, local contractions of the uterine wall in the second trimester, retroplacental leiomyoma, blood sinus in the placenta, placenta previa, and threatened rupture of the uterus.

2.6.4 Placental Tumor

2.6.4.1 Basic Concepts

The placental tumor is rare and can be divided into primary tumors and metastatic tumors. Primary tumors are chorioangioma and teratoma, etc. The metastatic tumors are extremely rare, most of which are malignant melanomas caused by hematogenous metastasis.

Placenta Hemangioma

Chorioangioma, also known as placental hemangioma, is a benign tumor with morbidity of 0.5% to 1%. Placenta hemangioma, single or multiple, locates on the surface of the placenta in most cases and some lie in the placental parenchyma. The tumor size varies with the gestational age.

Placental hemangioma affects fetal growth and development by changing the placental blood flow and disrupting normal blood supply. Small placental hemangioma, less than 5 cm in diameter, has no effect on the development of fetus or the pregnant women. If the placental hemangioma is larger than 5 cm, it may cause compression symptoms, polyhydramnios, prenatal bleeding, pregnancy-induced hypertension syndrome, premature delivery, fetal heart enlargement, stillbirth, etc.

Placenta Teratoma

Placenta teratoma is extremely rare, with less than 10 cases reported in literature. The tumors are mostly located on the fetal surface of the placenta, between the amnion and chorionic membrane, or on the fetal membrane at the edge of the placenta. Placenta teratoma is round or oval in shape, with a conspicuous boundary, and 5–8 cm in diameter.

2.6.4.2 Ultrasonic Diagnosis

Placenta Hemangioma

1. The tumor is a round mass with a conspicuous boundary. The larger placental hemangioma often protrudes into the fetal surface. The hemangioma lying on the maternal surface or parenchyma is usually small with solid isoechoic.
2. Part of the large hemangioma has pattern-shaped and strip calcification, accompanied by polyhydramnios, or fetal development abnormalities (Figs. 2.164 and 2.165).
3. Abundant blood flow signals in the placental hemangioma are visible (Fig. 2.166).

Placenta hemangioma with hyperechoic calcification.

Placenta Teratoma

1. Placenta teratoma is characterized by a cystic and solid mass with a smooth surface (Fig. 2.167).
2. Calcification is visible in 40% of the cases, showing hyperechoic mass with posterior attenuation.
3. Color Doppler shows no blood flow signals in most of the masses.

2.6.4.3 Special Tips

1. The placental hemangioma should be differentiated from uterine leiomyoma. Uterine leiomyoma is mostly located in the uterine muscle wall, closely related to the uterine wall, with surrounding annular blood flow. Uterine leiomyoma has no relation to the placental blood flow (Fig. 2.168).
2. As the placental hemangioma grows fast, we should recheck the placental hemangioma regularly to observe its size dynamically.

2.6.5 Umbilical Cord Abnormality

2.6.5.1 Basic Concepts

The umbilical cord is the link connecting the placenta to the fetus, and the link of blood circulation between the mother

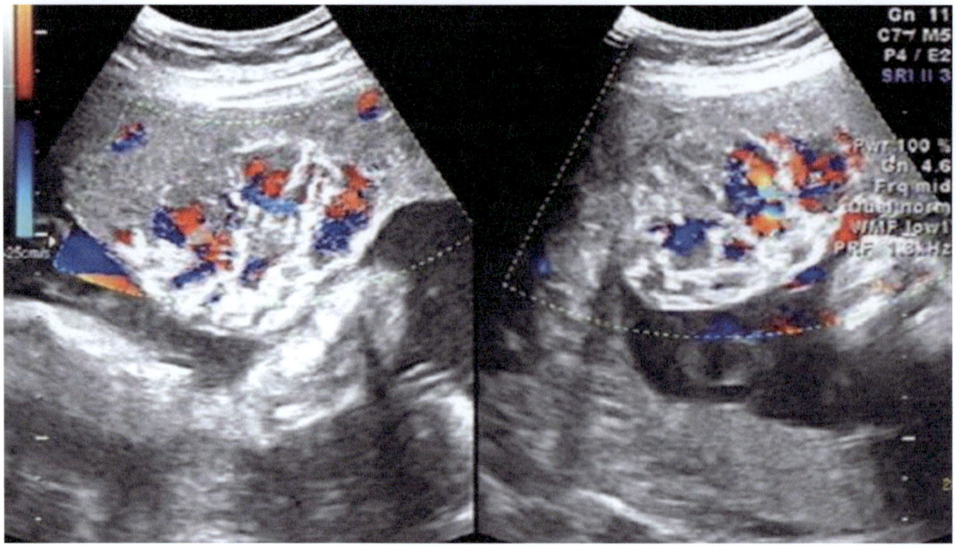

Fig. 2.164 Placenta hemangioma(I)

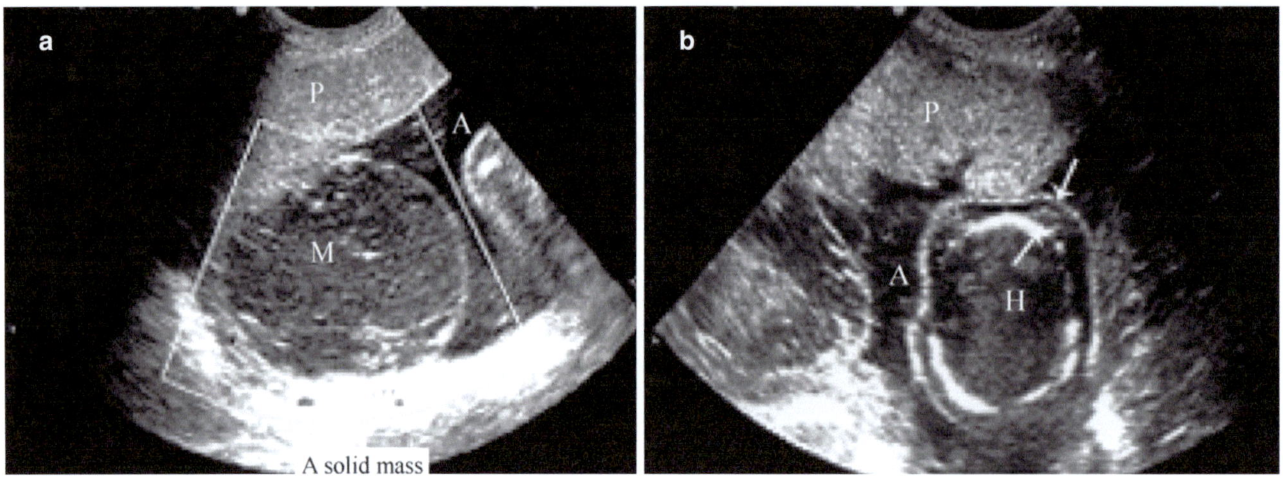

Fig. 2.165 Placenta hemangioma (II). (**a, b**). The patient is 20 years old, at 25 weeks of gestation. The fetus has died. The placenta is near the fundus of the uterus. A solid hypoechoic mass with conspicuous boundaries on the placental fetal surface is visible, protruding into the amniotic cavity. Fetal scalp edema is shown. M represents the hemangioma

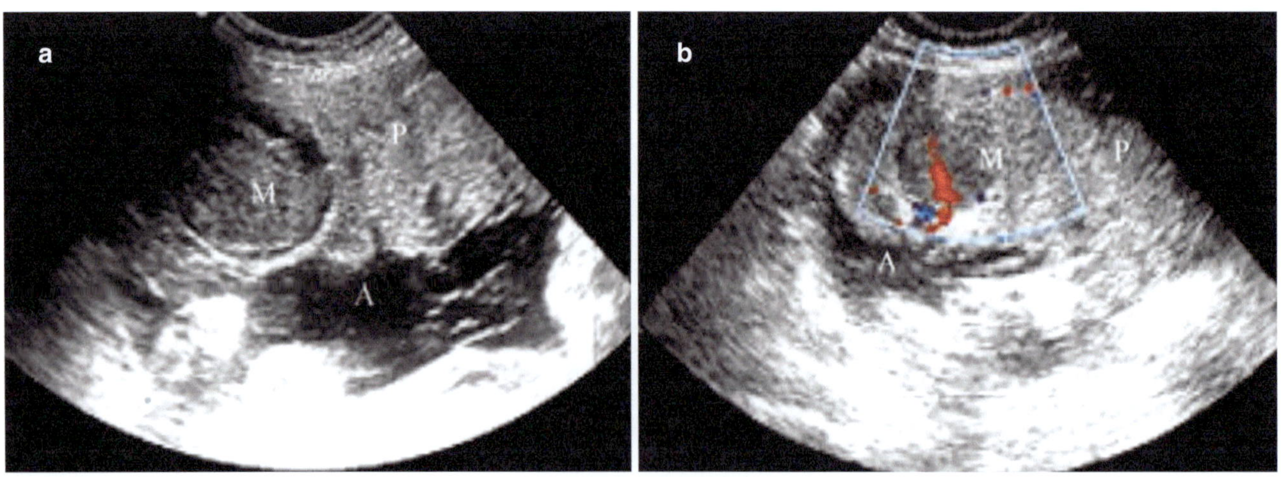

Fig. 2.166 Placenta hemangioma (III). (**a, b**). The same patient is 29 years old, 32 + 4 weeks gestation, and the placenta is located in the anterior wall. Sonogram shows a 4.8 cm × 3.8 cm × 4.8 cm hypoechoic mass in the parenchyma, with visible color blood flow. The reexamination one month later shows that the placenta mass is larger, with a size of 6.8 cm × 5.4 cm × 6.3 cm. M shows hemangioma

and the fetus. The umbilical cord of a term fetus is 40–60 cm in length, 1.5–2.0 cm in diameter, which is approximately the same as the length of the fetus. Excessively short umbilical cord refers to the umbilical cord is shorter than 30 cm, while those longer than 70 cm in excessively long umbilical cord cases. The umbilical cord is curved and floats in the amniotic cavity.

Umbilical Cord Coiling

The incidence is 13.7%–20%. Nuchal umbilical cord is the most common, which occurs in 25% of pregnancies, followed by umbilical cord coiling of the trunk and limbs. 1 to 2 loops of the nuchal cord are common; multiple loops of the nuchal cord are rare.

Umbilical Cord Twist

The umbilical cord twist can be up to 6 to 7 loops under physiological conditions, and it may endanger the fetal life when the umbilical cord twists more than 11 loops.

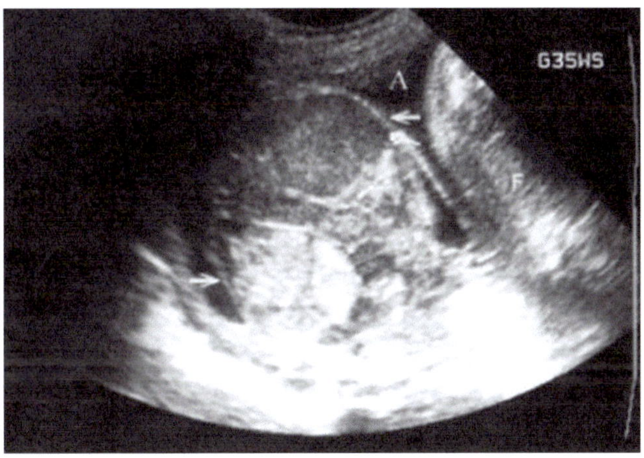

Fig. 2.167 Placenta teratoma

Single Umbilical Artery

Single umbilical artery happens in about 1% of pregnancies, 25%–30% of which combined with a variety of severe visceral malformation. The perinatal mortality is 20%.

Umbilical Cord Cyst

Umbilical cord cysts are divided into pseudocyst and true cyst. Pseudocyst, without capsule, is a kind of cyst with different sizes, caused by focal hydropic or metamorphosed Wharton jelly. A true cyst is the remains of an embryo with a layer of epithelial cells lining the cyst wall, formed by a yolk or allantoic sac.

The Umbilical Cord Insertion into the Placenta

The umbilical cord normally inserts to the center of the placenta or the eccentric position in about 90% cases. Marginal cord insertion is defined as the cord insertion is less than 2 cm away from the edge of the placenta. Velamentous cord insertion refers to the condition that the umbilical cord inserts into the fetal membrane beyond the edge of the placenta, and the blood vessels enter the placenta between the chorionic and amniotic membranes, in fan-shaped and distributed like sails.

2.6.5.2 Ultrasonic Diagnosis

Umbilical Cord Coiling

1. The 2-D ultrasound image is characterized by a "U" or "W" shaped or serrated impression of the neck skin on the longitudinal section of the fetus.
2. Color Doppler flow imaging (CDFI) shows the red and blue garland-like umbilical cord around the neck of the fetus. Appropriately slant the probe to show a complete multicolor umbilical cord around the neck.
3. A "U" or "W" shaped impression on the fetal surface is visible if the umbilical cord twists around the fetal body (Fig. 2.169).

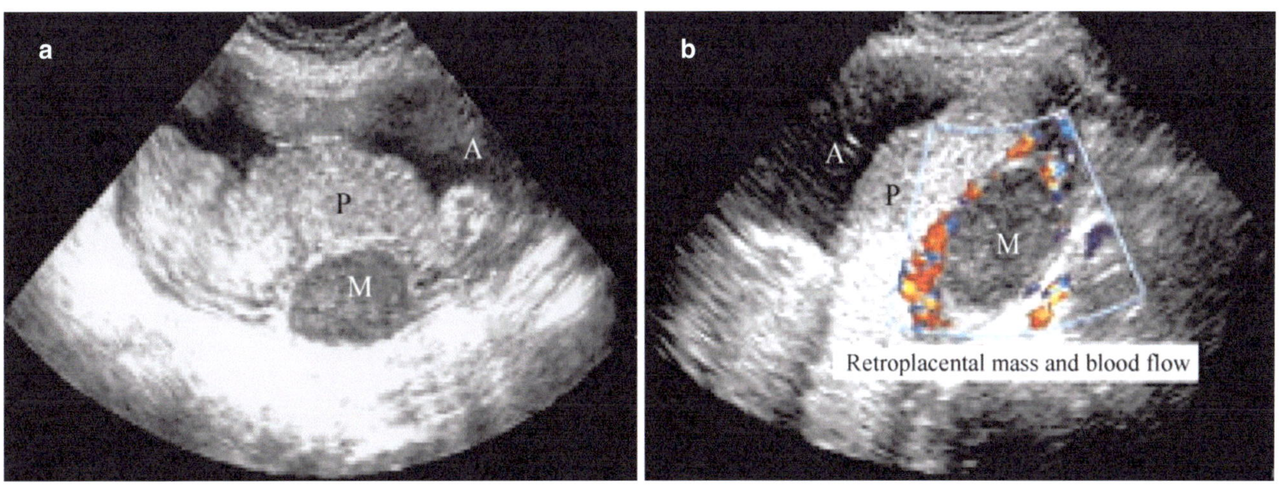

Fig. 2.168 Myoma of uterus. (**a**, **b**). The patient is 30 years old and at 28 weeks of pregnancy. Sonogram shows solid hypoechoic mass between the posterior placenta and the muscle wall, with a conspicuous boundary and surrounding blood flow. M represents the myoma

Umbilical Cord Twist

CDFI of the normal umbilical cord is a red-and-blue structure in the shape of a Chinese fried dough twist. In the absence of a cord helix, the shape of twist disappears, and the red-and-blue blood flow in cord vessels are parallel.

Single Umbilical Artery

1. The transverse view of the cord shows only one umbilical artery and one umbilical vein, representing two parallel circles in the shape of the Chinese character "吕" (Fig. 2.170).
2. On the longitude view, only one umbilical artery can be found under multidirectional scanning, and its inner diameter is larger than the normal umbilical artery.
3. CDFI shows two circular structures, one is in red color, and the other is blue.

Umbilical Cord Cyst

1. The cyst is a round anechoic area with a smooth surface. It protrudes to one side of the umbilical cord, floating in amniotic fluid with the umbilical cord (Fig. 2.171).

   The cyst protrudes to one side of the umbilical cord.
2. Umbilical cord cyst mostly occurs in the umbilical ring or the beginning part of placenta of the fetus, generally 3–4 cm in diameter. Once the blood vessel is compressed, the fetus may die.
3. CDFI shows no blood flow signal inside the cyst.

Abnormal Umbilical Cord Insertion into the Placenta

Abnormal umbilical cord insertion includes marginal cord insertion and velamentous cord insertion (Fig. 2.172).

2.6.5.3 Special Tips

1. In the second trimester, the umbilical cord, twisting around the neck or limbs, can be self-released. The fetus is endangered in multiple loops twisting cases, with deep impression around the neck.
2. In single umbilical artery cases, observe in detail to exclude the fetal malformation and IUGR.
3. The cord cyst wall is thin, floating in amniotic fluid, which is easy to be missed.

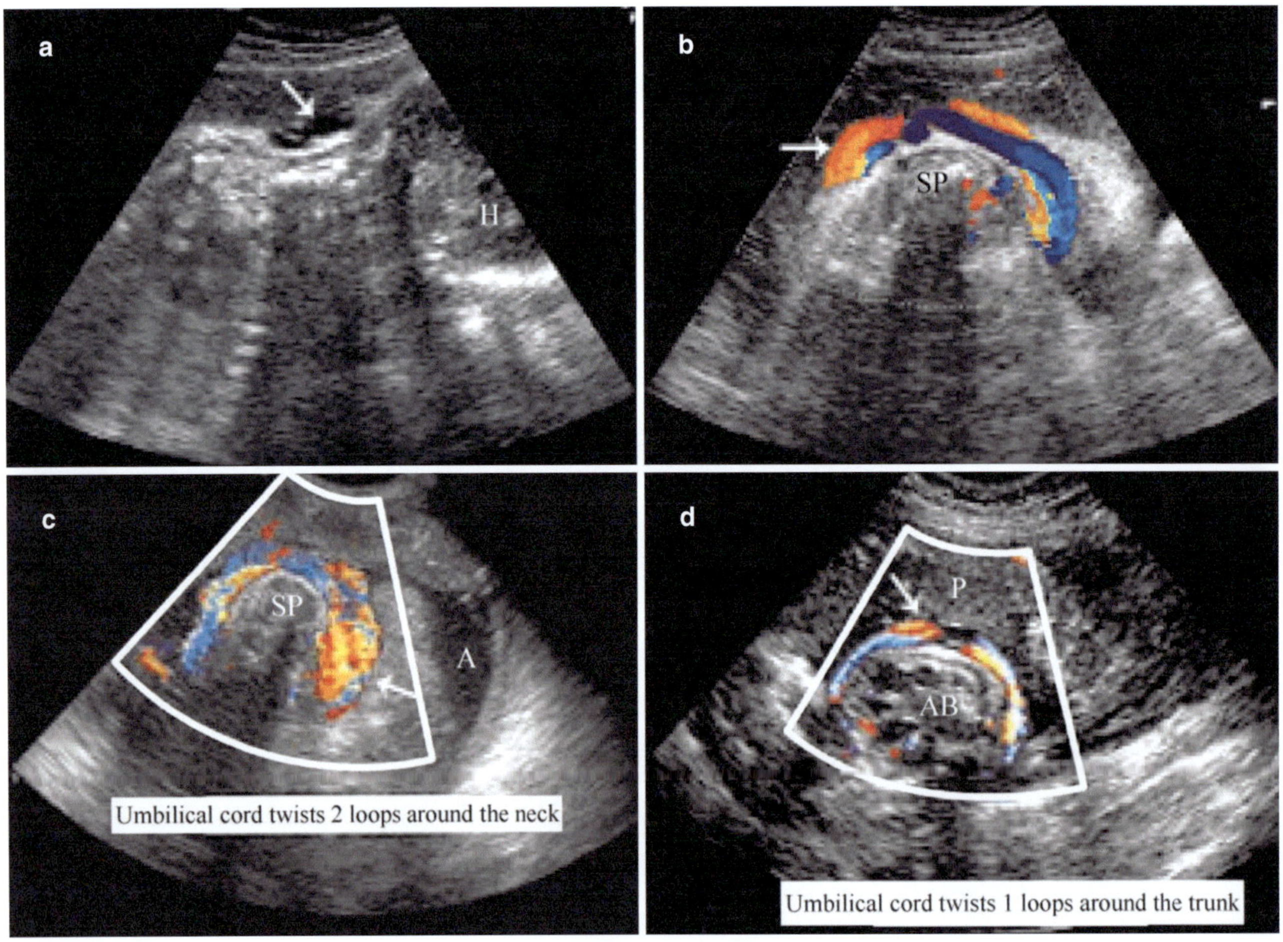

Fig. 2.169 The umbilical cord twists around the neck and trunk. a. There is a "W" shape impression on the neck of the fetus in a 2-D ultrasound image. b,c. CDFI shows the umbilical cord twists 1 and 2 loops. d. Umbilical cord twists one loop around the fetal body

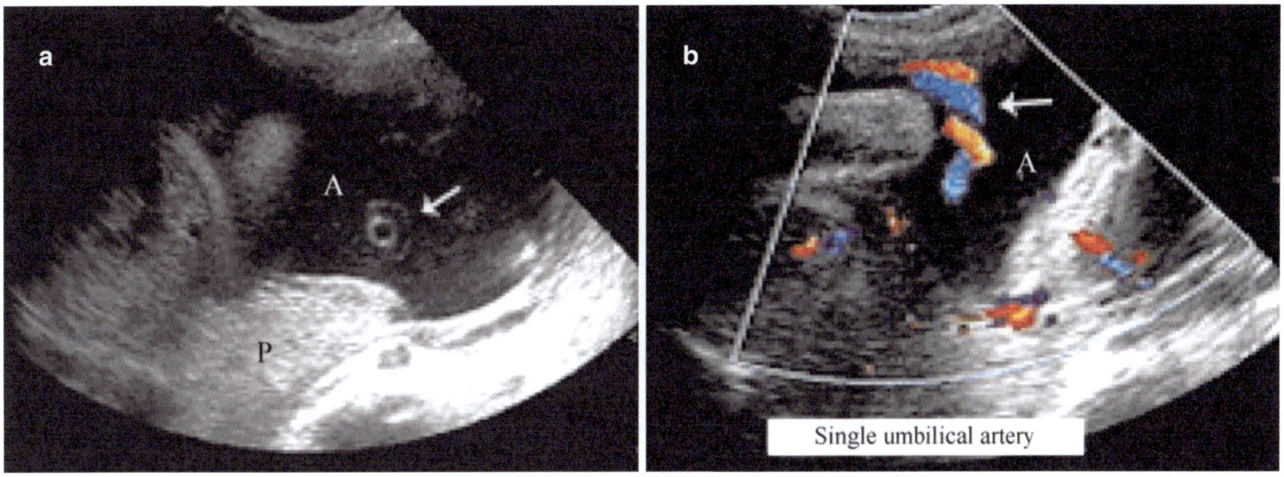

Fig. 2.170 Single umbilical artery. (**a, b**). The same patient 31 years old, at 37 + 1 week gestation. The image shows the umbilical cord in the shape of "吕" in amniotic fluid in the transverse view, and color blood flow shows only one artery and one vein. The arrow shows the single umbilical artery

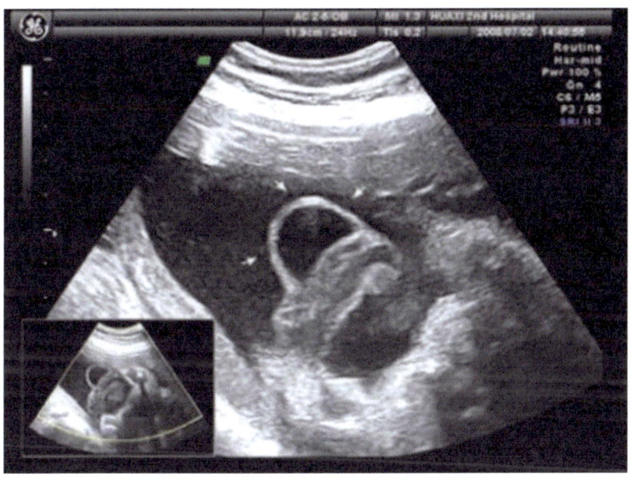

Fig. 2.171 Umbilical cord cyst

2.6.6 Polyhydramnios and Oligohydramnios

2.6.6.1 Basic Concepts

Polyhydramnios

Polyhydramnios is defined as the volume of the amniotic fluid more than 2000 ml in the third trimester, which can be divided into chronic polyhydramnios and acute polyhydramnios.

Oligohydramnios

Oligohydramnios refers to the volume of the amniotic fluid less than 300 ml at the term of pregnancy. Oligohydramnios always happens in the early or second trimester, leading to miscarriage.

Oligohydramnios is often accompanied by fetal urinary tract malformation, and the prognosis of the fetus is poor if oligohydramnios occurs in the early or second trimester of pregnancy.

2.6.6.2 Ultrasonic Diagnosis

1. Prenatal ultrasound can accurately diagnose polyhydramnios or oligohydramnios.
2. The ultrasonic diagnosis criteria of polyhydramnios and oligohydramnios are: the vertical depth of amniotic fluid is more than 8 cm in polyhydramnios cases, and the vertical depth of amniotic fluid is less than 2 cm in oligohydramnios. Amniotic fluid index (AFI) method: if the AFI is greater than 20 cm, it means polyhydramnios; if the AFI is less than 5 cm, it is oligohydramnios.
3. The fetus sinks to the posterior uterine wall in polyhydramnios cases, which makes it difficult to observe the fetal spine (Fig. 2.173).
4. The boundary between amniotic fluid and the fetal body surface cannot be seen well in oligohydramnios cases; the fetal structure is challenging to display (Fig. 2.174).

2.6.6.3 Special Tips

1. About 20% of pregnant women with polyhydramnios are combined with fetal dysplasia. Notice the fetal malformation during the ultrasound examination.
2. Pay attention to fetal urinary system abnormality in oligohydramnios cases.
3. During the ultrasound scanning, we should pay attention to the fetal malformation caused by the mechanical compression of oligohydramnios, such as Potter syndrome.

2.7 Ultrasonic Diagnosis of Cervical Insufficiency in Pregnancy

2.7.1 Basic Concepts

Cervical insufficiency of pregnant women, that is, the relaxation of the internal cervical os, is one of the major causes of

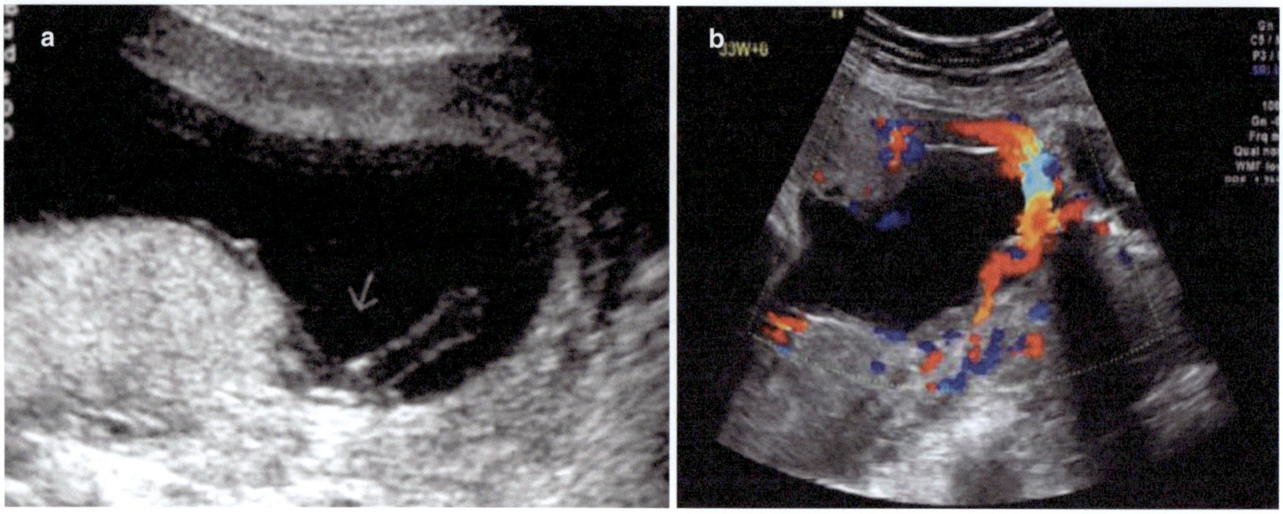

Fig. 2.172 Abnormal umbilical cord insertion. (**a**). Marginal cord insertion: it shows the cord insertion at the edge of the placenta. (**b**). Velamentous cord insertion: the cord inserts between the chorionic and amniotic membranes

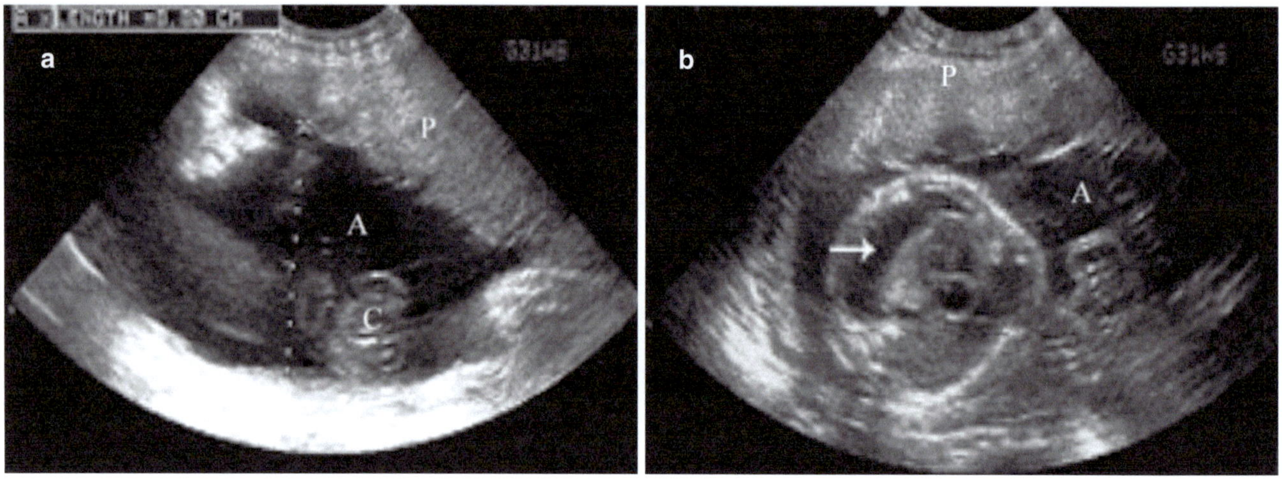

Fig. 2.173 Polyhydramnios. (**a, b**). The same patient, at 33 weeks of gestation. Polyhydramnios with fetal pleural effusion (arrow)

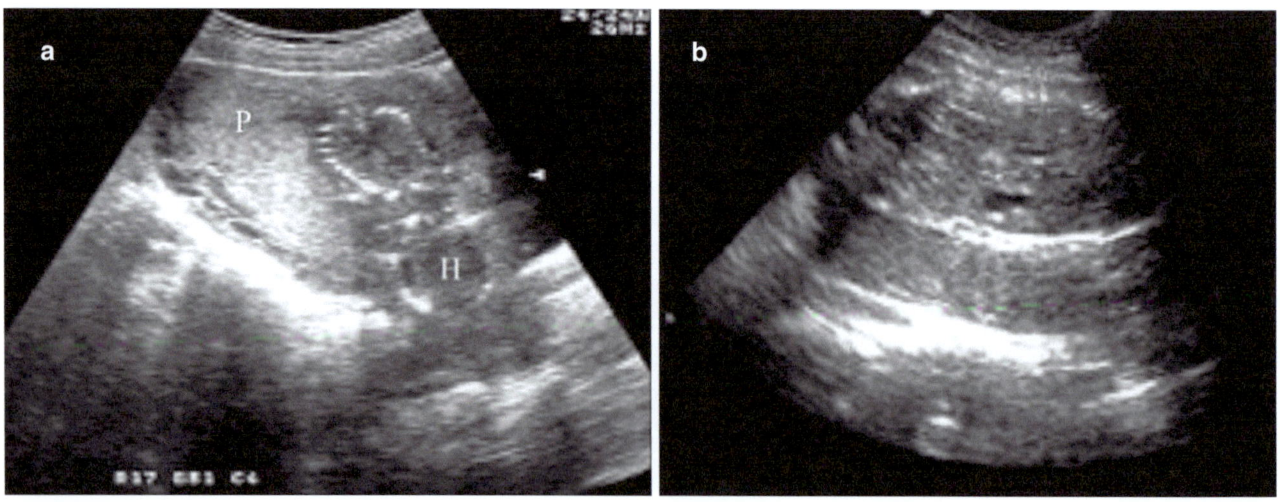

Fig. 2.174 Oligohydramnios. (**a**). At 3 months of gestation, there is extremely little amniotic fluid, and the fetus is close to the uterine wall and the placenta. (**b**). At 27 weeks of gestation, no amniotic fluid is visible

recurrent late miscarriage and premature birth. After the second and third trimesters of pregnancy, the fetus and its appendages grow fast, the pressure in the uterine cavity increases and the fetal sac protrudes into the internal cervical os, leading to abortion or premature delivery.

For pregnant women with threatened preterm delivery, cervical examination is often used to evaluate preterm delivery. However, multiple examinations may promote preterm delivery. Since the 1980s, ultrasound has been used to evaluate the cervical morphology, including length changes of the cervix during pregnancy and dilatation of the internal cervical os. Ultrasound is utilized to screen patients at risk of premature birth and monitor the treatment of threatened premature birth.

For pregnant women who have a history of habitual abortion or cervical insufficiency, ultrasound helps to choose clinical treatment or a proper position for cervical cerclage after the second trimester, providing a method to evaluate the prognosis after cerclage or fetal protection.

Ultrasound is used to measure the length of the cervix from the time of pregnancy or 2 weeks before the previous miscarriage, observing whether the internal cervical os is dilated and whether the fetal sac is protruded into the cervical canal. The common methods include transabdominal ultrasound and transvaginal ultrasound.

2.7.1.1 Transabdominal Ultrasound

Before the examination, the moderately filled bladder and amniotic fluid are used to form an acoustic window. Observe the length of the cervix, whether there is dilatation of the internal cervical os, and whether the amniotic fluid is embedded into the cervix on the sagittal view.

2.7.1.2 Transvaginal Ultrasound

The patient should empty the bladder before the examination, and take the bladder lithotomy position. After sterilizing the vulva, place the sterilized condom over the disinfected vaginal probe, and insert the vaginal probe into the vagina for longitudinal fan scanning. Observe the whole cervix and the amniotic cavity between the internal cervical os and the uterus, and observe whether the internal cervical os is dilated or whether amniotic fluid is embedded into the cervix.

2.7.2 Ultrasonic Diagnosis

1. Under the moderately filled bladder, the internal cervical os of the normal cervix in pregnancy is closed, the cervical canal is not dilated, and the cervical length is more than 3 cm (Fig. 2.175).

Transabdominal scanning shows the cervical length and the shape of the internal cervical os during pregnancy.

2. Using ultrasound to measure cervical length changes, and observe the internal cervical os if there is dilatation, and the width and depth of the dilatation should be measured to evaluate the prognosis of preterm labor. The cervical length of 131 normal women in early, middle, and late pregnancy was measured in our hospital. The results confirmed that the cervical length was significantly shortened after term pregnancy, which was consistent with the cervical physiological changes during pregnancy. In another study, TVS was chosen to measure the cervical length and observe the shape of the internal cervical os of 52 pregnant women, who had been clinically diagnosed as threatened preterm delivery. According to the ROC curve, taking the cervical length of 17 mm as the critical value, was the best choice to predict the outcome of preterm delivery (Figs. 2.176, 2.177, and 2.178).
3. The dilatation of the internal cervical os and amniotic sac embedding into the cervix are reliable indications for preterm birth.
4. The nonpregnant cervix and the internal cervical os are closed, and there is no individual morphological change on the ultrasound image. It is almost impossible to determine whether the internal cervical os is dilated or not, and there is no objective criterion for dilatation. Therefore, the clinical gynecological examination is a unique method. In non-pregnancy, cervical insufficiency should be considered when the cervical dilator (7–8 mm), can easily get through the internal cervical os; cervical relaxation is suspected when feeling the external cervical os is relaxed with bimanual examination.

At 33 $^{+5}$ weeks of gestation, clinical diagnosis: threatened preterm labor. Ultrasound shows that the cervical length is 2.1 cm, without amniotic fluid embedded in the internal cervical os. Keep on fetal protection treatment until term delivery.

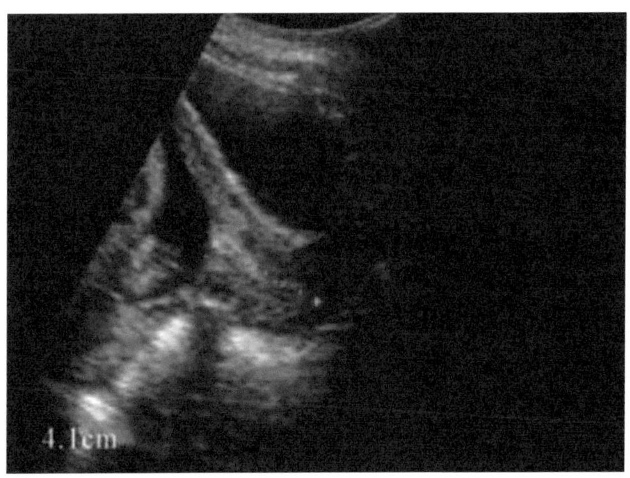

Fig. 2.175 Normal cervix during pregnancy

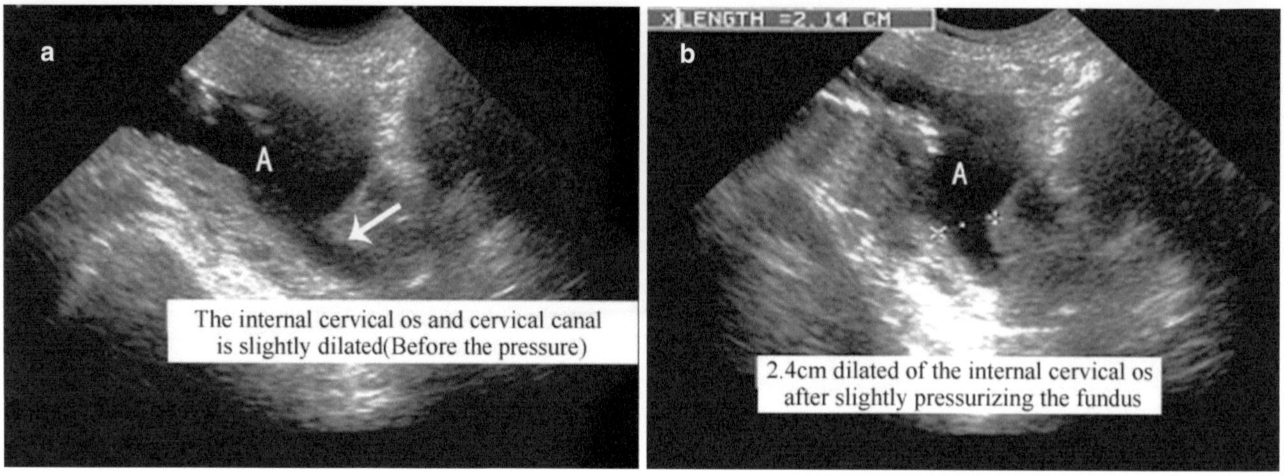

Fig. 2.176 Cervix dilatation(I). (**a**). The patient had recurrent miscarriage for 3 times. At 34 weeks of gestation, the clinical diagnosis is threatened preterm birth, the cervical length is less than 2.0 cm, and the internal cervical os is slightly dilated by 1.0 cm. (**b**). The amniotic fluid was embedded into the cervical canal and 2.4 cm dilated after slightly pressurizing the fundus. Preterm labor occurred 3 days later

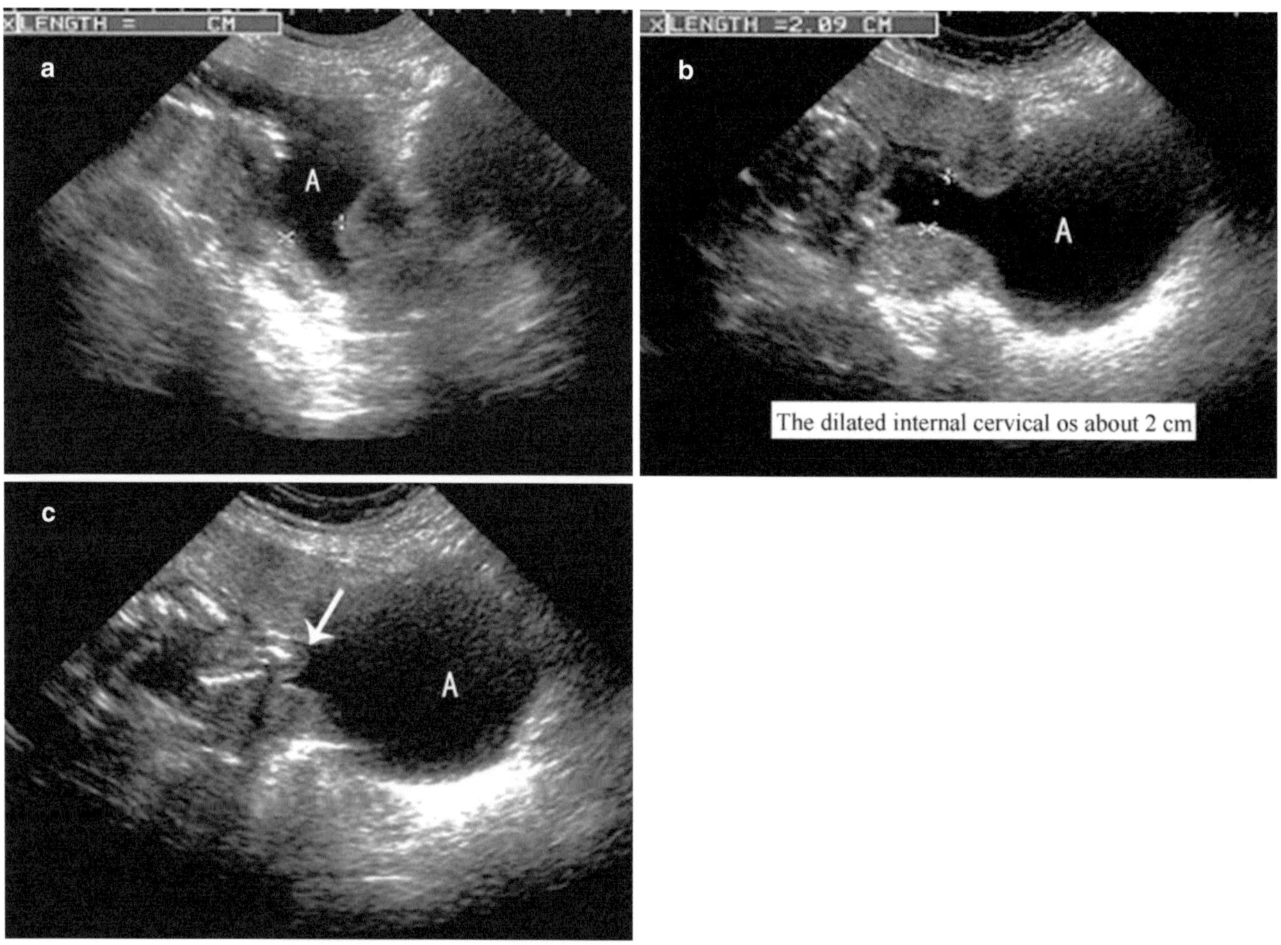

Fig. 2.177 Cervix relaxation (II). (**a**). The patient had 5 pregnancies with spontaneous abortion. At 26 weeks of the sixth pregnancy, the sonogram shows the shortened cervix and the dilated internal cervical os, about 1.5 cm. (**b, c**). The cervical canal is obviously dilated after 2 days, the amniotic sac has protruded into the vagina, and premature delivery occurred once more

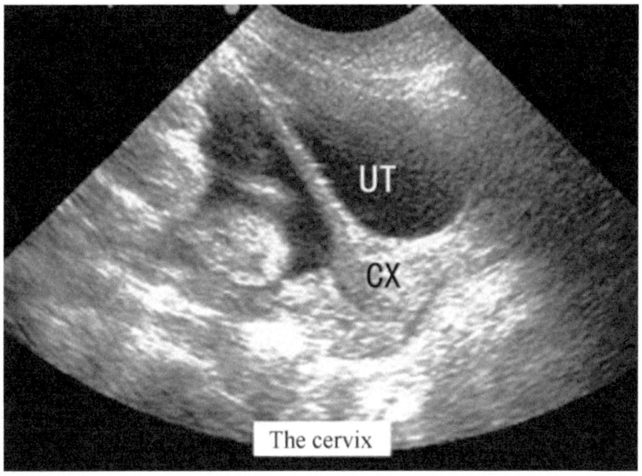

Fig. 2.178 Threatened preterm birth

2.7.3 Special Tip

1. The moderately filled bladder is necessary for pregnant women to observe the relaxation of the internal cervical os with transabdominal ultrasound.
2. In order to observe whether there is dilatation in the internal cervical os, we can compress the uterine fundus when there is no uterine contraction.
3. Transvaginal ultrasound can show more details of the cervix. Be gentle and careful to avoid excessive pressure. Affected by the probe pressure, the dilated cervix may contract and close, resulting in missed diagnosis of cervical insufficiency.
4. The length of the cervix may change spontaneously during examination (Fig. 2.179).

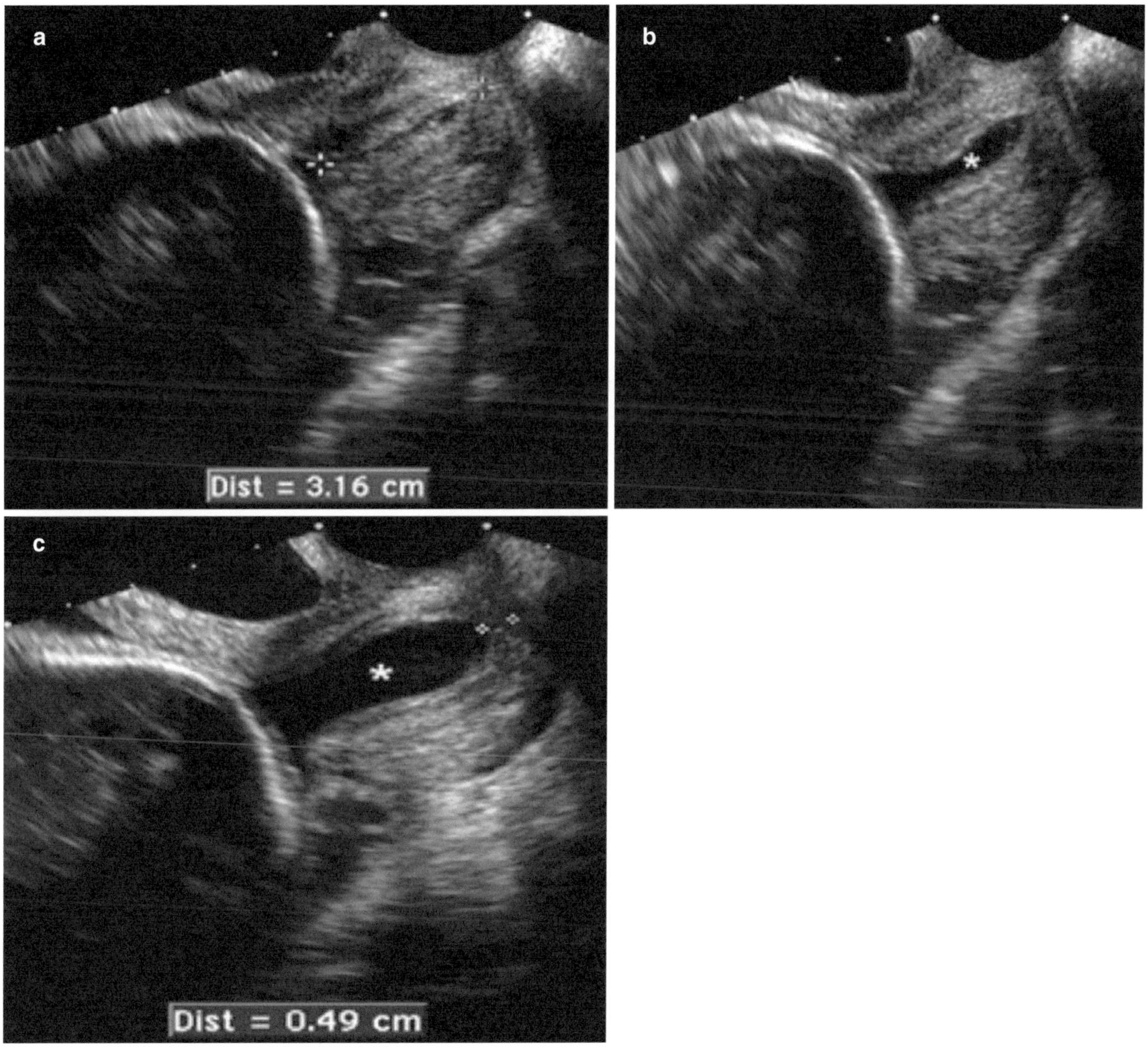

Fig. 2.179 Cervical spontaneous change. (**a**). The vaginal sagittal view shows the cervix with normal length, which is about 3.16 cm. (**b**). About 20 seconds later, cervical canal is moderately dilated (*). (**c**). Twenty more seconds later, the cervix dilates further, and the remaining closed part is only 0.49 cm in length

2.8 Ultrasonic Diagnosis of Abnormal Puerperium

2.8.1 Basic Concepts

Puerperium refers to the process from the delivery of placenta to the recovery of all organs of the whole body to the normal prepregnancy state, generally 6 weeks. During the puerperium, the maternal reproductive organs may undergo genital infection, bleeding, poor recovery, and other abnormalities, because of childbirth, trauma, decreased body resistance, and the invasion of some pathogenic bacteria in the body.

The clinical manifestation of puerperal abnormality is varied, common puerperal infectious diseases are as follows: acute vulvitis, acute vaginitis, acute cervicitis, acute endometritis, myositis, acute pelvic peritonitis, diffuse peritonitis, acute pelvic connective tissue inflammation, acute salpingitis, postpartum hemorrhage, placenta residue or implantation, incision infection of the abdominal wall or uterus, etc.

Ultrasound cannot diagnose all abnormal diseases in the puerperium, but provide a reference for clinical diagnosis and treatment through some abnormal ultrasound images of the genitals. Ultrasound is utilized to locate and qualitatively diagnose inflammatory mass, abscess, and intrauterine residue.

2.8.2 Ultrasonic Diagnosis

2.8.2.1 Acute Endometritis

The uterus of the patients with poor involution is larger than that of the normal puerperal uterus. Heterogeneous speckled echo and strong strip echo in the dark area of effusion are visible in the uterine cavity. The uterine cavity line is not apparent or hypoechoic (Fig. 2.180).

2.8.2.2 Acute Pelvic Parametritis and Abscess

The uterus is larger than the normal puerperal uterus, the outline is indistinct, and echo of the myometrium is nonuniform. Irregular, inhomogeneous, and hypoechoic area and fluid echolucent area without boundaries are visible beside the uterus or in the pelvic cavity. There are complex echoes or cystic masses on both sides or posterior to the uterus, some of which even surround and adhere to the uterus, leading to an indistinguishable uterine boundary (Figs. 2.181 and 2.182).

2.8.2.3 Gestational Residual Pregnancy Tissue

The uterus is large, with poor involution. The hyperechoic strip in the uterine cavity represents residual membranes. Residual placenta is characterized by irregular, heterogeneous, hyperechoic solid tissue of different sizes in the uterine cavity. Color Doppler image shows a little blood flow around the residual placenta (Fig. 2.183).

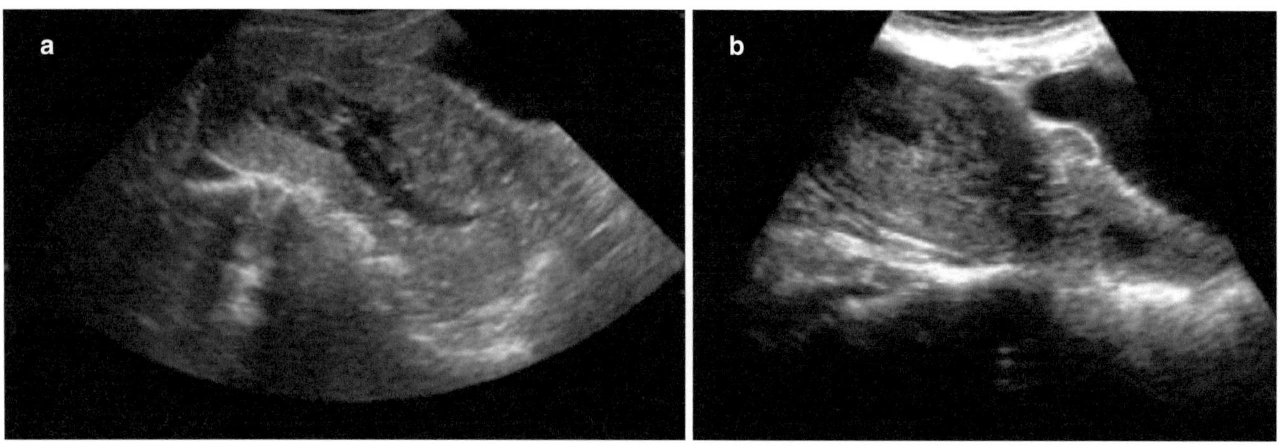

Fig. 2.180 Acute endometritis. (**a**). Large uterus, inhomogeneous, and hypoechoic endometrium. (**b**). Endometritis after induced labor, inhomogeneous endometrium with some liquid echolucent area

2.8.2.4 Postpartum Placenta Implantation

Complete placenta implantation shows the enlarged uterus, and the hyperechoic mass occupied the whole uterine cavity. Partially placental implantation is characterized by a part of the myometrium missing or interrupted, without a distinct boundary between the placenta and uterus. The placenta implants to the serosa layer, with surrounding blood flow (Fig. 2.184).

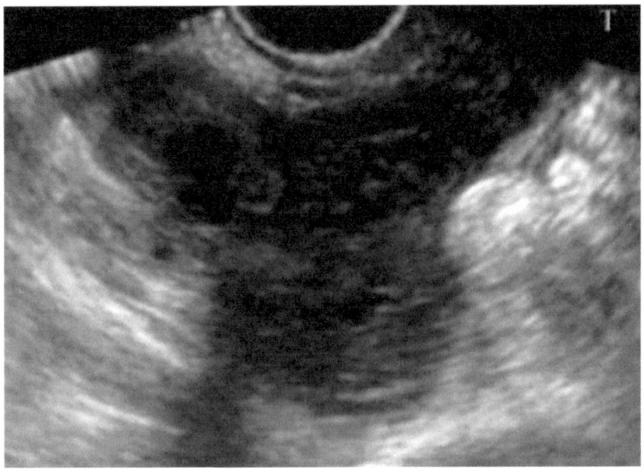

Fig. 2.181 Acute pelvic parametritis. On the eighth day after delivery, the patient has pain in the lower abdomen, with increased body temperature and increased white blood cells. Sonogram shows the indistinguishable uterus contour and surrounding irregular hypoechoic tissue

2.8.2.5 Abnormal Uterine Incision after Cesarean Section

Transabdominal or transvaginal scan shows the enlarged uterus, hypoechoic, anechoic, or hyperechoic anterior uterine wall incision, protruding to the bladder. The cloudy-shaped and flocculent echo can be seen in the mass. In severe cases, the continuous echo of serosa layer on the lower part of the anterior uterine wall is interrupted, even with anechoic diverticulum (Fig. 2.185).

2.8.2.6 Abdominal Wall Hematoma and Pelvic Hematoma

Irregular spindle-shaped hypoechoic lesion is visible under the abdominal incision. The hematoma forms a mass, locates under the peritoneum, and protrudes into the abdominal cavity. Pelvic hematomas are mostly located in the incision of the anterior wall and the side of the uterus. The hematoma shows homogeneous hypoechoic spots, and hyperechoic mass in the long duration hematoma (Fig. 2.186).

2.8.2.7 Foreign Body of the Abdominal Cavity

The foreign body mass with posterior attenuation is visible in the abdominal cavity or pelvic cavity. The mass is extremely hyperechoic in the near field, with a waterfall-like posterior attenuation shadow (Fig. 2.187).

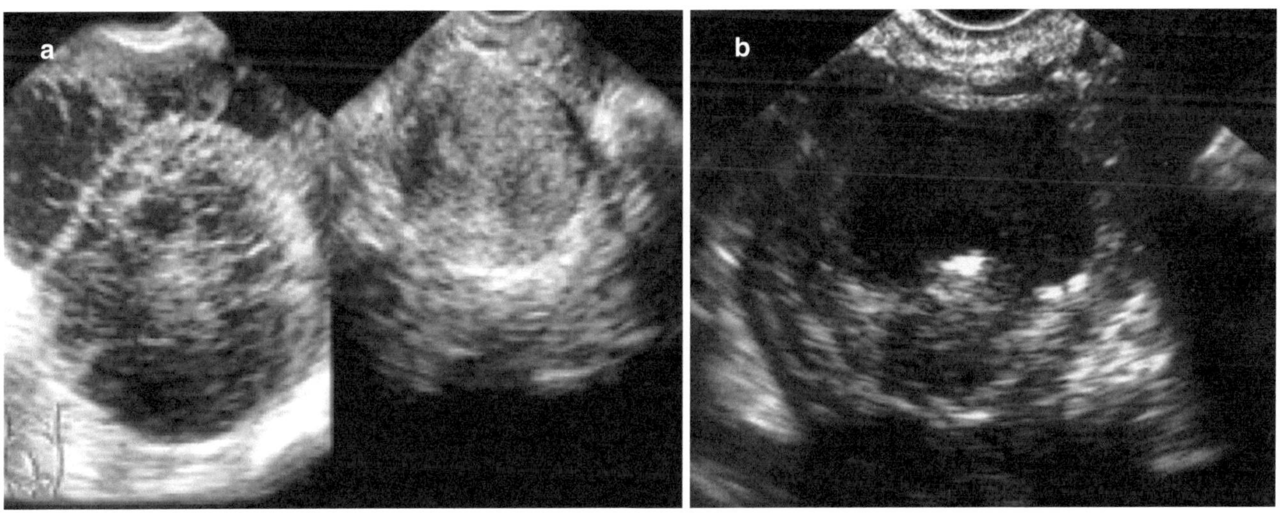

Fig. 2.182 Postpartum pelvic inflammatory mass. (**a**). 11 days after labor induction, the patient has a fever and abdominal pain. Ultrasonography examination shows the heterogeneous, irregular masses on the right side of the pelvic cavity without a conspicuous boundary. (**b**). On the 20th day after delivery, the patient has abdominal pain. Ultrasonography shows a cyst in the pelvic cavity, with unclear fluid and flocculent hyperechoic

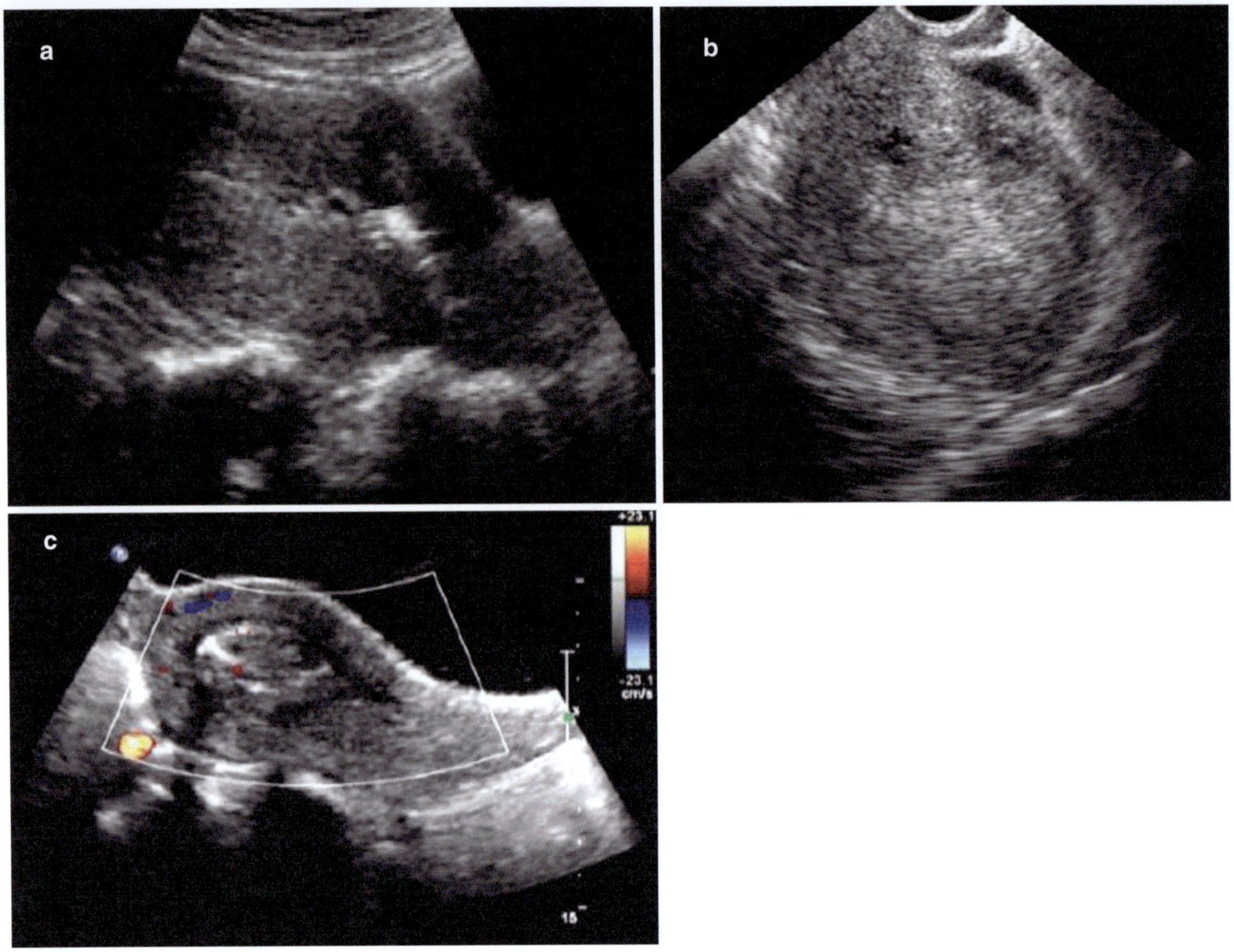

Fig. 2.183 Intrauterine pregnancy residue after delivery. (**a**). On the sixth day after delivery, area of increased echogenicity is found in the lower segment of the uterine cavity. The discharged mass is residual fetal membrane; (**b, c**). The space-occupying lesion is found in the intrauterine cavity, **b** shows a homogeneous mass of increased echogenicity in the uterus, c shows the echo enhancement of the intrauterine residue with posterior attenuation, and the discharged mass is the residual placenta and organized tissue

2.8.3 Ultrasound Findings

1. The patients with postpartum hemorrhage or puerperal infection should be routinely examined by ultrasound.
2. Pay attention to whether there are space-occupying lesions and liquid echolucent areas in the pelvic cavity, and observe the size of the uterus, the echo of the muscle wall, and residue in the uterine cavity. Note the healing of the uterine incision and abdominal wall incision in cesarean section cases.
3. Expand the scope of scanning to the above pelvic parts, which is conducive to detect lesions other than uterine appendages.

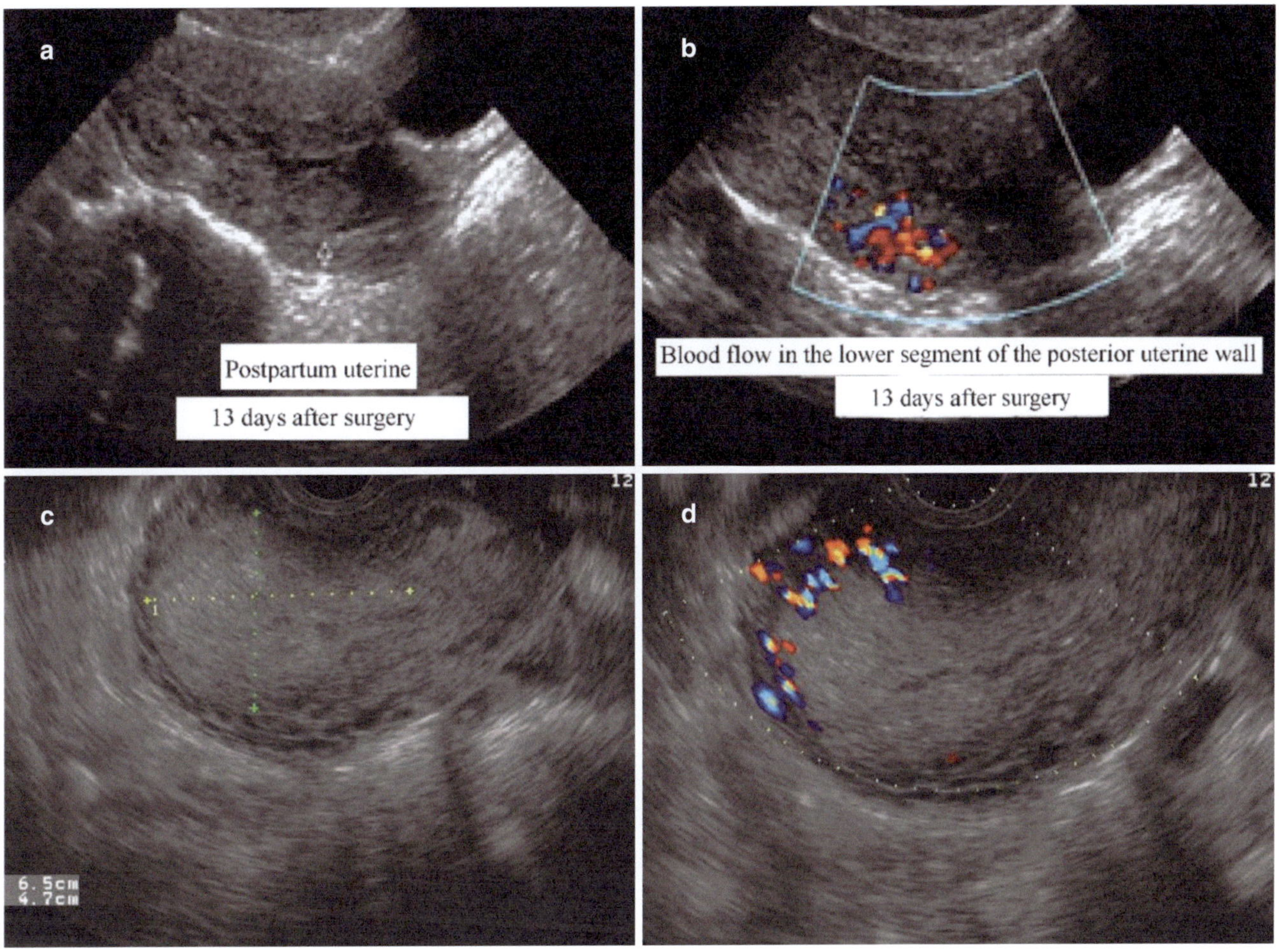

Fig. 2.184 Postpartum partial placenta implantation. (**a, b**). The patient is diagnosed with placenta implantation by ultrasound before the operation and confirmed by cesarean section. After 2 weeks of fetal preservation treatment, a mass in the lower segment of the posterior uterine wall is shown, with surrounding blood flow; (**c, d**). Incomplete placental abruption after induced labor. A hyperechoic mass is visible, at the right corner of the uterine cavity, 6.5 cm in diameter, which is connected with the uterine cavity, and without surrounding blood flow. No residue is scraped out after two times of curettage, and finally the placenta is removed by laparotomy

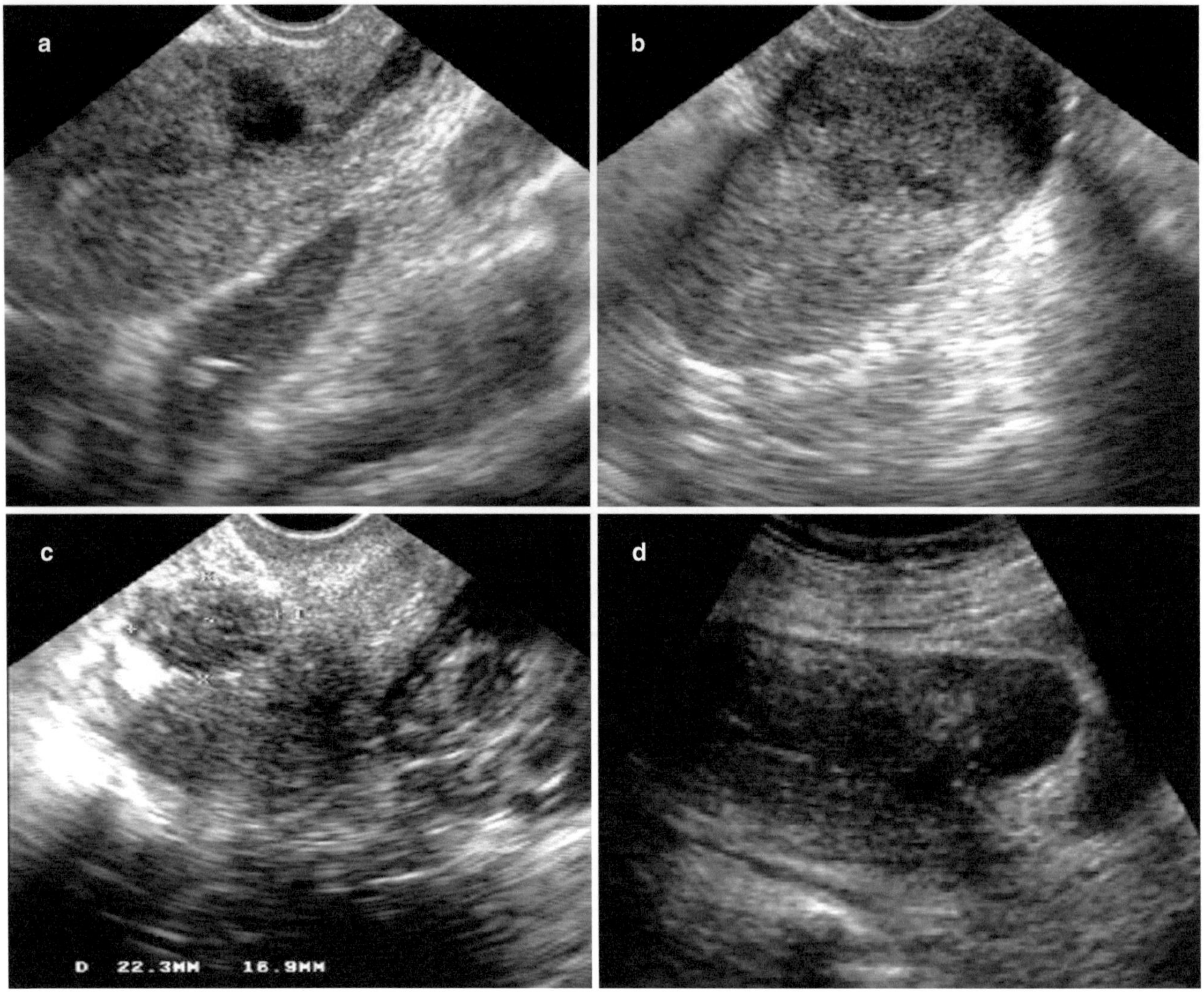

Fig. 2.185 Abnormal anterior wall incision of the postpartum uterus. (**a**). At 50 ⁺ days after delivery, the puerpera has vagina bleeding. Sonogram shows irregular hypoechoic mass at the incision of the anterior uterine wall, with a diameter of about 2.0 cm. (**b**). On the 40th day after delivery, the hypoechoic mass is found in the incision of the lower segment of the anterior uterine wall, with unclear boundary. (**c**). On the 18th day after delivery, a hypoechoic mass with a diameter of 2.0 cm is visible under the serous membrane of the anterior uterine wall, which is a hematoma. (**d**). On the 17th day after delivery, the puerpera has vaginal bleeding and fever. Transabdominal scan shows a hypoechoic mass, 3.0 cm in diameter, at the incision of the lower segment of the anterior uterine wall, with the liquid echolucent area inside

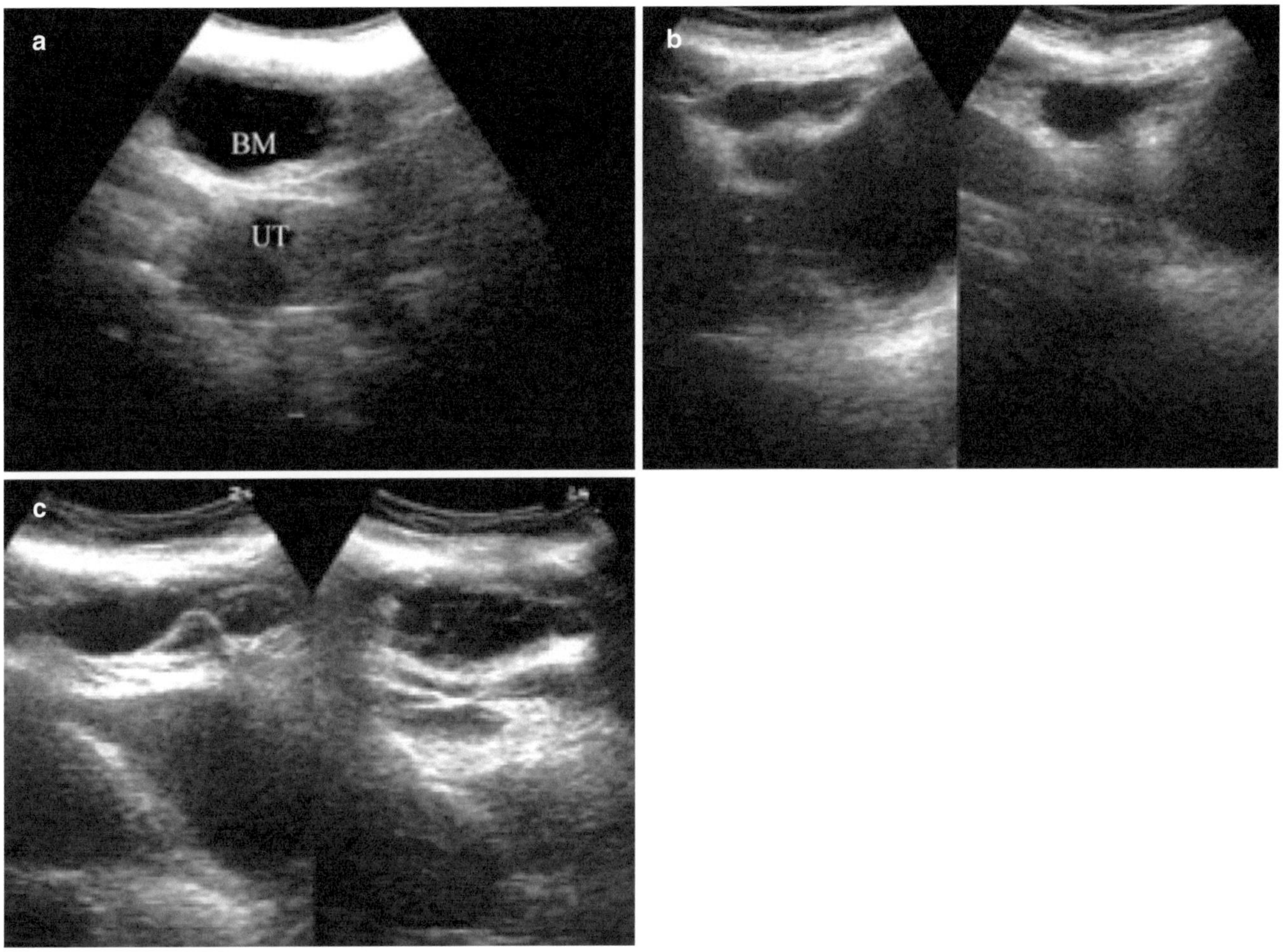

Fig. 2.186 Hematoma under the abdominal incision. After cesarean section, irregular anechoic or hypoechoic masses are visible under the abdominal wall

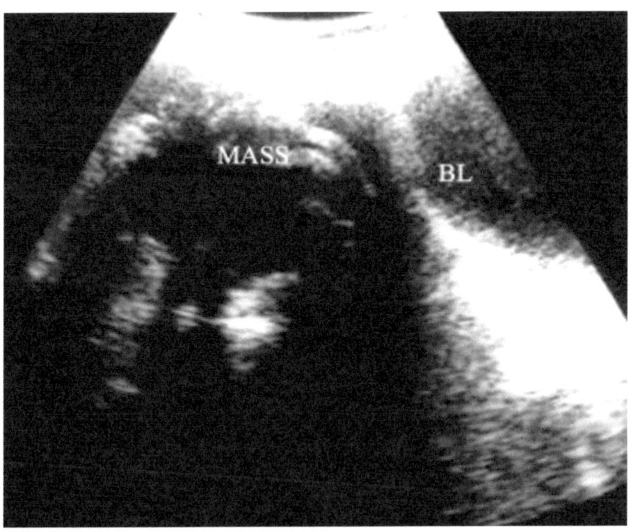

Fig. 2.187 Foreign body in the abdominal cavity (gauze). Three weeks after delivery, the patient has obvious abdominal pain, accompanied by fever. Sonogram shows an irregular hyperechoic mass, about 8.0 cm in diameter in the middle abdomen, without an obvious boundary. A posterior waterfall-like attenuation shadow is visible. It is confirmed as residual gauze by laparotomy

2.9 Ultrasonic Diagnosis of Brain Diseases in the Neonate

2.9.1 Anatomy of the Brain

The brain tissue is composed of the skull, meninges, brain, and ventricle.

2.9.1.1 The Skull

The skull consists of the frontal bone, parietal bone, temporal bone, and occipital bone, with bony suture and fontanelle formed at the junction. Fontanelle includes anterior fontanelle, posterior fontanelle, temporal fontanelle, and mastoid fontanelle. The anterior fontanelle is closed at 1.5–2 years old, and the temporal fontanelle is closed about 2 months after birth. The anterior fontanelle and temporal fontanelle are the main acoustic windows of ultrasonic examination.

2.9.1.2 Meninges

The meninges are divided into three layers from outside to inside: dura, arachnoid, and pia mater.

2.9.1.3 The Brain

The brain includes the cerebrum, diencephalon, brain stem, and cerebellum. The brain stem is composed of midbrain, pons, and medulla oblongata.

1. Cerebrum:
   (a) The cerebrum is divided into two hemispheres by the falx cerebri. From front to back, they are the frontal lobe, parietal lobe, occipital lobe, and the temporal lobe on both sides.
   (b) The left and right cerebral hemispheres are connected by the corpus callosum.
   (c) The surface layer of the cerebral hemisphere is the cortex—also known as gray matter, and the deep part is the medulla—also known as white matter. There are many gray matter cell masses in the medulla, called basal ganglia, which are caudate nucleus, zonal nucleus, lenticular nucleus, and amygdala.
   (d) The caudate nucleus is divided into head, body, and tail. The head is located under the anterior horn of the lateral ventricle. There is embryonic germinal layer between the head and the ependyma of lateral ventricle, and rich vascular network, which is the predilection site of intracranial hemorrhage.
2. Diencephalon: Located between the cerebral hemisphere and the brainstem.
3. Brainstem: Connecting the diencephalon upward and spinal cord downward.
4. Cerebellum: Located in the dorsal side of the brainstem and inferior to the occipital lobe of the brain, and composed of left and right expanded cerebellar hemispheres and narrow vermis in the middle.

2.9.1.4 Ventricles

Ventricles include the left and right lateral ventricles, the third ventricle, and the fourth ventricle.

1. Lateral ventricle: ①The lateral ventricle has anterior horn, body, posterior horn, and inferior horn. The junction of the posterior horn, inferior horn, and body is the trigone of lateral ventricle. ② The choroid plexus is formed by the pia mater of the top cerebral artery and ependyma, protruding into the ventricles, which is located in the middle and lower part of the lateral ventricle. The choroid plexus is well displayed at the trigone of the lateral ventricle. ③ The lateral ventricle is connected with the third ventricle through the interventricular foramen. ④ The lateral ventricle is filled with cerebrospinal fluid and is the largest anechoic area in the brain.
2. The third ventricle: Located between the thalamus on both sides, showing a small space. The third ventricle is connected with the fourth ventricle through the aqueduct of the midbrain.
3. Fourth ventricle: Located between brain stem and cerebellum.

2.9.1.5 Blood Vessels of the Brain

1. Cerebral artery: The blood supply of the brain mainly comes from the internal carotid artery and vertebral artery, constituting a rich vascular network in the brain to supply brain tissue. The circle of cerebral artery, Willis Circle, is located at the bottom of the brain. It is composed of the branches of the bilateral internal carotid arteries and vertebral arteries, and the starting part of the anterior, middle, and posterior cerebral arteries, and connected by the anterior and posterior communicating branches.
2. Cerebral vein:

The venous return is divided into two groups: Superficial vein and deep vein. The cerebral vein does not accompany the artery.

2.9.2 Neonatal Brain Examination

2.9.2.1 Examination Conditions of Neonatal Brain

1. 2-D high frequency curved transducer, 5-7 MHz, is commonly used.
2. It should be carried out in a quiet environment, and sedatives are necessary sometimes.
3. Choose the anterior fontanelle and temporal fontanelle as the acoustic window for neonatal brain examination.

2.9.2.2 Examination Method of Neonatal Brain

Scanning Method of the Anterior Fontanelle

1. Coronal view: Let the neonate lie in the supine position, then place the probe on the anterior fontanelle. The anterior fontanelle is the right niche, which is the best acoustic window for neonatal brain examination. A series of coronal views of the brain can be obtained by fan scanning from the anterior to the posterior coronal section.

2. Sagittal view: Rotate the probe 90 ° from coronal direction at the anterior fontanelle, scanning from left to right in a fan-shaped, and a series of sagittal views of the brain can be obtained.

Scanning Method of Temporal Fontanelle

1. Place the probe on the temporal fontanel and scan from front to back or from top to bottom, by which a series of transection images of the brain can be obtained. It is mainly used to measure the ratio of lateral ventricle diameter to cerebral hemisphere.
2. The blood flow of the cerebral artery and the Willis Circle is shown.

In addition, other fontanelle and bony suture can be used as an acoustic window for brain examination, but it is rarely used because of its small size and inconvenient operation.

2.9.3 Ultrasonogram of Normal Neonatal Brain

2.9.3.1 2-D Manifestations of Neonatal Brain Tissue

1. The skull shows a thick bright linear echo.
2. The brain tissue represents homogeneous and diffuse hypoechoic; only the echo of the cerebellum is slightly stronger.
3. The cerebrospinal fluid in the ventricles is anechoic.
4. The walls of ventricles and the falx cerebri show bright linear echoes, and bilateral structures of the midline are symmetrical.
5. The normal choroid is hyperechoic, bilaterally symmetrical, and less than 12 mm in width.

2.9.3.2 Ultrasonic Measurement of Neonatal Brain

1. The body width of the lateral ventricle in normal neonates is less than 5 mm. The standard measurement is the vertical distance between the lateral ventricle wall and the contralateral side of the caudate nucleus. According to the measured width, the lateral ventricular dilatation and hydrocephalus are divided into mild, medium, and heavy degrees. The width of the lateral ventricle body is 5-10 mm in mild cases, 10-15 mm in moderate cases, and more than 15 mm in severe cases.
2. Ventricular ratio is the ratio of the distance between the external wall of the lateral ventricle and the brain midline to the diameter of the ipsilateral cerebral hemisphere, which is not more than 0.35 normally.

2.9.3.3 Examination Technique of Neonatal Brain

Coronal View

1. Coronal view through the anterior horn of lateral ventricle: The bilateral anterior horn of lateral ventricles is in "V" shape, and the hypoechoic horizontal zonal corpus callosum is above the bilateral ventricles anterior horns. The anechoic transparent septum locates between the two anterior horns.
2. The coronal view through the interventricular foramen: The anterior horn of bilateral ventricles and the third ventricle form a "Y" shape, which is used as the level to measure the width of the lateral ventricle and the third ventricle.
3. Coronal view of the trigonometry of lateral ventricle: The bilateral choroid plexus is hyperechoic in the shape of the Chinese character "八," and the inferior cerebellum is visible (Fig. 2.188).

Sagittal View

1. Median-sagittal view: Arcuate corpus callosum can been seen, above and at the lateral of which are cingulate gyrus, frontal lobe, parietal lobe, and occipital lobe, in the inferior of which are the septum pellucidum, third ventricle, brainstem, and cerebellum.
2. Paramedian sagittal view: The arcuate anechoic area in the middle is the lateral ventricle, which is divided into anterior horn, body, posterior horn, and inferior horn; the frontal lobe, parietal lobe, and occipital lobe can be seen above and outside the lateral ventricle; the hyperechoic choroid plexus is in the trigonometry of lateral ventricle; caudate nucleus, thalamus, and thalamic sulcus of caudate nucleus are in the internal side of lateral ventricle; and cerebellar tissue is visible under the lateral ventricle (Fig. 2.189).
3. The transverse section shows the midline of the brain and bilateral symmetrical thalamus. Measure the ratio of the ventricle to the ventricle and observe the blood flow of circle Willis (Fig. 2.190).

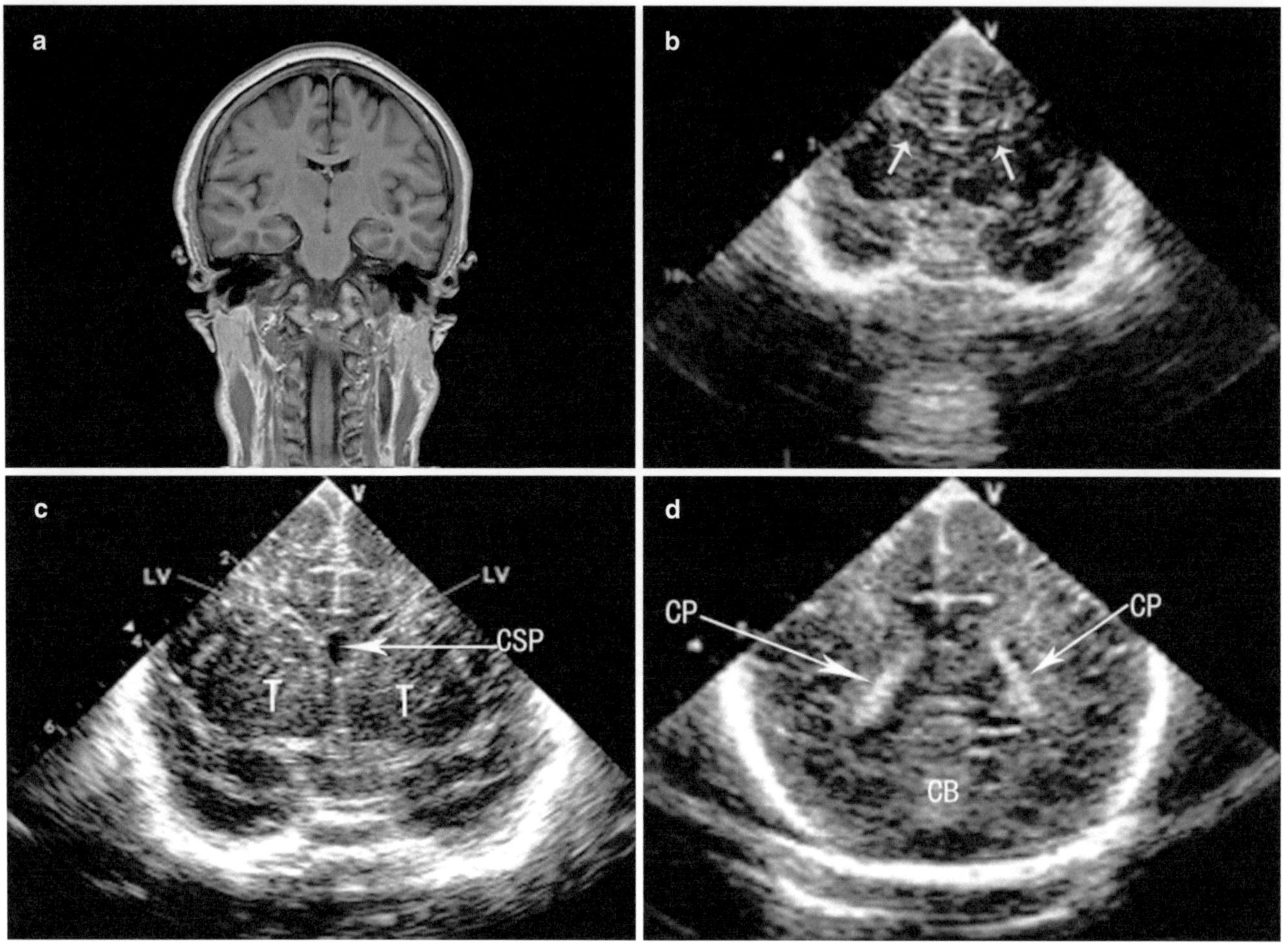

Fig. 2.188 Coronal section of the neonatal brain. (**a**). Coronal view of the brain. (**b**). Coronal view through the anterior horn of the lateral ventricle. (**c**). Coronal view through the interventricular foramen. (**d**). Hyperechoic choroid plexus in coronal view of the trigonometry of lateral ventricle presents "八" (arrow)

2.9.3.4 Color Doppler Ultrasound of the Neonatal Brain

Scanning through the Anterior Fontanelle

The internal carotid artery, basilar artery, and cerebral artery are visible on the sagittal view. The basilar artery travels toward the probe, and mostly appears in red color. The intracranial vein travels away from the probe and usually appears in blue. Based on this, we can get information on the blood flow of the arteries and veins, and measure S/D, PI, and RI (Fig. 2.191).

Scanning through the Temporal Fontanelle

The middle cerebral artery and the circle of Willis can be obtained on the transverse view.

Color Doppler ultrasound is utilized to identify the tubular structure as vessel or cyst, or to discriminate between normal vessel and the abnormal one, such as arteriovenous malformations (Fig. 2.192).

2.9.4 Abnormal Neonatal Brain Sonography

2.9.4.1 Hypoxic-Ischemic Encephalopathy

Basic Concepts

Neonatal hypoxic-ischemic encephalopathy (HIE) refers to the perinatal hypoxic-ischemic brain damage caused by asphyxia and hypoxia. HIE often occurs in term infants, leading to brain edema, periventricular leukomalacia,

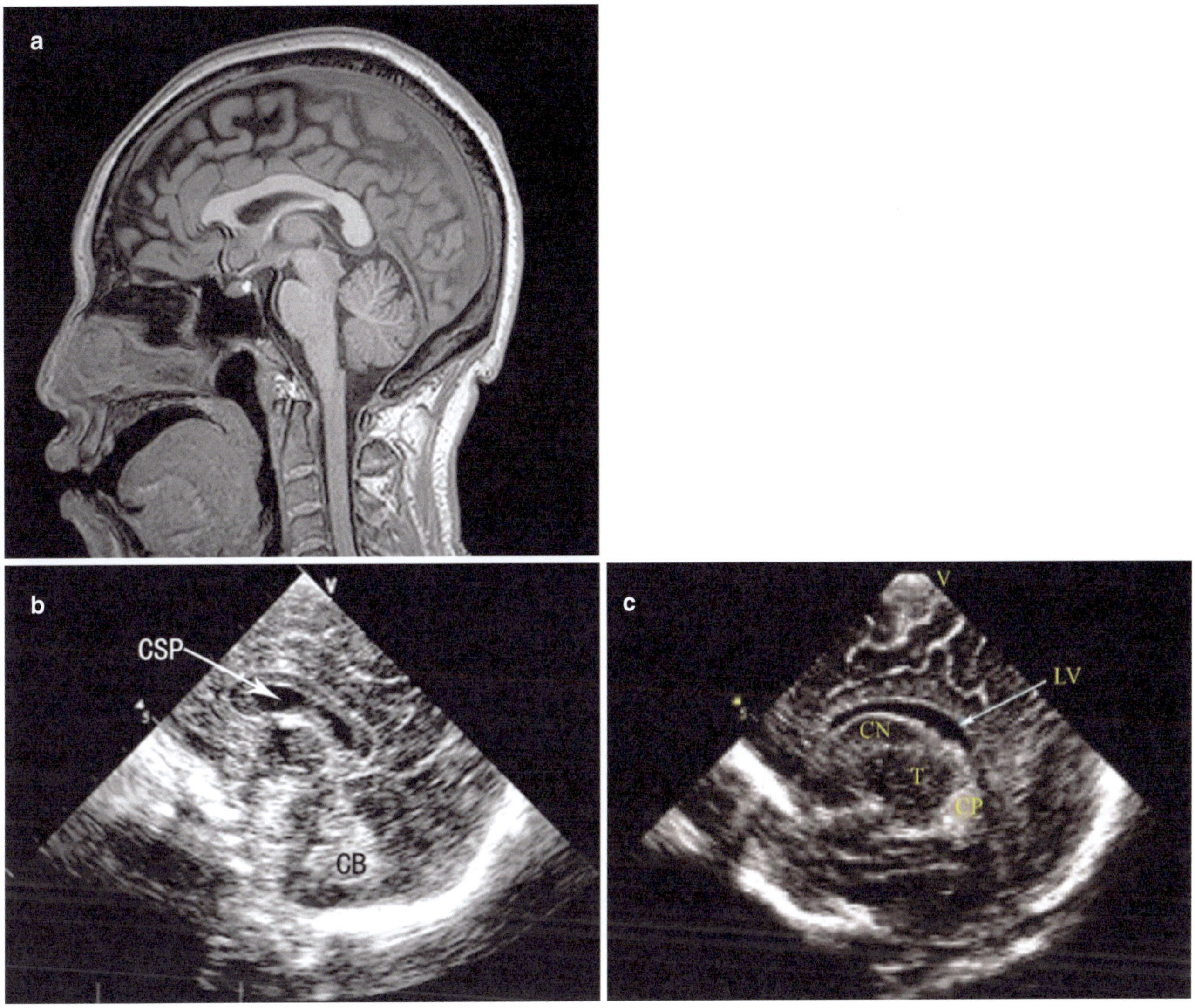

Fig. 2.189 Sagittal view of the neonatal brain. (**a**). Median-sagittal section of brain. (**b**). Median-sagittal view. (**c**). Paramedian sagittal view

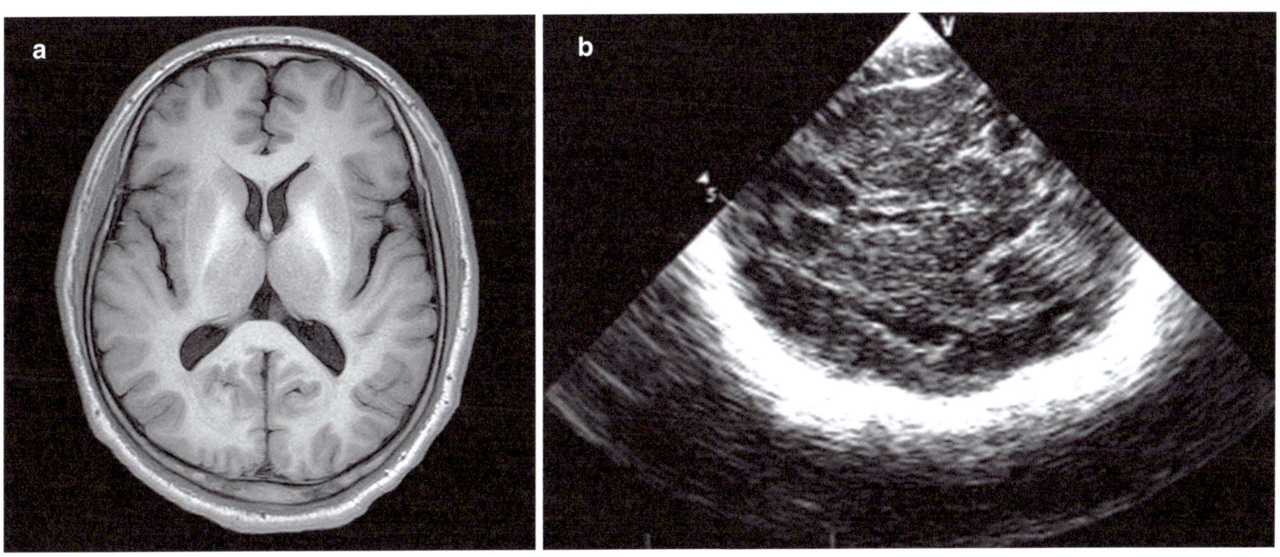

Fig. 2.190 The transverse view of the neonatal brain. (**a**). The transverse section of the neonatal brain. (**b**). The transverse view

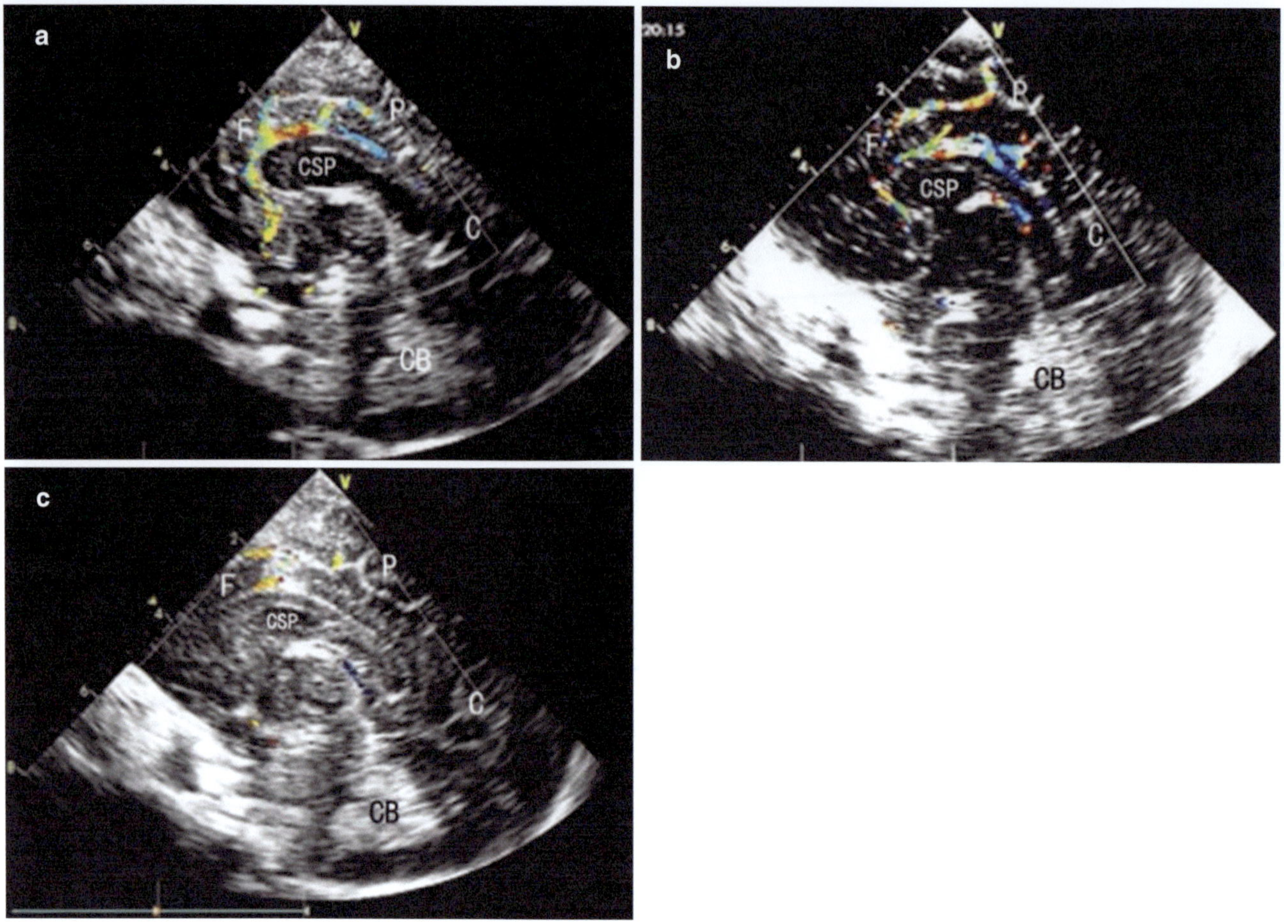

Fig. 2.191 Doppler imaging of the fetal cerebral artery and vein

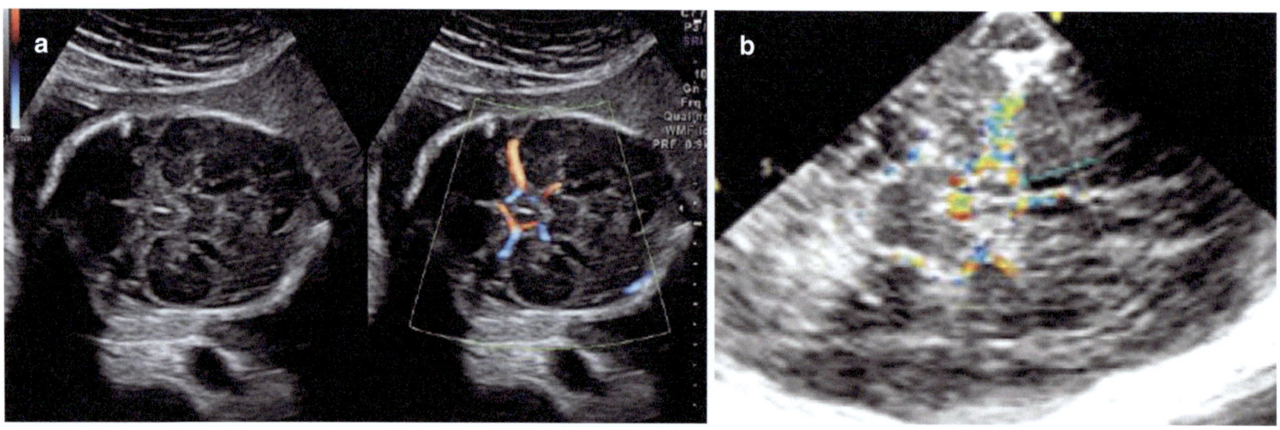

Fig. 2.192 CDFI of the fetal cerebral artery and Willis's circle. (**a**). CDFI of the fetal cerebral artery and Willis's circle. (**b**). Neonatal middle cerebral artery and Willis's circle

cerebral infarction, and basal ganglia and thalamus damage. The clinical manifestation is hyperactivity or depression within 12 hours after birth, with muscle tension changes—enhanced or weakened.

Ultrasound Diagnosis

1. Brain edema is characterized by mildly enhanced echo widely distributed in the brain parenchyma, narrowing or absent lateral ventricle, the unclear boundary of the sulcus gyrus, etc. (Fig. 2.193).
2. Periventricular leukomalacia is a bilateral and hyperechoic inverted triangle superolateral to the anterior horn of the lateral ventricle in the coronal section, and an area of irregular increased echogenicity superolateral to the lateral ventricle in the sagittal section. 2–3 weeks later, multiple small cysts are formed (Fig. 2.194).
3. Cerebral infarction shows localized hyperechoic reflection in the distribution area of the cerebral artery.
4. The injury of basal ganglia and thalamus represents bilaterally symmetric hyperechoic reflection.

Ultrasonic Classification

Some scholars classify the HIE by its sonographic changes.

1. Localized type: ① Scattered and unsymmetrical dot, strip, or fused hyperechoic area around the lateral ventricle and thalamus area is visible on the coronal view, with a diameter less than 1 cm; ② On the sagittal view, radiated hyperechoic area, forward from the triangle area, is shown.
2. Diffuse type: The whole brain is diffusely echo enhanced, presenting fuzzy structure and other manifestations of brain edema.

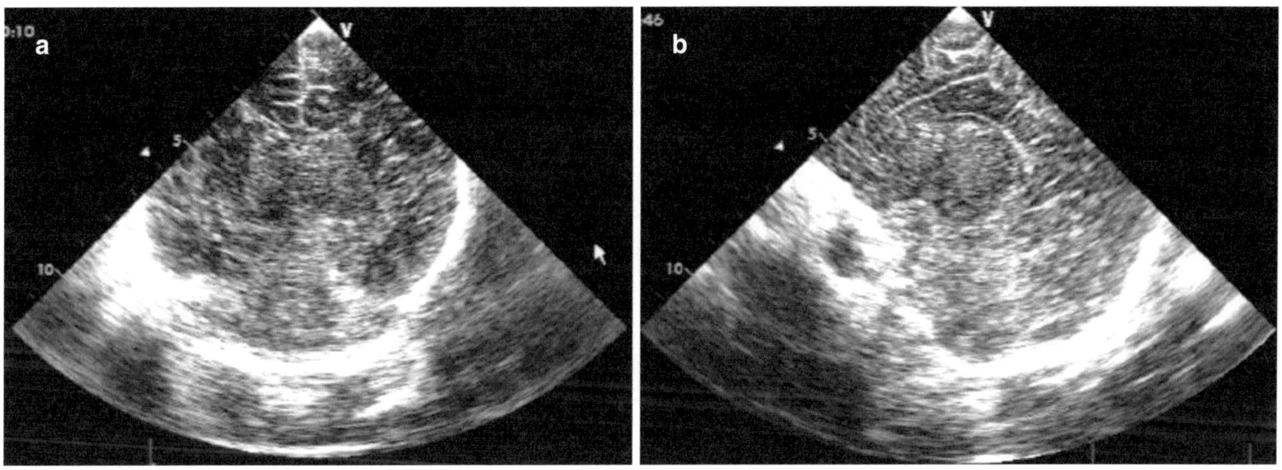

Fig. 2.193 Fetal brain edema. (**a**). Diffusely and slightly enhanced echo in the brain parenchyma of the fetal head in the coronal view. (**b**). The image shows diffusely and slightly enhanced echo in brain parenchyma in the sagittal section, narrowed lateral ventricle, and the sulcus gyrus with unclear boundary

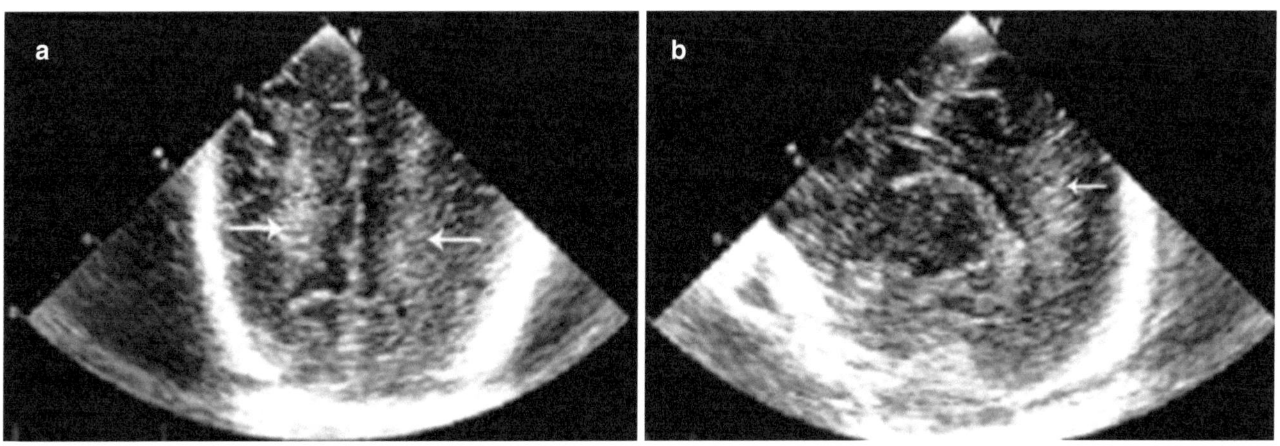

Fig. 2.194 Periventricular leukomalacia. (**a**). Coronal section: Bilateral periventricular echo is enhanced (arrow). (**b**). Sagittal view: Periventricular echo enhancement (arrow)

In mild cases, the echo of the lesion is lower than that of the choroid plexus; in a moderate degree, the echo of the lesion area is equal to that of the choroid plexus; in severe cases, the echo of lesion area is stronger than that of the choroid plexus.

Special Tips

1. Cranial ultrasound is the first choice for the diagnosis of neonatal HIE. CT is sensitive to early cerebral hemorrhage. MRI is an important supplement to ultrasound and CT, especially for the evaluation of mild HIE (Fig. 2.195).

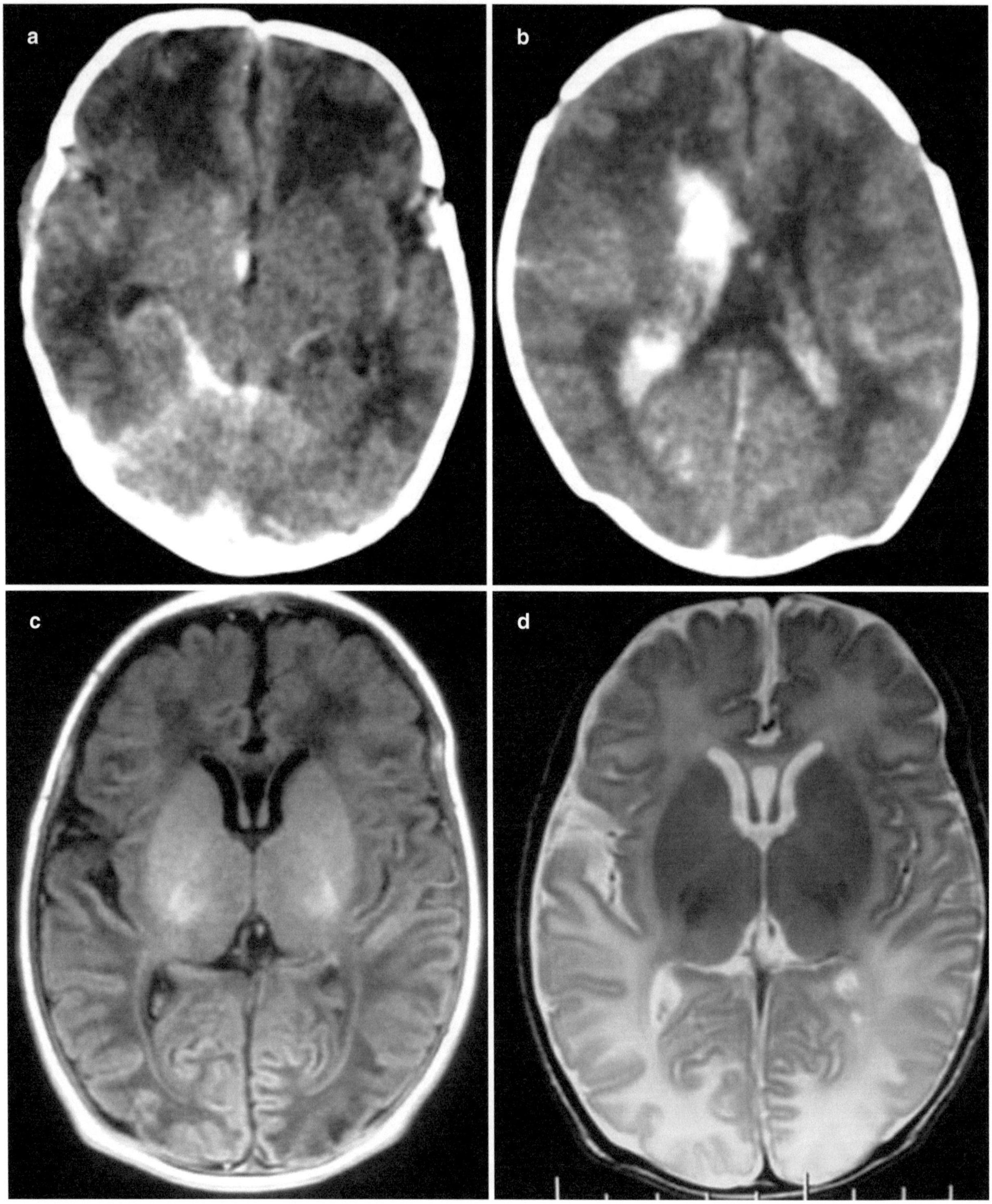

Fig. 2.195 CT and MRI findings of HIE. (**a, b**). CT shows intraventricular hemorrhage and subarachnoid hemorrhage. (**c, d**). MRI manifestations of the acute phase, a wide area of brain edema

2. HIE can be accompanied by intracranial hemorrhage, especially subarachnoid hemorrhage.
3. The lesions persist for 3 to 4 weeks in dynamic observation, and the prognosis is poor.

2.9.4.2 Intracranial Hemorrhage

Basic Concepts

Intracranial hemorrhage (IH), common in birth injury, hypoxia, hemorrhagic diseases, and so on, is the most common neonatal brain disease, especially in premature infants. Severe cases may cause death or neurological sequelae.

Clinical manifestations: Mild IH may be asymptomatic, and the prognosis is good. Severe IH with the following symptoms has a poor prognosis: irritability, convulsion, reduced reaction, low muscle tension, disturbance of consciousness, coma, and apnea.

Bleeding sites are subependymal, choroid plexus, brain parenchyma, subdural, subarachnoid space, and cerebellum. The morbidity and mortality of severe hemorrhage are high.

IH is generally divided into 4 grades: Grade I, subependymal hemorrhage; grade II, intraventricular hemorrhage; grade III, intraventricular hemorrhage with ventricular dilatation; grade IV, ventricular dilatation and intracerebral hemorrhage.

Ultrasonic Diagnosis

1. Subependymal hemorrhage.
   (a) Sonogram shows a focal hyperechoic mass under the anterior horn of lateral ventricle, unilateral, or bilateral.
   (b) Combine the abnormalities on the coronal and sagittal views for further diagnosis.
   (c) Subependymal cyst is formed after the hemorrhage is absorbed (Fig. 2.196).

2. Intraventricular hemorrhage.
   (a) Intraventricular hemorrhage is caused by subependymal hemorrhage broke into the lateral ventricle, or choroid plexus hemorrhage flowed into the lateral ventricle.
   (b) Sonogram shows hyperechoic masses in the ventricle with irregular distribution; the choroid plexus is thickened, enlarged, and lengthened, with a rough surface (Fig. 2.197).

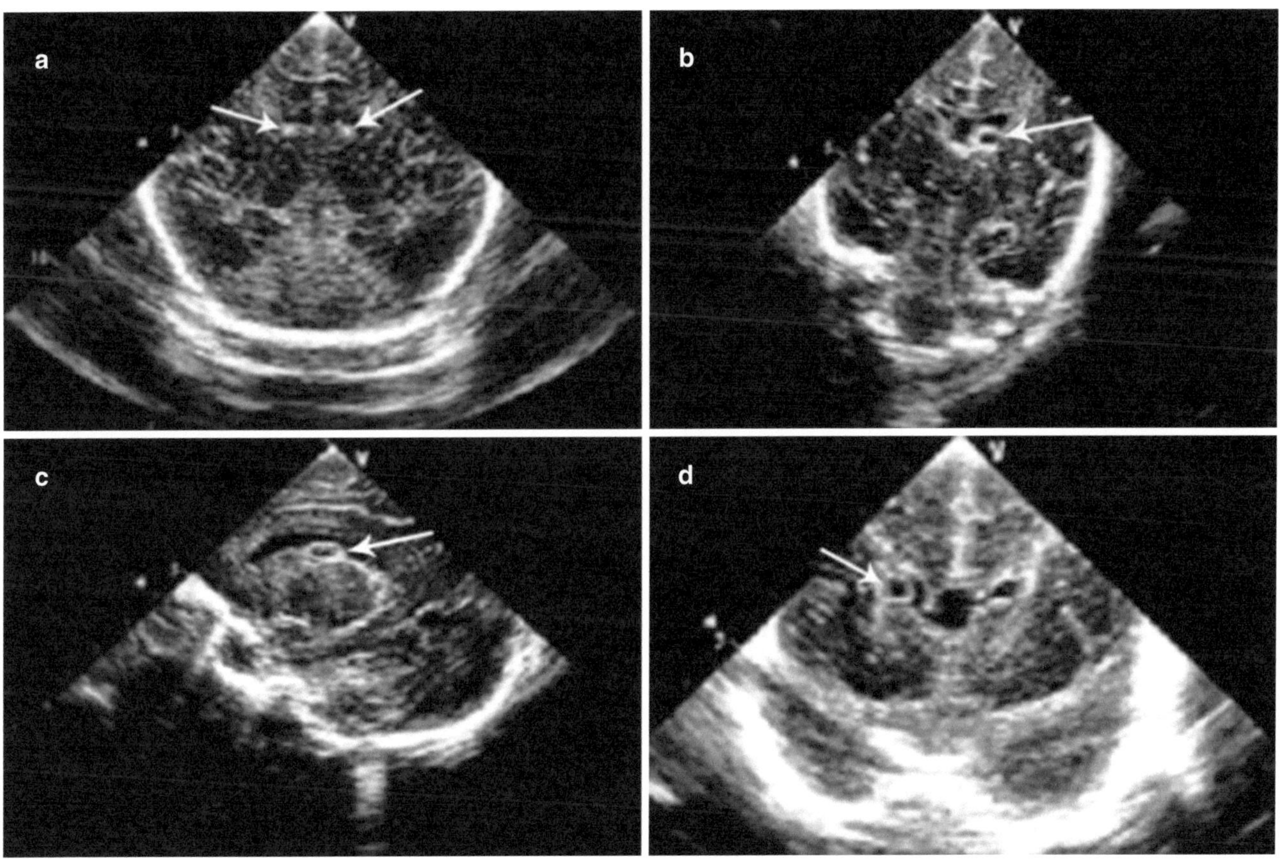

Fig. 2.196 Subependymal hemorrhage. (**a**). The coronal view of the neonatal head shows subependymal hemorrhage under the anterior horn of bilateral ventricles (grade I). (**b**). The coronal view of the neonatal head shows the formation of the left ependymal cyst in the late stage of hemorrhage (arrow). (**c**). The sagittal view of the neonatal head shows the left ependymal cyst in the later stage of hemorrhage (arrow). (**d**). Coronal view of the neonatal head shows the right ependymal cyst in the late stage of hemorrhage (arrow)

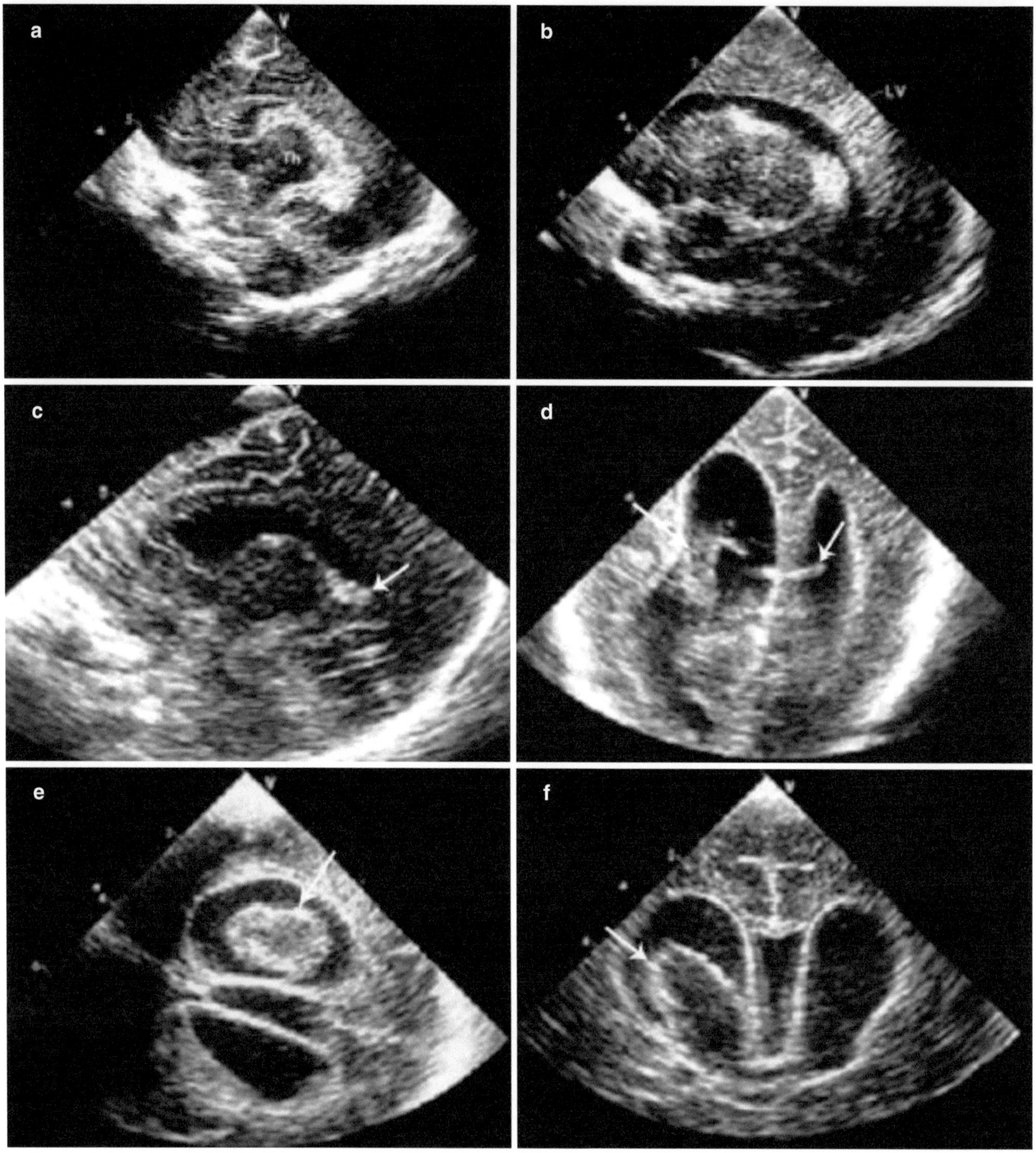

Fig. 2.197 Intraventricular hemorrhage. (**a**). On the sagittal view, the right ventricle is filled with irregular hyperechoic mass, combining with lateral ventricular dilatation. (**b**). In the sagittal view, lateral ventricular dilatation and irregular hyperechoic mass at thalamic sulcus of the caudate nucleus are shown. (**c**). Lateral ventricular dilatation and hyperechoic mass (arrow) at the choroid plexus are visible in the sagittal section. (**d**). The coronal view shows bilateral ventricular dilatation and bilateral intraventricular hyperechoic mass (arrow). (**e**). The transverse view shows bilateral ventricular dilatation and hyperechoic mass in the right ventricle (arrow), indicating intracranial hemorrhage (grade III). (**f**). The coronal view shows the bilateral ventricular dilatation, and a mass with relatively hyperechoic edge (arrow), which is formed by the liquefied blood clot in the late stage of hemorrhage. (**g**). The transverse view shows the dilated bilateral ventricles, shifted midline, and a mass with relatively hyperechoic edge (arrow), which is formed by the liquefied blood clot in the late stage of hemorrhage. (**h, i**). The coronal view shows the dilated bilateral ventricles, and a mass with relatively hyperechoic edge (arrow), which is formed by the liquefied blood clot in the late stage of hemorrhage

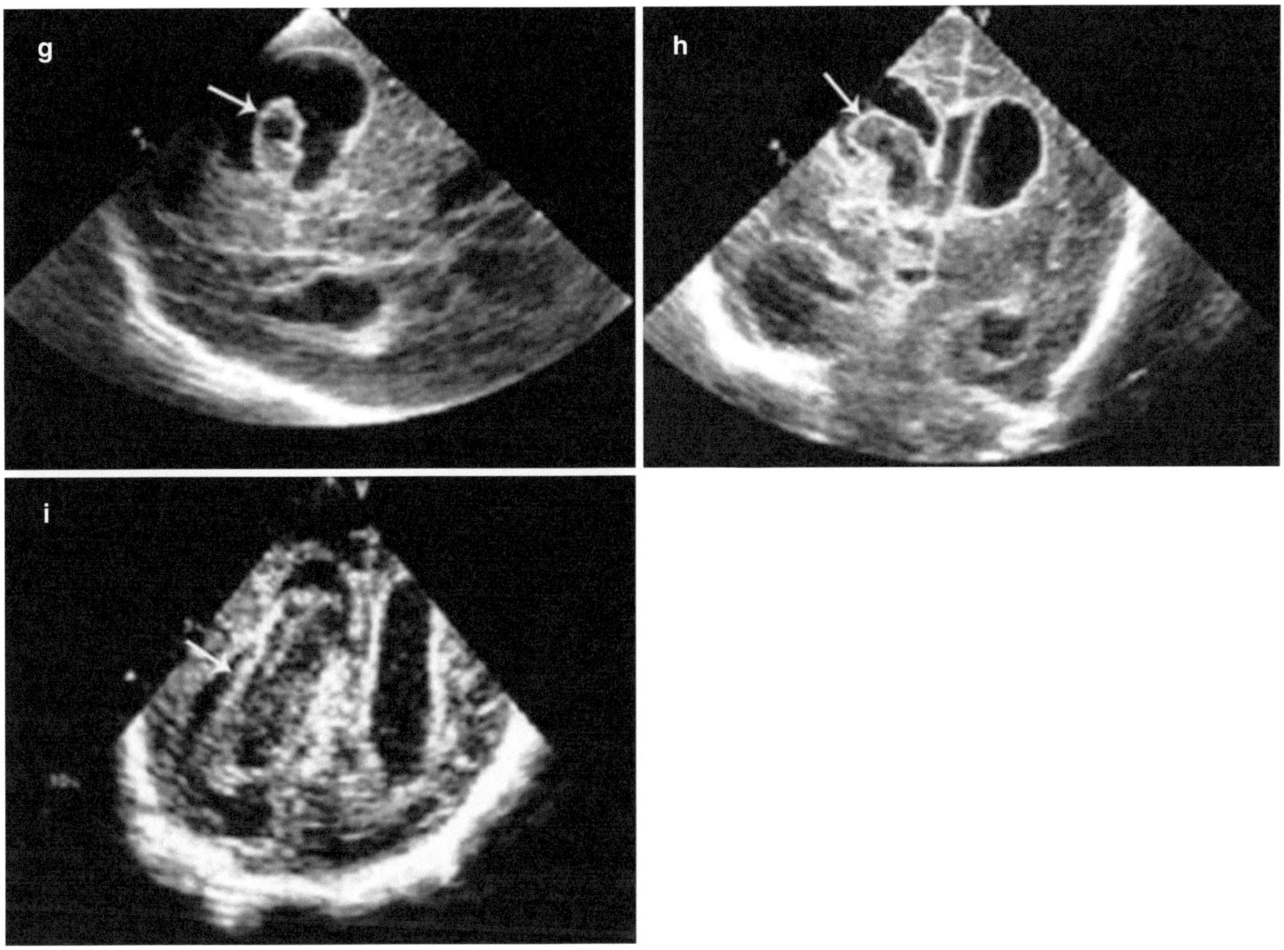

Fig. 2.197 (continued)

(c) In the late stage of hemorrhage, the echo intensity gradually become weakened or absorbed to form a cyst.

3. Hemorrhage of cerebral parenchyma.
1. Hemorrhage of cerebral parenchyma is the most serious type of intracranial hemorrhage, and the mortality rate is as high as 75%. Survivors often have neurological sequelae, such as cerebral palsy, epilepsy, growth retardation, mental or motor disorders. It happens in the frontal lobe, occipital lobe, or parietal lobe, especially in premature cases.
2. Sonogram shows the focal increased echogenicity or complex echoic mass in the cerebral parenchyma, regular or irregular, with a conspicuous boundary. When the mass is large, the cerebral midline will be shifted to the healthy side (Fig. 2.198).
4. Subdural hemorrhage: Subdural hemorrhage is caused by the rupture of the tentorium cerebelli or falx cerebri. The distance between the skull and brain tissue increases, representing an anechoic area with scattered points echo inside. If a large clot forms, it could be hyperechoic (Fig. 2.199).
5. Subarachnoid hemorrhage: The widened horizontal or vertical part of the lateral fissure or the enlarged cistern is visible in the sonogram.
6. Cerebellar hemorrhage: Sonogram shows abnormal area of increased echogenicity in the cerebellum, with irregular margins.

Special Tips

1. Meningitis, brain tumor, and brain abscess may also exhibit t areas of increased echogenicity, enlarged ventricular, echo enhanced choroid plexus, anechoic, and complex echo areas. It is necessary to combine the history and clinical manifestations for further diagnosis.
2. Under ultrasound examination, it is difficult to show small subdural hemorrhage, subarachnoid hemorrhage, and cerebellar hemorrhage.
3. Generally, ultrasound is the first choice for routine screening of neonatal intracranial hemorrhage. When there are

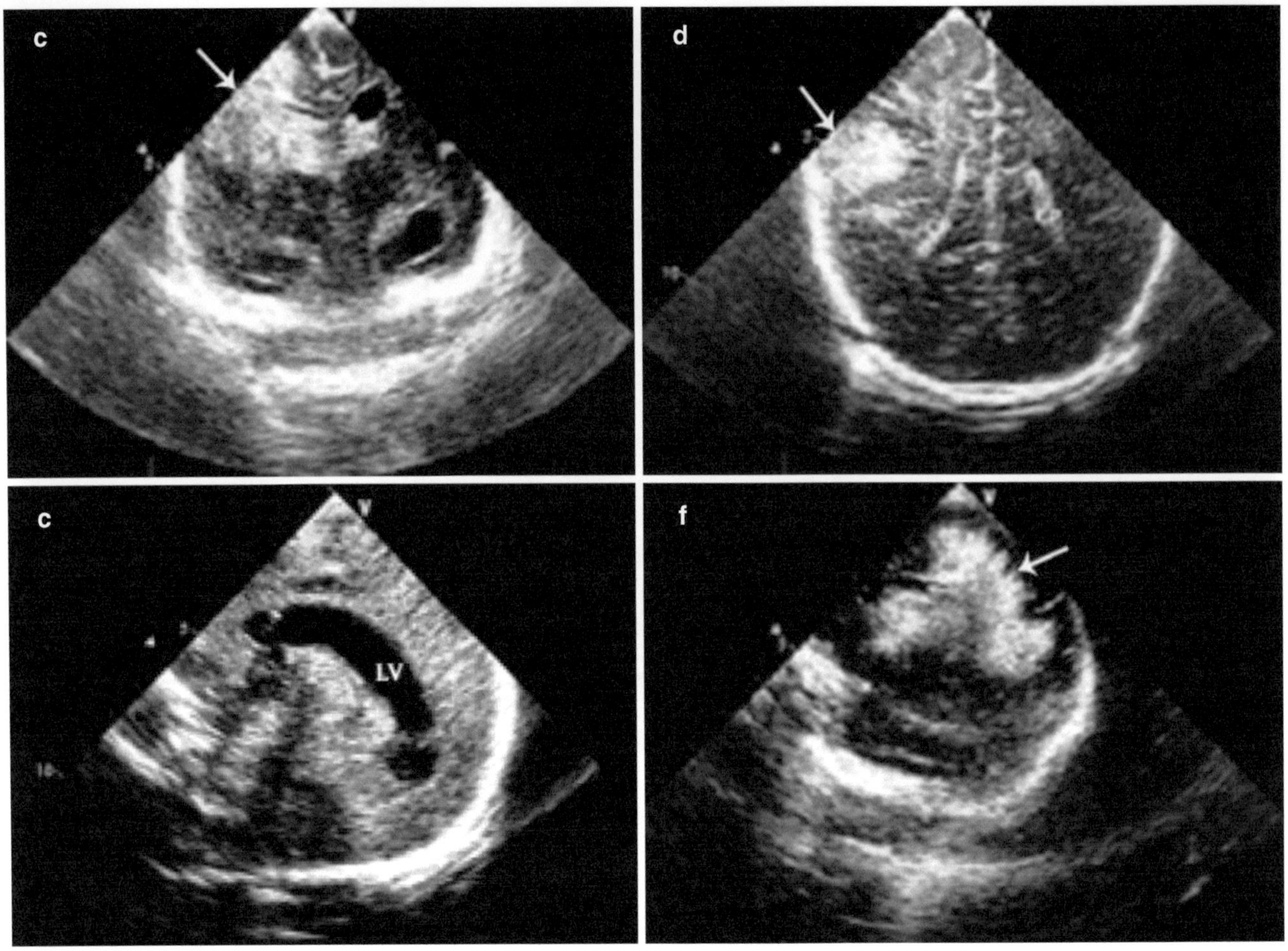

Fig. 2.198 Parenchymal hemorrhage. (**a**). The transverse view shows the enhanced echo in the right brain parenchyma and midline deviation. (**b**). The coronal view shows the enhanced echo in bilateral parenchyma. (**c**). The coronal view shows the enhanced echo in bilateral parenchyma, mainly on the right side. (**d**). The coronal view shows the enhanced echo in the right brain parenchyma (arrow). (**e**). The sagittal view shows the dilated lateral ventricle and the hyperechoic mass in the thalamus. (**f**). The sagittal view shows the enhanced echo in the left parenchyma, indicating intracranial hemorrhage (grade IV)

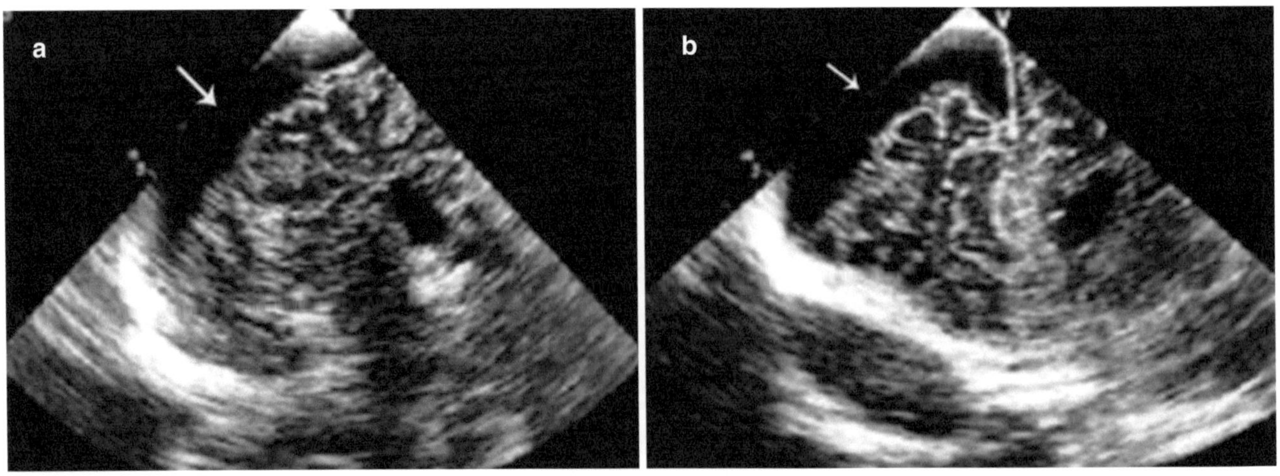

Fig. 2.199 Subdural hemorrhage. (**a**). The coronal view shows the right subdural hemorrhage (arrow). (**b**). The lateral transverse view shows the subdural hemorrhage (arrow)

no positive findings by ultrasound while highly suspected abnormal in clinical, CT, or MRI is recommended to detect subdural hemorrhage, hemorrhage in posterior fossa and other marginal locations, and brain parenchyma point hemorrhage. If the condition of neonate keeps stable and accessible to MRI, it is better to choose MRI than CT. MRI is superior to CT and ultrasound in assessing the prognosis (Fig. 2.200).

2.9.4.3 Periventricular Leukomalacia

Basic Concepts

Periventricular leukomalacia (PVL) refers to the ischemic coagulation necrosis of periventricular white matter, which mostly involves the optic radiation area of the lateral ventricular triangle and the white matter area outside the anterior horn. PVL often occurs in premature infants, and can be divided into four stages: ① enhanced echo phase; ② relatively normal phase; ③ cyst formation phase; and ④ cyst disappearance phase.

Ultrasonic Diagnosis

1. In the early stage of PVL, sonogram shows the enhanced echo around the ventricle, manifested as bilaterally symmetrical and rough echo enhanced areas (Fig. 2.201).
2. At the late stage (2–3 weeks), cysts are formed around the ventricles, accompanied by ventricular enlargement caused by white matter atrophy.

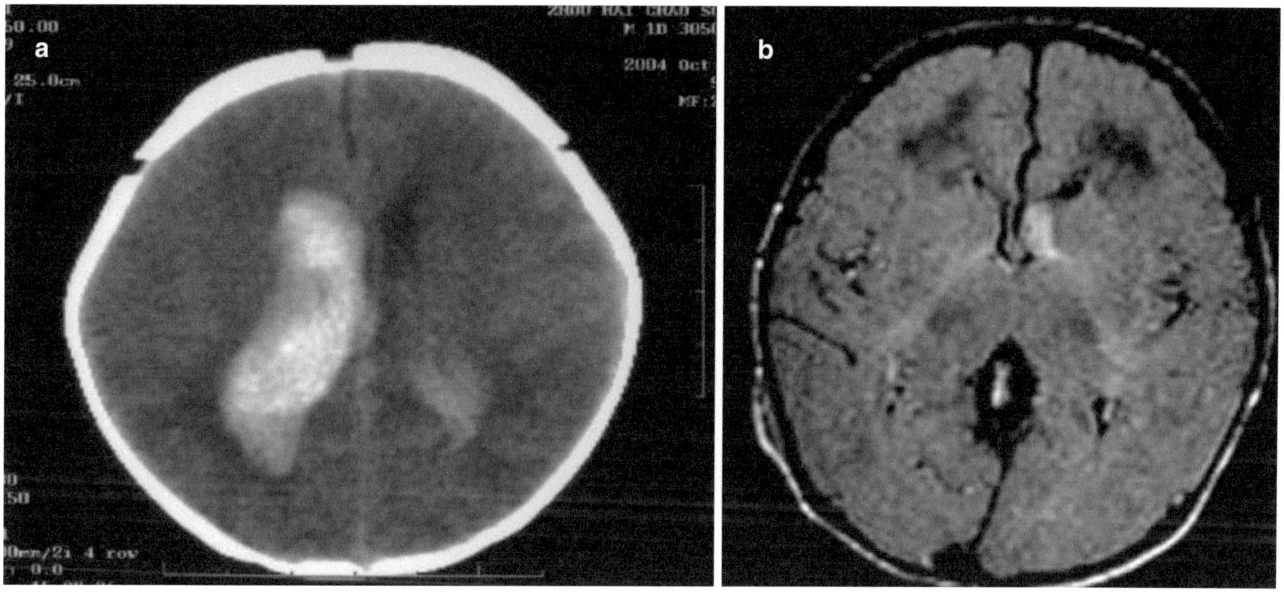

Fig. 2.200 CT and MRI manifestations of neonatal intracranial hemorrhage. (**a**). CT shows extensive hemorrhage in the right ventricle. (**b**). MRI (T1WI) shows hyperintense hemorrhage near the anterior horn of the left ventricle

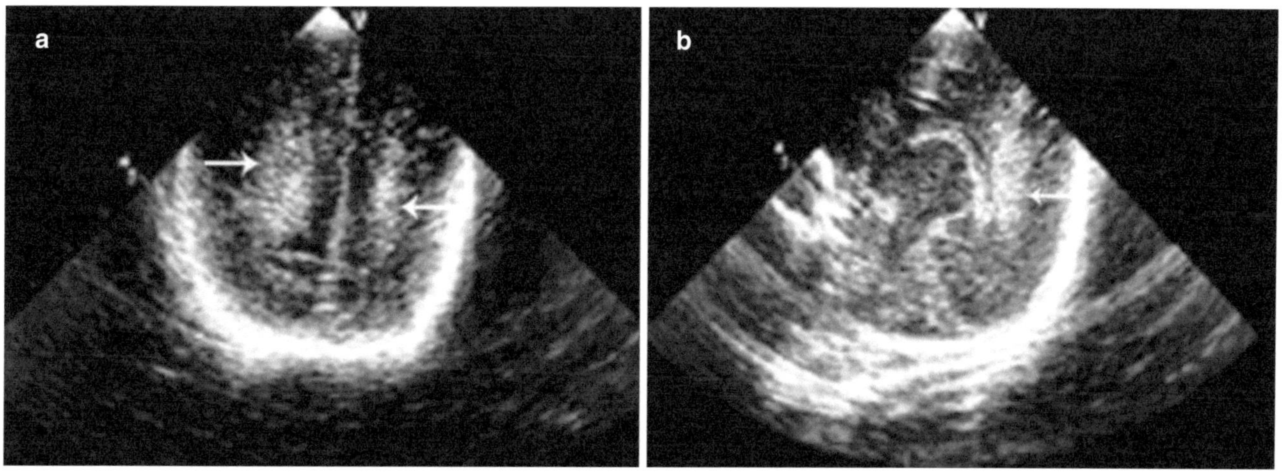

Fig. 2.201 Periventricular leukomalacia. (**a**). The coronal view shows bilateral periventricular echo enhancement (arrow). (**b**). The sagittal view shows periventricular echo enhancement (arrow)

Special Tips

1. The sensitivity of ultrasonography in the diagnosis of PVL is low.
2. MRI is of poor specificity in the diagnosis of early lesions of focal PVL, but it is more valuable in the diagnosis of late PVL. In MRI images, PVL represents decreased white matter volume, enlarged ventricle, irregular ventricle wall, gliosis, and delayed myelination (Fig. 2.202).

2.9.4.4 Neonatal Hydrocephalus

Basic Concepts

Neonatal hydrocephalus refers to the ventricular dilatation or accumulation because of the excessive increase of cerebrospinal fluid and accumulation in the ventricular system, caused by the obstruction of cerebrospinal fluid circulation, excessive secretion of cerebrospinal fluid, or disorder of cerebrospinal fluid absorption. The cerebrospinal fluid circulation is affected by midbrain aqueduct stenosis, intracranial hemorrhage, and infection.

Generally, ventriculomegaly is characterized by an enlarged ventricle without head circumference enlargement. In contrast, enlarged ventricular with head circumference enlargement is hydrocephalus.

Ultrasonic Diagnosis

1. Sonogram shows ventricular enlargement or hydrocephalus (Fig. 2.203).
2. According to the size of the lateral ventricle, hydrocephalus is divided into mild, medium, and severe degrees. The width of the lateral ventricle is 4–6 mm in mild cases, 7-10 mm in moderate cases, and more than 10 mm in severe cases.
3. It may be accompanied by brain tissue compression and atrophy.

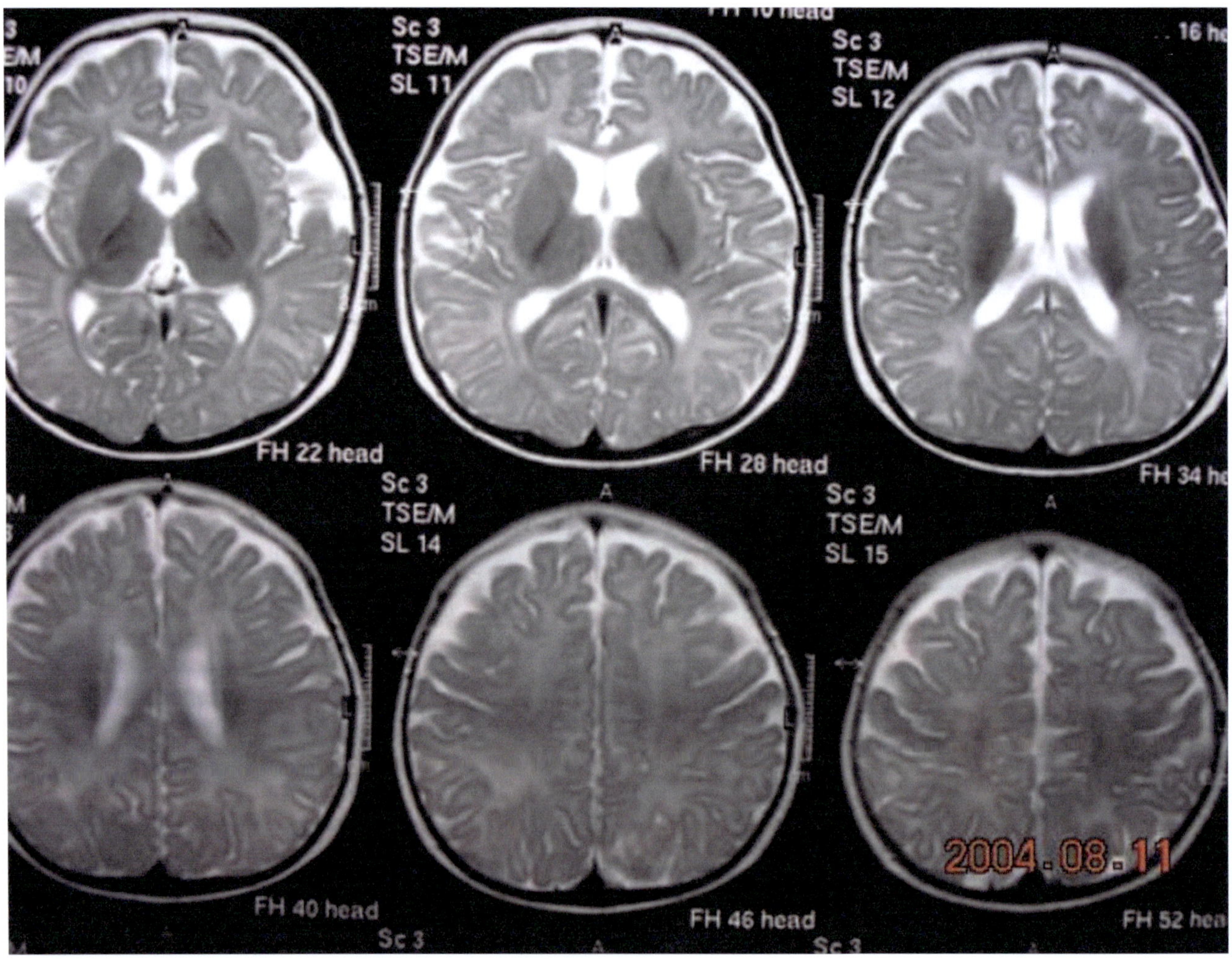

Fig. 2.202 MRI findings of PVL

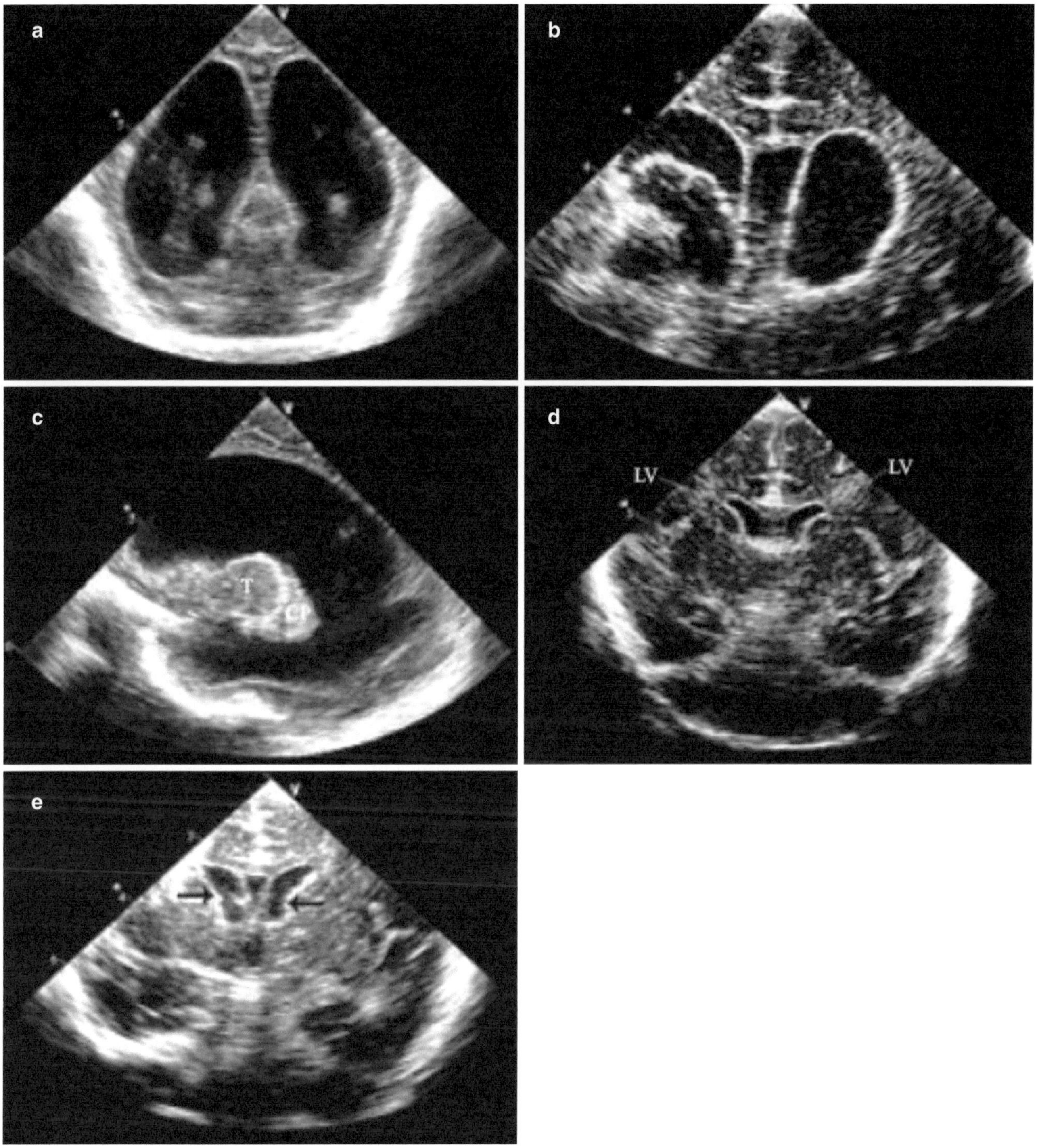

Fig. 2.203 Neonatal hydrocephalus. (**a, b**). The coronal view shows massive hydrocephalus in bilateral ventricles (severe). (**c**). The sagittal view shows massive hydrocephalus in left ventricle (severe). (**d, e**). The coronal view shows the dilation of bilateral anterior horn of ventricles with remote blood clots in the right ventricle

Special Tips

It is easy to diagn'ose ventricular dilatation and hydrocephalus.

1. Dynamic observation shows that most of the progressive ventricle expansion cases are hydrocephalus.
2. In some brain atrophy cases, the ventricles are also enlarged, but the sulcus, cistern, and hemispheric fissure are widened significantly.

Suggested Reading

1. Salomon LJ, Alfirevic Z, Bilardo CM, et al. ISUOG praction guideline: performance of first-trimester fetal ultrasound scan[J]. Ultrasound Obstet Gynecol. 2013;41(1):102–13. https://doi.org/10.1002/uog.12342.
2. Nardozza LM, Caetano AC, Zamarian AC, et al. Fetal growth restriction: current knowledge. Arch Gynecol Obstet. 2017;295(5):1061–77.
3. International Society of Ultrasound in Obstetrics and Gynecology, Carvalho JS, Allan LD, et al. ISUOG practice guidelines (updated): sonographic screening examination of the fetal heart[J]. Ultrasound Obstet Gynecol. 2013;41(3):348–59.
4. Birch PK, Hoffmann E, Rifbjerg LC, et al. Cesarean scar pregnancy:a systematic review of treatment studies [J]. Fertil Steril. 2016;105(4):958–67.
5. Witters I, Sieprath P, Van Holsbeke C, Deraedt K. Prenatal diagnosis of multiple large subchorionic placental cysts with intracystic hemorraghe. Facts Views Vis Obgyn. 2017 Dec;9(4):223–5.
6. Song B, Wei ZL, Xu XF, Cao YX. Prevalence and risk factors of monochorionic diamniotic twinning after assisted reproduction: a six-year experience base on a large cohort of pregnancies. PLoS One. 2017;12(11):e0186813.
7. Sun L, Guo C, Yao L, et al. Quantitative diagnostic advantages of three-dimensional ultrasound volume imaging for fetal posterior fossa anomalies: preliminary establishment of a prediction model. Prenat Diagn. 2019;39(12):1086–95.
8. Syngelaki A, Hammami A, Bower S, et al. Diagnosis of fetal non-chromosomal abnormalities on routine ultrasound examination at 11-13 weeks' gestation. Ultrasound Obstet Gynecol. 2019;54(4):468–76.
9. Altmann R, Schertler C, Scharnreitner I, et al. Diagnosis of fetal posterior Fossa malformations in high-risk pregnancies at 12-14 gestational weeks by transvaginal ultrasound examination. Fetal Diagn Ther. 2019;5:1–6.
10. Gallardo AM, Lvarez RM, De Luis E, et al. Antenatal ultrasound diagnosis and neonatal results of the congenital cystic adenomatoid malformation of the lung. Rev Chil Pediatr. 2018;89(2):224–30.
11. Bentur L, Gur M, Pollak M, et al. Early prenatal ultrasound diagnosis of congenital thoracic malformations. J Matern Fetal Neonatal Med. 2019;32(21):3531–6.
12. Gerscovich EO, Sekhon S, Loehfelm TW, et al. Fetal ultrasound: early diagnosis and natural evolution of proximal femoral focal deficiency. J Ultrason. 2017;17(71):294–8.
13. Millischer AE, Grevent D, Rousseau V, et al. Fetal MRI compared with ultrasound for the diagnosis of obstructive genital malformations. Prenat Diagn. 2017;37(11):1138–14.
14. Das R, Subedi N, Gurung G. Chorioangioma of placenta. J Nepal Med Assoc. 2017;56(208):472–4.
15. House M, Feltovich H, Hall TJ, Stack T, Patel A, Socrate S. Three-dimensional, extended field-of-view ultrasound method for estimating large strain mechanical properties of the cervix during pregnancy. Ultrason Imaging. 2012;34(1):1–14. https://doi.org/10.1177/016173461203400101.
16. Bohîlțea RE, Munteanu O, Turcan N, et al. A debate about ultrasound and anatomic aspects of the cervix in spontaneous preterm birth. J Med Life. 2016;9(4):342–7.
17. Jeremejeva J, Orro T, Valdmann M, Kask K. Bacteriological and cytological findings during the late puerperal period after two different treatments of retained placenta followed by acute puerperal metritis. Acta Vet Scand. 2010;52(1):41. Published 2010 Jun 15. https://doi.org/10.1186/1751-0147-52-41.
18. Gupta N, Grover H, Bansal I, et al. Neonatal cranial sonography: ultrasound findings in neonatal meningitis-a pictorial review. Quant Imaging Med Surg. 2017;7(1):123–31.
19. Lalzad A, Wong F, Schneider M. Neonatal cranial ultrasound: are current safety guidelines appropriate? Ultrasound Med Biol. 2017;43(3):553–60.
20. Tann CJ, Nakakeeto M, Hagmann C, et al. Early cranial ultrasound findings among infants with neonatal encephalopathy in Uganda: an observational study. Pediatr Res. 2016;80(2):190–6.
21. Shen W, Pan JH, Chen WD. Comparison of transcranial ultrasound and cranial MRI in evaluations of brain injuries from neonatal asphyxia. Int J Clin Exp Med. 2015;8(10):319–26.
22. Narchi H, Mahmoud-Ghoneim D, Skinner A, et al. Texture analysis of periventricular echogenicity on neonatal cranial ultrasound predicts periventricular leukomalacia. J Neonatal-Perinatal Med. 2013;6(2):117–24.
23. Resch B, Kaltenberger Z, Resch E, et al. Interobserver reliability of neonatal cranial ultrasound scanning regarding white matter disease. Pediatr Neonatol. 2013;54(3):214–5.
24. Himpens E, Oostra A, Franki I, et al. Predictability of cerebral palsy and its characteristics through neonatal cranial ultrasound in a high-risk NICU population. Eur J Pediatr. 2010;169(10):1213–9.
25. ISUOG. Practice guidelines: intrapartum ultrasound. Ultrasound Obstet Gynecol. 2018;52(1):128–39.
26. Popowski T, Porcher R, Fort J, et al. Influence of ultrasound determination of fetal head position on mode of delivery: a pragmatic randomized trial. Ultrasound Obstet Gynecol. 2015;46(5):520–5.
27. Sherer DM, Miodovnik M, Bradley S, et al. Intrapartum fetal head position I: comparison between transvaginal digital examination and transabdominal ultrasound assessment during the active stage of labor. Ultrasound Obstet Gynecol. 2002;19(3):258–63.
28. Ramphul M, Kennelly M, Murphy DJ. Establishing the accuracy and acceptability of abdominal ultrasound to define the fetal head position in the second stage of labour: a validation study. Eur J Obstet Gynecol Reprod Biol. 2012;164(1):35–9.
29. Ramphul M, Ooi PV, Burke G, et al. Instrumental delivery and ultrasound: a multicentre randomised controlled trial of ultrasound assessment of the fetal head position versus standard care as an approach to prevent morbidity at instrumental delivery. BJOG. 2014;121(8):1029–38.
30. Dupuis O, Ruimark S, Corrine D, et al. Fetal head position during the second stage of labor: comparison of digital and vaginal examination and transabdominal ultrasonographic examination. Eur J Obstet Gynecol Reprod Biol. 2005;123(2):193–7.
31. 张波, 杨太珠.三维超声在胎儿肺容积生理测值中的应用.四川大学学报(医学版), 2011, 42(1):141–143 (无英文摘要).
32. Wen X, Luo H, Shaoyu A, et al. The correlation analysis of fetal skeletal anomalies with chromosome abnormality by prenatal systematic ultrasonography examination. Chin J Med Ultrasound (Electronic Edition). 2015;12(2):54–6.
33. Bo Z, Yang T-z, Luo H. Combination of ultrasound and MRI in the diagnosis of fetal posterior fossa anomalies. J Chin Clin Med Imaging. 2015;26(2):111–3.
34. He G, Luo H, Yang J. Prenatal ultrasonography for fetal limb malformation screening at 11-13+6 weeks of gestation. Chin J Med Imaging. 2014;22(8):634–7.

35. He G, Luo H, Yang J, et al. Prenatal ultrasonographic diagnosis of fetal absent pulmonary valve syndrome. Chin J Med Ultrasound (Electronic Edition). 2014;11(10):816–9.
36. Bo Z, Yang T-z, Qi Z, et al. Clinical prognosis of isolated absence of septum pellucidum diagnosed with prenatal ultrasonography. J Chin Clin Med Imaging. 2013;24(12):866–8.
37. Cai-yun Z, Luo H. Waveform and spectrum parameters of ductus venosus in fetus with congenital heart disease. Chin J Med Imaging Technol. 2013;29(4):599–603.
38. Cai-yun Z, Hong L. Analysis of normal fetal ductus venosus spectrum at 11-40 weeks of gestation. West Chin Med J. 2013;28(2):244–8.
39. 周彩云, 罗红, 超声产前诊断双胎输血综合征38对分析, 四川大学学报(医学版), 2012,43(2):302—304(无英文摘要).
40. Cai-yun Z, Luo H. Prenatal color Doppler ultrasonography in diagnosis of prune-belly syndrome. Chin J Med Imaging Technol. 2011;27(8):1647–50.
41. Ying T, Yang T-z, Hong L, et al. Prenatal ultrasound diagnosis and prognosis of fetal persistent right umbilical vein. Chin J Obstet Gynecol Pediatr (Electron Ed). 2010;6(3):165–7.

3 Ultrasonic Diagnosis of Pathological Obstetrics

Taizhu Yang and Hong Xu

3.1 Ultrasonic Diagnosis of Early Abortion

3.1.1 Basic Concepts

1. Abortion is defined as the pregnancy is terminated before 28 weeks and the fetus weight is less than 1000 g. Early abortion refers to the abortion occurred before 12 weeks of pregnancy, and late abortion occurred at 12–28 weeks of pregnancy. The spontaneous abortion accounts for about 15% of all pregnancies, and the majority is early abortion.
2. The causes of early abortion are as follows: abnormal chromosome number and structure in genetic defects; excessive exposure to harmful chemical and physical factors in environmental factors; maternal factors include systemic diseases, reproductive organ diseases, endocrine disorders, trauma, etc.; hypofunction of the placenta endocrine, immune factors between the embryo and mother, and mechanical reasons.
3. The pathological change of early abortion is that the embryos die, followed by decidual hemorrhage. The villi of the embryo separated from the decidua, causing uterine contraction, and evacuated from the uterine cavity. Due to the incomplete development of villi, the implantation is not firm, and the pregnancy tissue can be completely evacuated. At 8–12 weeks of gestation, the placental villi develop luxuriantly and are firmly connected with the decidua. When abortion occurred, the pregnancy tissue is not easy to be evacuated completely. After 12 weeks of pregnancy, abdominal pain is the earliest clinical symptoms of abortion, and then the fetus and placenta are evacuated.
4. According to the different stages of the abortion, it is clinically divided into threatened abortion, inevitable abortion, incomplete abortion, complete abortion, missed abortion, infectious abortion, and recurrent abortion. The intrauterine gestational sac changes in different types of early abortion: gestational sac deformation, pregnancy failure, pregnancy sac downward movement.
5. The clinical presentations of different types of abortion are diverse. Most of the patients with threatened abortion have amenorrhea history, morning sickness, vaginal bleeding, and slight abdominal pain. The patients with inevitable abortion or incomplete abortion have paroxysmal lower abdominal pain or back pain after amenorrhea, with amount of vaginal bleeding. In the late abortion cases, the fetus or part of placental tissue has been evacuated, and some fetal material remains in the uterine cavity, which affects uterine contraction and causes massive bleeding and even shock. The abdominal pain and bleeding stop when the embryonic tissue is completely evacuated from the uterus. Missed abortion is the result of failed evacuation of the dead embryo, most of them used to undergo threatened abortion. The embryo in missed abortion cases no longer grows and develops, and the uterus will stop growing. The hCG in urine or blood is positive or weakly positive in majority abortion cases, which may be negative for patients with prolonged dead embryo.

3.1.2 Ultrasonic Diagnosis

1. The echo of gestational sac and embryo in threatened abortion is the same as that of the normal pregnancy. The embryo survives and continues to grow (Fig. 3.1).
2. In incomplete or inevitable abortion cases, the deformed and collapsed gestational sac in the uterine cavity moves to the cervical internal os. No embryo or indistinct embryo without heartbeat is visible in the pregnancy sac. In patients with incomplete abortion, residual pregnant

This chapter was translated by **Miaoqian Wang** and **Qiubo Lv**. Department of Obstetrics and Gynecology, Beijing Hospital, National Center of Gerontology, Beijing, China

T. Yang (✉) · H. Xu
Department of Ultrasonography, West China Second University Hospital, Sichuan University, Chengdu, China

T. Yang, H. Luo (eds.), *Practical Ultrasonography in Obstetrics and Gynecology*, https://doi.org/10.1007/978-981-16-4477-1_3

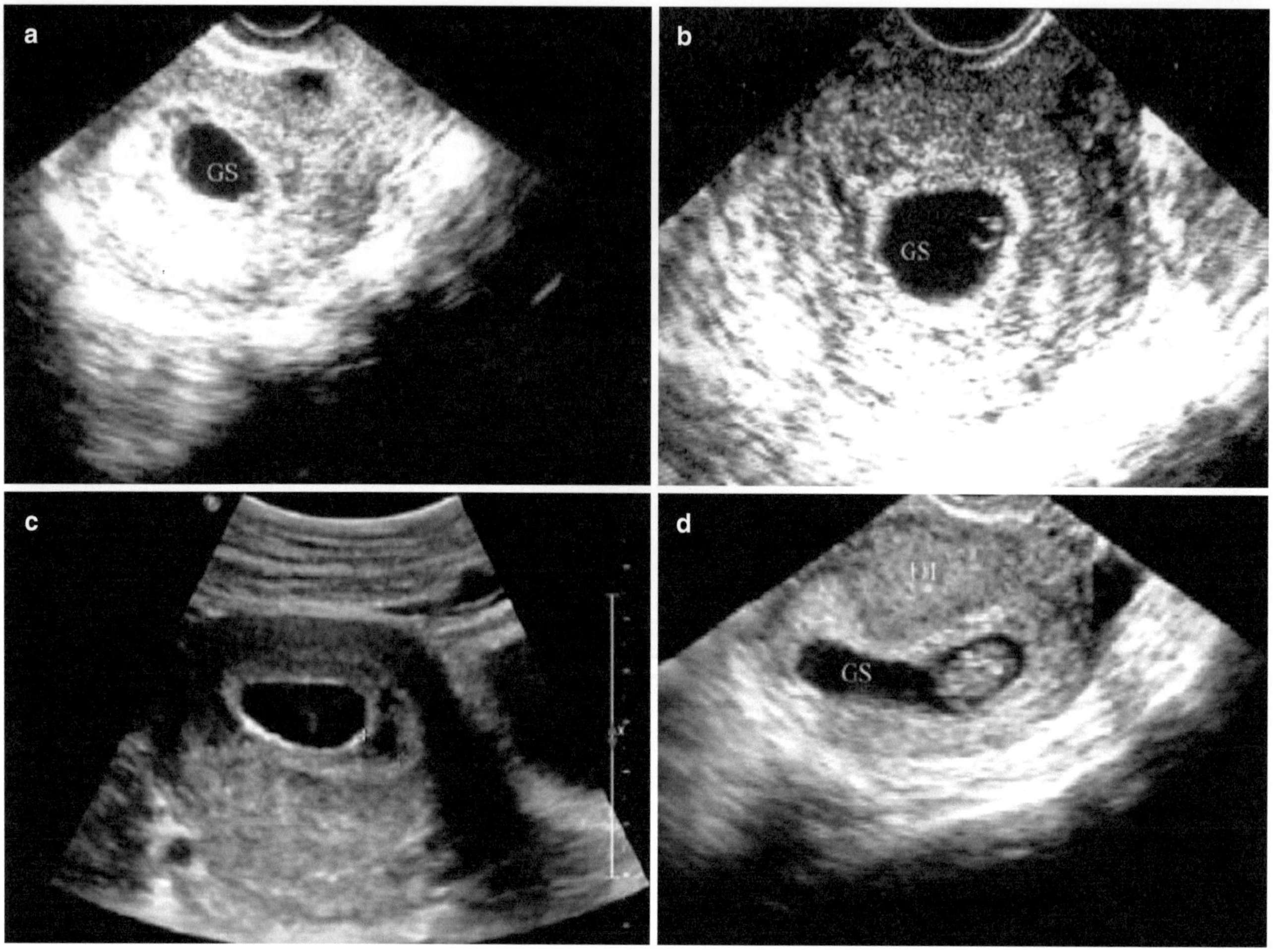

Fig. 3.1 Threatened abortion. (**a**). On the 46th day of pregnancy, the patient has a little vaginal bleeding, and the sonogram shows the gestational sac and embryo; (**b**). On the 42nd day of pregnancy, the patient has abdominal pain accompanied with vaginal bleeding, and the sonogram shows the normal yolk sac and embryo with heartbeat; (**c**). On the 50th day of pregnancy, the patient has more vaginal bleeding with abdominal pain, and the sonogram shows the normal yolk sac, embryo with visible heartbeat, and hematocele in the uterine cavity; (**d**). On the 50th day of gestation, the patient has abdominal pain accompanied with vaginal bleeding, and the sonogram shows the normal yolk sac and embryo

tissue or blood clots represent irregular strong echo in the uterine cavity (Fig. 3.2).

3. The uterus of patients with missed abortion no longer grows or even gradually retract, the placenta tissue is organized with abnormal shape, and there is no embryo or fetus in the uterine cavity. Some of the intrauterine pregnancy sac is round and full, but no embryo or only withered embryo without heartbeat is visible (Fig. 3.3).
4. After complete abortion, the uterus is in normal size or slightly enlarged, without pregnant tissue in the uterine cavity, and the echo of uterine cavity line is clear (Fig. 3.4).

3.1.3 Special Tips

1. Combined with the clinical history and symptoms, pay attention to differentiate abortion from the ectopic pregnancy (Fig. 3.5).
2. Observe the size and echo changes of yolk sac in the pregnancy sac. It is of great significance to identify whether the yolk sac is healthy or not for further prediction of prognosis of early pregnancy.
3. The accurate diagnosis of abortion type using ultrasound is vital for clinical treatment (Fig. 3.6).

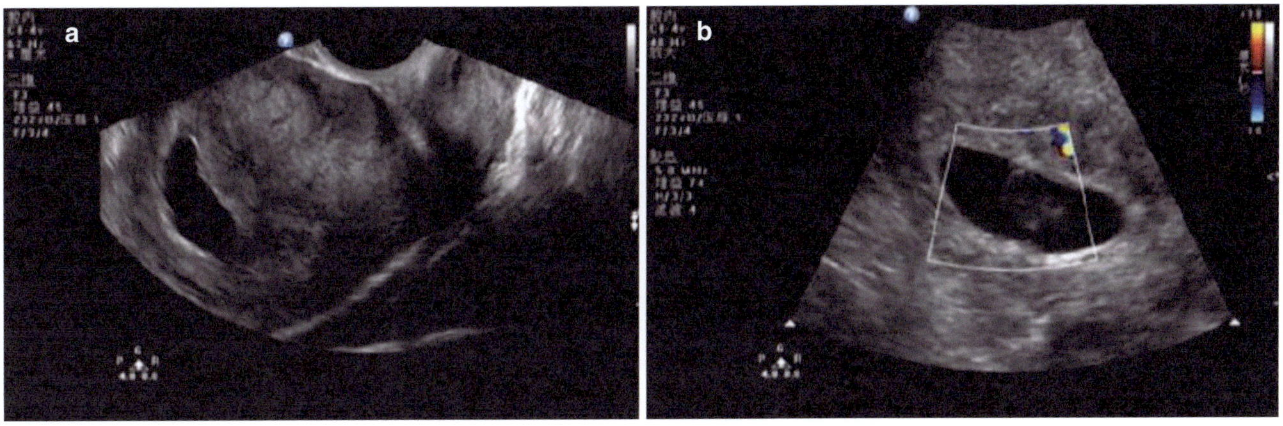

Fig. 3.2 Inevitable abortion. (**a**). On the 58th day of gestation, the gestational sac in the uterus is visible, without evident decidual reaction and embryo; (**b**). On the 63th day of pregnancy, the intrauterine gestational sac is deformed without evident decidual reaction, the embryo shape is irregular without heartbeat

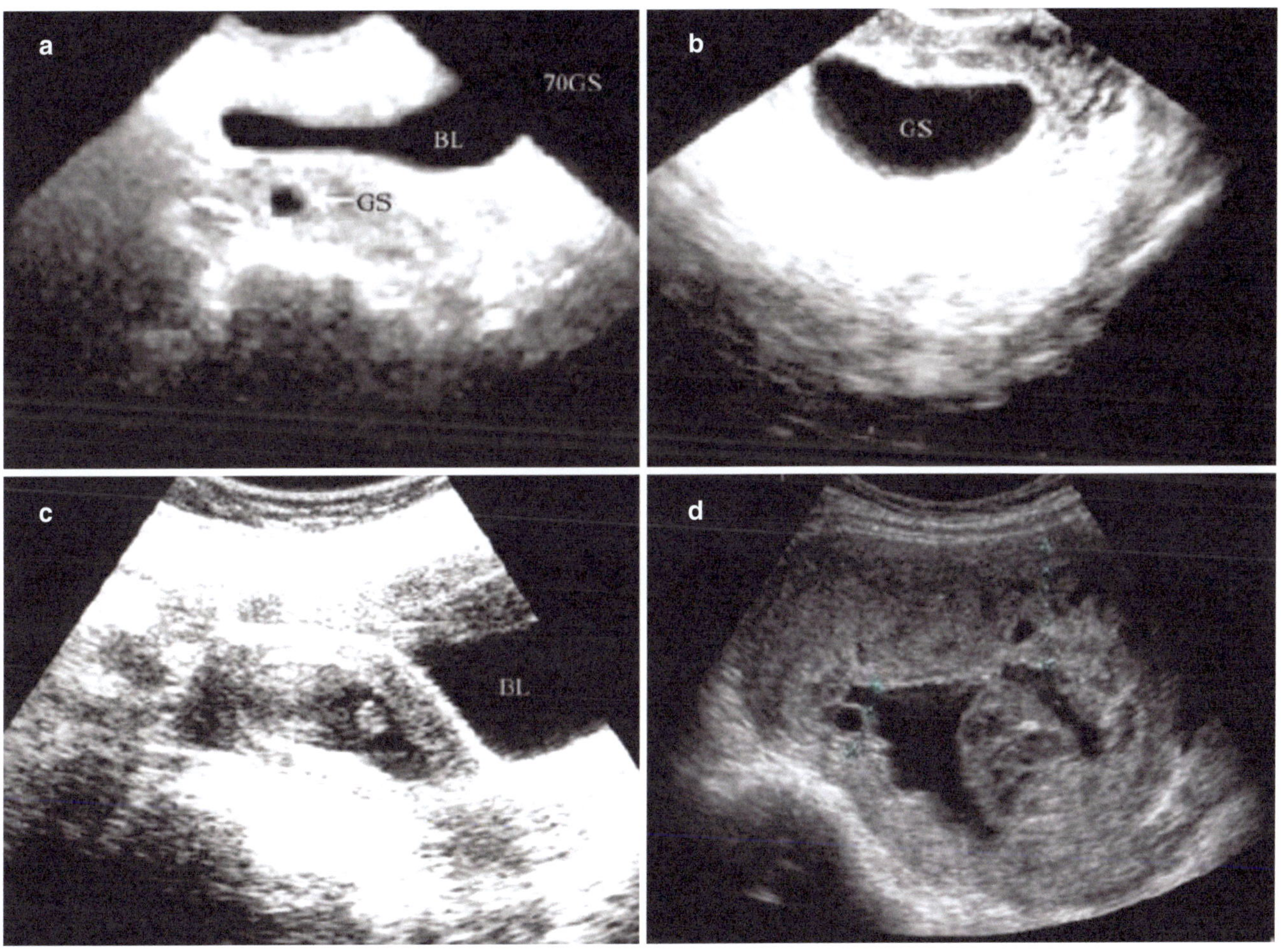

Fig. 3.3 Missed abortion. (**a**). The diameter of the gestational sac is only 1.1 cm on the 70th day of pregnancy; (**b**). On the 57th day of gestation, the sonogram shows a gestational sac in the uterus, without an embryo; (**c**). On the 61th day of pregnancy, the sonogram shows a deformed embryo in the gestational sac, without heartbeat and evident decidual reaction; (**d**). On the 83th day of pregnancy, the formed placental is in an abnormal shape, with inhomogeneous echo. No fetus is found in the uterus

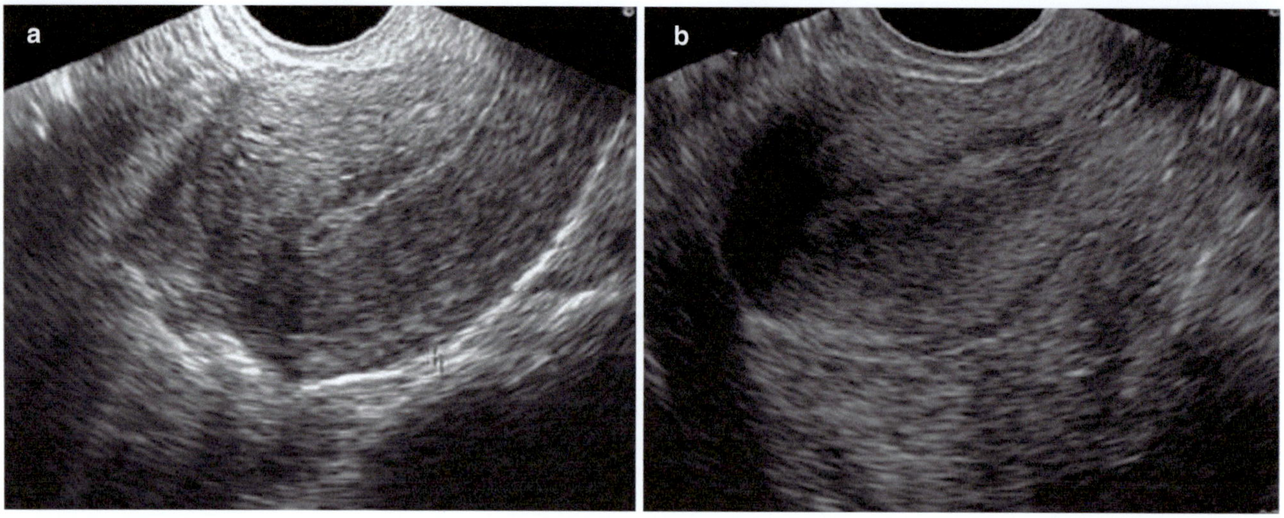

Fig. 3.4 Complete abortion. (**a. b**). After complete spontaneous abortion in early pregnancy, the uterus is slightly enlarged, without pregnant tissue in the uterine cavity, and the echo of uterine cavity line is obvious

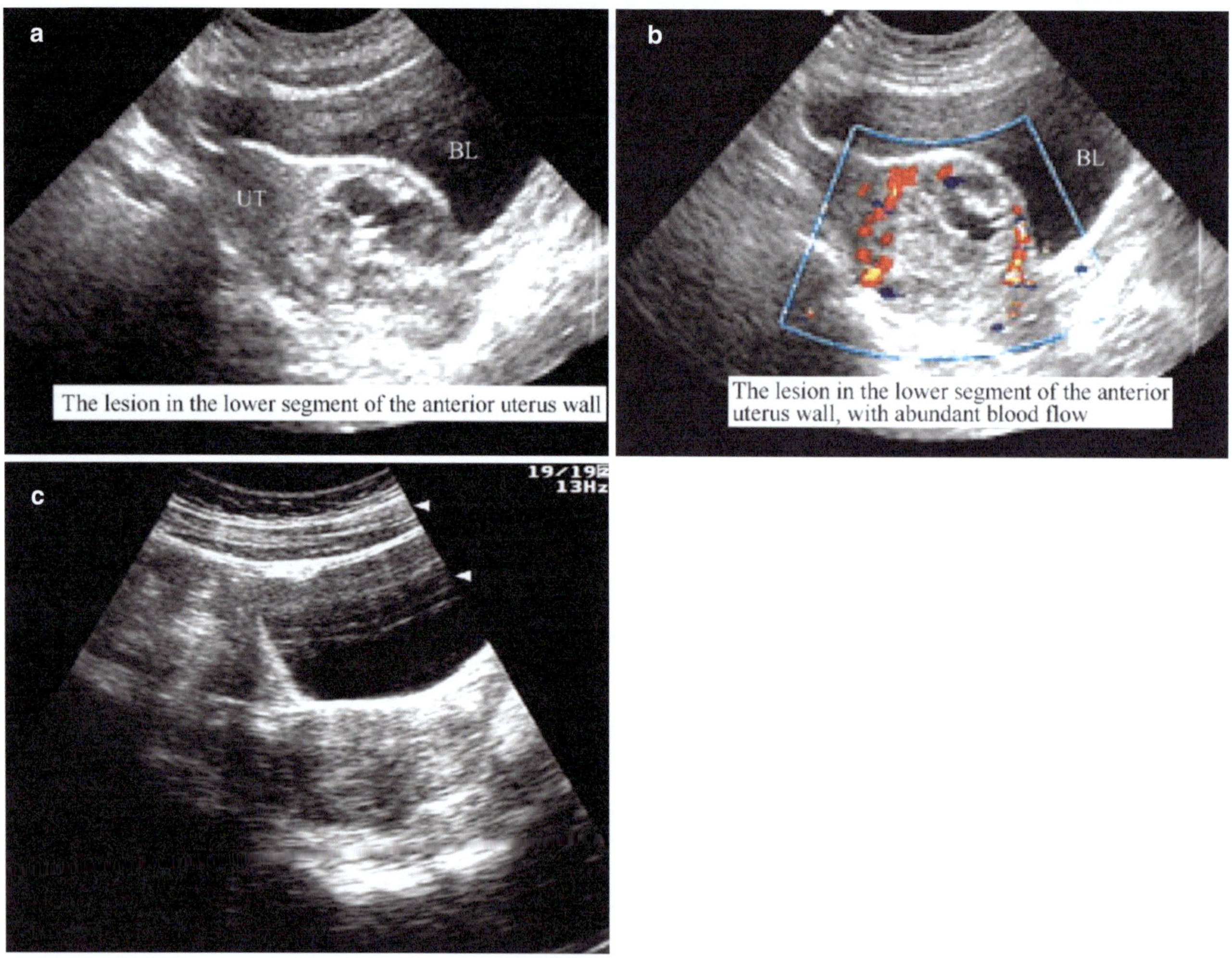

Fig. 3.5 Identification of incomplete abortion. (**a. b**). The cesarean scar pregnancy is misdiagnosed as incomplete abortion. After several times of curettage, serum hCG was positive. Via ultrasound examination, the lesion in the lower segment of the anterior uterus wall is visible, with abundant blood flow. After clinical conservative treatment, hCG decreased; (**c**). The cesarean scar pregnancy is cured after treatment

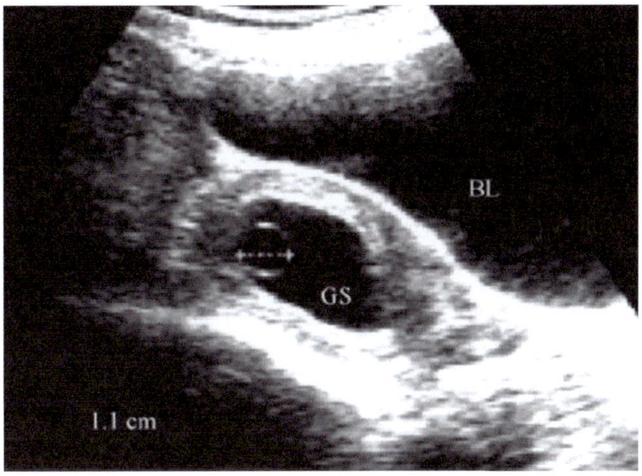

Fig. 3.6 The diameter of the yolk sac is more than 1.0 cm and no embryo is visible at 58 days of amenorrhea

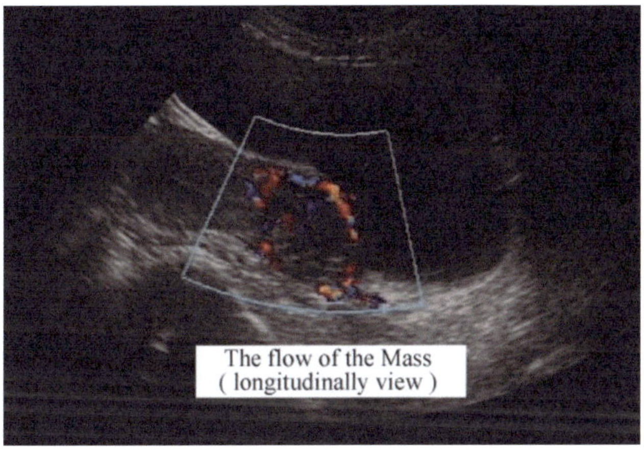

Fig. 3.7 Isthmus pregnancy (I)

3.1.4 Typical Cases

Following are the cases and images of isthmus pregnancy, cornual pregnancy, or interstitial pregnancy, misdiagnosed as incomplete abortion for multiple times of curettage (Figs. 3.7 and 3.8).

The patient, 31 years old, has undergone contraceptive operation twice after amenorrhea for 43 days.

Sonogram shows a weak echo mass in the lower part of the anterior uterine wall, with a diameter of 3.0 cm, surrounded by color blood flow. No space-occupying lesion in the uterine cavity, while serum hCG is positive.

The same patient with Fig. 3.7, is diagnosed as isthmus pregnancy. After treatment, the surrounding blood flow decreases significantly and hCG is weakly positive.

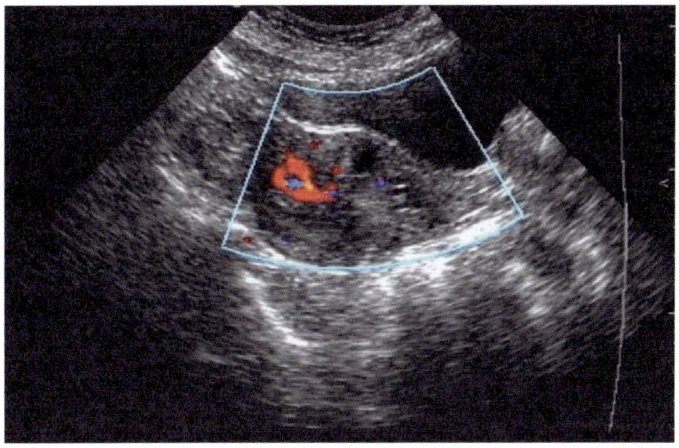

Fig. 3.8 Isthmus pregnancy (II)

3.2 Ultrasonic Diagnosis of Ectopic Pregnancy

3.2.1 Basic Concepts

1. The ectopic pregnancy (EP), also known as exfetation, is defined as the oosperm implanted outside the uterine cavity. According to the location of the fertilized eggs, EP is divided into tubal EP, ovarian EP, abdominal EP, broad ligament EP, cervical EP, etc. Other unusual EP includes cornual EP, uterine muscular EP, rudimentary horn EP, isthmic EP, and so on.
2. According to the domestic reports, the incidence of EP is increasing progressively, and the ratio of ectopic pregnancy to normal pregnancy increased from 1:167 to 1:(56–93). Tubal EP is the most common, accounting for more than 95% of EP.
3. The main factors of EP are: tubal inflammation, tubal surgery history, tubal dysplasia, tubal dysfunction, assisted reproductive technology, contraceptive failure (intrauterine device), fertilized egg migration, uterine fibroids, ovarian mass compression, and myomectomy.
4. The tubal cavity is narrow, and the tube wall is thin and lacks submucosal tissue. When the embryo is implanted in the fallopian tube or other rare parts, it fails to form intact decidua to adapt to the development of the embryo. With the development of pregnancy, pregnancy abortion, pregnancy rupture, and secondary abdominal pregnancy may occur.
5. Amenorrhea, abdominal pain, and vaginal bleeding are major symptoms of typical EP. The clinical manifestation is related to the location, rupture, abortion,

bleeding, and the duration of EP. 20% - 30% of the patients have no obvious history of amenorrhea, representing irregular menstruation, abdominal distension, and anal bearing-down pain. Pelvic mass is detected in some patients, and the positive rate of serum hCG is 80% - 100%. Clinical signs include anemia, rapid and weak pulse; cervical staining, lifting pain or rocking pain, pelvic mass, and uterine floating. The blood punctured form posterior fornix is not coagulated.

6. With the wide application of transvaginal ultrasound, the diagnostic accuracy of ectopic pregnancy can reach 95%. For other rare EP, such as cornual EP, uterine muscular EP, rudimentary horn EP, isthmic EP, the diagnostic accuracy rate is higher than before.

3.2.2 Ultrasonic Diagnosis

1. Ultrasound scanning shows the enlarged or plump uterus, without gestational sac and embryo in the uterine cavity. The thickened endometrium may be accompanied by liquid dark area, irregular hyperechoic, reticular echo, linear echo, and pseudogestational sac. Abnormal uterine echo is related to decidual reaction and bleeding (Fig. 3.9).
2. Depending on the ultrasonic manifestations, tubal EP is divided into live EP (unruptured EP with gestational sac), mass EP, ruptured EP (EP with uterine floating), and old EP.

① Live EP with a complete extrauterine gestational sac is usually detected in early pregnancy. The embryo with heartbeat is visible in some cases. There is no obvious hematoma in the rectouterine pouch. ② Mass EP is due to the fallopian tube abortion or rupture. The gestational sac and the blood clot accumulating around the fallopian tube, forming adnexal hematoma. The adnexal mass represents hyperechoic, complex, or attenuated echo, and gestational sac-like structure accompanied by surrounding nourishing vessels is visible in some cases. Free fluid can be detected in the rectouterine pouch, iliac fossa, and abdominopelvic cavity. The echo of

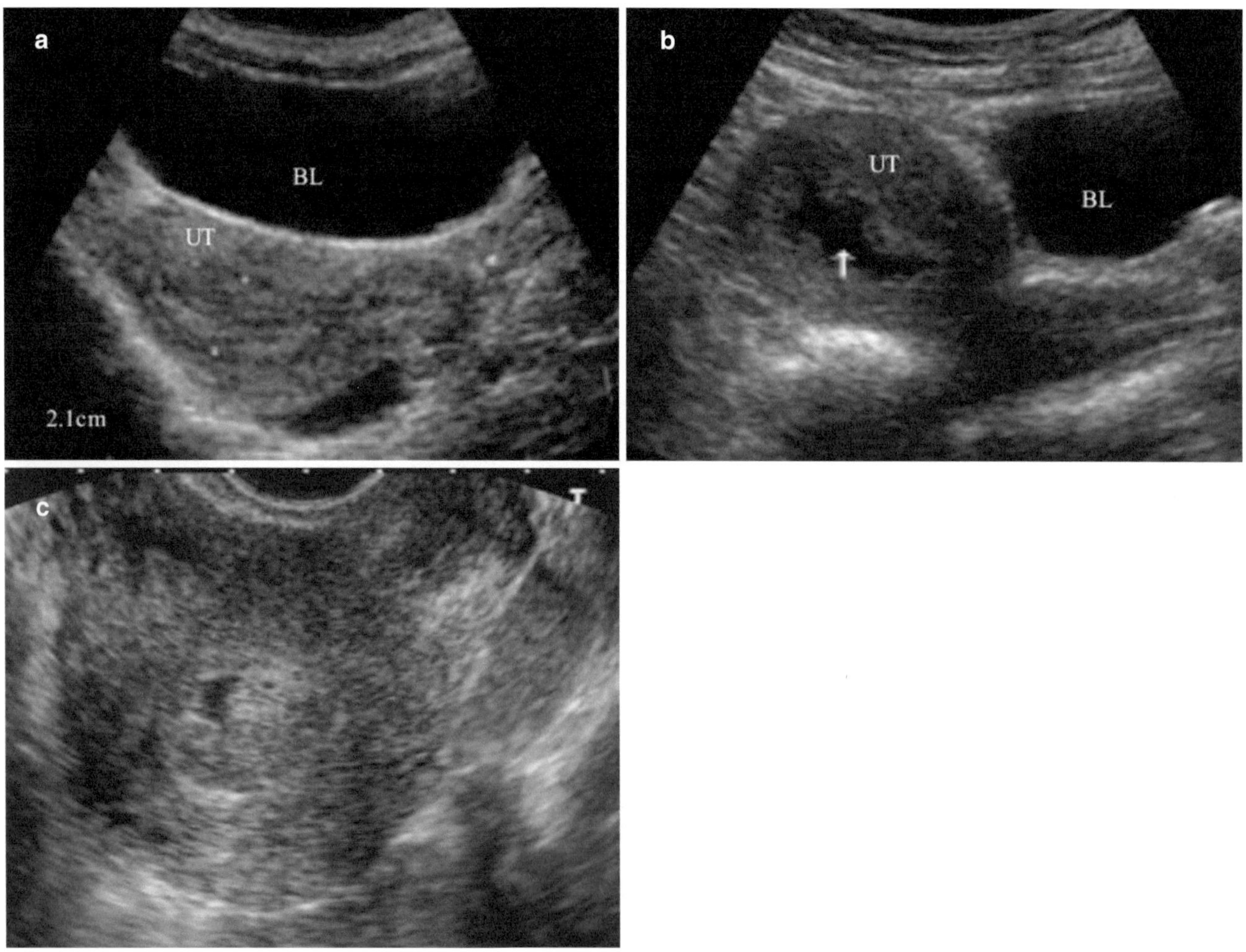

Fig. 3.9 Ectopic pregnancy. (**a–c**). The sonogram shows the enlarged uterus, thickened endometrium, uterine cavity hematocele, and intrauterine pseudogestational sac

the mass is complex and mixed over time. ③Most of the old EP mass is solid, which is easily misdiagnosed as ovarian solid mass. ④ Ruptured EP is an emergency case in clinical, which is caused by the rupture of isthmic EP, and shows a large amount of liquid areas surrounding the uterus in the pelvic cavity (Figs. 3.10, 3.11, and 3.12).

3. Cervical EP, isthmic pregnancy, rudimentary horn EP, ovarian EP, uterine muscular EP, and abdominal EP are rare clinical pregnancy. Cervical EP is characterized by the empty uterine cavity, abnormal enlarged cervix, with the internal cervical os closed, irregular hyperechoic space-occupying mass, and the gestational sac can be seen occasionally in the cervical canal. The color Doppler ultrasound shows abundant blood flow along the inner cervical wall or the pregnancy tissue. Cesarean scar ectopic pregnancy occurs in women with a history of cesarean section. Ultrasound shows gestational sac-like structure or irregular enhanced echo at the internal cervical os, next to the anterior wall of the lower uterine segment and the bladder wall. Color Doppler ultrasound shows a circular blood flow around the mass (Figs. 3.13, 3.14, 3.15, 3.16, 3.17, 3.18, and 3.19).

3.2.3 Special Tips

1. It is vital to collect the history of amenorrhea, symptoms, signs, and serum hCG test results, combined with the characteristics of ultrasound images for the diagnosis of ectopic pregnancy.
2. If the patient has more than two of the three symptoms of amenorrhea, abdominal pain, and vaginal bleeding, and the hCG test is positive, and there is no obvious pregnancy in and outside the uterine cavity, it is strongly recommended to follow-up with ultrasonography regularly.
3. During ultrasound scanning, change the patient's position and rotate the probe to the left and right adnexal area to obtain satisfied images. Notice small ectopic pregnancy lesions around the ovary and the presence of the free fluid in the rectouterine pouch and iliac fossa.
4. Pay attention to differentiate ectopic pregnancy from the corpus luteum rupture, follicle rupture, intrauterine pregnancy abortion, appendicitis, uterine or cervical fibroids, ovarian masses, cervical cancer, pelvic inflammatory disease, and other diseases (Figs. 3.20, 3.21, 3.22, and 3.23).

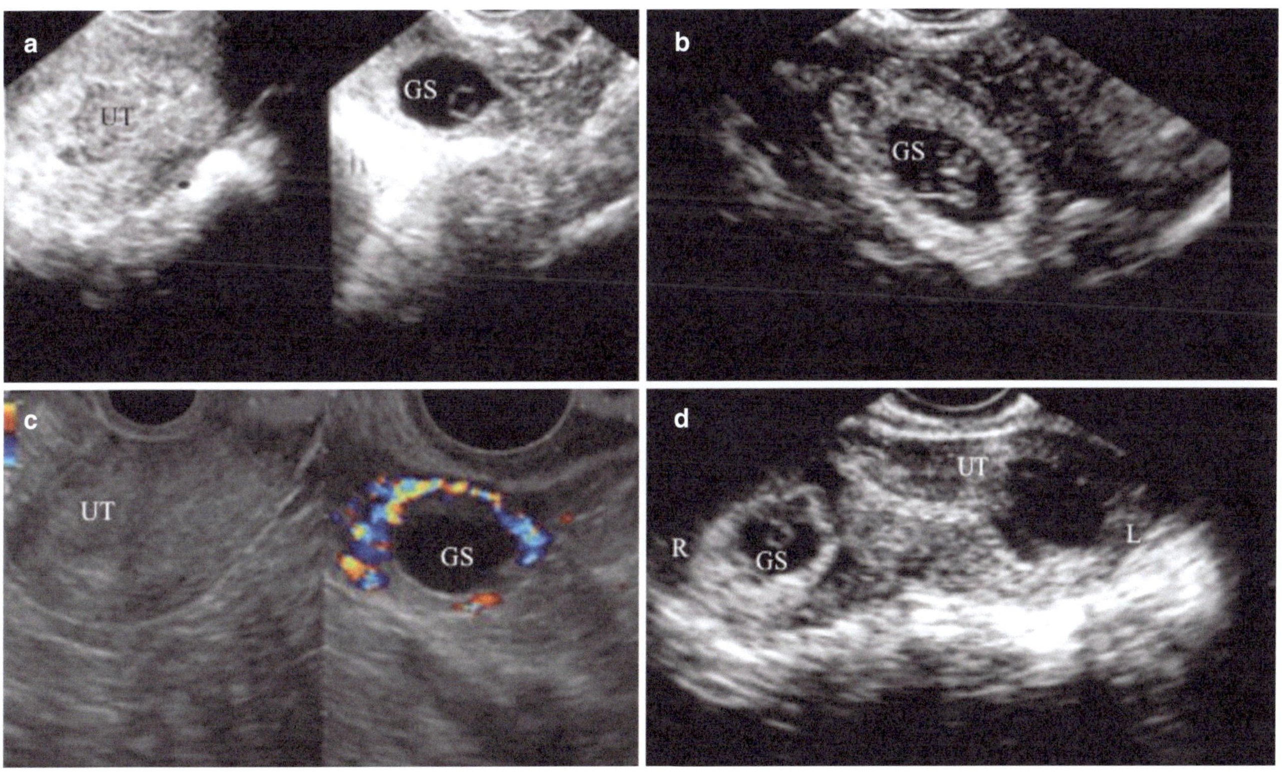

Fig. 3.10 Live ectopic pregnancy. (**a**). On the 44th day of gestation, the uterine cavity is empty, and an extrauterine gestational sac with yolk sac is visible; (**b**). On the 48th day of pregnancy, there is no gestational sac in the uterus, and the gestational sac with embryo and heartbeat is found on the right side of the uterus. The decidual reaction is distinct. (**c**). On the 48th day of pregnancy, there is no gestational sac in the uterus, and a gestational sac-like echo is found on the left side of the uterus, and the color Doppler ultrasound shows surrounding trophoblastic blood flow. (**d**). After 50 days of amenorrhea, there is no gestational sac in the uterus, only fluid is visible in the uterine cavity. The gestational sac with embryo and heartbeat is found on the right side of the uterus

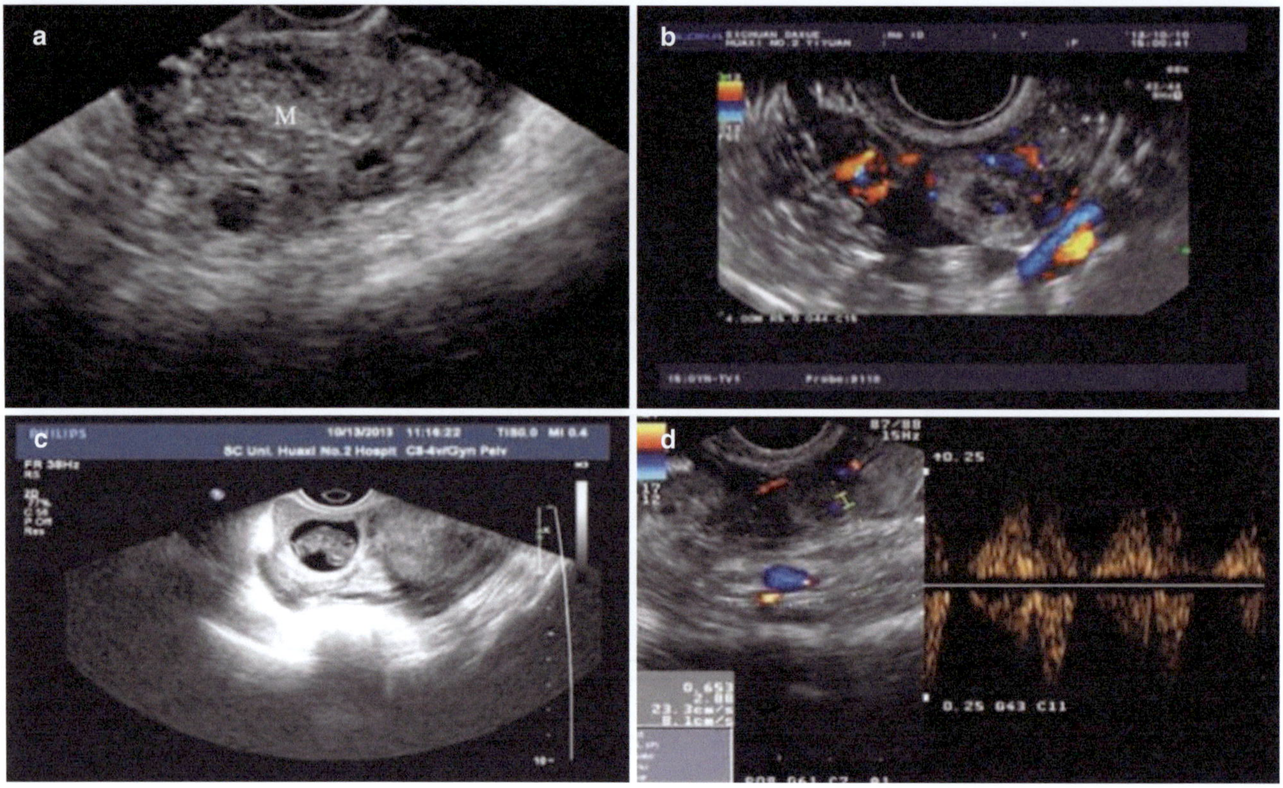

Fig. 3.11 Mass ectopic pregnancy. (**a**). On the 34th day of gestation, the patient has irregular vaginal bleeding for 6 days, with abdominal pain and positive hCG. The ultrasound examination shows a parauterine hypoechoic mass with a diameter of about 5.0 cm. A gestational sac-like echo is visible in the mass, with yolk sac and surrounding decidua-like enhanced echo. No embryo is detected. (**b**). On the 46th day of pregnancy, the patient has vaginal bleeding for 4 days and abdominal pain for 1 day, with positive hCG. Sonogram shows the irregular hypoechoic mass, 3.0 cm in diameter, on the right side of the uterus. In the mass, there is an atypical gestational sac-like echo and an embryo inside. The pelvic hematocele is shown. (**c**). On 57 days of gestation, irregular vaginal bleeding for 8 days. A mass of 3.1 cm in diameter is found in the left adnexal area, with a gestational sac-like echo and a 2.0 cm long embryo inside. (**d**). The shape of the blood flow spectrum in the EP mass likes a "tropical fish"

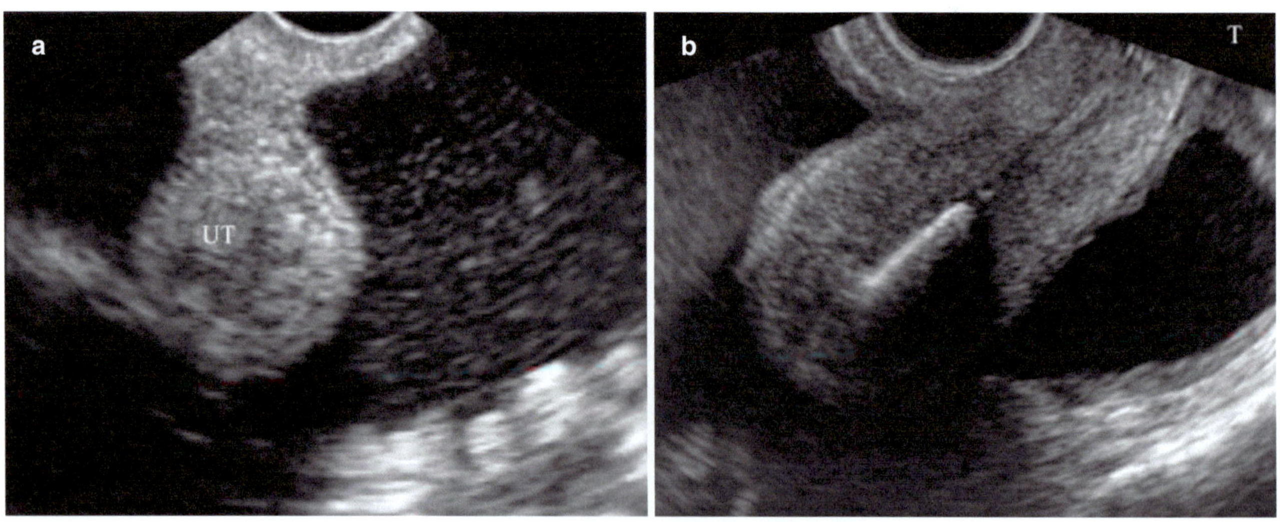

Fig. 3.12 Ruptured ectopic pregnancy (EP with floating uterus). (**a, b**). After 37 and 43 days of amenorrhea, the patient under sudden lacerate pain at the lower abdomen. Ultrasound scan shows a lot of liquid areas around the uterus, and floating dot echoes are visible in the dark area. The patient is diagnosed as ruptured ectopic pregnancy, with massive hematocele in the pelvic cavity

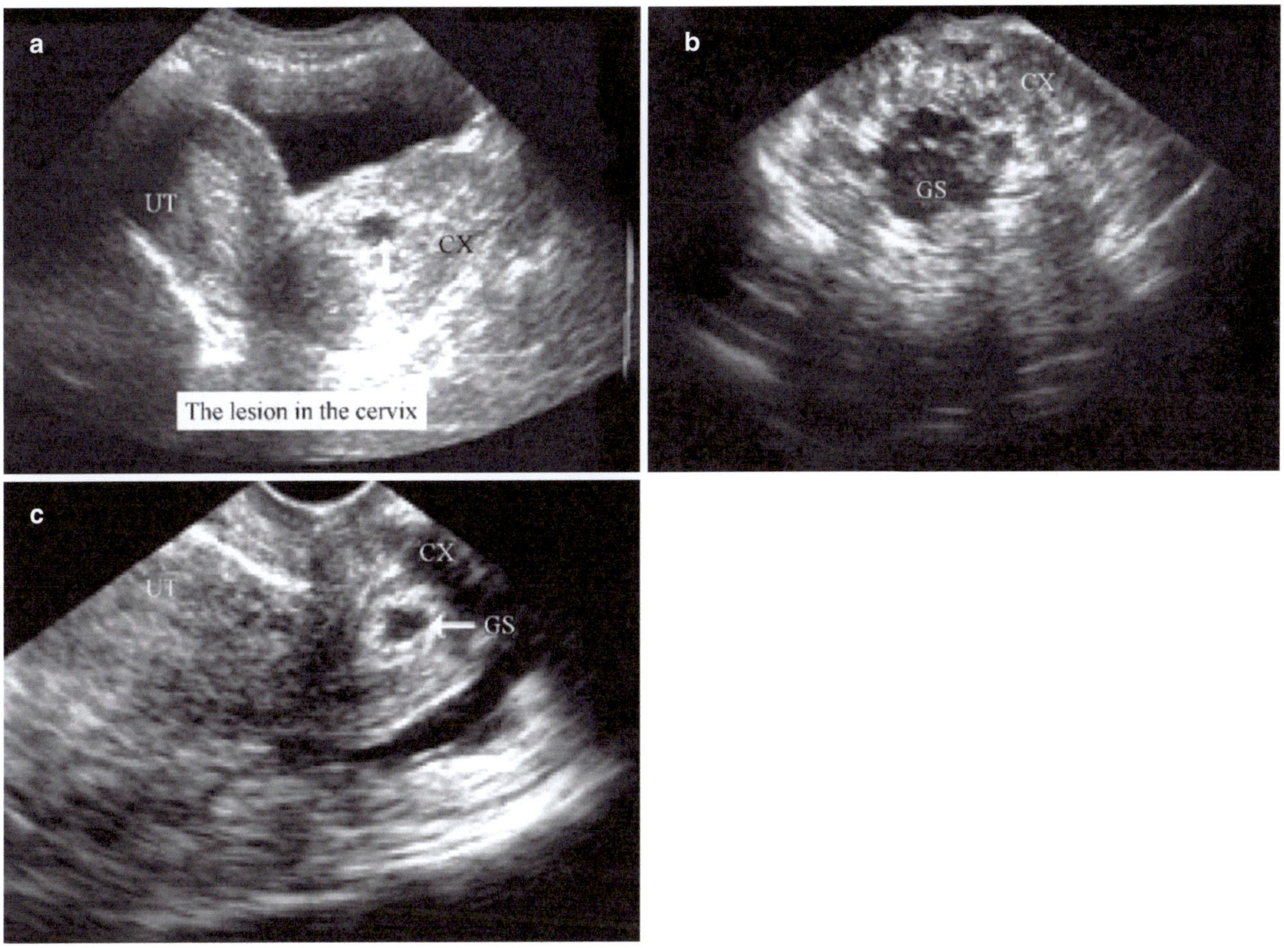

Fig. 3.13 Cervical ectopic pregnancy. (**a**). At 46 days of amenorrhea, ultrasound shows no pregnancy tissue in the uterine cavity, and the cervix is "barrel-shaped" enlarged with a gestational sac-like echo (0.8 cm in diameter), which is diagnosed as cervical ectopic pregnancy. (**b**). After 49 days of amenorrhea, there is no pregnancy in the uterine cavity. On the anterior wall of the lower uterine segment, heterogeneous hyperechoic mass with a diameter of about 5.0 cm is found, which protruding toward the bladder. A gestational sac-like echo, with embryo and heartbeat, is visible in the anterior wall of the lower uterine segment. And the patient is diagnosed as isthmic pregnancy. (**c**). Cervical ectopic pregnancy:on the 34th day of amenorrhea, no gestational sac is found in the uterine cavity. The gestational sac echo is detected in the cervical canal, and serum hCG is positive

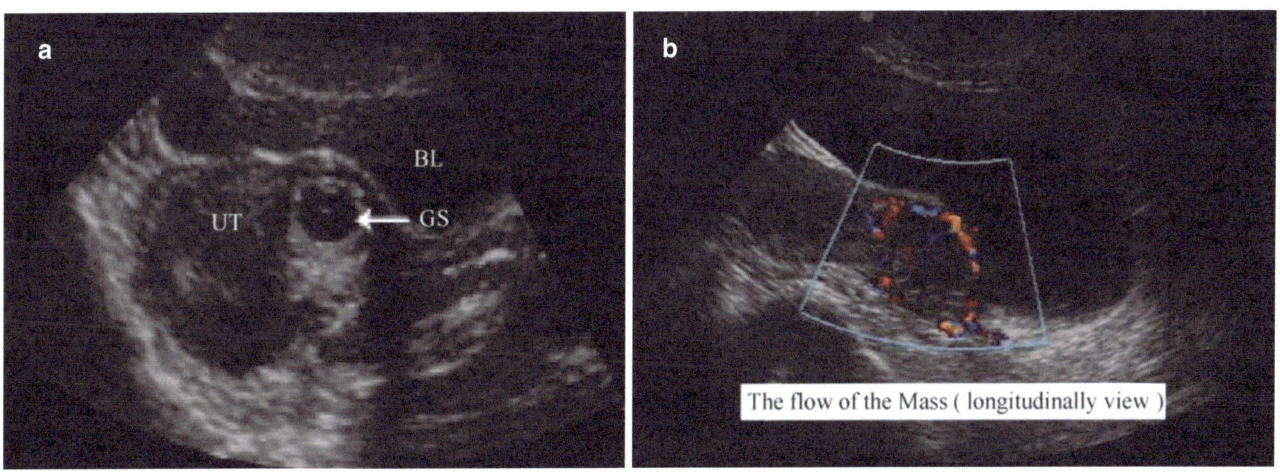

Fig. 3.14 Isthmic ectopic pregnancy. (**a**). After 43 days of amenorrhea, there is no gestational sac in the uterus, and the gestational sac is found in the isthmus of uterus; (**b**). Color Doppler shows the circular blood flow around the ectopic pregnancy in the uterine isthmus

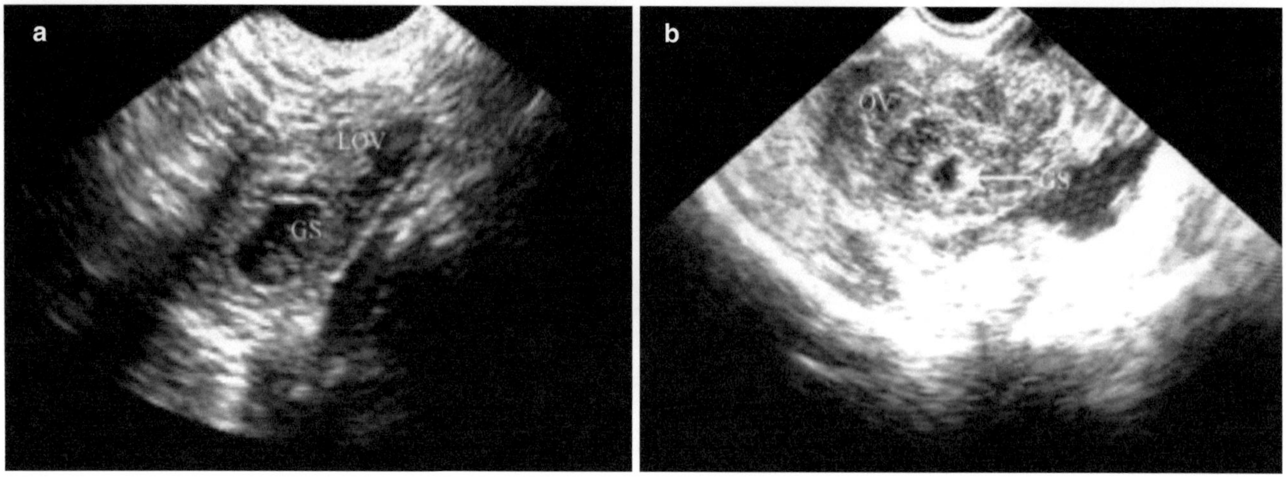

Fig. 3.15 Ovarian ectopic pregnancy. (**a**). Unruptured gestational sac is found in the left ovary, with embryo and heartbeat; (**b**). The gestational sac with a diameter of 1.0 cm is visible in the ovary, with decidual reaction

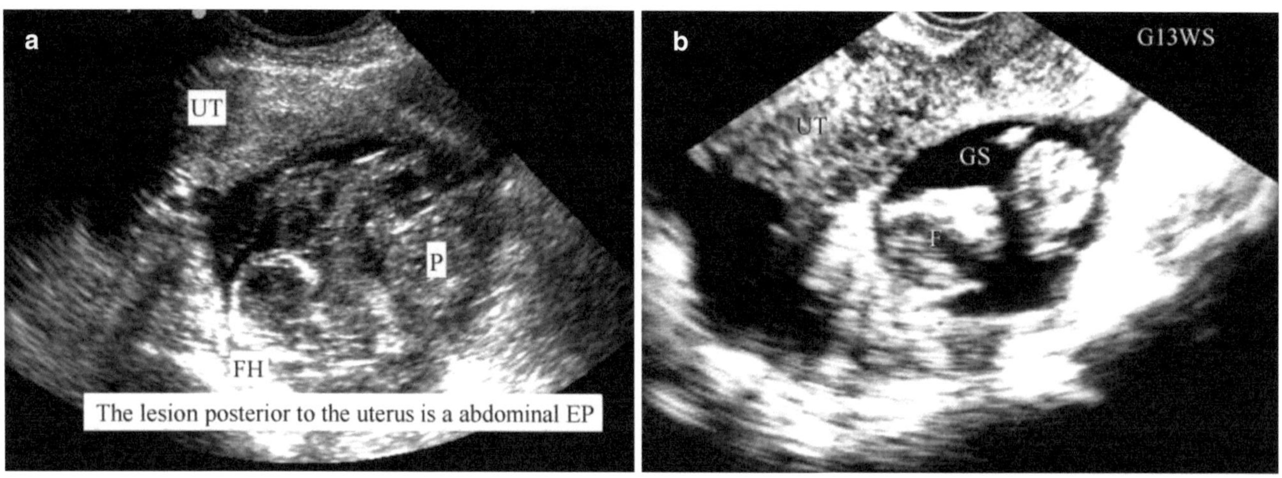

Fig. 3.16 Abdominal ectopic pregnancy. (**a**). At 11 weeks of gestation, the uterine cavity is empty, and the fetus with heartbeat is detected posterior to the uterus, which is diagnosed as abdominal EP; (**b**). At 13 weeks of pregnancy, there is no fetus in the uterine cavity, and the fetus with heartbeat and movement is detected posterior to the uterus in the pelvic cavity

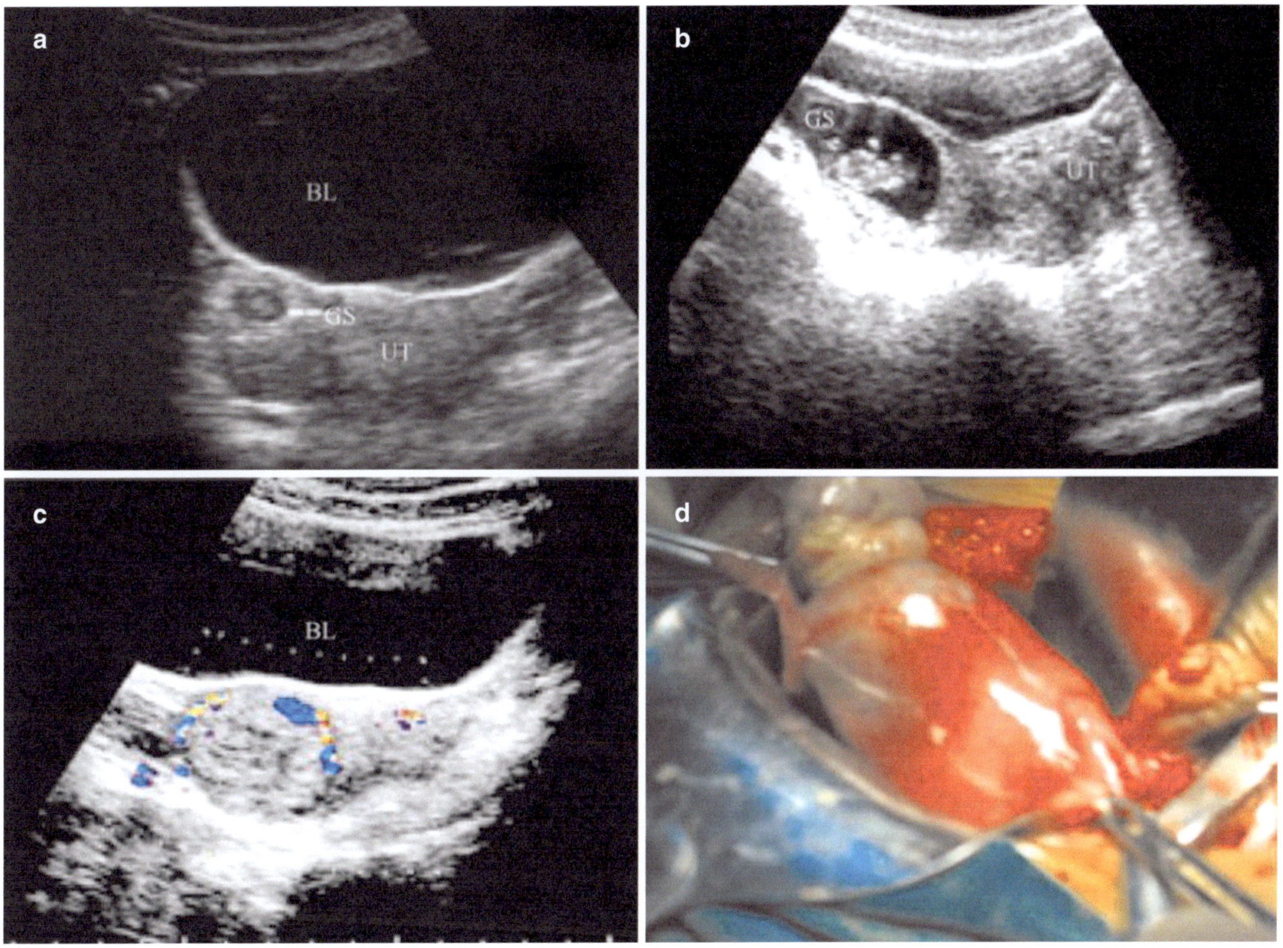

Fig. 3.17 Interstitial pregnancy. (**a**). After 47 days of menopause, the patient had underwent contraceptive operation. After the operation, she had irregular vaginal bleeding for half a month. After three times of uterine curettage, she went to hospital for abdominal pain. Ultrasound examination shows a 3.0 cm × 4.3 cm × 4.1 cm hyperechoic mass in the right corner of the uterus, with a 0.8 cm diameter bubble-like anechoic area. Serum hCG is positive. (**b**). After 54 days of amenorrhea, there is no gestational sac in the uterine cavity. A gestational sac, protruded to the right, is visible in the right corner of the uterus, with embryo and heartbeat. (**c, d**). After 59 days of amenorrhea, pregnancy residue is suspected after contraceptive operation. After curettage twice, space-occupying mass remains visible in the uterine cavity. Sonogram shows the area of increased echogenicity with a diameter of 3.6 cm at the right corner of the uterine cavity. The color Doppler ultrasound shows surrounding blood flow. It is interstitial pregnancy, confirmed by operation

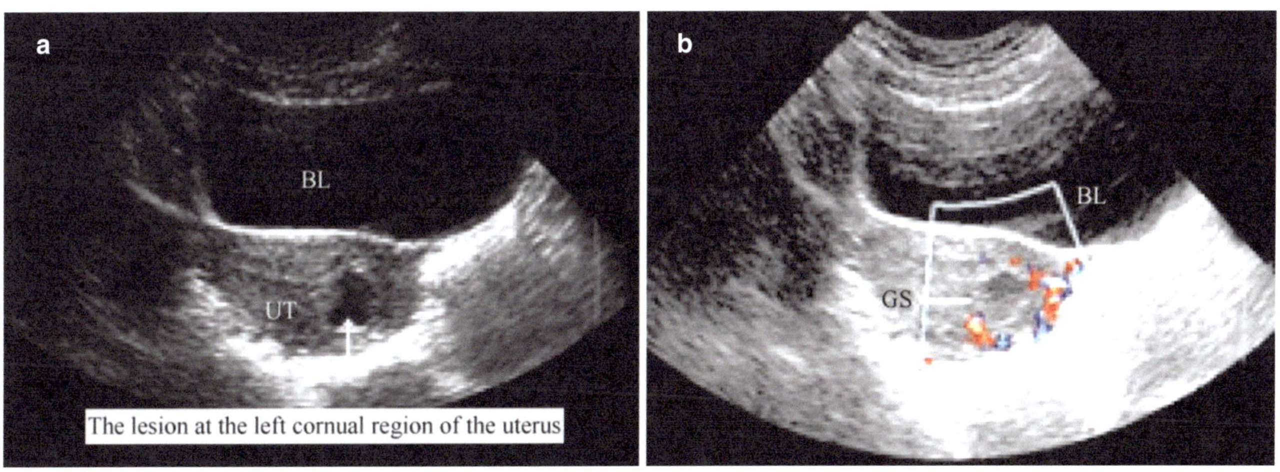

Fig. 3.18 Cornual pregnancy. (**a**). After 42 days of amenorrhea, contraceptive operation failed. Ultrasound scan shows the pregnancy sac at the left cornual region of the uterus. The echo of uterine serosa layer is continuous, and the shape of the uterus is normal; (**b**). Color Doppler ultrasound shows abundant blood flow around the cornual pregnancy, and then the pregnancy tissue is cleared up under ultrasonic monitoring

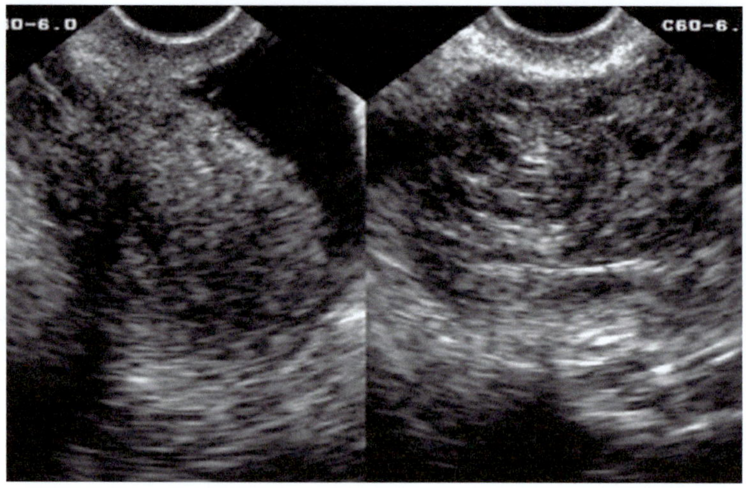

Fig. 3.19 Old ectopic pregnancy. After 48 days of amenorrhea, irregular vaginal bleeding for 20 + days. hCG is suspected to be positive. Ultrasonography shows the normal uterus and a hypoechoic mass beside the uterus, without obvious velamen. A small amount of liquid is visible in the rectouterine pouch

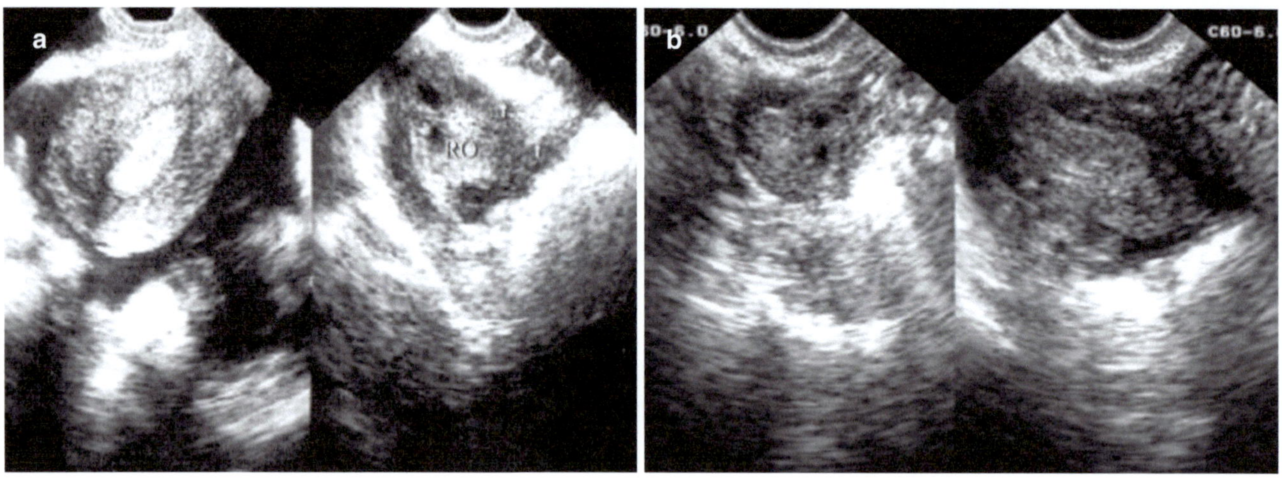

Fig. 3.20 Differentiation between follicle rupture, corpus luteum rupture, and ectopic pregnancy. (**a**). A hyperechoic mass, 3.0 cm in diameter, is visible in the left ovary, with liquid area posterior to the uterus. Serum hCG is negative; (**b**). 48 days after amenorrhea and irregular vaginal bleeding for 10$^+$days, the area of increased echogenicity with a diameter of 2.4 cm is visible in the left adnexal area, and hCG is positive

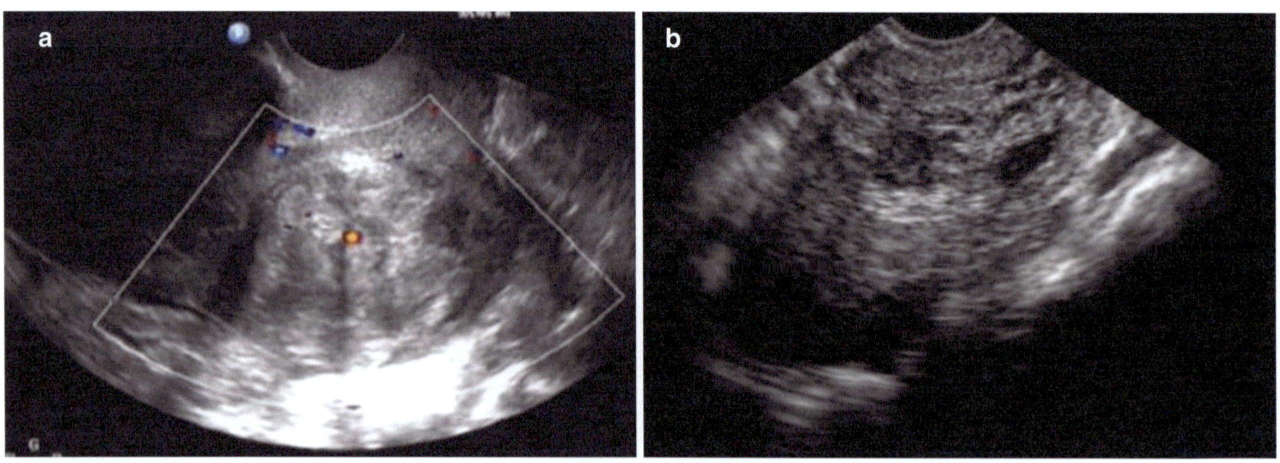

Fig. 3.21 Differentiation of cervical leiomyoma and cervical pregnancy. (**a**). The cervical leiomyoma is a round hypoechoic mass, with a clear boundary; (**b**). After 44 days of amenorrhea, hCG is positive and the cervix is enlarged and inhomogeneous

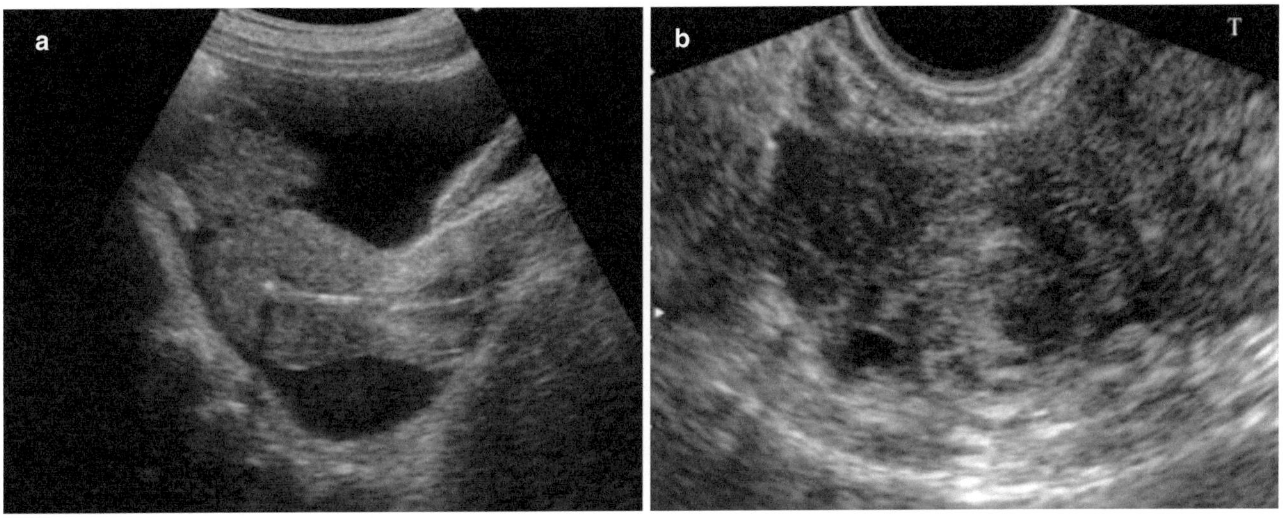

Fig. 3.22 Differential diagnosis of ovarian mass and ectopic pregnancy. (**a**). 38 years old patient with abdominal distension for more than one month. Sonogram shows normal uterus and an irregular mass with diameter of 3.0^{+}cm in right adnexal area. Serum CA125 is increased and hCG is negative; (**b**). 33 years old patient with 42 days of amenorrhea, 3 days of abdominal pain, and 8 days of vaginal bleeding. Serum hCG is positive. A heterogeneous mass of 4.0 cm in diameter is visible in right adnexa area

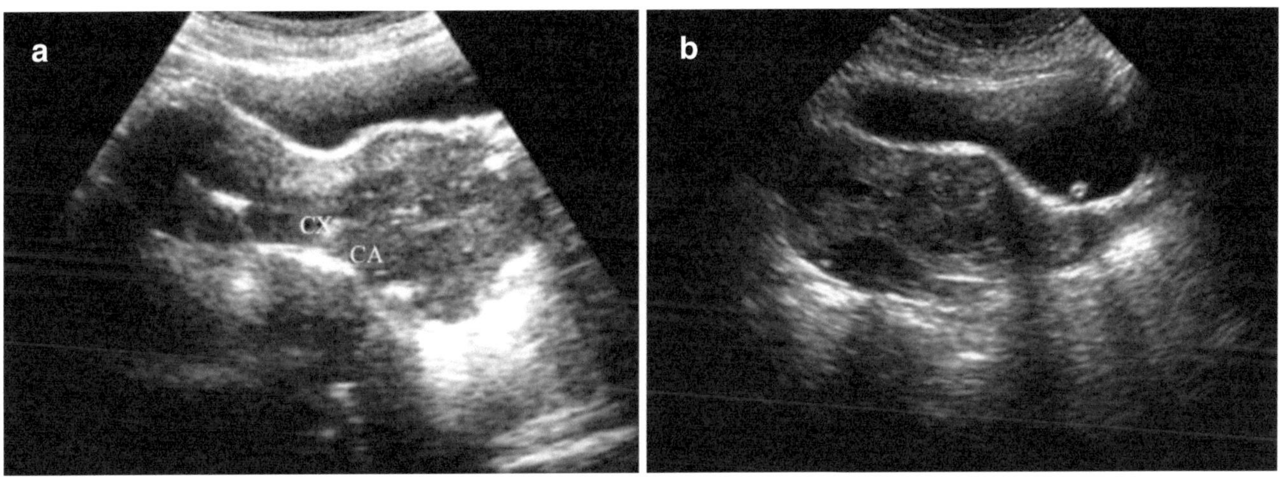

Fig. 3.23 Differential diagnosis of cervical cancer and cervical pregnancy. (**a**). The 43 years old patient had vaginal bleeding for half a year. Ultrasound scan shows abnormal cervical morphology and a hypoechoic mass with a diameter of 4.0 cm. The pathological diagnosis is cervical cancer. (**b**). The 29 years old patient, who had a history of cesarean section, has irregular vaginal bleeding after 46 days of amenorrhea. Ultrasound examination shows a heterogeneous hypoechoic mass, 3.0 cm in diameter, at the junction of the anterior cervical body and neck. Serum HCG is positive

3.3 Ultrasonic Diagnosis of Gestational Trophoblastic Disease

3.3.1 Basic Concepts

1. Gestational trophoblastic disease (GTD) is a spectrum of diseases stemming from the placental villous trophoblastic cells, including hydatidiform mole, invasive hydatidiform mole, choriocarcinoma, and rare placental-site trophoblastic tumor.
2. Hydatidiform mole is classified as complete hydatidiform mole and partial hydatidiform mole. The high-risk factors of hydatidiform mole include the region, nutritional status, social economy, cell genetics, etc. There is an increased risk of hydatidiform mole in women under the age of 20 and over the age of 40 years. The recurrence rate in women with a history of mole pregnancy is 4 to 5 times higher than that of the patients without relative history. The incidence of hydatidiform mole in women over 40 years old is 7.5 times higher than young women.

3. The pathological features of hydatidiform mole are villous interstitial edema, vascular absence, and trophoblastic proliferation. Invasive hydatidiform mole, secondary to hydatidiform mole, occurs within 6 months after hydatidiform mole evacuation. Mole tissue can penetrate the myometrium, leading to tissue damage or complicated with extrauterine metastasis. Choriocarcinoma, secondary to normal or abnormal pregnancy, is a malignant trophoblastic tumor. The absence of formed villi or hydatidiform structure is the pathological feature of choriocarcinoma. Both the invasive hydatidiform mole and choriocarcinoma can have blood metastasis, most frequently affecting the lung, followed by the vagina, liver, and even the whole body. The tumor can invade the myometrium or blood vessels of the uterus, and even penetrate the uterine wall and expand into the broad ligament or abdominal cavity, causing internal bleeding.
4. Amenorrhea history and severe morning sickness are the clinical features of the GTD. During pelvic examination, the uterus is softened and significantly larger than the gestational week, failing to feel the fetal body and fetal heartbeat. After the last pregnancy, the patient suffers from irregular vaginal bleeding and metastasis symptoms, such as expectoration, hemoptysis, headache, vomiting, convulsion, coma, etc. Serum hCG is abnormally increased or continuously positive.

3.3.2 Ultrasonic Diagnosis

3.3.2.1 Hydatidiform Mole (HM)

1. Sonogram shows the enlarged uterine body without normal gestational sac and embryo in the uterine cavity and the disappeared uterine cavity line. The uterine cavity is filled with dense honeycomb liquid dark areas of different sizes. The myometrium is thin, and the boundary between myometrium wall and intrauterine vesicle is identifiable.
2. One third of hydatidiform mole complicates with intrauterine hemorrhage. Ultrasound scan shows liquid dark areas, homogeneous weak echo, or hyperechoic clots in the uterine cavity.
3. More than half of hydatidiform mole patients had unilocular or multilocular theca lutein cysts with different sizes in one or both adnexal areas. The ultrasonographic features of the theca lutein cysts include thin and clear capsule, thin septum, and clear fluid.
4. The uterine enlargement of partial hydatidiform mole patients is consistent with the gestational age. The fetus in the amniotic cavity is visible, and multiple small cystic spaces are seen in the normal placenta (Figs. 3.24, 3.25, and 3.26).

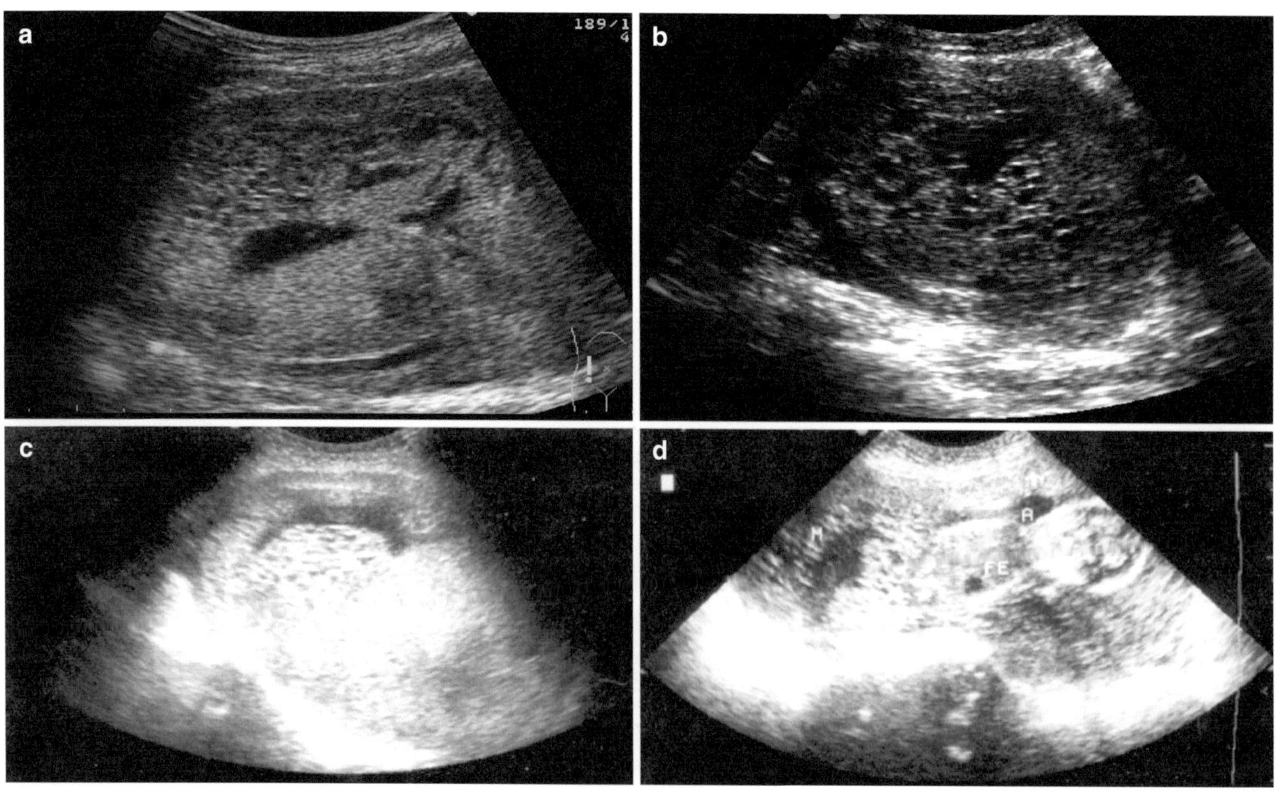

Fig. 3.24 Hydatidiform mole (I). (**a**–**c**). complete hydatidiform mole, uterus is enlarged than the gestational age, with intrauterine "honeycomb" echo; (**d**). 14 weeks of amenorrhea, sonogram shows a normal fetus and part of the placenta appears the "honeycomb" echo

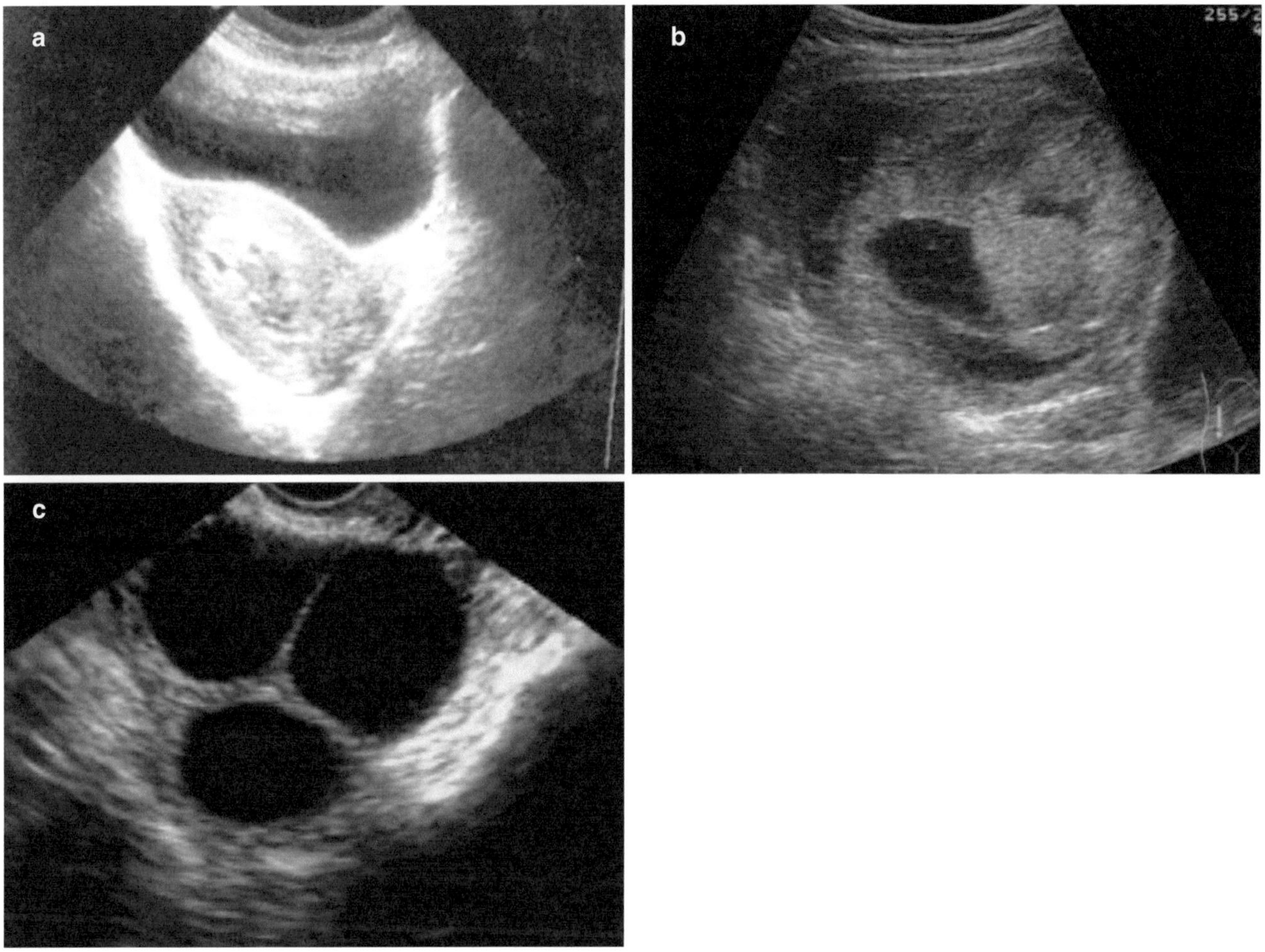

Fig. 3.25 Hydatidiform mole (II). (**a**). After 13 weeks of amenorrhea, no normal fetus and placenta in the uterus. Heterogeneous hyperechoic mass is found in the uterine cavity, which is suspected of missed abortion by ultrasound, and it is pathologically diagnosed as hydatidiform mole; (**b**). After 10 weeks of amenorrhea, hydatidiform mole complicated with intrauterine hemorrhage, with inside blood clot and liquid dark area; (**c**). The same patient as **b**, complicated with left adnexal theca lutein cysts

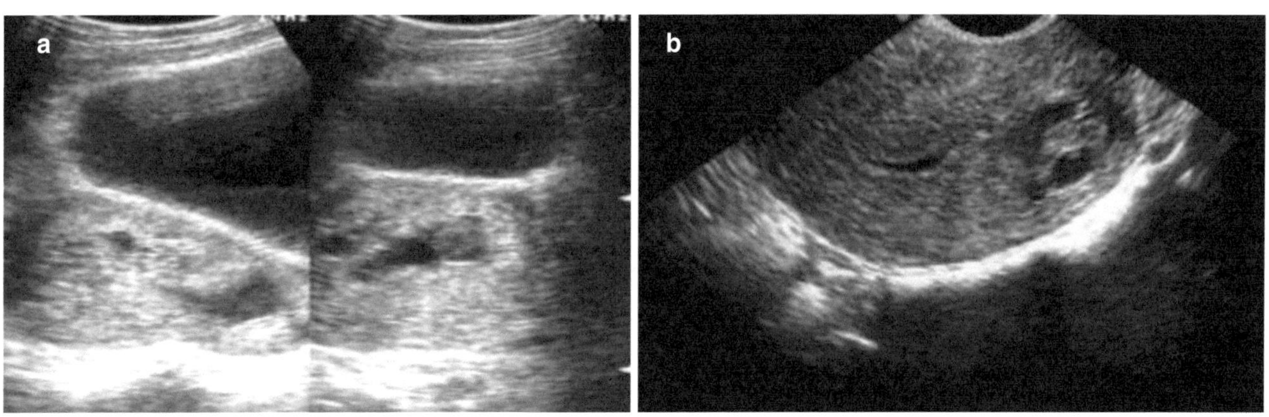

Fig. 3.26 Atypical hydatidiform mole. (**a**). Amenorrhea for 63 days with vaginal bleeding. Intrauterine heterogeneous enhanced echo with liquid dark area is visible. No embryo is detected, and hCG is significantly increased. The patient is diagnosed as hydatidiform mole after curettage; (**b**). The patient has irregular vaginal bleeding, without definite history of amenorrhea, hCG is gradually increased, and diagnosed as malignant trophoblastic tumor in clinical. Ultrasonography shows cystic masses with inside septum near the uterine fundus, with a diameter of 3.0^{+}cm. After curettage, hydatidiform mole is confirmed

3.3.2.2 Invasive Hydatidiform Mole and Choriocarcinoma

1. Except for the pathological microscope represents, the clinical symptoms, signs, hCG changes, and treatment principles of invasive hydatidiform mole and choriocarcinoma are basically the same. It is difficult to distinguish between invasive hydatidiform mole and choriocarcinoma on sonogram. When there are eroded lesion, bleeding, and necrosis tissue in the uterine muscle wall, ultrasound images represent the inhomogeneous echo of uterine muscle wall, with focal or diffuse honeycomb echo and unclear boundary, which looks like marshland. No endometrial echo is visible. The eroded focus lesion gradually expands and penetrates the serosa layer of uterus, leading to an abnormal morphology and even pelvic hemorrhage.
2. Color Doppler flow imaging shows increased number of blood vessels of the eroded focus lesion. The color blood flow spectrum: ① abundant venous spectrum; ② low resistance arterial spectrum, RI < 0.4; ③ arteriovenous fistula like blood flow spectrum.
3. In the chemotherapy of malignant trophoblastic tumor, ultrasound can continuously monitor the location and regression of uterine lesions to avoid the adverse consequences of blind chemotherapy, which is vital for the treatment guideline and the prognosis judgement (Figs. 3.27 and 3.28).

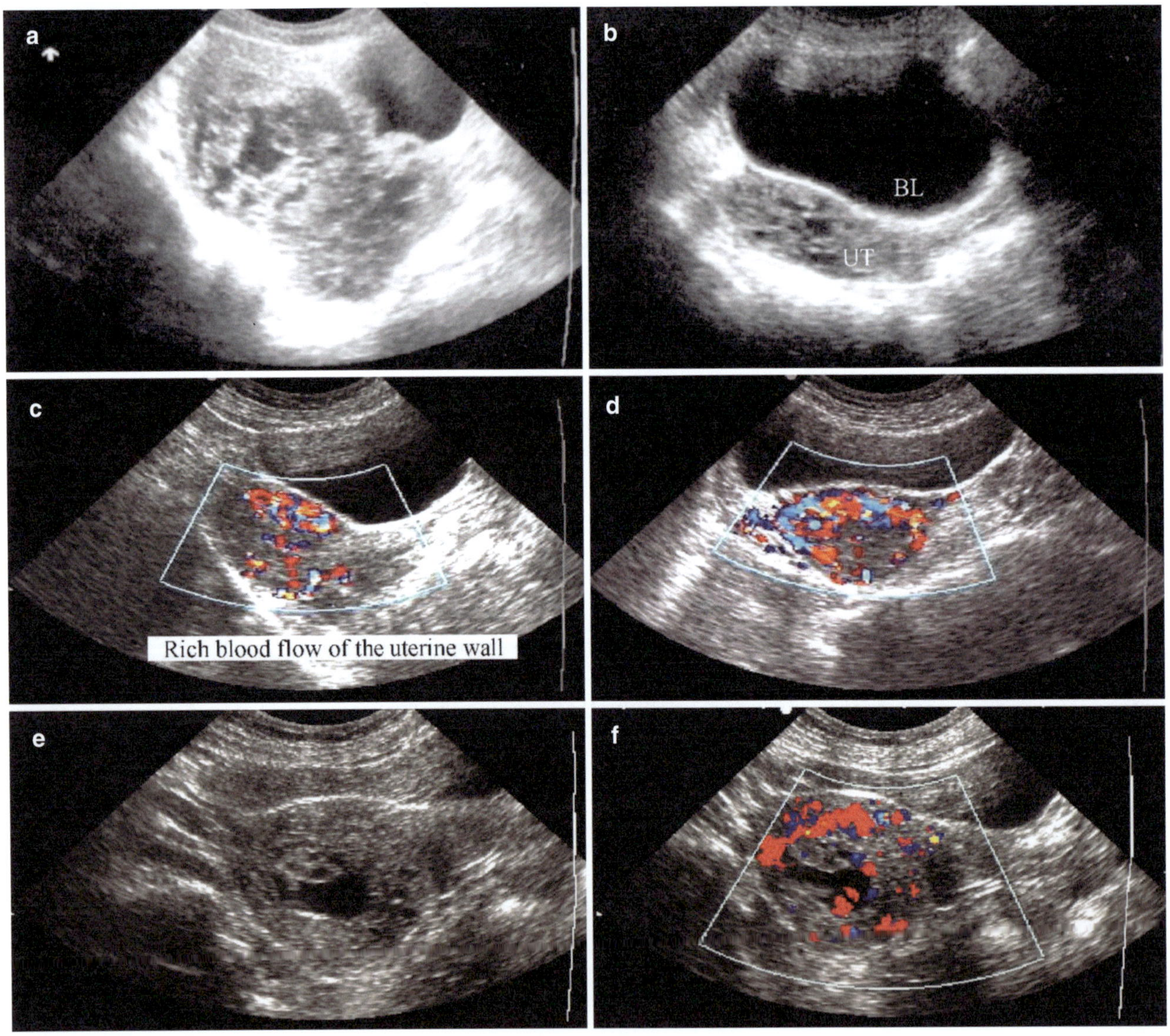

Fig. 3.27 Invasive hydatidiform mole. (**a**). 4 months after the operation of hydatidiform mole, the uterus is enlarged with abnormal shape, the endometrium is disappeared, and hCG is high. Multiple "honeycomb" echo is shown in the uterine body and cervix. (**b**). The patient has irregular vaginal bleeding for half a year, with significantly increased hCG, and clinical diagnosis is choriocarcinoma. Ultrasound shows the absent endometrium and the inhomogeneous uterine body muscle wall with several irregular small liquid dark areas. (**c, d**). In the same patient, the clinical diagnosis of invasive hydatidiform mole, color ultrasound shows extremely rich blood flow of the uterine wall. (**e, f**). 3 months after the operation of hydatidiform mole, the uterus is enlarged, and the endometrium is disappeared. Sonogram shows the inhomogeneous space-occupying mass in the posterior uterine wall, about 4.0 cm in diameter, with abundant blood flow

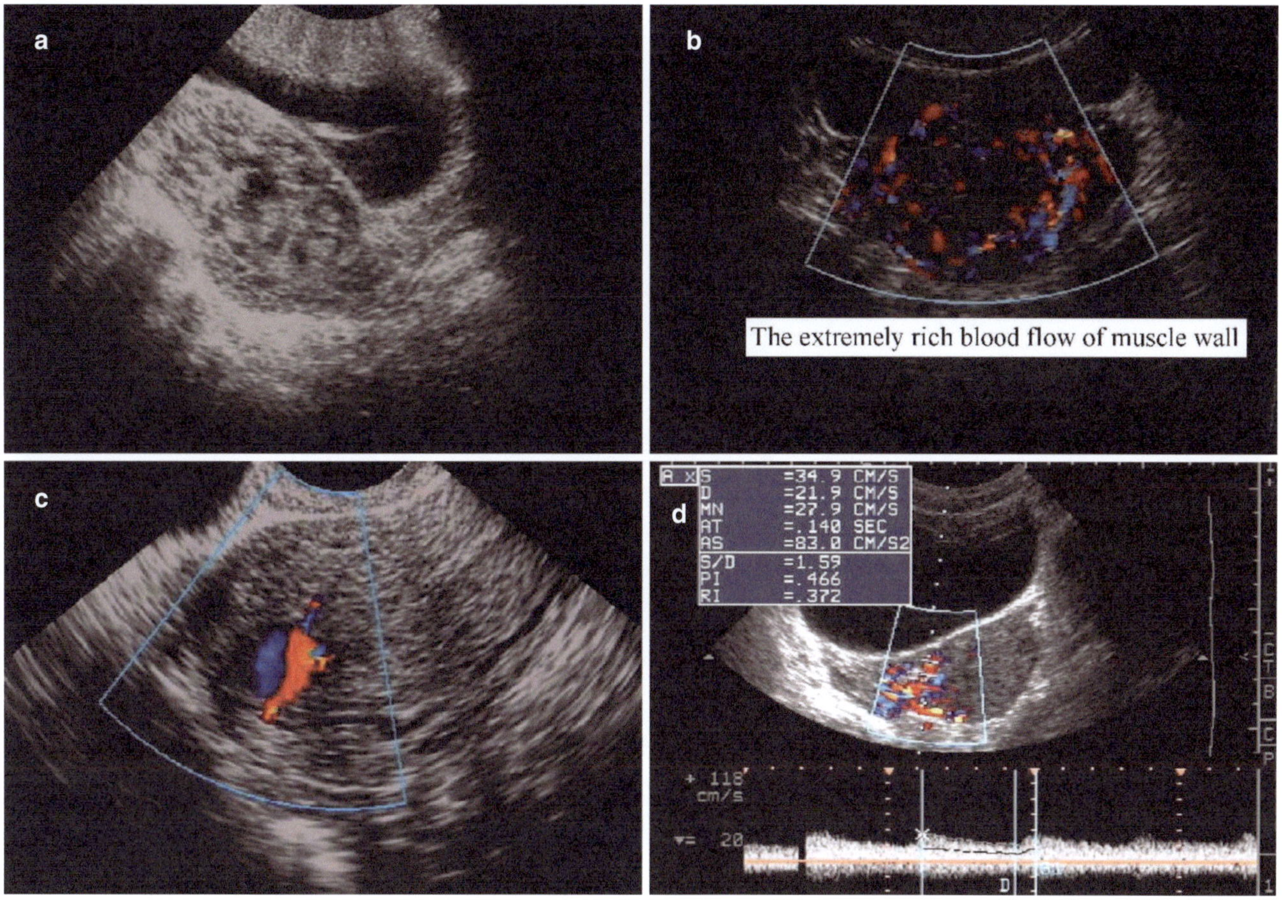

Fig. 3.28 Malignant trophoblastic tumor. 7 months after the operation of hydatidiform mole, a 32 years old patient is diagnosed as invasive hydatidiform mole, with irregular vaginal bleeding and high hCG level. (**a**). Ultrasound scan shows the enlarged uterus without endometrial echo, and the muscle wall represents "honeycomb" echo; (**b**). The extremely rich blood flow of muscle wall shows like a "color ball"; (**c**). After four courses of chemotherapy, the uterus is slightly enlarged, a hypoechoic mass with a diameter of 2.0 cm is seen in the muscle walls, and inside blood flow is visible. (**d**). The blood flow spectrum shows RI = 0.37

3.3.3 Special Tips

1. Combining the clinical data and serum hCG value, pay attention to differentiate atypical hydatidiform mole from missed abortion, hysteromyoma, endometrial carcinoma, and endometrial hyperplasia.
2. The erosion lesions in the uterine muscle walls should be differentiated from myoma degeneration and adenomyosis. When the blood flow is visible in the erosion lesions, it should be differentiated from uterine vascular malformation, adenomyosis, placenta residue after abortion, uterine muscle wall EP, cornual EP, and interstitial EP (Figs. 3.29, 3.30, 3.31, and 3.32).

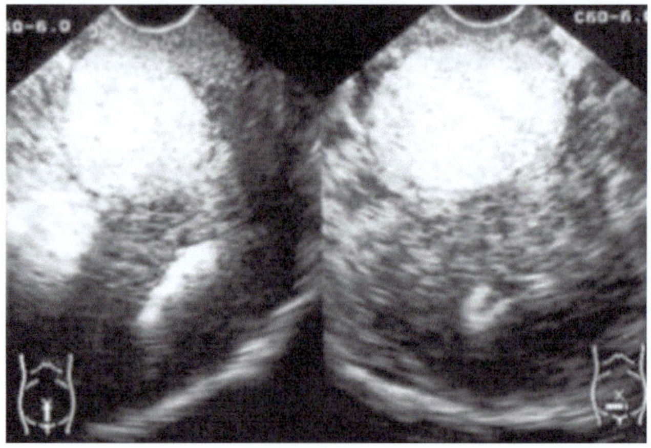

Fig. 3.29 Uterine hemangioma. A homogeneous enhanced echo mass with clear boundary is visible in the muscle wall. The patient has no bleeding and hCG is negative

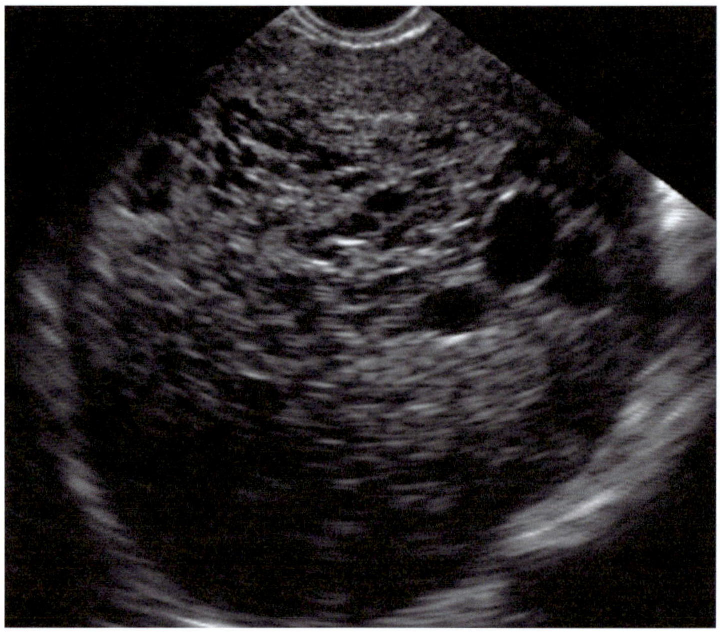

Fig. 3.30 Myoma degeneration. The patient has a history of myoma for 8 years. Ultrasound shows that the diameter of the inhomogeneous myoma is more than 8.0 cm, and there are several liquid dark areas in the myoma. hCG is negative

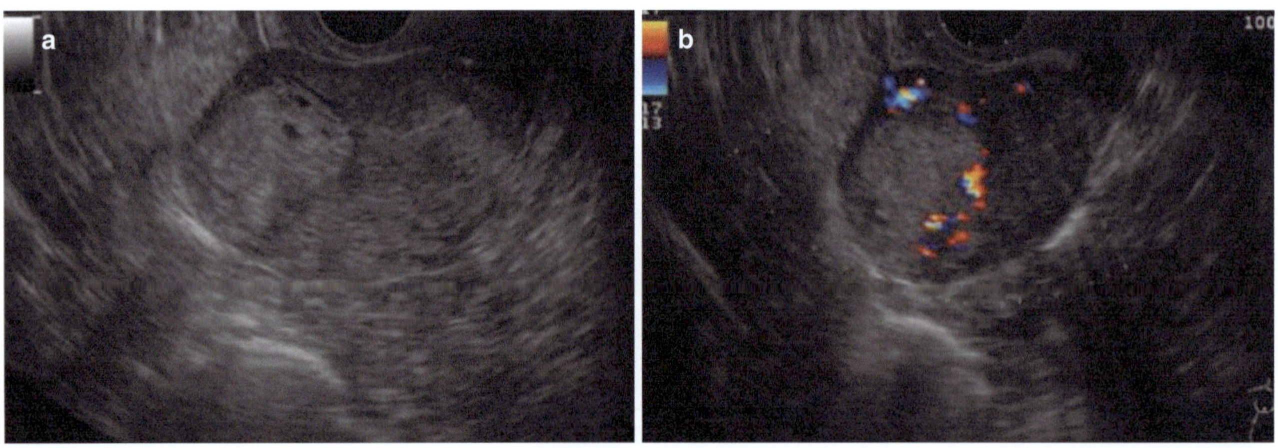

Fig. 3.31 Interstitial pregnancy. After 51 days of amenorrhea, the patient has irregular vaginal bleeding after contraceptive operation. Multiple ultrasound scans show the space-occupying mass at the uterine fundus. hCG is positive, and no tissue is scraped out of the uterus, invasive hydatidiform mole is clinically suspected. (**a, b**). There is no space-occupying mass in the uterine cavity. The hyperechoic mass with a diameter of 2.5 cm is found at the right uterine fundus, and surrounding blood flow is visible. It is confirmed by surgery as interstitial pregnancy

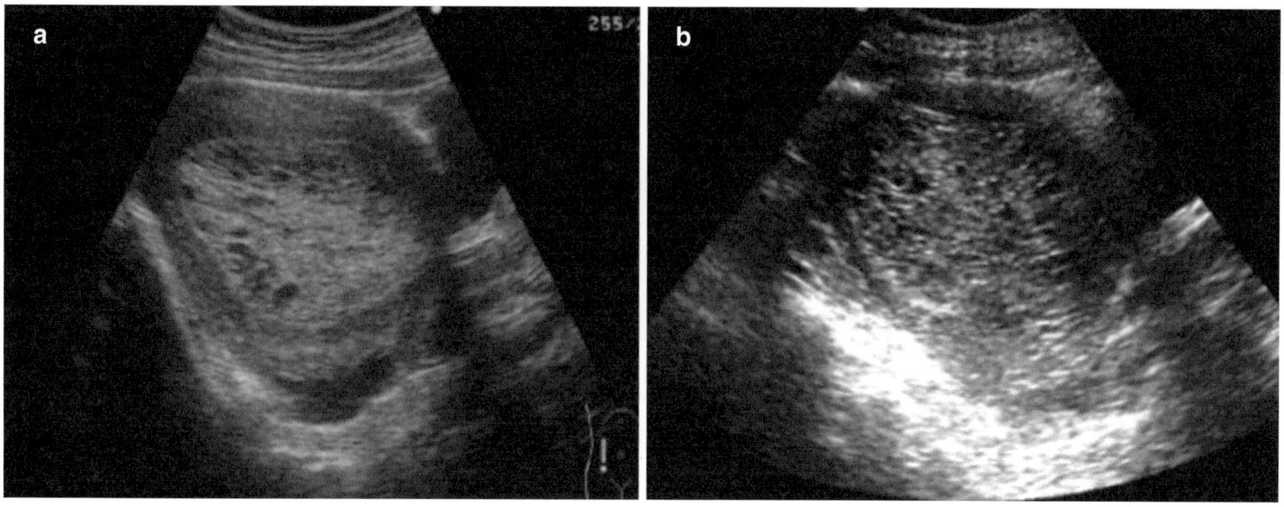

Fig. 3.32 Endometrial hyperplasia. The patient suffers menstrual disorder for nearly one year. (**a**). Ultrasound examination shows the enlarged uterus and a hyperechoic mass with a diameter of 4.0 cm in the uterine cavity, with small bubble-like dark areas. Hydatidiform mole is suspected. hCG is negative, and endometrial hyperplasia is confirmed after curettage. (**b**). Image of hydatidiform mole

Suggested Reading

1. Young L. Barnard. The diagnostic performance of ultrasound in the detection of ectopic pregnancy. N Z Med J. 2017 Mar 24;130(1452):17–22.
2. Goettler S, Zanetti-Dällenbach R. Heterotopic pregnancy. N Engl J Med. 2016 Nov 17;375(20):1982.
3. Gardyszewska A. Non-simultaneous two-stage detection of spontaneous bilateral isthmic tubal pregnancy. Ginekol Pol. 2016;87(10):728.
4. Xin C, Luo H. The value of transvaginal color Doppler ultrasound in the diagnosis and treatment of cesarean scar pregnancy. Technicla Acoustics. 2013;32(4):339–41.

4 Ultrasonic Diagnosis of Fetal Heart

Qi Zhu, Jiao Chen, and Nan Guo

Congenital heart disease (CHD) is a common congenital malformation in children, with an incidence of approximately 8 per 1000 live births. According to statistics, more than 100,000 CHD occurs in China every year, which seriously affects the physical and mental development of children, leading to the decline of children's quality of life. Also, CHD is an important cause of the perinatal death of birth defects. At present, some kinds of CHD can be treated by operation or catheterization. Sad to say, there are still some severe heart malformation cases that cannot be cured by operation and some cases with unsatisfied therapeutic effect. It is important to take the routine sonographic evaluation and prenatal fetal malformation screening. Moreover, during the perinatal health care period, systematic fetal echocardiography is necessary for pregnant women with cardiac teratogenic factors to identify cardiac abnormalities.

4.1 Characteristics of Cardiovascular Development and Blood Circulation in Normal Fetus

4.1.1 Fetal Cardiovascular Development

At the end of the third week of embryonic development, fetal cardiovascular system begins to develop, and the heart is formed at the eighth week. Atriums, ventricles, atrial and ventricular septum, mitral valve, tricuspid valve, aortic valve, pulmonary valve, aorta, pulmonary artery, superior vena cava (SVC), inferior vena cava (IVC), and pulmonary veins are present. If there is abnormal development in any part of the heart during this period, various types of congenital heart disease will occur.

4.1.2 Characteristics of Fetal Circulation

Fetal lungs have no respiratory function. The respiratory, metabolism, and nutrition functions are completed by the blood circulation between the fetal heart and the placenta. The umbilical artery of the fetus sends the blood with low oxygen and metabolites to the placenta for gas and material exchange with the blood of the mother. After the blood gains high oxygen saturation and nutrition, it travels through the umbilical vein to the fetus. The umbilical vein is divided into two branches in front of the portal of the liver of the fetus, one enters through the portal vein, the hepatic sinus and the hepatic vein into the inferior vena cava, accounting for about 40% of the blood; the other enters the inferior vena cava directly through the ductus venous, accounting for about 60% of the blood.

The blood from the umbilical vein into the inferior vena cava together with the blood from the fetal trunk, viscera, and lower extremity, enter the right atrium (RA). Most of the blood enters the left atrium (LA) via the foramen ovale, and then to the left ventricle (LV) and the aorta, supplying the fetal head, neck, and upper limbs. Part of the blood pass through the tricuspid valve and the right ventricle (RV) to the pulmonary artery, together with the blood from SVC returned into the RA. The rest, except a few nourishing pulmonary tissues, flows into the descending aorta through the ductus arteriosus, nourishing the fetal trunk, viscera, and lower limbs. Most of the blood from the descending aorta flow back to the placenta through two umbilical arteries and then the next circulation begins. Therefore, foramen ovale, ductus arteriosus, ductus venous, as well as umbilical artery and vein are necessary to maintain fetal blood circulation. The diagram of fetal blood circulation is as follows:

This chapter was translated by **Mingchun Zhi**, and **Miaoqian Wang** Department of Obstetrics and Gynecology, Beijing Hospital, National Center of Gerontology, Beijing, China

Q. Zhu (✉) · J. Chen · N. Guo
Department of Ultrasonography, West China Second University Hospital, Sichuan University, Chengdu, China

T. Yang, H. Luo (eds.), *Practical Ultrasonography in Obstetrics and Gynecology*, https://doi.org/10.1007/978-981-16-4477-1_4

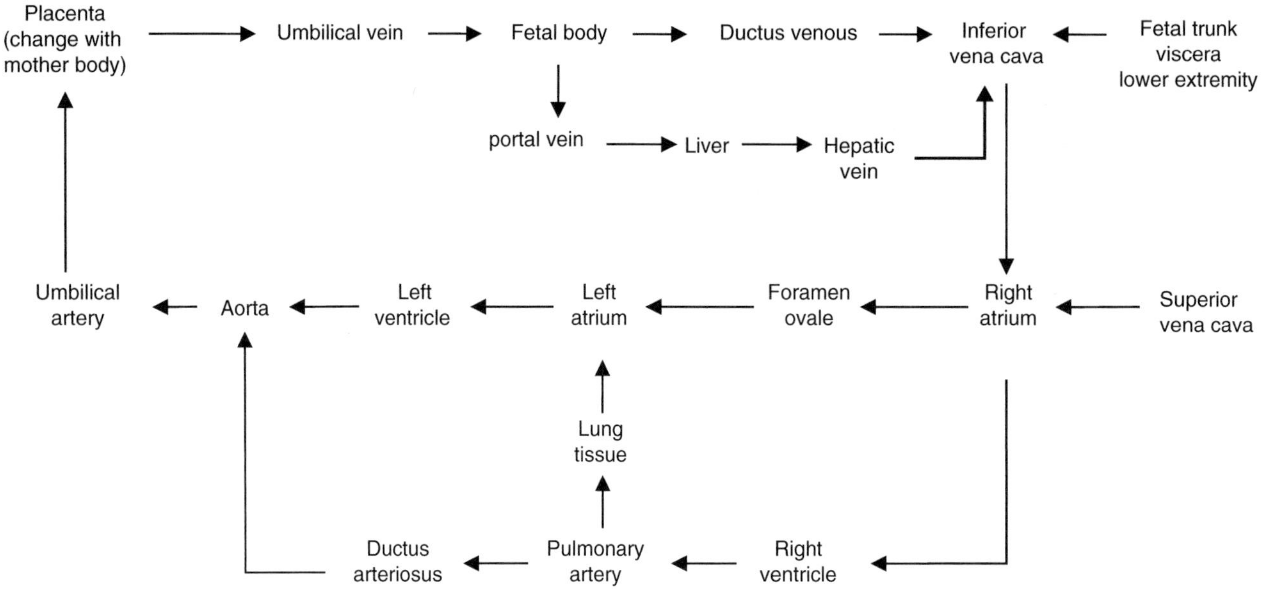

4.2 Echocardiographic Scanning of Fetal Heart

4.2.1 Indications for Fetal Echocardiography

- Mother aspect
  - Maternal infection during pregnancy (rubella, herpes, varicella, influenza, cytomegalovirus, etc.). Autoimmune diseases (systemic lupus erythematosus, hyperthyroidism, rheumatism, Sjogren's syndrome, etc.). Metabolic and endocrine diseases (diabetes, phenylketonuria, etc.).
  - The pregnant age is more than 35. History of CHD children or abnormal pregnancy such as abortion, intrauterine stillbirth.
  - Family history (CHD).
  - Teratogenic drugs, fetal alcohol syndrome (long-term drinking), fetal tobacco syndrome (long-term smoking).
  - Contact history of harmful environment and substances (harmful gases, radiation, chemicals, etc.).
- Fetal aspect
  - Fetal chromosomal anomalies, fetal arrhythmia (especially bradycardia), polyhydramnios, oligohydramnios, single umbilical artery, intrauterine growth retardation (IUGR), etc.
  - Fetal cardiovascular malformations often coexist with extracardiac anomalies, such as hydrocephalus, gastrointestinal atresia, omphalocele, diaphragmatic hernia, visceral ectropion, limb or facial malformations, renal hypoplasia, systemic edema, and ascites.
  - The incidence of CHD in artificial insemination and in vitro infants is three times higher than that in the healthy population. About 50% of heart structural abnormalities come from low-risk pregnant women. According to the literature, there is no significant statistical difference between the incidence of fetal CHD in the low-risk population and the high-risk population. Therefore, fetal echocardiography should be used as routine prenatal screening.

4.2.2 Fetal Echocardiography

- Fetal echocardiography techniques
  - Two-dimensional (2-D) ultrasound
  - M-mode echocardiography
  - Color Doppler imaging and spectral Doppler ultrasound
  - Three-dimensional (3-D) and four-dimensional (4-D) ultrasound
  - The 2-D ultrasound is still the primary method of fetal echocardiography at present.
- Exam conditions of fetal echocardiography
  - The frequency of the 2-D ultrasonic probe is 3–5 MHz.
  - Transabdominal ultrasonography is performed at 16 weeks of gestation. Fetal echocardiography is best accomplished at about 24 weeks of gestation. It is easy to obtain a satisfactory image as the structure of the heart is clear during this period. Moreover, the amount of amniotic fluid is moderate, the size of the fetal heart is appropriate, and the sound shadow of the spine and rib is inconspicuous.

  - In some special cases, transvaginal ultrasound can be performed as early as about 12 weeks of pregnancy, only for those with severe cardiac structural abnormalities.
- Content of fetal echocardiography
  - Morphology, structure, and blood flow of fetal heart
  - It contains heart axis, position, visceral and atrial situs, AV connection, ventricular-arterial connection, ventricular wall thickness, inner diameter of heart cavity and great arteries, septal morphology, valve structure and movement, great artery relationship, space-occupying lesions, blood flow velocity, and abnormal blood flow, etc.
  - Fetal arrhythmia
  - It contains sinus tachycardia, supraventricular tachycardia, ventricular tachycardia, atrial flutter, atrial fibrillation, sinus bradycardia, atrioventricular block, atrial premature beat, ventricular premature beat, tachyarrhythmia with atrioventricular block, etc.
  - Fetal heart function
  - EF, FS; E/A; Tei index; cardiovascular profile score.
- Common views of fetal echocardiography
- Standard views are four-chamber view; the long axis of left ventricular outflow tract (LVOT); the long axis of right ventricular outflow tract (RVOT); short-axis view of the great artery; three-vessel view; three-vessel and trachea view; long-axis view of the aortic arch and arterial catheter arch; long-axis view of SVC and IVS, and a transverse view of abdomen. Observe the heart structure by demonstrating different exam views.
- We can take other standard or nonstandard views when observing the anatomic structure in the region of interest, such as the long-axis view of the right ventricular inflow canal and the short-axis view of the LV, etc.
- Scanning techniques of fetal echocardiography
  - Tilting: The long-axis of the LVOT and the RVOT can be obtained by tilting the probe to the fetal cephalic direction in the four-chamber view.
  - Rotation: The long-axis of the LVOT and RVOT and biventricular short axis and short-axis of the great artery can be obtained by continuously rotating the probe to the left side of the fetus in the four-chamber view.
  - Parallel movement: Three-vessels and three-vessels and trachea views can be obtained by moving the probe to the cephalic direction parallelly from the four-chamber view.
  - The specific manipulation should be flexible according to the fetal position.
- Position of fetal heart
- We can determine the fetal orientation by 2-D ultrasound, according to the position of the fetal head and spine. Along the long axis of the fetal spine, the probe rotates 90° at the fetal chest and gets the transverse view of the chest. The direction of the probe should be consistent with the fetus. Pay attention to distinguish the situs inversus.
- Usually, the thoracic and abdominal aorta is located to the left of the spine with pulsation. In contrast, the inferior vena cava is to the right of the spine without pulsation. The gastric bubble locates on the left side, which is one of the indicators of the left and right side of the fetus.
- The orientation of the four-chamber heart and the apex are used to determine the position of the heart.
- The position of the fetal heart in the thoracic cavity
  - Situssolitus, the heart locates in the left chest with apex pointing to the left, and the viscera situs is normal (the stomach bubble locates on the left side of the spine, and IVC is on the right side).
  - Levocardia, the heart locates in the left chest with apex pointing to the left, and the viscera is situs inversus (the stomach bubble locates on the right side of the spine and the IVC on the left side).
  - Mesocardia, the heart locates in the middle of the chest with apex pointing to the front, and the viscera is normal (the stomach bubble locates on the left side of the spine and the IVC on the right side).
  - Dextrocardia, the heart locates in the right chest with apex pointing to the right, and the viscera is situs inversus (the stomach bubble locates on the right side of the spine and the IVC on the left side).
  - Dextroversion, the heart locates in the right chest with apex pointing to the right, and the viscera is normal (the stomach bubble locates on the left side of the spine and the IVC on the right side).
  - The heart displaces to the right, the heart locates in the right chest with apex pointing to the left, usually seen in cases of the mediastinal tumor, left diaphragmatic hernia, and massive pleural effusion.
  - The heart outside the chest, the sternum is partially or entirely absent. The heart is partially or entirely outside the chest.

4.2.3 Normal Fetal Echocardiography

- 2-D echocardiography
  - Four-chamber view

    The probe is placed parallelly to the spine along the long axis of the spine. Rotate the probe about 90 ° when the heart appears in the chest. When a relatively complete rib is displayed, the standard four-chamber view is obtained (Fig. 4.1).

    Normally, the RV is close to the sternum. There is a moderator band near the apex of the heart. The LA is close to the descending aorta and spine, and there

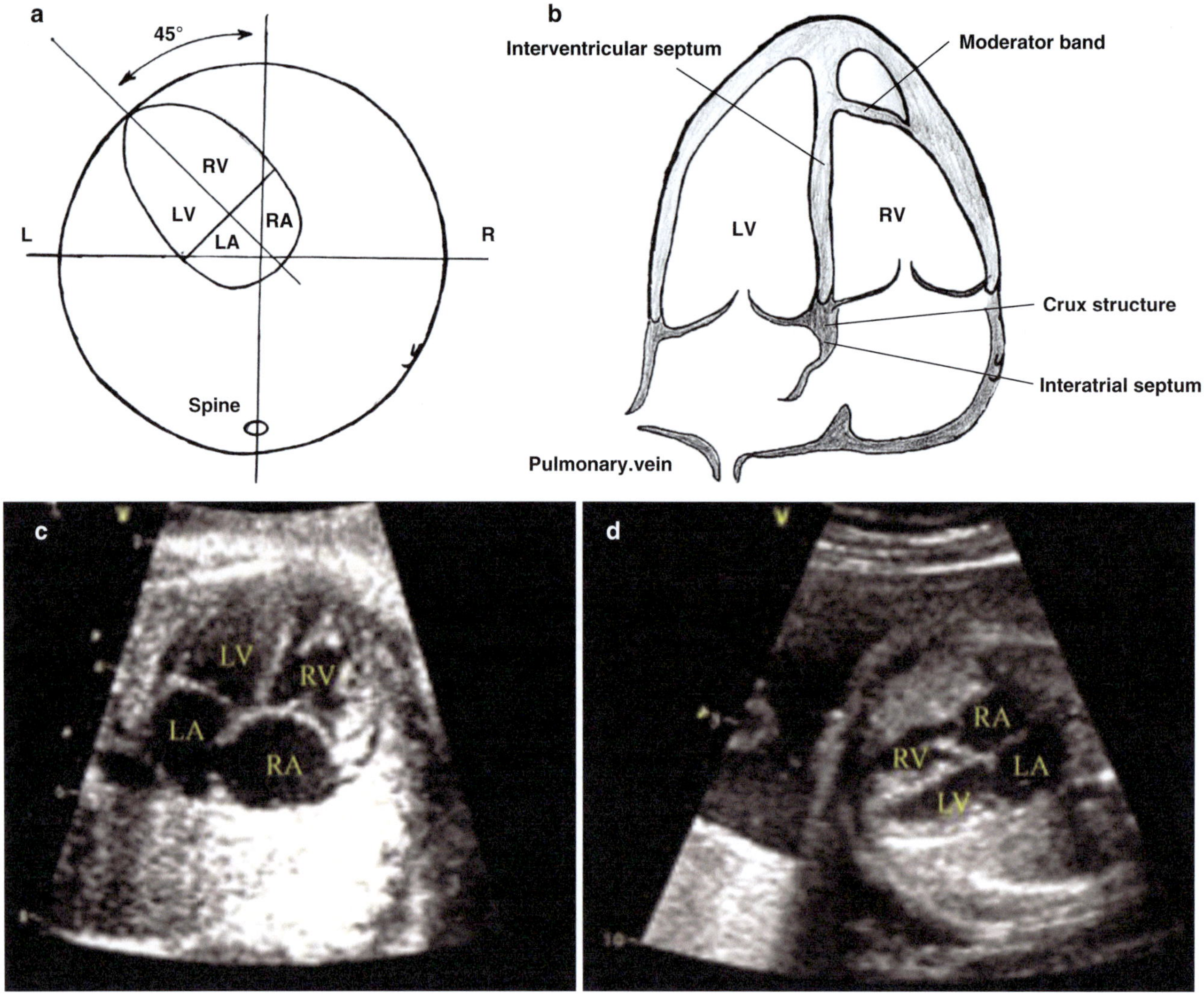

Fig. 4.1 Four-chamber view of fetal heart. (**a**) Axial of fetal heart; (**b**) Four-chamber diagram of fetal heart; (**c**) four-chamber heart in the supine position; (**d**) four-chamber heart with the fetal position of left occipital anterior

is a connection between the pulmonary veins and the LA. The valve of foramen ovale is open to the LA. The vena cava is connected to the RA. The position of tricuspid valve attachment to the ventricular septum is lower than that of the anterior bicuspid valve. The tricuspid valve is open to the RV, and the mitral valve is open to the LV. The above characters can be used to distinguish the left and right atria/ventricle.

Usually, the size of the fetal left and right chambers are balanced in the four-chamber view. Sometimes, the RA and RV are slightly larger. The ratio of heart area to the chest area in this section view can be used to judge the size of the heart. The ratio ranges from 0.25 to 0.33.

We should observe the following aspects: whether there is any defect in the atrium and ventricular septum; the development and opening of valve of foramen ovale; whether there is an abnormality in mitral valve, tricuspid valve, and accessory devices; the size of each chamber; whether there is a lesion in the heart chamber; the thickness of the ventricular wall; the connection of pulmonary veins, etc.

Enhanced echogenic dots are found on the left and right ventricular chordate tendineae or papillary muscles in about 25% of pregnant women in the second trimester, with uncertain causes. With the progress of the pregnancy, the enhanced echogenic dots may shrink or disappear gradually, which is a variation or acoustic phenomenon with an unknown cause. However, it has been reported that a few of

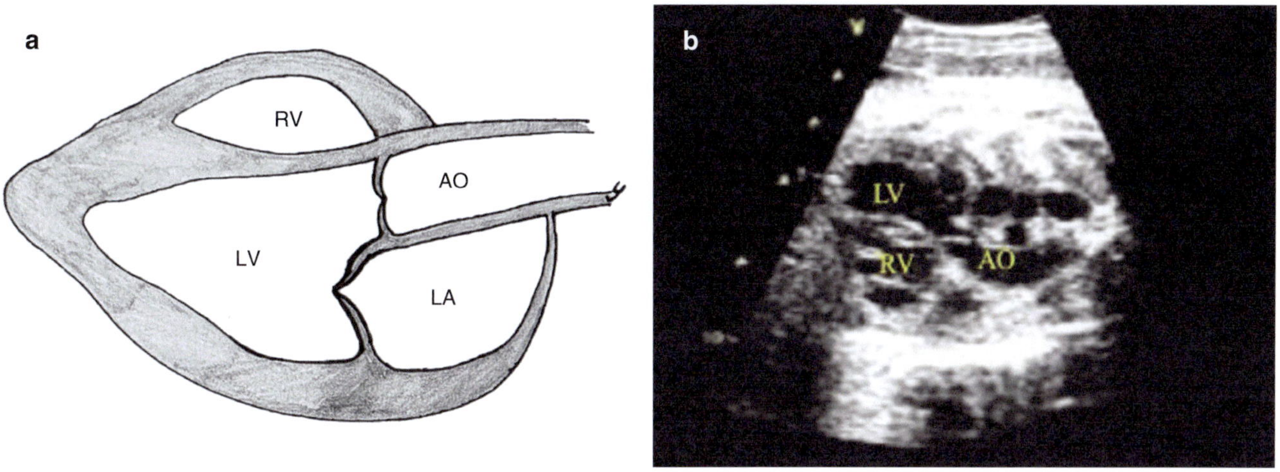

Fig. 4.2 Long-axis view of LVOT of fetal heart (**a**) Long-axis diagram of LVOT. (**b**) Long-axis view of fetal LVOT

them are related to fetal chromosomal abnormalities.

- Long-axis view of LVOT

  (The long-axis view of LVOT can be obtained by inclining the probe slightly to the fetal head (Fig. 4.2).

  In most normal individuals, the blood vessel ascending from the middle of the heart is the aorta, and the great vessel around the edge of the heart is the pulmonary artery.

  We should observe the following aspects: whether there are pathological changes of the aortic orifice (including subvalvular, valvular and supravalvular), whether the inner diameter is normal; whether the aortic and ventricular septum is continuous; whether the aorta has straddle sign; the connection between the aorta and the ventricle; the left heart development condition and whether there are lesions in cavity.

  Is color Doppler blood flow imaging normal?

- Long-axis view of RVOT

  After showing the long-axis view of the LVOT, incline the probe to the fetal cephalic side slightly to show the long-axis of the RVOT. Pay attention to the origin and relationship of the two major arteries. Normally, the two outflow channels are crossed (Fig. 4.3).

  We should observe following aspects: whether there is a pathological change in the pulmonary orifice (including subvalvular, valvular and supravalvular); whether the pulmonary artery and interventricular septum is continuous; the connection between pulmonary artery and ventricle; the development of right ventricle; and whether there is a lesion in the chambers.

  Is color Doppler blood flow normal?

- Short-axis view of the great artery

  The short-axis view of the great arteries can be obtained by rotating the probe about 50° clockwisely from the four-chamber view (Fig. 4.4).

  We should observe following aspects: whether the position of the great artery is normal; whether the RVOT and pulmonary valve have lesions; whether the inner diameter of the pulmonary artery and branches are normal; whether there is continuous interruption of subvalvular interventricular septum of pulmonary artery. The inner diameter of the pulmonary artery is generally 15–20% larger than that of the aorta.

  Is color Doppler blood flow normal?

- Ductal and aortic arch long axis view

  Parallel the probe to the thoracic spine of the fetus and slightly tilt to the left on the middle anterior abdomen and the back, the view of aortic arch may be seen in the shape of a "crutch handle." Moving the probe slightly to the left and right, we can see the view of the "hockey stick" shape of the ductal arch (Fig. 4.5).

  The inner diameter of the ascending aorta, the aortic arch, and the descending aorta are observed in the long-axial view of the aortic arch. We should pay attention to the development of transverse arch, whether there is coarctation, atresia or interruption. We can also observe the three brachial arteries.

  We should observe whether there is stenosis or premature closure in the long-axial view of the ductus arteriosus arch. Premature closure of ductus arteriosus affects fetal development, leading to right heart failure. The inner diameter of the ductus arteriosus is similar to that of the descending aorta.

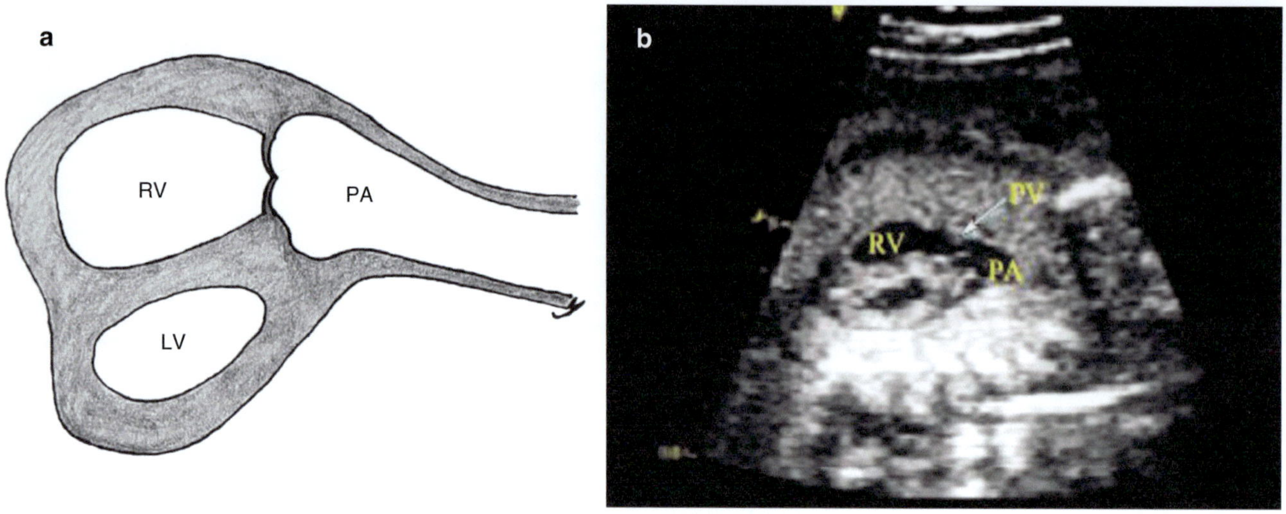

Fig. 4.3 Long-axis view of fetal RVOT. (**a**) Long-axis diagram of fetal RVOT. (**b**) Long-axis of fetal RVOT

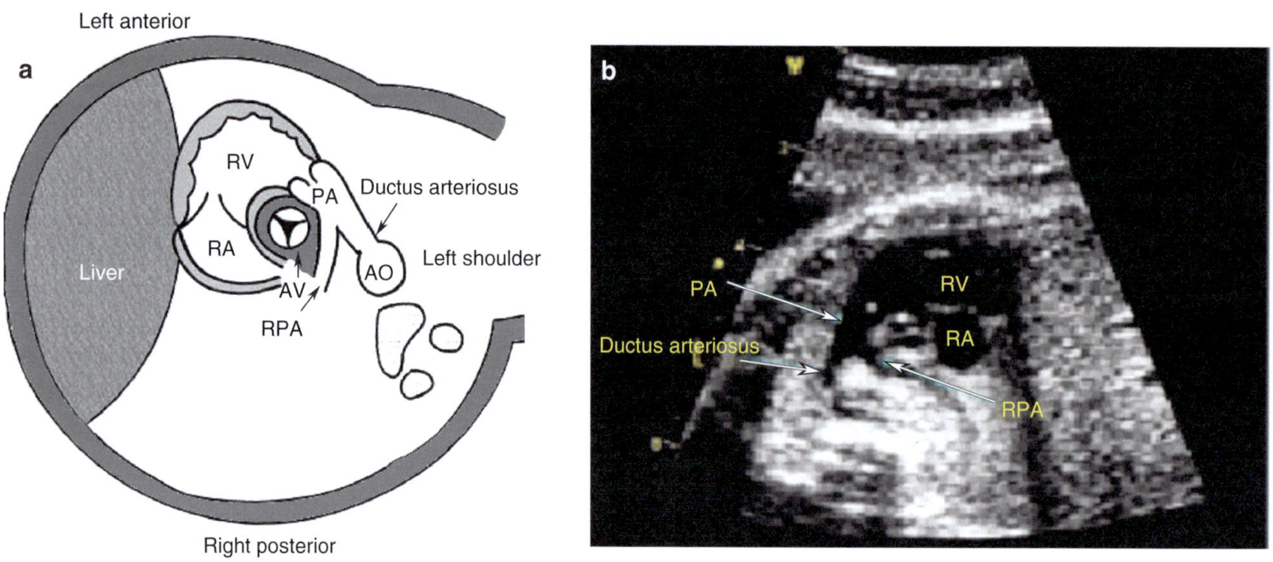

Fig. 4.4 Short-axis view of fetal great arteries. (**a**) Diagram of short-axis view of fetal great arteries (**b**) short-axis view of fetal great arteries

Is color Doppler flow imaging normal?

- Long-axis view of vena cava

  The long-axis view of the vena cava can be obtained by moving the probe slightly to the right of the aortic arch view, showing the connection of the SVC and IVC with the RA (Fig. 4.6).

  Is color Doppler flow imaging normal?
- Three-vessel view, three vessel and trachea view
- From the four-chamber view, move the probe to the cephalic side of the fetus to obtain the three-vessel view. And continuously move up slightly to obtain the three-vessel and trachea view. These two sections show anatomical information about the aorta, pulmonary artery, ductus arterosus, right SVC, and trachea, providing the basis for screening and diagnosing the structural abnormalities of above-mentioned.

  Observe the number of large blood vessels. Usually, three blood vessels are shown in the view of three blood vessels. From left to right of the fetus are pulmonary artery, aorta, and right SVC, respectively (Fig. 4.7). The trachea is shown between the aorta and the right SVC in the view of three-vessel and trachea (Fig. 4.8).

  Observe the spatial arrangement. The three blood vessels are arranged in a line. During the dynamic scanning from three-vessel view to the three-vessel

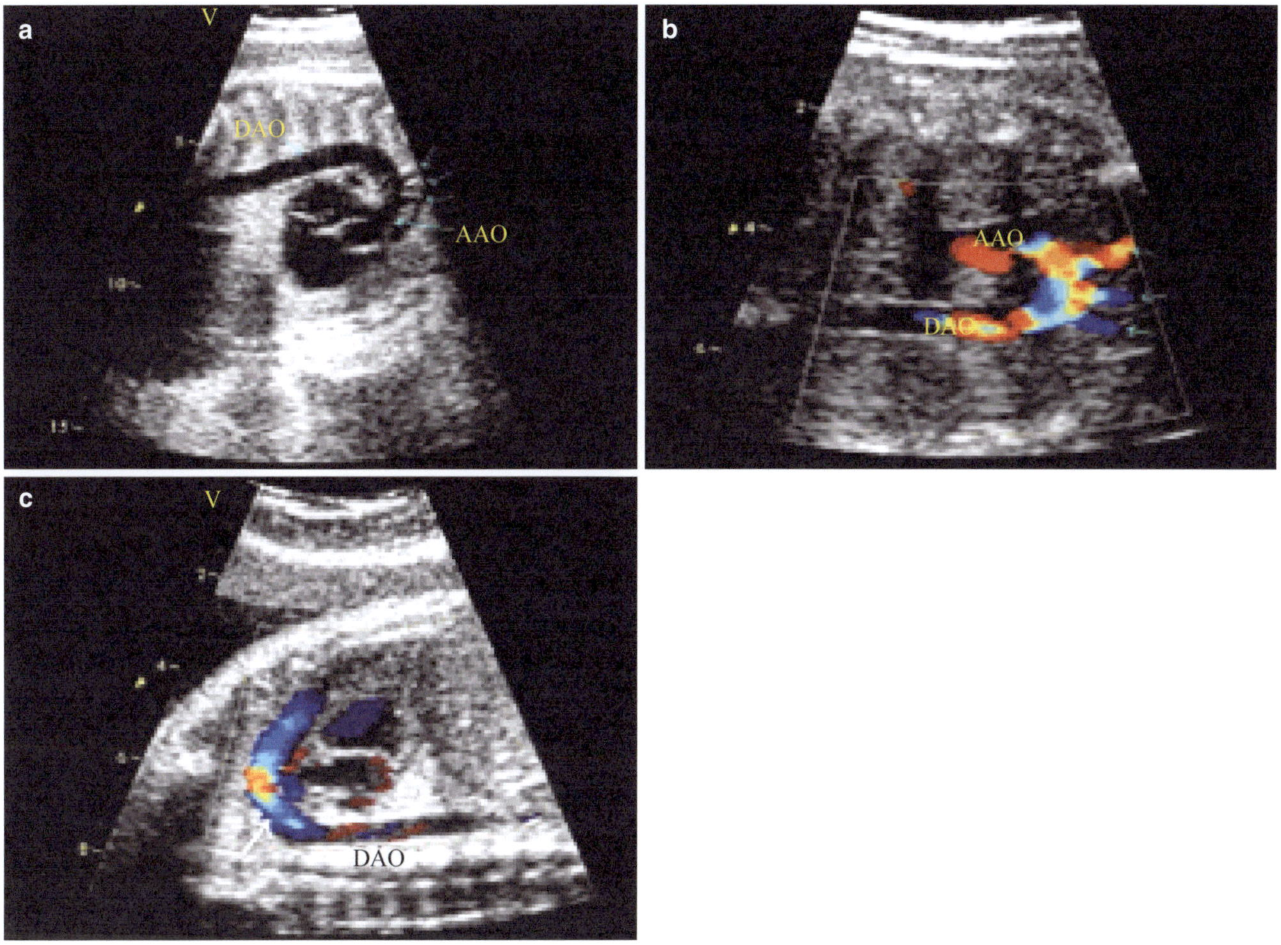

Fig. 4.5 Long-axis view of fetal ductal and aortic arch. (**a**) 2-D imaging of the fetal aortic arch in the prone position, arrow shows the three brachiocephalic arteries; (**b**) Color Doppler imaging of the fetal aortic arch in the supine position, with arrows showing three brachiocephalic arteries; (**c**) Color Doppler imaging of the ductal arch in the supine position

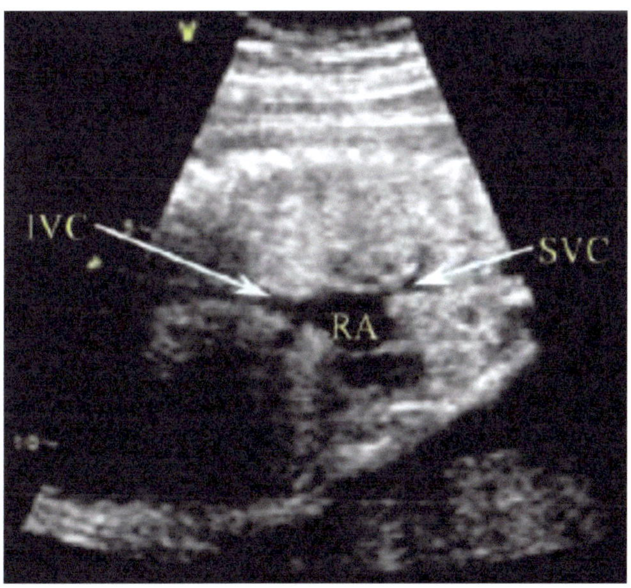

Fig. 4.6 Long-axis view of fetal SVC and IVC

and trachea view, we can determine the type of blood vessels and find out the abnormality in the spatial arrangement.

Observe the diameter of the great vessels. The three-vessel view shows that the diameter of the pulmonary artery is slightly wider than that of the aorta. The inner diameter of the aorta is slightly wider than that of the right SVC. The inner diameter of blood vessels decreases from left to right.

Observe the color Doppler imaging of vessels. In most normal individuals, the directions of flow in the pulmonary artery and aorta are the same in the three-vessel view, without obvious accelerated flow. We can get a comprehensive examination of the morphology, structure, and blood flow of the fetal heart through the above views. The four-chamber view is the most essential among all the views, in which many congenital heart diseases will have

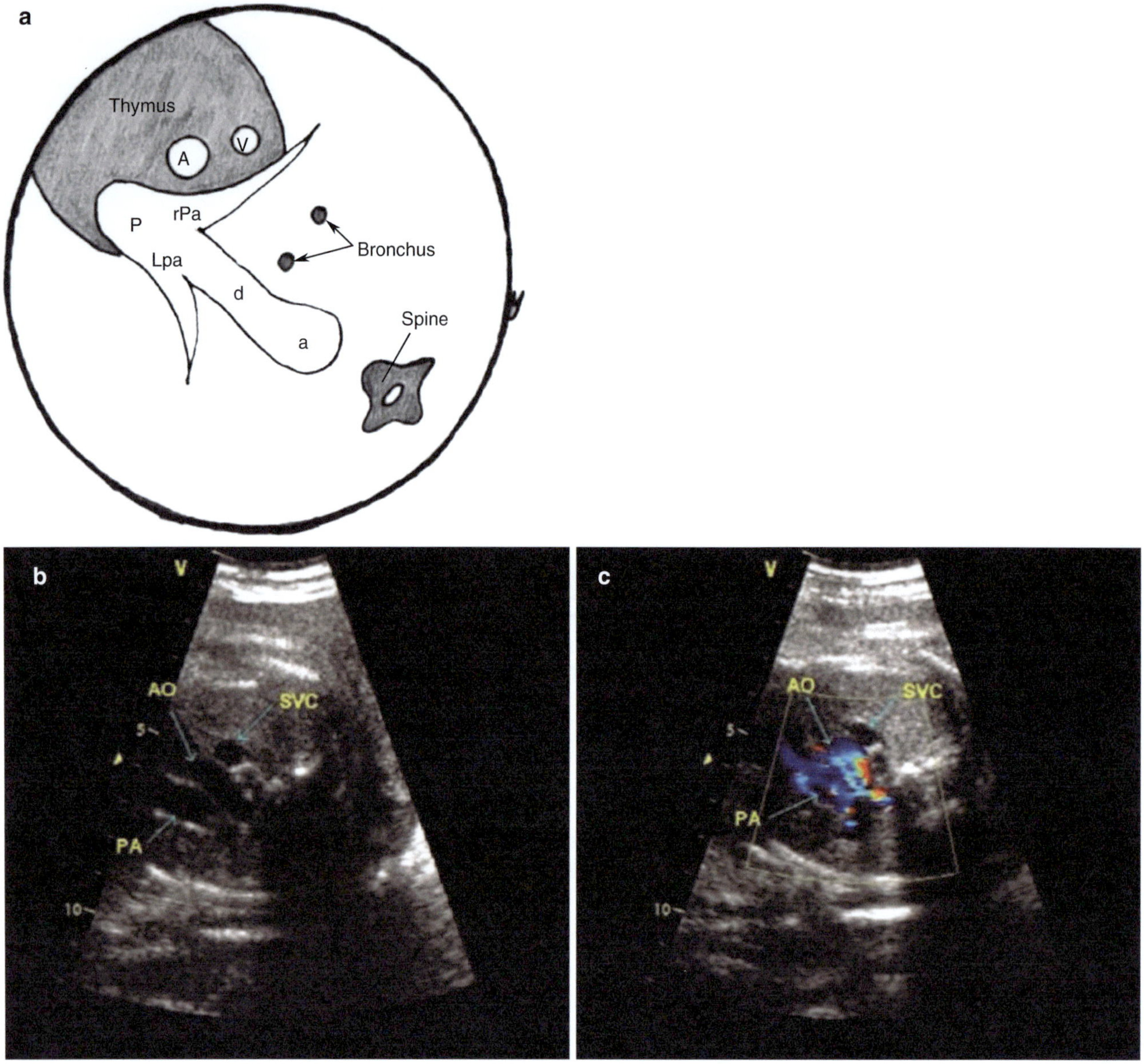

Fig. 4.7 Three-vessel view. (**a**) Diagram of the three-vessel view. (**b**) 2-D sonography of three-vessel view. (**c**) Color Doppler flow imaging of three-vessel view

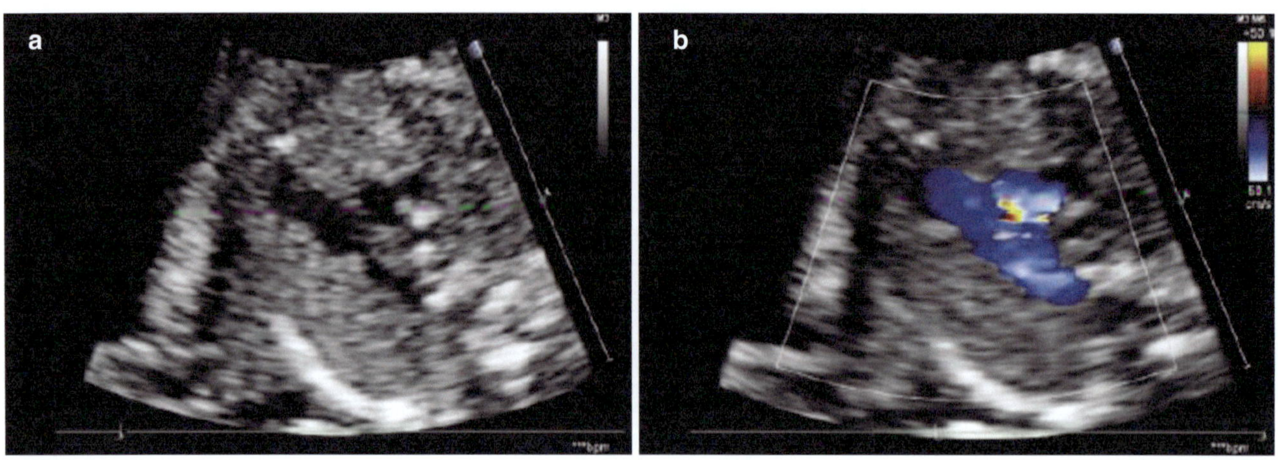

Fig. 4.8 Three-vessel and trachea view and color Doppler flow imaging. (**a**) 2-D sonography of three-vessel trachea view. (**b**) Color Doppler flow imaging of three-vessel trachea view

abnormal manifestations and 70–80% of CHD can be ruled out by observing this view alone.

- M-mode echocardiography
  - Under the guidance of two-dimensional ultrasound, m-mode image shows clear anatomical structures when the sampling line is placed through the four-chamber view, the long-axis view of the LV, the short-axis view of the ventricle, and the short-axis view of the great artery (Fig. 4.9).
  - The M-mode motion curves of the atrial and ventricular walls, atrioventricular and semilunar valves can be obtained at the same time when the sampling line is placed through these parts.
  - Distinguish the types of fetal arrhythmia according to the relationship of the motion curve between the atrial wall and the ventricular wall. Evaluate the systolic and diastolic conditions of the myocardium by evaluating the systolic and diastolic inner diameters of the ventricular cavity, which can help to evaluate the cardiac function. Ventricular Wall thickness, atrioventricular size, the diameter of large vessels, the width of pericardial fluid, and heart rate are measured.
  - M-mode echocardiography has a unique advantage to diagnose fetal arrhythmia. The motion curve relationship between atrial wall and ventricular wall contraction activity in each cardiac cycle is clear, which is of great help to analyze the type of arrhythmia.
- Color Doppler flow imaging (CDFI)
  - CDFI can display the phase and direction of blood flow in real time. And the location of accelerated blood flow, regurgitation, and abnormal shunting can be distinguished.
  - The observation sites are atrial septum, interventricular septum, mitral valve, tricuspid valve, aortic valve, pulmonary valve, aortic arch, and ductal arch.
  - In the fetal period, the foramen ovale is open. In the four-chamber view, CDFI shows the shunting flow through the foramen ovale at the atrial level, from right to left, and the width of the blood flow is generally no more than 8 mm.
  - Commonly, we cannot detect shunt through the ventricular septum.
  - Commonly, there is no obvious enhanced blood flow and reflux at each valve orifice.
  - According to the blood flow imaging at the arch of the aorta and ductus arteriosus, we can discover whether there are obvious abnormalities of the inner diameter and the direction of blood flow.
- Spectral Doppler ultrasound
  - Spectral Doppler ultrasound can be used to detect the flow velocity through the valves, the atrial septum, and ventricular septum, then calculating the cross-valve or cross-septal pressure gradience.
  - Use spectral Doppler ultrasound to analyze fetal arrhythmia.
  - The doppler flow spectrum of mitral and tricuspid valves is a bimodal pattern. The first peak is E and the second peak is A. The difference between fetal spectrum and postnatal spectrum is that in fetus the A peak > E peak, A/E > 1 (Figure 4.10a, b).
  - The velocity and volume of blood flow at the tricuspid valve are more than that of the mitral valve.
  - The Doppler flow spectrum of the aorta is unimodal, similar to the pulmonary artery in shape (Figure 4.10c, d).

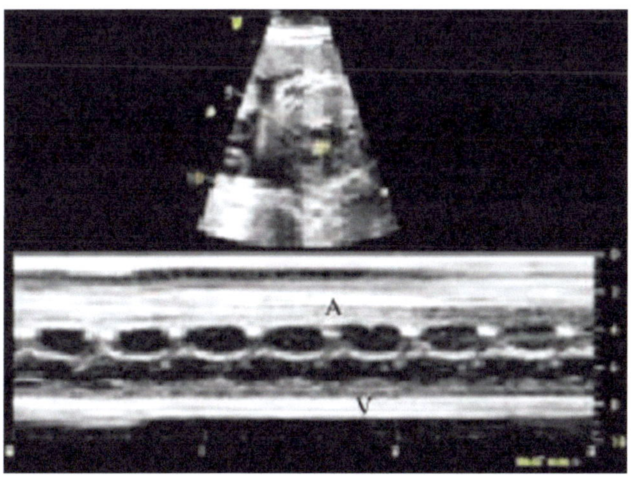

Fig. 4.9 Movement curves of atrial and ventricular walls. The upper curve of motion in the m-mode imaging refers to the movement of the atrial wall. The lower curve of motion refers to the movement of the ventricular wall, and the middle one refers to the movement of ventricular septum. Atrial rate = ventricular rate. The curves of atrial and ventricular walls are consistent

4.2.4 Abnormal Fetal Echocardiography

1. Septal defect
   - Atrial septal defect
     - Concepts

       Atrial septal defect (ASD) is a common type of CHD, accounting for 15–25% of postnatal CHD. It may exist alone or associate with other congenital cardiac anomalies.

       ASD is divided into ostium primum, ostium secundum, sinus venosus, and mixed type.

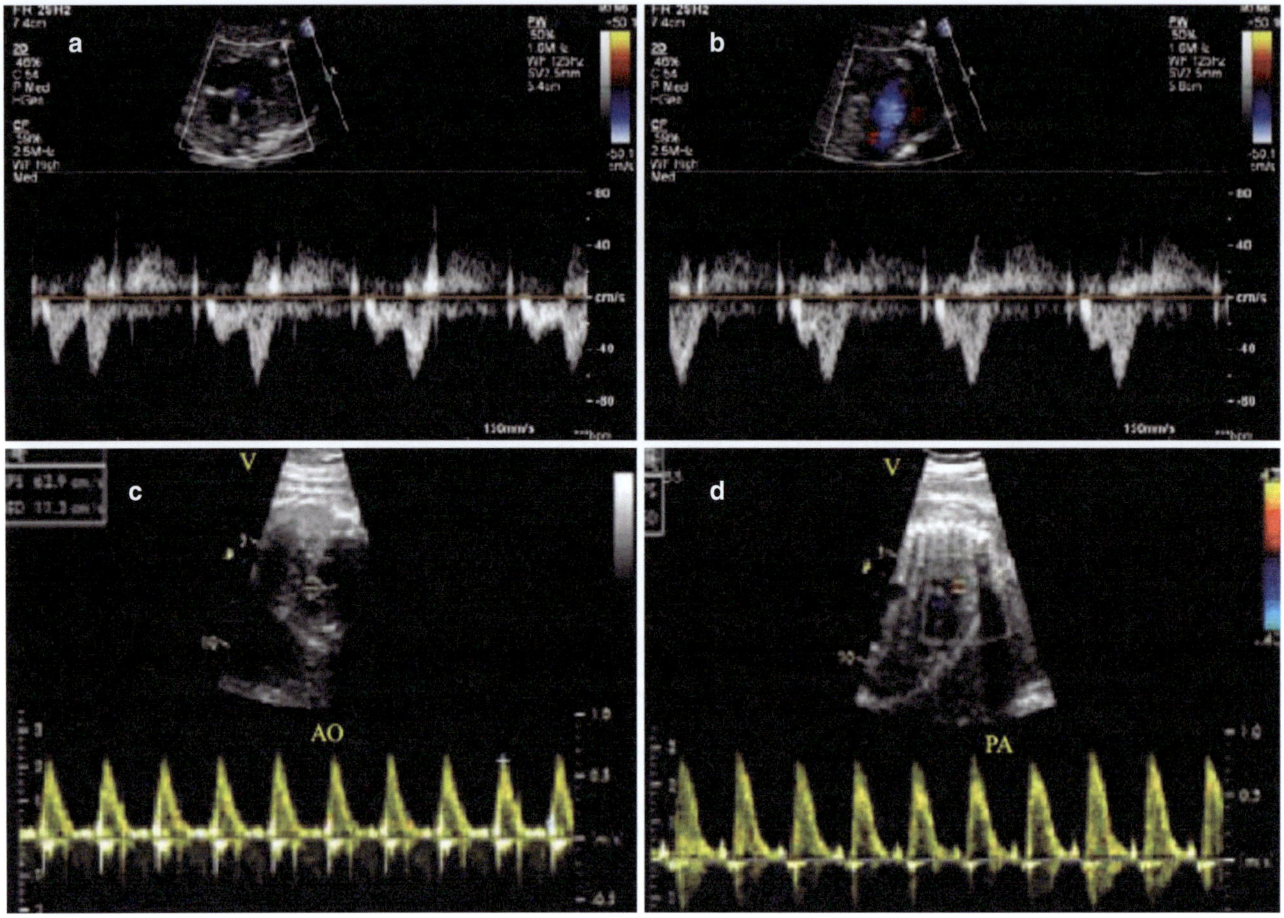

Fig. 4.10 Doppler flow spectrum of the fetal heart. (**a**) Blood flow spectrum of the mitral valve orifice; (**b**) Blood flow spectrum of the tricuspid valve orifice; (**c**) Blood flow spectrum of the aortic valve; (**d**) Blood flow spectrum of the pulmonary valve

– Ultrasonography

Observed the atrial septum in four-chamber view and short-axis view of the great artery.

ASD appears as an area of discontinuity in the atrial septum. The echo discontinuity of the atrial septum is more than 8 mm, with invisible valves of foramen ovale. The area of the defect of atrial septum is invisible even with increasing gain, and the top of the defect shows like a match head sign.

Determine the type of ASD according to its location. The ostium primum ASD is located in the lower part of atrial septum. The ostium secundum ASD locates in the middle part of the atrial septum. The sinus venosus ASD locates at the top and posterior of the atrial septum, near the opening of the vena cava. The defect of mixed type includes multiple sites involved above (Fig. 4.11).

– Tips

We can observe the blood flow at atrial level visually using color Doppler. The foramen ovale allows blood to flow from RA to LA prenatally, which is not helpful for prenatal sonographic diagnosis of ASD.

It may be extremely difficult to find out sinus venosus ASD by fetal echocardiography, which is almost impossible to diagnose.

The diagnosis of fetal ASD should be cautious. Generally, the diagnosis of ASD of septum secundum should be made after serious consideration prenatally.

Pay attention to identify the ultrasonographic images of the RA where the coronary sinus enters, and do not misdiagnose it as the ostium primum ASD.

The prognosis is good.

- Ventricular septal defect
  – Concepts

Ventricular septal defect (VSD) is a common CHD that can exist in isolation, accounting for 25% of postnatal CHD. VSDs are usually associated with other complex cardiovascular malformations, accounting for 50% of postnatal CHD.

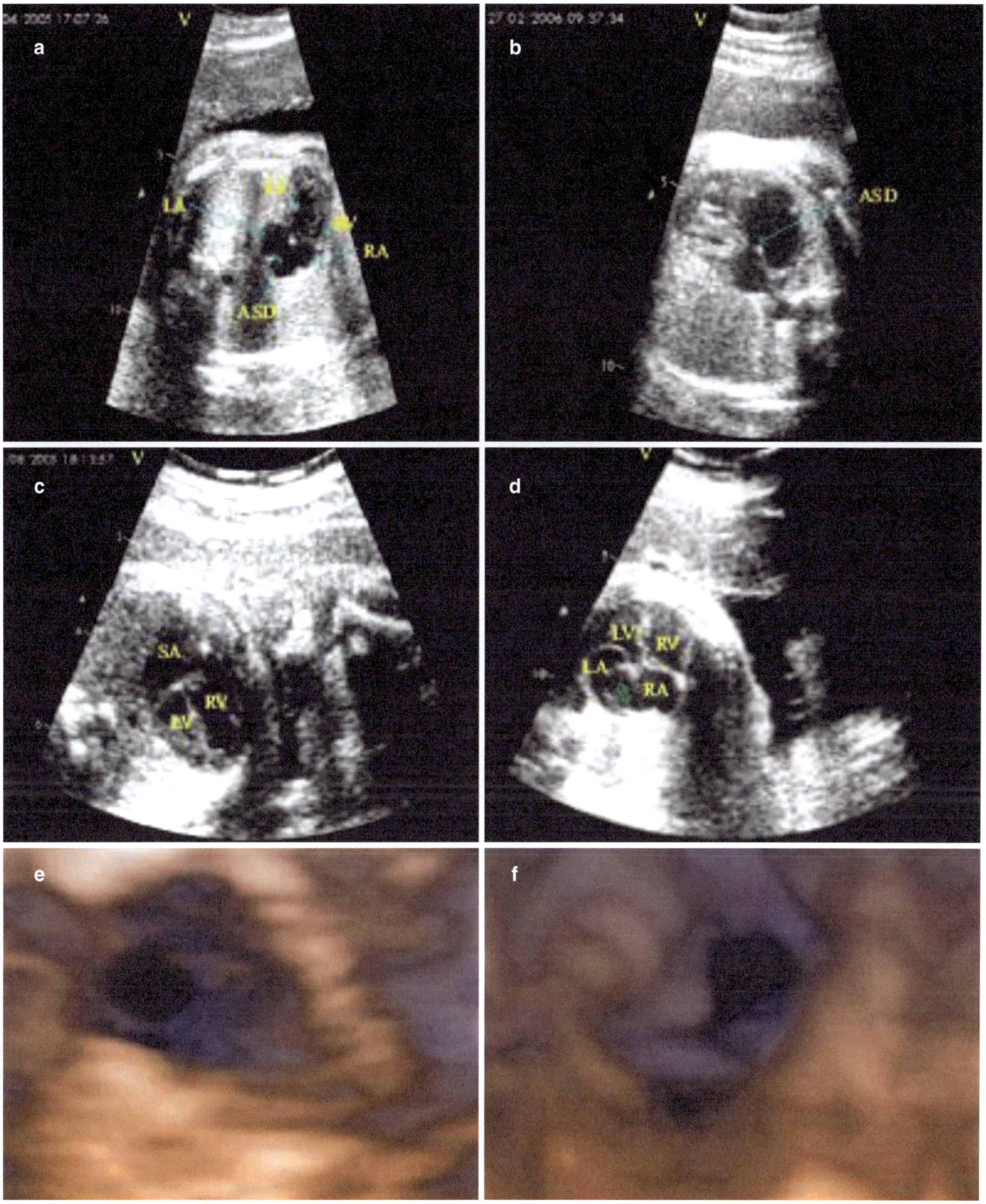

Fig. 4.11 Atrial septal defect. (**a**) Continuity is interrupted in the middle segment of the atrial septum of the fetus; (**b**) The continuity of the lower segment of the atrial septum is interrupted; (**c**) Complete absence of atrial septum in fetal heart; (**d**) Atrial septal excursion of the fetal heart (green arrows); (**e**) The foramen ovale of the fetus is a regular ellipse in shape in 3-D imaging; (**f**) Fetal heart with an irregular shape of foramen ovale in 3-D imaging. This baby has an atrial septal defect after birth

VSDs are divided into perimembranous VSD, muscular VSD, subarterial VSD and mixed type.

– Ultrasonic diagnosis

Observe the ventricular septum in the long-axis view of the left ventricular outflow, the four-chamber view, the short-axis view of the great artery, and the short-axis view of the ventricle. Distinguish the type of VSD according to the position and size of the defect (Fig. 4.12).

Observe the blood flow across the ventricular septum under the color doppler ultrasound at ventricular level, and it helps to determine the type of the defect according to the position and width of the blood flow.

– Tips

The detection rate of ventricular septal defect is very low by prenatal imaging, accounting for about only 10% of the CHD diagnosed in utero, significantly lower than that after birth.

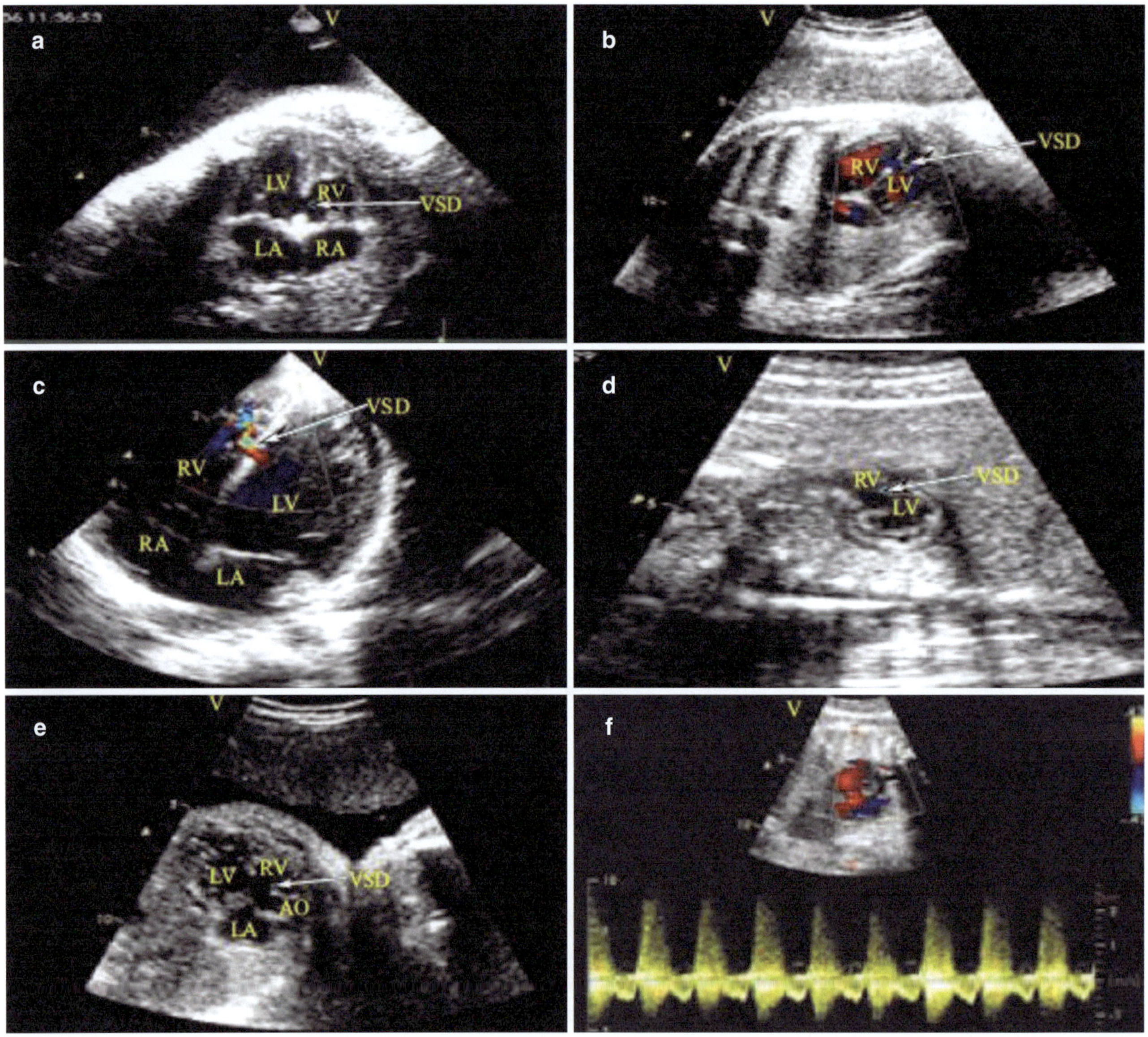

Fig. 4.12 Ventricular septal defect. (**a**) 2-D four-chamber view demonstrates the defect of the ventricular septal muscle; (**b**) Color Doppler imaging of a right-to-left shunt in four-chamber view, at the part of muscular part at ventricular level; (**c**) Left-to-right shunt in four-chamber view of the same child after birth, at the part of muscular part at ventricular level; (**d**) 2-D ultrasound shows the defect of muscular part of interventricular septum in the ventricular short-axis view of the fetus; (**e**) Perimembranous defect of interventricular septum in the left ventricular long-axis view; (**f**) Spectral imaging of blood shunt at the ventricular level; (**g**) 3-D imaging of the normal intact ventricular septum of the fetal heart; (**h**) 3-D imaging of VSD of the fetal heart

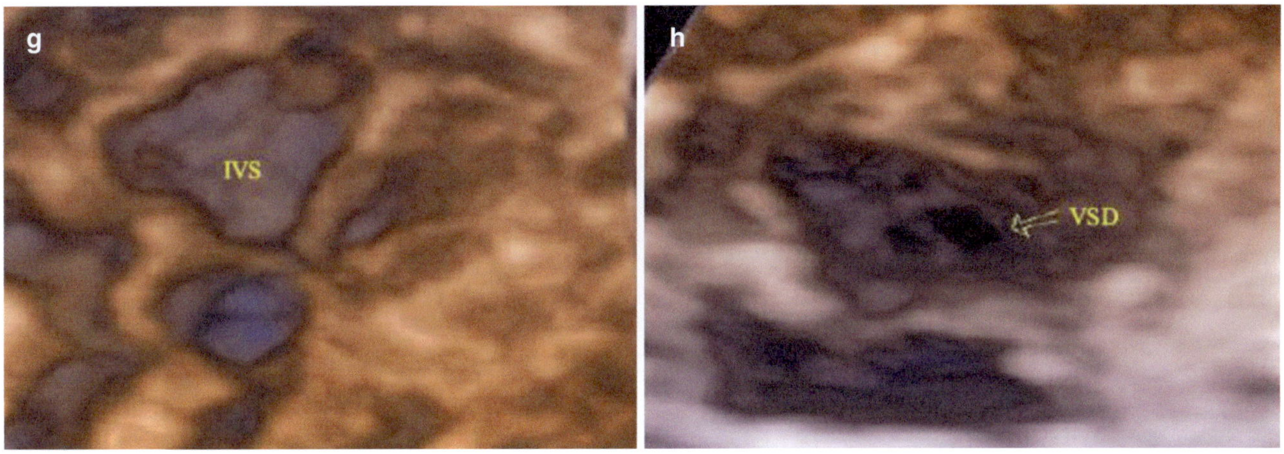

Fig. 4.12 (continued)

It is difficult to show the ventricular septal defect by 2-D ultrasound or color Doppler ultrasound when the size of the ventricular septal defect is less than 3 mm. Furthermore, an improper fetal position makes it harder.

Ventricular septal defect with higher location is difficult to observe, which is often missed by prenatal imaging.

The membranous and muscular VSDs may close spontaneously, which should be observed regularly.

Pay attention to other cardiac malformations.

Prognosis of isolated VSDs is good.

- Atrioventricular septal defect
  - Concepts

    Atrioventricular septal defect (AVSD) is defined as hypoplasia or absence of the septal tissue near the atrioventricular valve, associated with some degrees of atrioventricular valve dysplasia. AVSD is also known as an endocardial cushion defect, atrioventricular tube malformation, common atrioventricular channel, and so on. It accounts for 4–5% of postnatal CHD.

    Fetal AVSDs are divided into partial AVSDs and complete AVSDs.

    Complete AVSD is classified into A, B, and C types according to the attachment site of the valve or chordae tendineae. In type A, the valve or chordae tendineae attaches directly to the interventricular septal ridge or interventricular septum. In type B, the chordae tendineae attached to the right ventricular septum or right ventricular papillary muscle. In type C, the chordae tendineae are attached to the anterolateral papillary muscle of the LV and RV, respectively.
  - Ultrasonic manifestations

    Observe the atrial septum and interventricular septum in four-chamber view.

    A partial AVSD refers to a defect of the inferior portion of atrial septum, complicated with abnormal atrioventricular valves. The defect of the lower portion of atrial septum and the superior portion of interventricular septum, and the absence of intracardiac cross structure suggests a complete AVSD (Fig. 4.13).

    Determine the type of AVSD by the attachment locations of valves and chordae tendineae.

    Systolic regurgitation may be visible at the point of mitral and tricuspid valves by color Doppler.
  - Tips

    It is easy to detect antenatal AVSDs.

    Pay attention to differentiate AVSD with mitral valve atresia or tricuspid valve atresia, which is complicated with ventricular hypoplasia. Color Doppler ultrasonography shows no blood flow at the site of atresia.

    Pay attention to other concomitant heart malformations.

    The prognosis of the partial AVSD is better than that of the complete AVSD.

2. Left cardiac system malformation
   - Hypoplastic left heart syndrome
     - Concepts

       Hypoplastic left heart syndrome (HLHS) refers to the hypoplasia of the LV, caused by severe valve lesions, foramen ovale lesions, aorta or pulmonary vein lesions of the left heart.

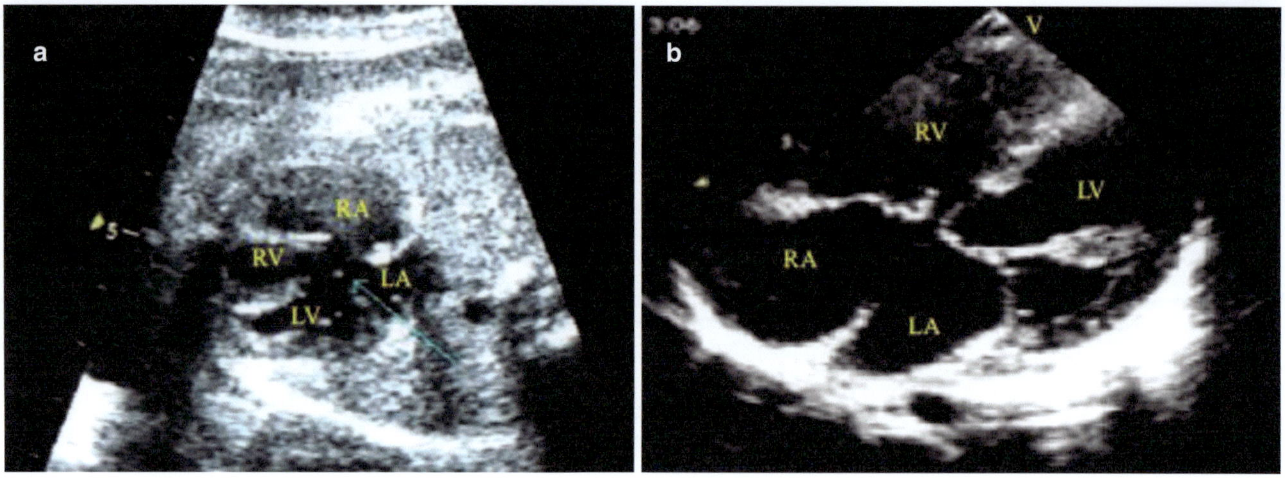

Fig. 4.13 Atrioventricular septal defect. (**a**) Image of the defect of inferior part of the atrial septum and the superior part of the ventricular septum. The cardiac crux structure is invisible. (**b**) Image of the same baby after birth shows the defect of inferior part of the atrial septum and the superior part of the interventricular septum. The cardiac crux structure is invisible

Actually, it is a severe lesion at the inlet and outlet of the LV. HLHS constitutes 1.3% ~ 7.5% of postnatal CHD.

The abnormalities include aortic or mitral valve stenosis, atresia, stenosis or premature closure of the foramen ovale, severe pulmonary vein stenosis or atresia, hypoplasia of the ascending aorta, etc.

– Ultrasonic manifestation

The mitral valve is thickened, and the mitral annulus is stenosed in the four-chamber view and the long axis of the LVOT. The movement of the mitral valve is limited or missing. The left ventricular cavity is small, and the right heart is enlarged (resulting bilateral asymmetry). The echo of the interventricular septum is discontinuous (Fig. 4.14).

The aortic valve is thickened, restricted, or atresia in the view of the long axis of the LVOT and the long axis of the aortic arch. The ascending aorta is smaller than average, and the arch may be constricted, detached, or atresia.

Color Doppler ultrasound shows the absence of flow through the atresia valves. When the mitral valve is severely stenosis or atresia, the blood flow travels from left to right at the atrial level (normally from right to left). The blood flow reversing from the ductus arteriosus is detected in the ascending aorta when the aortic valve is severely stenosis or atresia.

– Tips

High intrauterine detection rate.

The concurrent severe lesions of the inlet and outlet of the LV, such as severe mitral stenosis or atresia with severe aortic stenosis or atresia, suggests left ventricular dysplasia syndrome.

It is not appropriate to diagnose the HLHS if the ventricular septal defect is large and the left ventricular structures are not significantly small enough. We should make a qualitative diagnosis, such as severe mitral stenosis or atresia, severe aortic stenosis or atresia with left ventricular dysplasia, and ventricular septal defect.

The prognosis of HLHS is extremely poor.

- Aortic stenosis
  – Concepts

Aortic stenosis includes subvalvular, valvular and supravalvular types. Valvular stenosis is the most common, accounting for 1.9% ~ 7.6% of the postnatal CHD.

It may occur at single or multiple sites, also can coexist with other cardiac malformations.

– Ultrasonic manifestation

Observe the subvalvular, valvular and supravalvular stenosis in the long axis of LVOT, with the manifestation of reduced diameter of aorta and the dilation after stenosis.

Color doppler ultrasound and spectral Doppler ultrasound show accelerated blood flow at the stenosis site (Fig. 4.15).

– Tips

The detection rate of severe stenosis prenatally is relatively high. The diagnosis of mild to moderate stenosis is difficult because it is difficult to observe the restricted opening of the aortic valve by 2-D ultrasound. We cannot make a diagnosis when there is no obvious

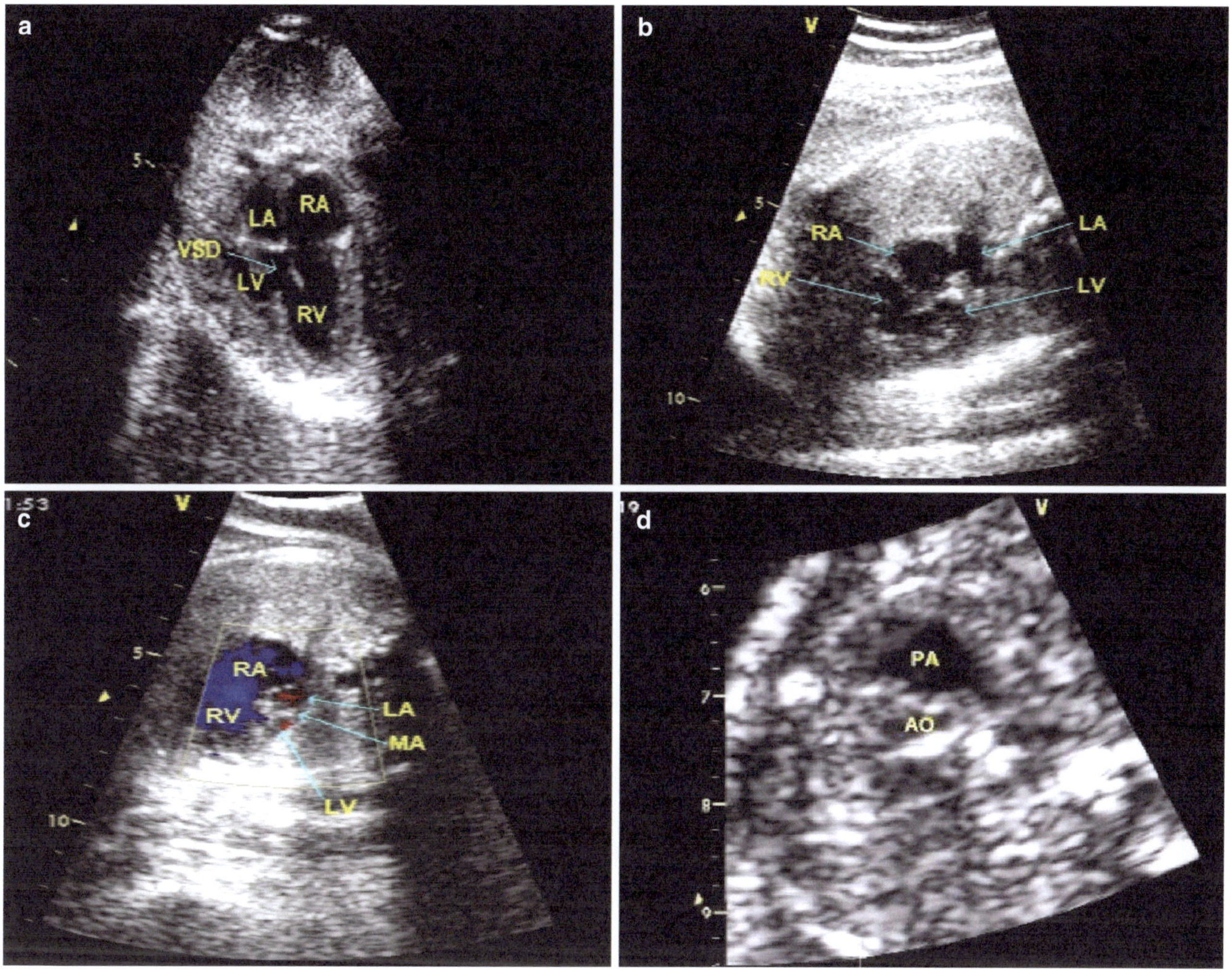

Fig. 4.14 Hypoplastic left heart syndrome. (**a**) Fetal mitral atresia: mitral valve did not open during diastole; small LA and LV; (**b**) The structural abnormality is the same as Fig. 4.14a. (**c**) Color Doppler flow imaging of the heart of the same fetus: no blood flow through the mitral valve orifice was detected. (**d**) Aortic stenosis in the three-vessels view

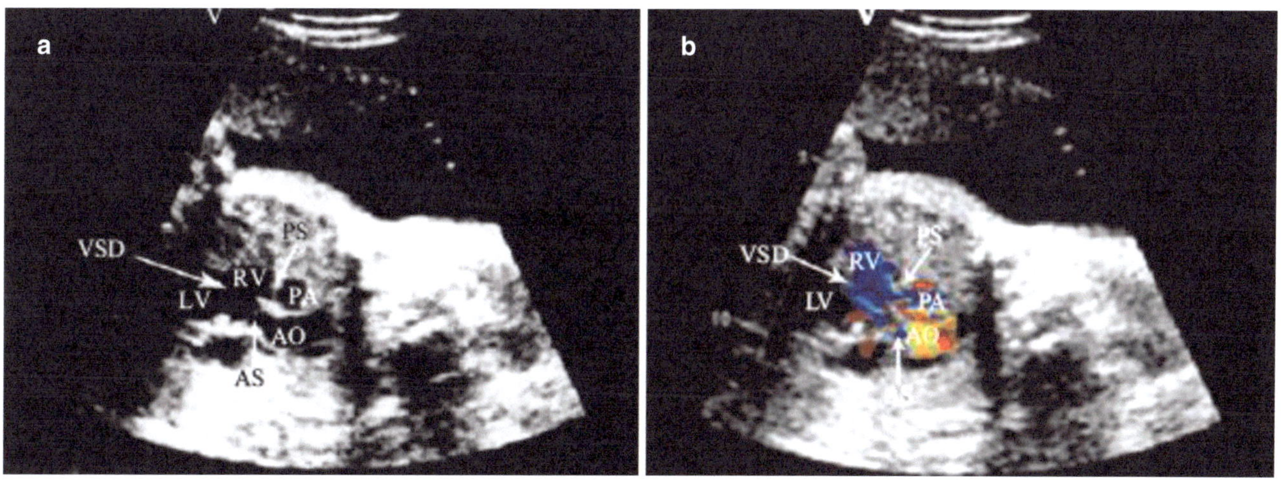

Fig. 4.15 Aortic stenosis. (**a**) Fetal heart: aortic stenosis with pulmonary stenosis and VSD; (**b**) Color flow imaging of the same fetus: enhanced blood flow at the valves of aorta and pulmonary artery

accelerated blood flow in the color Doppler flow imaging of mild to moderate stenosis.
Valvular stenosis is a CHD that can progress during pregnancy and should be followed up.
Pay attention to other abnormalities of the fetal heart.
The prognosis of severe aortic stenosis with hypoplasia of left heart is poor.

- Coarctation of the aorta
  - Concepts

    Coarctation of aorta refers to the localized narrowing of the aorta, owing to that the thickening and infolding aortic intima protrudes into the aortic lumen. The aortic arch and descending aorta above the renal artery are the most common lesion sites. It accounts for 2.2% of congenital heart disease.

    Coarctation of the aorta is usually detected at the descending of the aortic arch, also known as the isthmus of aortic arch.

    Coarctation of the aorta is classified into three types: preductal type (the most common one), postductal type, and juxtaductal type.
  - Ultrasonic manifestation

    The shape of the aortic arch changes in the long axis view, with decreased curvature and inner diameter, indicating transverse arch hypoplasia. The distance between the brachiocephalic artery branches increases (Fig. 4.16).

    The four-chamber view shows the asymmetric ventricular size, with a more visible RV and relatively small LV.

    The view of the RVOT and the view of the ductal arch shows the enlarged inner diameter of pulmonary artery and ductus arteriosus.

    Color Doppler image shows increased velocity or narrowed blood flow at the coarctation.
  - Tips

    Despite echocardiographic screening, prenatal diagnosis of mild or moderate aortic coarctation remains difficult. It is relatively easy to diagnose severe ones. It is difficult to make a diagnosis when color Doppler flow imaging shows no distinct increased color flow.

    The diagnosis of aortic coarctation is excluded when the diameter of the aortic arch isthmus is larger than that of the left subclavian artery.

    Aortic coarctation is a congenital cardiovascular structural anomaly that may progress during pregnancy and should be followed up.

    The prognosis of preductal type is poor.

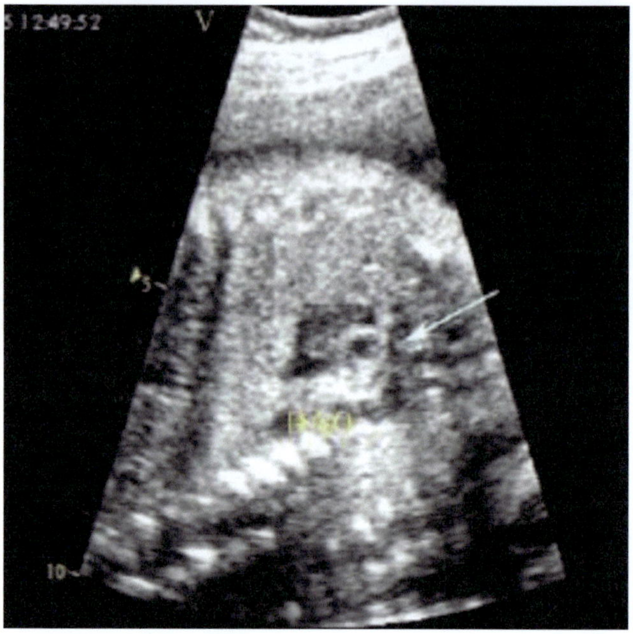

Fig. 4.16 Coarctation of the aorta. The shape of the fetal aortic arch changes abnormally, with decreased curvature, transverse arch hypoplasia. The distance betweenthe brachiocephalic artery branches increases

- Interruption of the aortic arch (IAA)
  - Concepts

    Interruption of the aortic arch (IAA) is defined as a complete interruption between the aortic arch and the descending aorta, accounting for 1% of postnatal CHD. Blood in descending aorta comes from the ductus arteriosus.

    IAA is divided into three types: type A, type B, and type C. Type A: It is interrupted distal to the left subclavian artery. Type B: Interruption locates between the left common carotid artery and the left subclavian artery. Type C: Interruption locates between the brachiocephalic artery and the left common carotid artery.
  - Ultrasonic manifestation

    The long axis of the aortic arch shows no connection between the aortic arch and the descending aorta.

    Determine the type according to the site of interruption.

    The four-chamber view shows the imbalance in size of the left and right chambers, with larger right chambers and relatively small left chambers.

    The view of the RVOT and the view of the ductal arch show the enlarged inner diameter of pulmonary artery and ductus arteriosus.

- Tips

  Pay attention to the other malformations, as IAA is usually associated with other cardiovascular defects.

  The prognosis of IAA is relatively poor.

- Mitral stenosis or mitral regurgitation
  - Concepts

    Mitral stenosis refers to abnormal development of the valve, annulus, chordae tendineae, and papillary muscles, accounting for 0.2% of the postnatal CHD.

    Mitral regurgitation is caused by valve cleft, valve prolapse, annulus dilatation, chordae tendineae rupture, or papillary muscles rupture. Mitral regurgitation accounts for 0.5% of the postnatal CHD.

    Severe mitral stenosis can lead to left heart hypoplasia. Severe mitral regurgitation may result in left heart dilatation and heart failure.
  - Ultrasonic manifestation

    The four-chamber view shows enhanced echo of the mitral valves, restricted orifice (Fig. 4.17), or only one enlarged papillary muscle, a parachute mitral valve for example. Cleft or inaccurate shutting of the mitral valves could result in mitral regurgitation.

    Color Doppler ultrasound shows enhanced blood flow at the stenosis, and supravalvar regurgitation of the mitral regurgitation (Fig. 4.18).
  - Tips.

    Mitral valve lesion can rarely be isolated; it is often associated with other cardiac malformations.

    The prognosis of severe mitral stenosis or mitral regurgitation is poor.

    Mitral stenosis and mitral regurgitation may progress during pregnancy; the fetus should be followed up.

- Mitral atresia
  - Concepts

    No valvular tissue is visible at the site of the mitral valve, resulting in the absence of an atrioventricular connection.

    Mitral atresia is often associated with left ventricular dysplasia.
  - Ultrasonic manifestation

    The four-chamber view shows a band-like echo at the site of the mitral valve, without normal motion. The two ventricles are imbalanced in size, with more enlarged right cham-

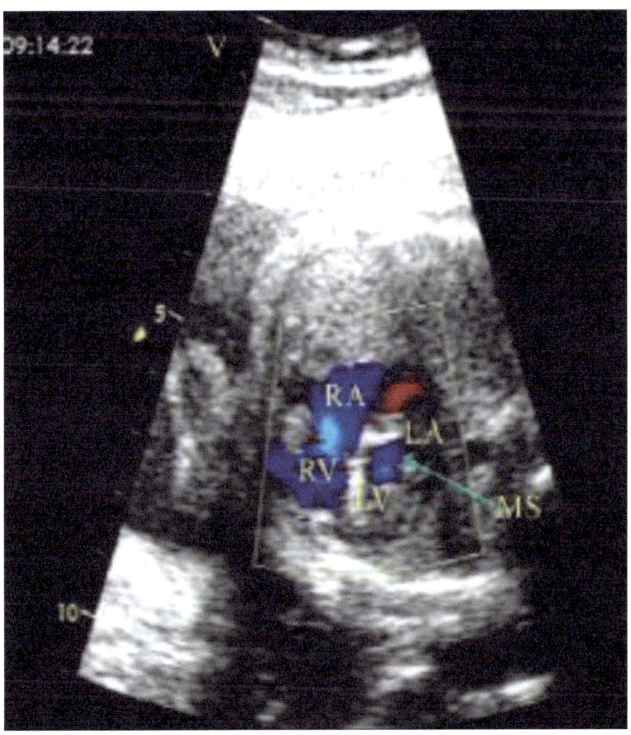

Fig. 4.17 Mitral stenosis. The diastolic image of the fetal heart shows minor blood flow through the valve. Arrow shows the stenosed mitral valve and small LV

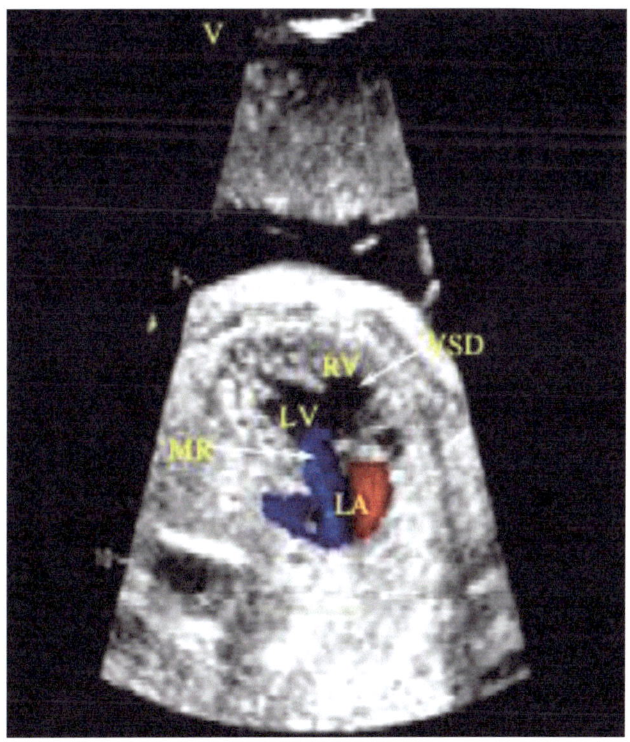

Fig. 4.18 Mitral regurgitation. Mitral regurgitation in the long axis of fetal left ventricle

bers and relatively small left chambers (Fig. 4.19).

There is a ventricular septal defect.

Color Doppler ultrasound shows no blood flow through the valve atresia, with a left to right shunt at the atrial level and right to left shunt at the ventricular level.

– Tips

High intrauterine detection rate.

Mitral atresia is often associated with other cardiac malformations.

The prognosis of mitral atresia is extremely poor.

3. Malformation of the right cardiac system
   • Hypoplastic right heart
     – Concepts

Severe lesions of the valves or blood vessels of the right heart lead to right ventricular dysplasia.

Lesions including tricuspid valve stenosis or atresia, pulmonary artery stenosis, or atresia, results in right ventricular dysplasia.

– Ultrasonic manifestation

The tricuspid valve is thickened without normal motion and narrowing annulus in the four-chamber view. The RV is shrinked, and the left heart is enlarged (Fig. 4.20).

The view of the long axis of the RVOT and the short axis of the great artery demonstrates severe pulmonary valve stenosis or atresia, and a small pulmonary artery.

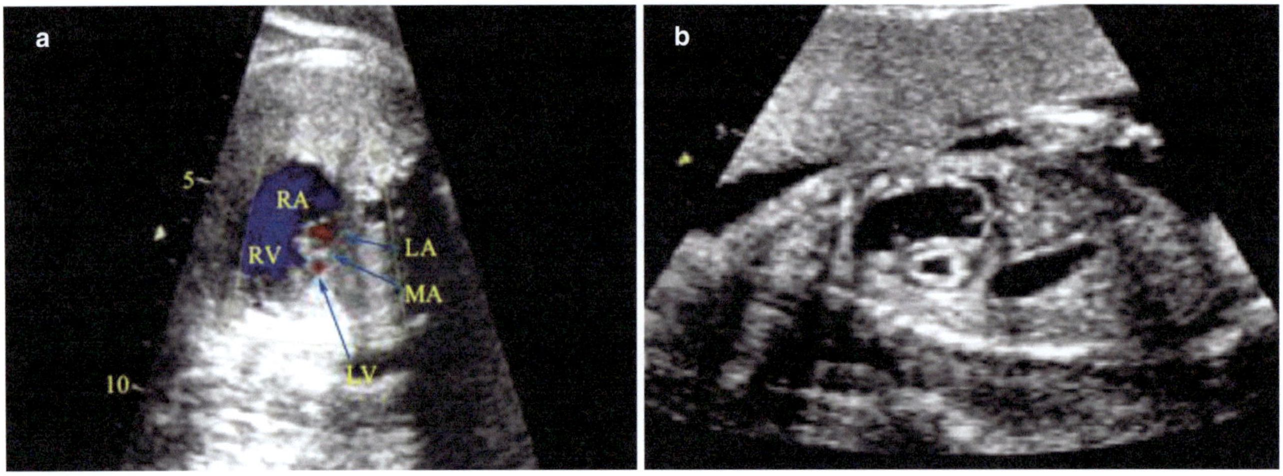

Fig. 4.19 Mitral atresia. (**a**) The four-chamber view shows mitral valve atresia, left ventricular dysplasia, and ventricular septal defect. (**b**) The short axis of the fetal ventricle shows a marked narrowing of the LV

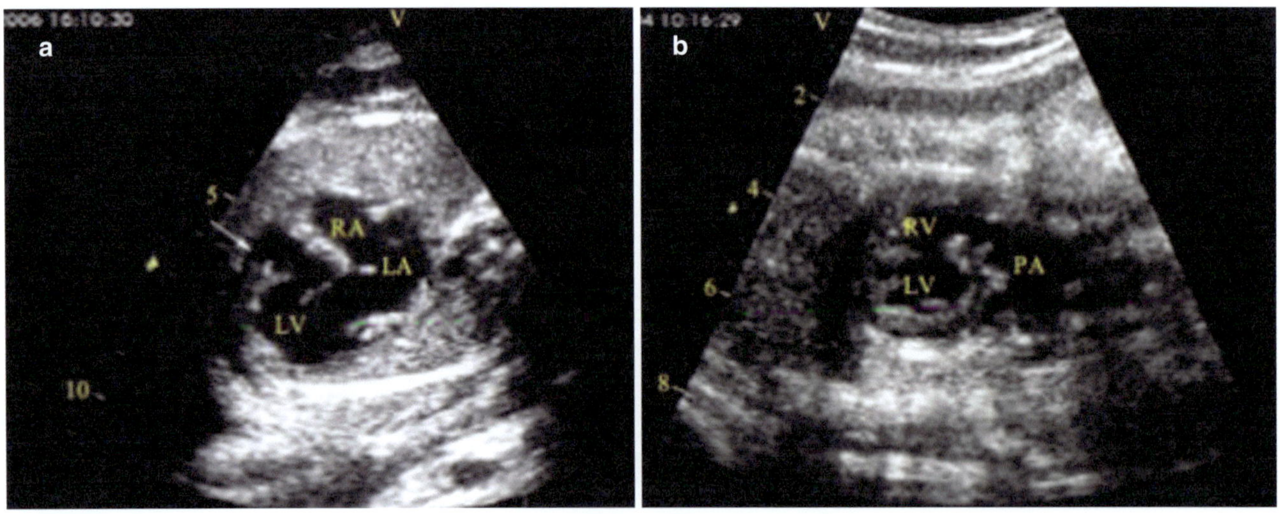

Fig. 4.20 Hypoplastic right heart. (**a**) In the diastolic period, the mitral valve is open, and the tricuspid valve is atretic without motion. (**b**) Restricted opening of the pulmonary valve during systolic period, suggests right ventricular dysplasia (tricuspid atresia + pulmonic stenosis)

Narrowed blood flow is detected at the severe stenosis and no blood flow at the atresia by color Doppler ultrasound.

- Tips

  High intrauterine detection rate.

  The presence of severe lesions of both the right ventricular inlet and outlet, such as severe stenosis or atresia of the tricuspid valve and pulmonary artery, suggests a right ventricular dysplasia syndrome.

  A qualitative diagnosis should be confirmed if there is an isolated severe tricuspid stenosis/atresia or pulmonary artery stenosis/atresia.

  The prognosis of hypoplastic right heart is poor.

- Pulmonary stenosis
  - Concepts

    Pulmonary stenosis is the stenosis of the RVOT, pulmonary valve, pulmonary artery and branches, accounts for approximately 10% of postnatal CHD. Valvular stenosis is the most common type.

    Pulmonary stenosis can be an isolated defect, but it may also coexist with other cardiac defects.

  - Ultrasonic manifestation

    In the long axis of the RVOT and the short axis of the great arteries, the pulmonary valve is thickened and restrictive. The inner diameters of the RVOT, pulmonary annulus, and pulmonary artery are significantly smaller than usual (Fig. 4.21).

    Local post-stenotic dilatation of the pulmonary artery is sometimes visible.

    Color Doppler ultrasonography demonstrates the enhanced acceleration of blood flow at the stenosis and tricuspid regurgitation.

  - Tips

    The intrauterine detection rate of severe stenosis is relatively high, and the diagnosis of mild and moderate stenosis is difficult.

    Valvular stenosis is a congenital cardiac structural anomaly that can progress during pregnancy and should be followed up.

- Pulmonary atresia
  - Concepts

    Pulmonary atresia refers to the atresia of pulmonary valve, pulmonary artery and branches, accounting for 1% of the postnatal CHD.

    It is divided into pulmonary atresia with VSD and pulmonary atresia without VSD.

    Pulmonary atresia with an intact interventricular septum will result in a residual cavity of RV (right ventricle dysplasia). The ASD or the patent foramen ovale is the only outlet of the right heart.

    In the cases of pulmonary atresia with large VSD, the RV can develop normally. The size of the RV depends on the amount of tricuspid regurgitation. The more regurgitation, the larger the RV is.

    The blood of pulmonary arteries mainly supplied by the left-to-right shunt of the ductus arterious.

  - Ultrasonic manifestation

    The short axis of the great artery and the long axis of the ROVT shows a linear echo at the pulmonary valve, without open-closed activity.

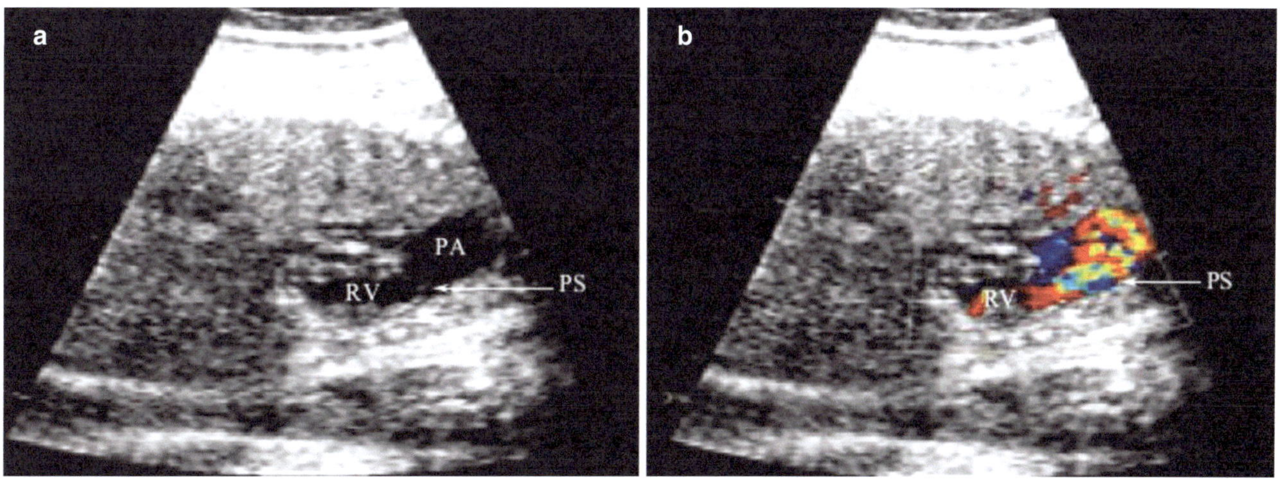

Fig. 4.21 Pulmonary stenosis. (**a**) In the view of the RVOT, it shows the restrictive pulmonary valve, post-stenotic dilatation, indicating pulmonary valve stenosis. (**b**) Enhanced blood flow can be seen in the view of RVOT of the same fetus, indicating forward acceleration of the blood flow

The inner diameter of the pulmonary artery is significantly smaller than normal (Fig. 4.22).

Observe the continuity of interventricular septum in the four-chamber view and the long axis of LVOT. The size of the LV and RV is imbalanced with a small RV and a large LV.

The inner diameter of pulmonary artery is usually smaller than that of aorta in the three-vessel view.

Color Doppler ultrasound shows no blood flow across the pulmonary valve. The short axis of the great artery and the long axis of the ductal arch show the left to right blood flow reverses to the pulmonary artery from the ductus arteriosus, which is usually right to left in fetal ductus arteriosus. The blood flow direction of the pulmonary artery is different from that of the aorta in the three-vessel view. Tricuspid regurgitation can be detected.

 – Tips

The intrauterine detection rate is relatively high.

Pulmonary atresia or severe stenosis should be considered if there is a left to right blood flow reverses to the pulmonary artery from the ductus arteriosus.

The prognosis is poor.

- Tricuspid insufficiency
  - Concepts

The tricuspid valve is dysplasia, with thickened leaflets. The surface of the leaflets is not smooth. Tricuspid valves cannot close well but can open normally.

Severe insufficiency of closure can result in right heart dilatation and failure.

 – Ultrasonic manifestation

Thickened tricuspid valve with closure insufficiency and enlarged right heart can be seen in the four-chamber view, short axis of the great artery and long axis of the right ventricular inflow tract (Fig. 4.23).

Color Doppler ultrasound shows blood regurgitation at the tricuspid valve.

 – Tips

The intrauterine detection rate is related to the fetal position.

It should be distinguished that the isolated tricuspid insufficiency is physiologic or pathologic. It is physiological if the blood flow velocity is less than 2 m/s with non-holosystolic period.

- Ebstein's anomaly of the tricuspid valve
  - Concepts

Ebstein's anomaly, accounting for 1% of congenital heart disease, is characterized by some or all of the tricuspid leaflets attached to the inferior interventricular septum and the right ventricular wall, but not the tricuspid annulus. It is common to see an inferiorly displaced septal leaflet or posterior leaflet, rarely of anterior leaflets.

The inferiorly displaced leaflets are dysplastic, manifesting as small, thickened, conglutinated or thin, even absent. The enlarged and elongated anterior leaflet maybe accompanied by clefts; it is unable to match the inferiorly displaced leaflet efficiently, resulting in incomplete closure.

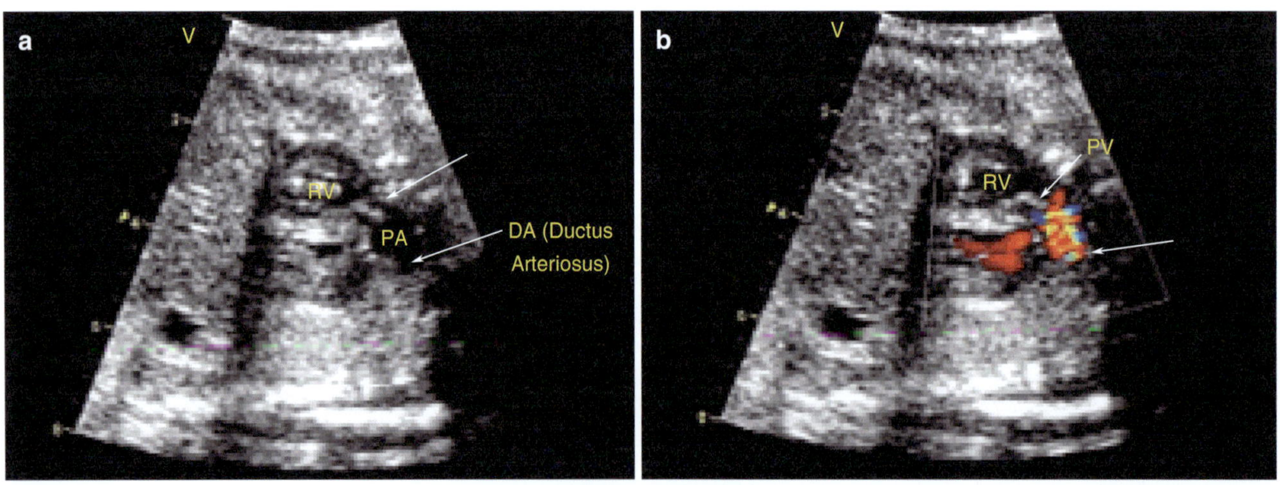

Fig. 4.22 Pulmonary atresia. (**a**) View of the fetal RVOT, arrows show the atretic pulmonary valve; (**b**) The same view of the same fetus shows no blood flow through the pulmonary valve. The arrows show the PV: pulmonary valve blood travels back to the pulmonary artery through Ductus Arteriosus

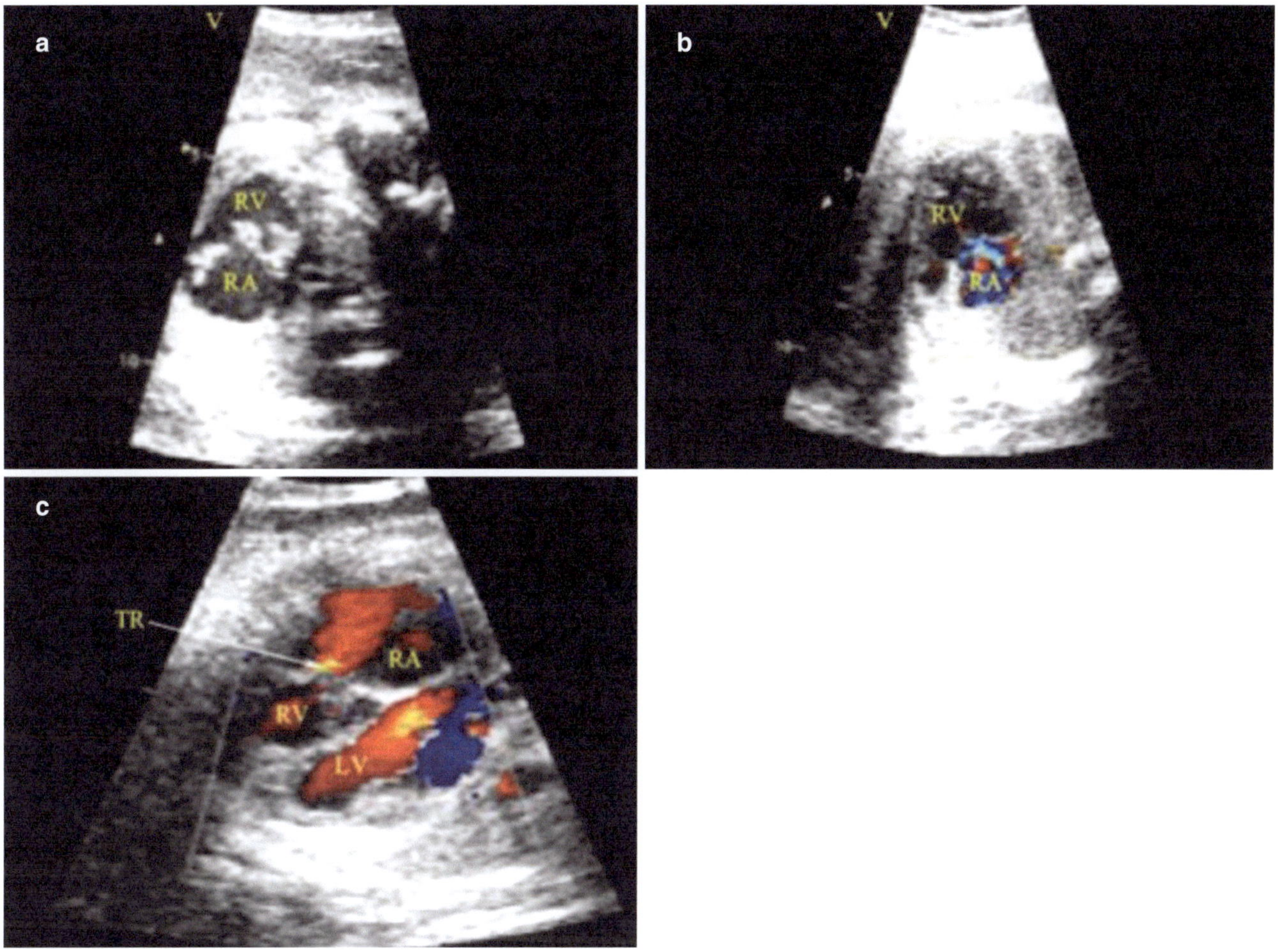

Fig. 4.23 Tricuspid insufficiency. (**a**) Fetal right ventricular inflow tract view shows tricuspid valve hypoplasia with thickening leaflets. (**b**) The right ventricular inflow tract view shows tricuspid regurgitation, indicating incomplete closure. (**c**) The fetal four-chamber view shows tricuspid regurgitation, indicating incomplete closure

Due to the inferiorly displaced leaflets, the RA is enlarged with an atrialized RV. The functional RV is small.

– Ultrasonic manifestation

The anterior leaflet, septal leaflet, and posterior leaflet of the tricuspid valve can be seen in the four-chamber view, the short axis of the great artery, and the long axis of the right ventricular inflow tract.

The inferiorly displaced leaflets and significantly enlarged RA (including the atrialized RV), indicate Ebstein's anomaly (Fig. 4.24).

Normally, the distance of the anterior mitral valve leaflet attachment to the apex of the heart is 1–1.2 times than that of the septal tricuspid valve leaflet attachment to the apex. In Ebstein's anomaly, the ratio reaches more than 1.8.

Ebstein's anomaly should be considered and followed up when the point that the anterior mitral valve leaflet attached to the ventricular septum is 4 mm away from that the septal tricuspid valve leaflet attached to the ventricular septum.

Tricuspid regurgitation can be detected.

– Tips

It can be diagnosed as Ebstein's anomaly when the inferior displacement of the septal tricuspid valve leaflet is more than half the length of the ventricular septum, or the posterior leaflet is not attached to the tricuspid annulus.

Severe Ebstein's anomaly has a relatively high detection rate in utero.

The prognosis is related to the degree of tricuspid valve inferiorly displacement.

- Tricuspid atresia
  – Concepts

Tricuspid atresia (TA) is a complete absence of the direct communication of the RA to the RV, resulting in hypoplasia of the RV. TA is often accompanied by other cardiovascular malformations, accounting for 1.4% of congenital heart disease.

TA is divided into muscular atresia, membranous atresia, and valvar atresia. Muscular atresia is the most common.

The VSD is the only entrance of the RV blood.

– Ultrasonic manifestation

The four-chamber view and the short axis of the great artery show the complete absence of the tricuspid valve. Thickened tissue at the atrioventricular annulus separates the RA from the RV, without movement. The LV is enlarged, while the RV is small (Fig. 4.25).

TA with a VSD is more frequently found. Sometimes, ASD or patent foramen ovale can be detected after birth.

Color Doppler ultrasound shows no blood flow through the tricuspid valve. Blood travels from right to left at the atrial level and left to right at the ventricular level.

– Tips

The detection rate of TA is high prenatally.

TA often accompanies other cardiac defects.

Prognosis: TA cases with normal great arteries arrangement have a relatively good prognosis, with a 15-year survival rate of 65–70%. The survival rate reduces in TA cases accompanied by transposition of great arteries or other malformations.

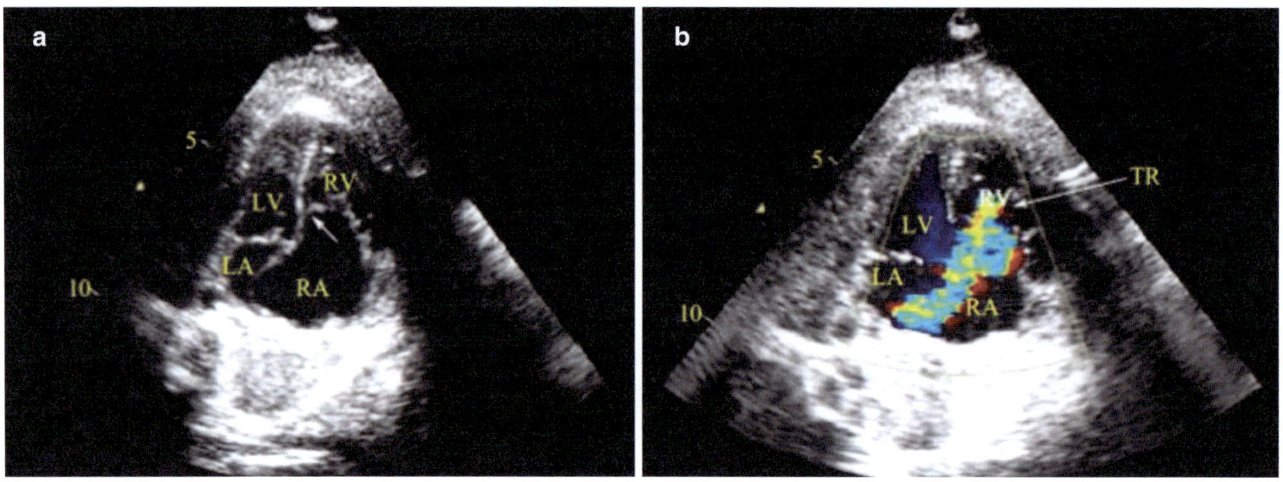

Fig. 4.24 Ebstein's anomaly. (**a**) The fetal four-chamber view shows the inferiorly displaced anterior leaflet of the tricuspid valve. (**b**) The fetal four-chamber view shows tricuspid regurgitation

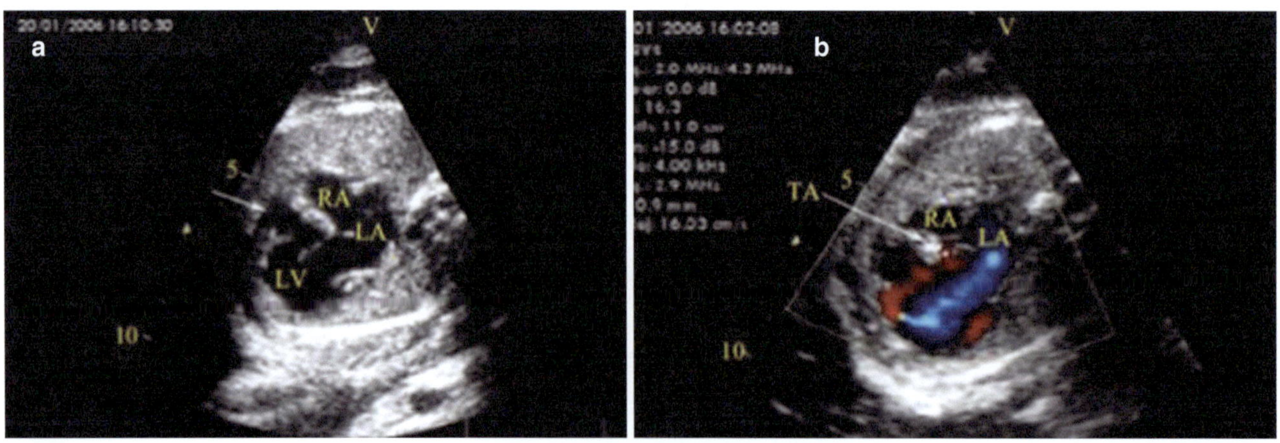

Fig. 4.25 Tricuspid atresia. (**a**) Fetal four-chamber view shows tricuspid atresia in diastole and right ventricular hypoplasia. (**b**) The four-chamber view of the same fetus shows nonobstructive blood flow of the mitral valve in diastole and right ventricular hypoplasia. No blood flow through the tricuspid valve is detected

4. Conotruncal defects
   - Tetralogy of Fallot
     - Basic concepts

       Tetralogy of Fallot (TOF) is the most common cyanotic CHD, accounting for 10% of postnatal CHD.

       TOF consists of pulmonary stenosis (including subvalvular type, valvular type, and supravalvular type), malalignment-type VSD, overriding aorta, and hypertrophy of the RV. The hypertrophy of the RV is not obvious in the fetal period.

       The spatial position of the two major arteries is normal in TOF cases. The pulmonary artery wraps the aorta.
     - Pathological anatomical classification

       Atypical TOF consists of pulmonary valve stenosis (mild or moderate), VSD, aortic overriding (mild), right ventricular hypertrophy (mild). Cyanosis is not obvious after birth.

       Typical TOF: pulmonary stenosis, VSD, aortic overriding, right ventricular hypertrophy (not obvious in the fetal period). Cyanosis is obvious after birth.

       Severe TOF (pseudo-truncus arteriosus): pulmonary atresia or severe infundibular hypoplasia, VSD, aortic overriding, right ventricular hypertrophy (not obvious in the fetal period). Some cases often have concomitant Patent ductus arteriosus and multiple aortopulmonary collateral arteries. Cyanosis is obvious after birth.
     - Ultrasonic manifestation

       The LVOT and the five-chamber view show VSD, overriding aorta with increased inner diameter. But no obvious thickened right ventricular wall is seen in the fetal period (Fig. 4.26).

       The long axis of RVOT, the short axis of the great artery, and the three-vessel view show the narrowed infundibular, narrowed pulmonary annulus and valve, narrowed pulmonary artery and branches, etc. The diameter of the aorta increases, which is out of proportion to that of the pulmonary artery. The inner diameter of the pulmonary artery is narrowed. The ratio of PA/AO is less than 1.

       Color Doppler ultrasound shows that biventricular blood flows into the aorta. Turbulence or fine blood flow can be seen at the stenosis of the right infundibular and valve.
     - Tips

       The intrauterine detection rate is relatively high.

       Double outlet of right ventricle should be considered when the rate of aorta straddling is greater than 50%.

       The conical structure between the semilunar valve and the atrioventricular valve of the double-outlet right ventricle cases is usually visible after birth, which is usually invisible in the fetus.

       In TOF, the spatial position of the two major arteries is normal, while is arranged in parallel in the double-outlet right ventricle cases.

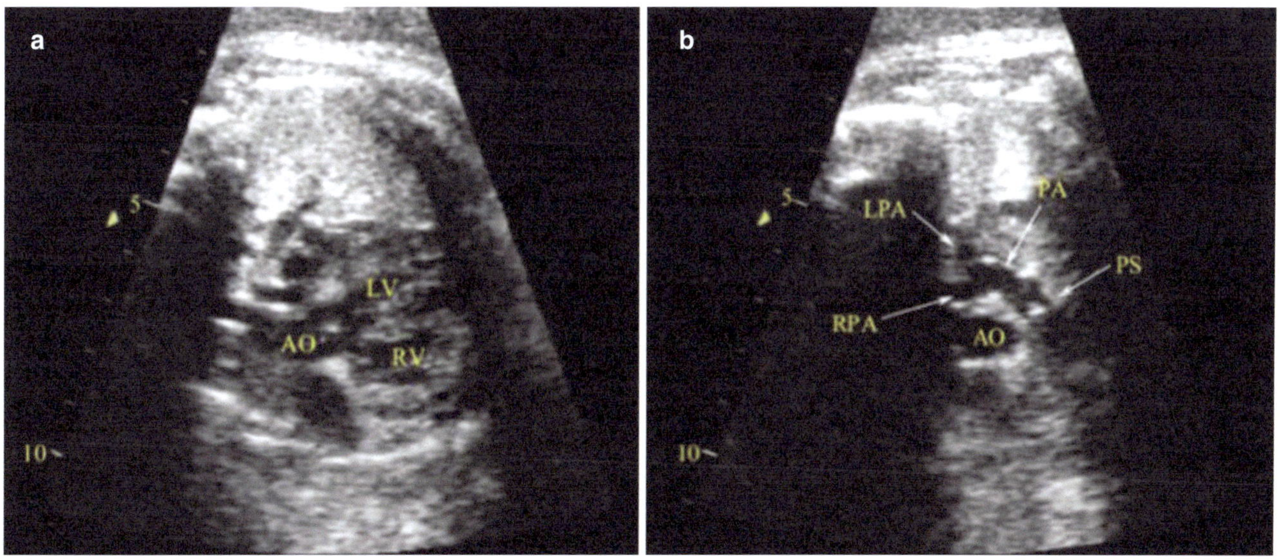

Fig. 4.26 Tetralogy of Fallot. (**a**) The long-axis view of left ventricle shows VSD and the aorta straddling across the ventricular septum. (**b**) The short axis of the great artery shows the pulmonary artery with a decreased inner diameter and an enlarged aorta. The ratio of PA/AO is less than 1

There is no significant right ventricular hypertrophy in the fetal period.

The prognosis is poor in cases of severe pulmonary artery stenosis or combined with extracardiac malformations (including chromosomal abnormalities).

- Double-outlet right ventricle
  - Concepts

    Double-outlet right ventricle (DORV) is defined as all or most of two major arteries arise from the RV, accounting for 5% of the postnatal CHD. On the contrary, it is called double-outlet left ventricle if all or most of two major arteries arise from the LV, which is one of cyanotic CHD.

    VSD is the only outlet of the left ventricle.

    The conical structure under the semilunar valve is visible after birth, which is usually invisible in the fetus.
  - Ultrasonic manifestation

    The long axis of the LVOT and the short axis of the great arteries show that the two great arteries arise from the RV in parallel (Fig. 4.27).

    VSD is visible in DORV cases.

    Color Doppler ultrasonography shows two parallel color blood flows from the RV and blood shunt at the ventricular level.
  - Tips

    The diagnosis of TOF should be considered when the rate of aorta straddling is greater than 50%, accompanied by pulmonary artery stenosis. The spatial position of the two major arteries is abnormal in DORV cases.

    When the rate of pulmonary artery straddling is less than 50%, transposition of the great arteries should be considered. Use the segmental analysis to determine the position of atrium, the position of ventricles and great arteries, the connection between atrium and ventricle, the relationship between ventricle and great arteries. According to the above analysis, identify whether the abnormity is DORV or transposition of major arteries.

    The subaortic conical structure is not obvious in fetus.

    The prognosis is poor.
- Truncus arteriosus
  - Concepts

    Truncus arteriosus is characterized by a single great artery arising from the base of the heart, which supplies the systemic circulations, pulmonary circulations, and coronary arteries, accounting for 2% of the postnatal CHD.

    There is only one set of semilunar valves in the truncus arteriosus, which can consist of two valves, three valves, four valves and more.

    There are four types of truncus arteriosus. Type I: the pulmonary artery, arising from the posterolateral ascending portion of the common truncal artery, then divides into the left and right branches. Type II: the left and right pulmonary arteries arise directly from the posterior or lateral truncus. Type III: one pulmonary artery directly arises from the truncus, while the other artery is absent (usually left pulmonary artery). Type IV: the pulmonary artery arises from the descending thoracic aorta or is absent.
  - Ultrasonic manifestation

    The large truncal artery overriding the ventricular septum is distinguished in the long axis of

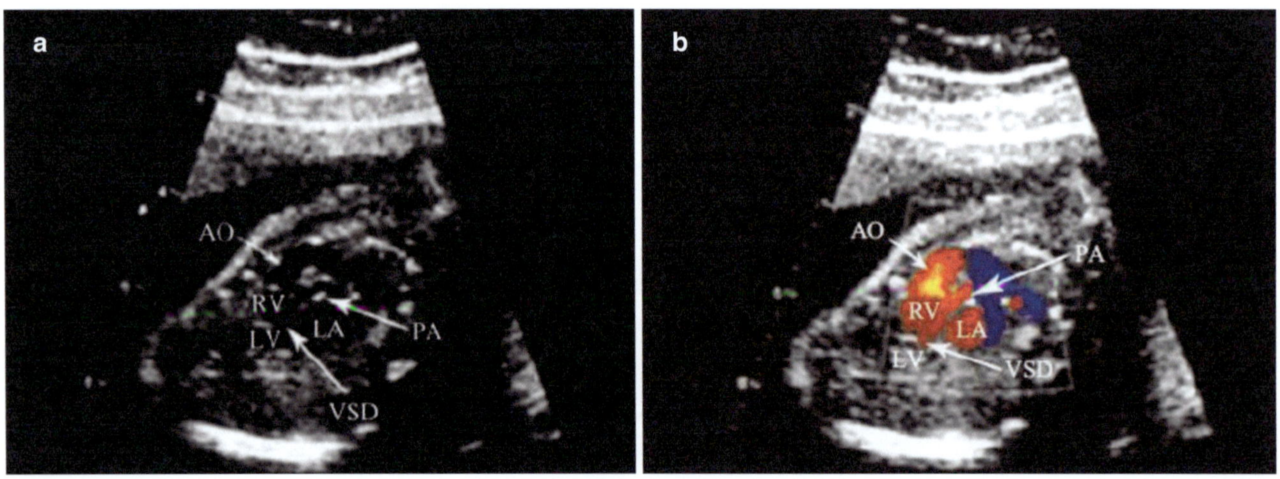

Fig. 4.27 Double-outlet right ventricle. (**a**) A nonstandard view of fetal heart shows that the pulmonary artery and the aorta arise from the RV. (**b**) A nonstandard view of the fetal heart shows that the color Doppler flow imaging of the two major arteries arises from the RV

the LVOT. The inner diameter of the truncal artery is significantly increased, forming a single outlet of both ventricles. The interruption between ventricular septum and the anterior truncal artery is visible. The anterior wall of the RV connects the anterior wall of the truncal artery (Fig. 4.28).

The short axis of the great artery shows "single-loop sign" and a set of semilunar valves, without normal RVOT and pulmonary artery.

There are two vessels in three-vessel view, one is the truncal artery, and the other is the superior vena cava. Sometimes only one enlarged artery is visible.

Color Doppler ultrasound shows that the blood from the left and right ventricular converges and flows into the great artery during the systolic period. Subvalvular regurgitation can be detected (Fig. 4.28).

  – Tips

    Only one great artery is visible in several views. The absence of RVOT indicates truncus arteriosus.

    Truncus arteriosus is diagnosed if four or more semilunar valves are observed in the great artery.

    Truncus arteriosus has a poor prognosis.

- Transposition of great arteries
  – Concepts

    Transposition of great arteries (TGA) is a cyanotic CHD, which is often associated with other cardiac anomalies, accounting for 7–9% of the postnatal CHD.

    TGA is divided into two types: Dextro-TGA (d-TGA) and congenitally corrected TGA (CCTGA). In both types, ventricular arterial discordance is visible.

    d-TGA is characterized by ventricular arterial discordance with atrioventricular concordance, no matter the atrium is in situs solitus or situs

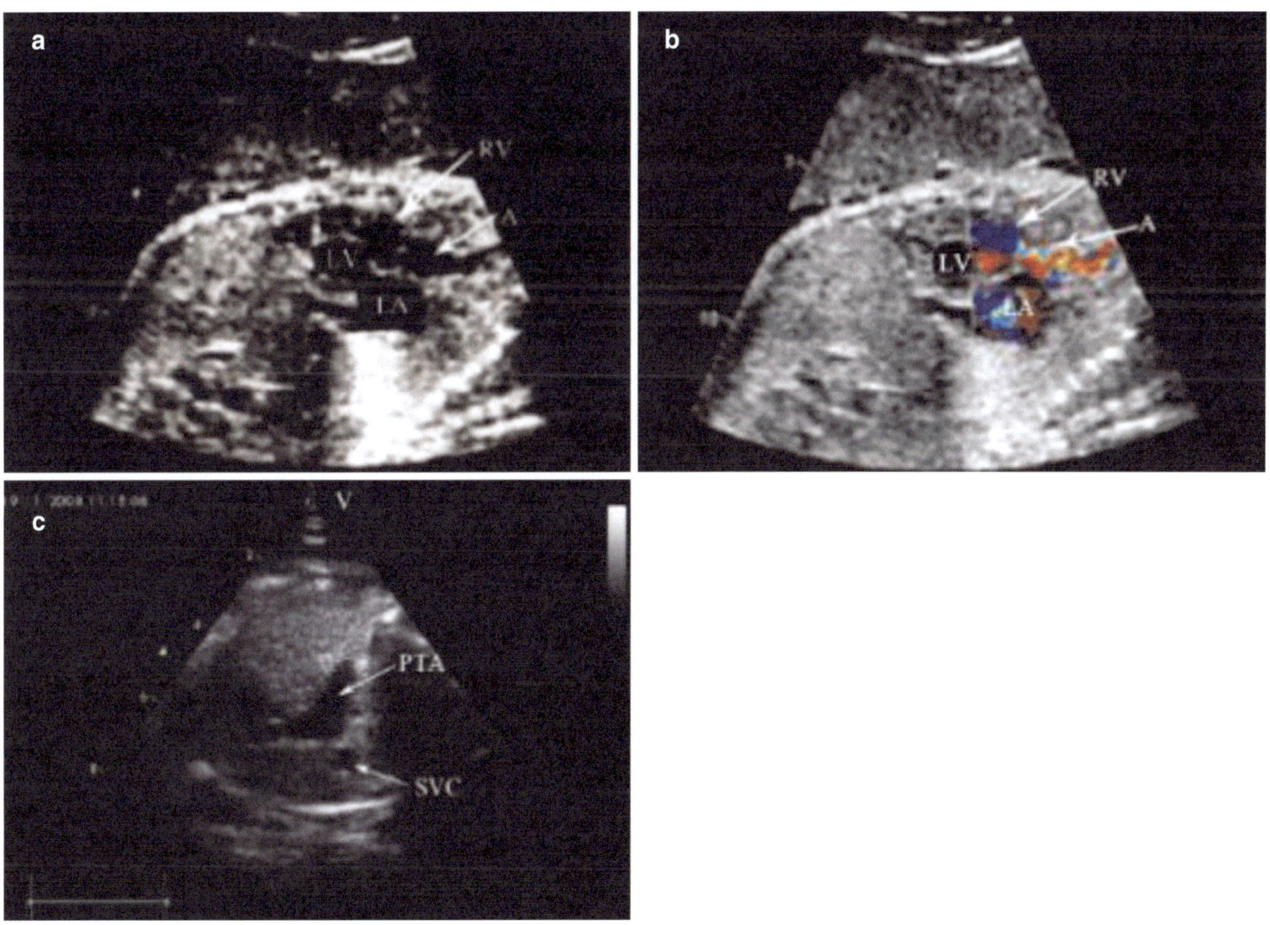

Fig. 4.28 Truncus arteriosus. (**a**) A nonstandard view of the fetal heart shows that a large artery arises from both ventricles. The anterior wall of the RV connects the anterior wall of truncal artery. (**b**) A nonstandard view of the fetal heart shows that the color flow of a large artery arises from both ventricles; (**c**) Three-vessel view shows the truncal artery and the superior vena cava

inversus. The pulmonary artery arises from the LV, and the LV connects with the LA. The aorta arises from the RV, and the RV connects with the RA.

CCTGA is characterized by both ventricular arterial discordance and atrioventricular discordance, regardless of the orientation of the atrium, the ventricles, and the great arteries. The pulmonary artery arises from the LV, and the LV connects with the RA. The aorta arises from the RV, and the RV connects with the LA. There are no hemodynamic changes in oxygenation, although the orientation of the blood flow through atrioventricular and great arteries is abnormal.

- Ultrasonic manifestation

  The short axis of the great artery shows the double-ring sign of two great arteries, with the absence of the pulmonary artery crossing the aorta.

  In the long axis of LVOT and RVOT, two large arteries are parallel to each other. The pulmonary artery connects with the LV, and the aorta connects with the RV. Identify the pulmonary artery according to the fact that the great artery divides into left and right branches. The arcuate large artery connecting with the brachiocephalic artery is identified as the aorta.

  The four-chamber view shows atrioventricular concordance in d-TGA and atrioventricular discordance in CCTGA (Fig. 4.29). Identify the LA and RA according to the direction of opening of foramen ovale valve and the connection of the pulmonary vein, vena cava, and atrium. Determine the LV and RV according to the site of attachment of the atrioventricular valve.

- Tips

  The heart structure is in a state of disorder in TGA cases. Use the segmental analysis to tell the following aspects sequentially: the position of atrium, ventricle, and great arteries, the connection between atrium and ventricle, the relationship between ventricle and great arteries.

  If the rate of pulmonary artery straddling is greater than 50%, a special type of DORV should be considered, known as Taussig–Bing syndrome.

  The spatial relationship of the two great arteries is abnormal.

  The prognosis is poor.

  Other congenital heart malformations.

- Single atrium
  - Concepts

    The single atrium is characterized by a common atrial cavity without atrial septum.

    The single atrium is a rare cyanotic CHD.
  - Ultrasonic manifestation

    No atrial septum is visible in the four-chamber view and the short axis of the aorta. (Fig. 4.30).

    Color Doppler ultrasound shows that the blood of vena cava and pulmonary vein mix in the common atrium.
  - Tips

    The intrauterine detection rate of the single atrium is high. Please pay attention to other accompanied cardiac malformations.

    The prognosis of the single atrium is poor.
- Single ventricle

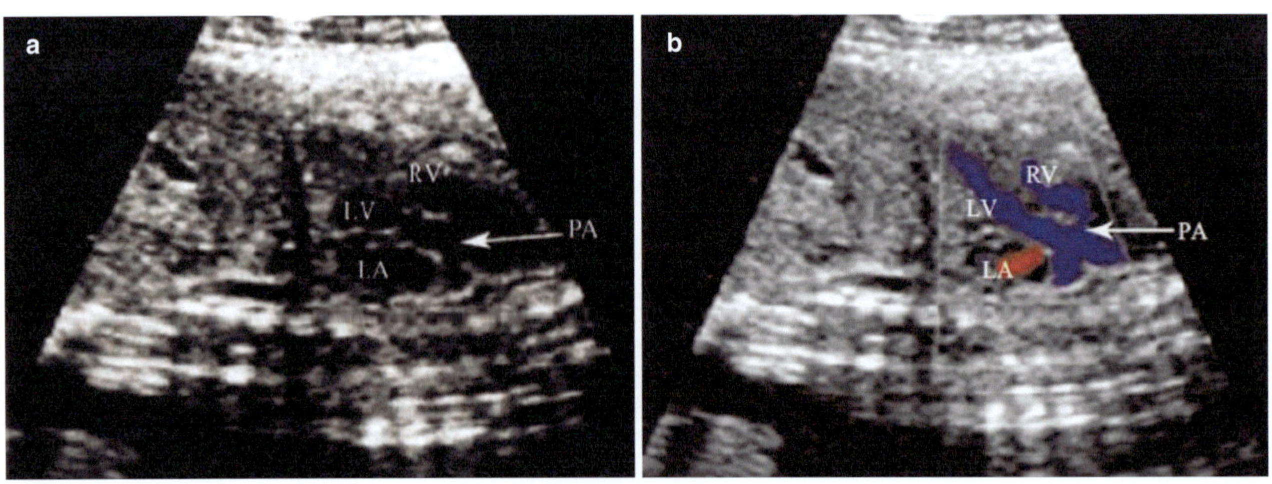

Fig. 4.29 Transposition of great arteries. (**a, b**) A nonstandard view of the long axis of the LV shows 2-D and color Doppler flow imaging shows ventricular arterial discordance with atrioventricular concordance, indicating d-TGA

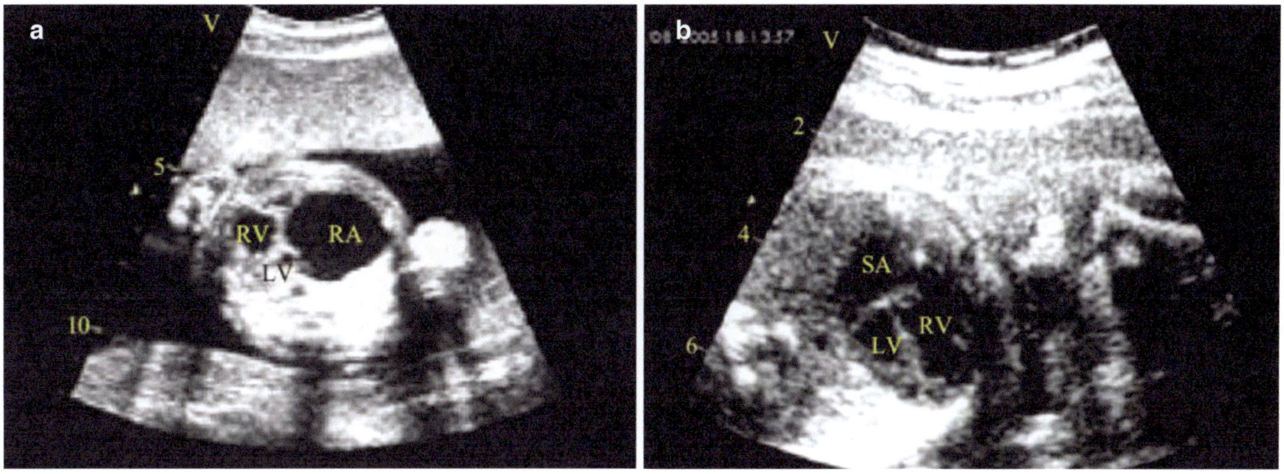

Fig. 4.30 Single atrium. (**a, b**) 2-D shows the absence of atrial septum in the atrial cavity

- Concepts

  The ventricular septum is completely absent or extremely dysplasia.

  Anatomic single ventricle: only one ventricular chamber, with one or two sets of atrioventricular valves connected with the ventricle abnormally.

  "Functional" single ventricle: there are two anatomic ventricles, and one of them is extremely small.

  It is a rare cyanotic CHD, accounting for 1% of postnatal CHD.

  It is often accompanied by ventricular arterial discordance and abnormal spatial relationships.
- Ultrasonic manifestation

  No ventricular septum is found. The four-chamber view shows only one common ventricle, with the absence of ventricular septum, communicating with the atrioventricular valves (Fig. 4.31).

  Color Doppler ultrasonography shows the atrial blood flows into the common ventricle from the left and right atrioventricular valves.
- Tips

  The intrauterine detection rate is high. Single ventricle is often accompanied by ventricular arterial discordance, atrioventricular discordance, and other cardiac malformations.

  The prognosis of single ventricle is extremely poor.

• Anomalous pulmonary venous connection
  - Concepts

    When an anomalous pulmonary venous connection is present, none or some of the pulmonary veins return to the LA. The pulmonary veins connect with the RA directly or indirectly by other paths.

    It can be divided into partial anomalous pulmonary venous connection (PAPVC), which is common, and total anomalous pulmonary venous connection (TAPVC). According to the pulmonary vein connection, both two types can be divided into intracardiac type, supracardiac type, and infracardiac type.
  - Ultrasonic manifestation

    Four-chamber view and nonstandard view shows none of the pulmonary veins drains into the left atrium.

    Usually, common vena cava can be detected in the lateral and posterior walls of LA (Fig. 4.32).

    The left atrium shrinks.
  - Tips

    The antenatal sonographic diagnosis of anomalous pulmonary venous connection is difficult. We should be cautious to improve the detection rate.

    Pay attention to other concomitant cardiac anomalies.

5. Cardiac tumors
   - Concepts
     - The fetal cardiac tumor is the abnormal mass in the heart, usually arising from the ventricular wall. The majority of cardiac tumors are benign tumors, and rhabdomyomas are the most frequently detected.
     - Rhabdomyomas account for 60% of cardiac tumors. It can be multiple or isolated. Larger tumors may result in hemodynamic disorders, leading to hydrops and fetal demise.
     - Other rare cardiac tumors include teratoma, fibroma, lipoma, hemangioma, and myxoma, etc.

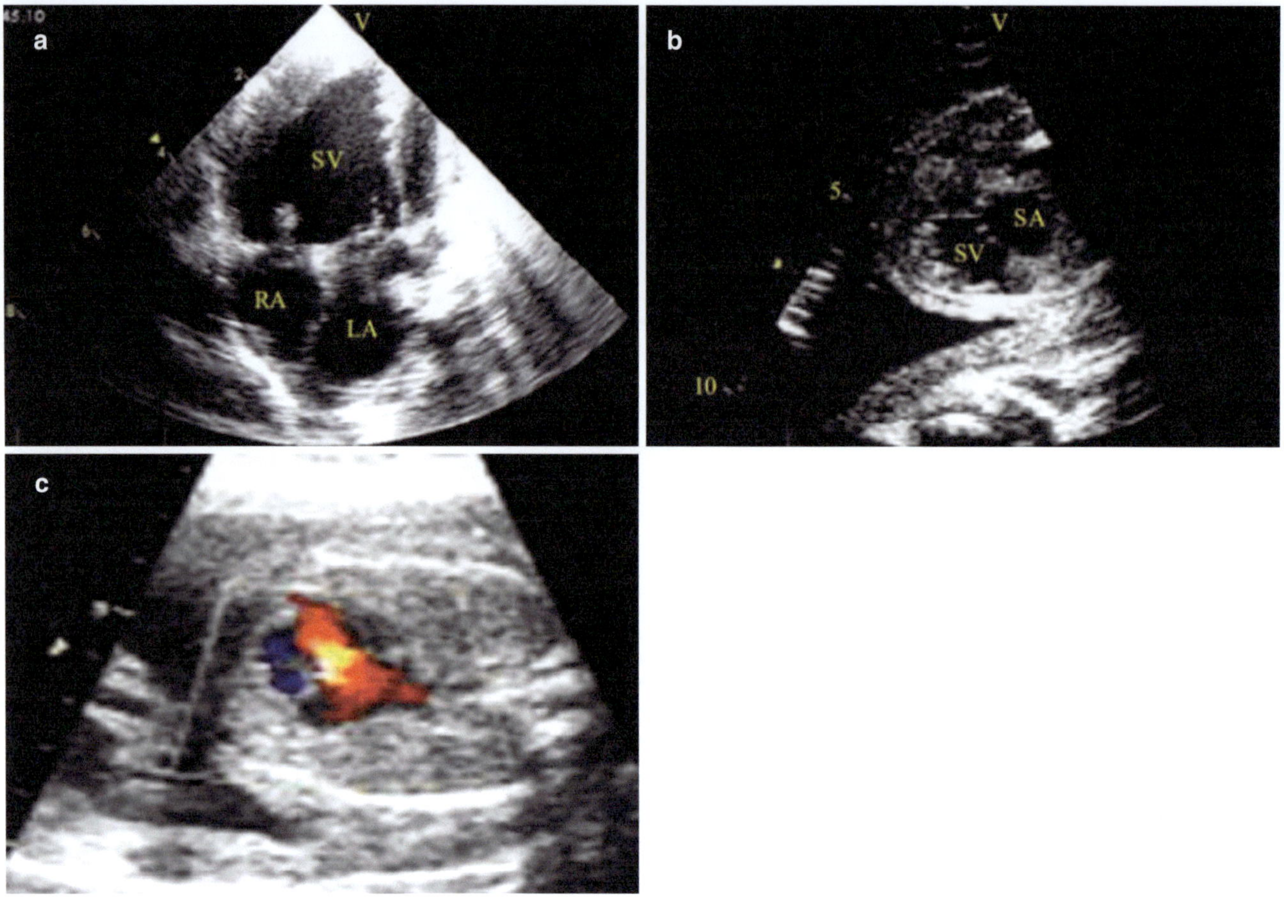

Fig. 4.31 Single ventricle. (**a**) The fetal four-chamber view shows the complete absence of ventricular septum—two sets of atrioventricular valves open to the common ventricle. (**b**) The four-chamber view shows a complete absence of the atrial septum and ventricular septum, indicating bilocular heart (single atrium and single ventricle). (**c**) Color blood flow imaging of the bilocular heart of the same fetus

- Ultrasonic manifestation
  - In the four-chamber view, rhabdomyomas appear as well-circumscribed, hyperechogenic masses.
  - Rhabdomyomas, multiple or single, may protrude into the heart cavity or locate in the ventricular wall mostly in the ventricular septum. Rhabdomyomas move with the systolic and diastolic cardiac movement (Fig. 4.33).
  - We should be cautious because of the various sonographic features in different cardiac tumors.
  - Color Doppler ultrasonography shows the blood flows between the tumor and the chamber's wall. In the cases with obstruction, accelerated blood flow will be detected.
- Tips
  - The intrauterine detection rate is high.
  - It is difficult to make a pathological diagnosis of cardiac tumors.
  - Once space-occupying lesions are detected, close observation should be followed. Some cardiac rhabdomyomas have been reported to shrink or completely regressed later.
  - Terminate the pregnancy if inflow or outflow tract obstruction is obvious.

6. Summary
   - Some CHDs are easy to be diagnosed by prenatal ultrasonic examination as follows: large VSD, ostium primum ASD, AVSD, single atrium, single ventricle, mitral valve atresia, tricuspid valve atresia, severe Ebstein's anomaly, left or right cardiac hypoplasia syndrome, etc.
   - Some CHDs are easy to be missed by prenatal ultrasonic examination as follows: high VSD, VSD that less than 3 mm, sinus venosus ASD, fenestrated ASD, anomalous pulmonary venous connection, valve stenosis, aortic coarctation, coronary artery disease, double-chamber right ventricular, myocardial disease, etc.
   - Some CHDs are difficult to be diagnosed by prenatal ultrasonic examination as follows: conotruncal defects, such as TOF, transposition of the great artery, DORV, TA.

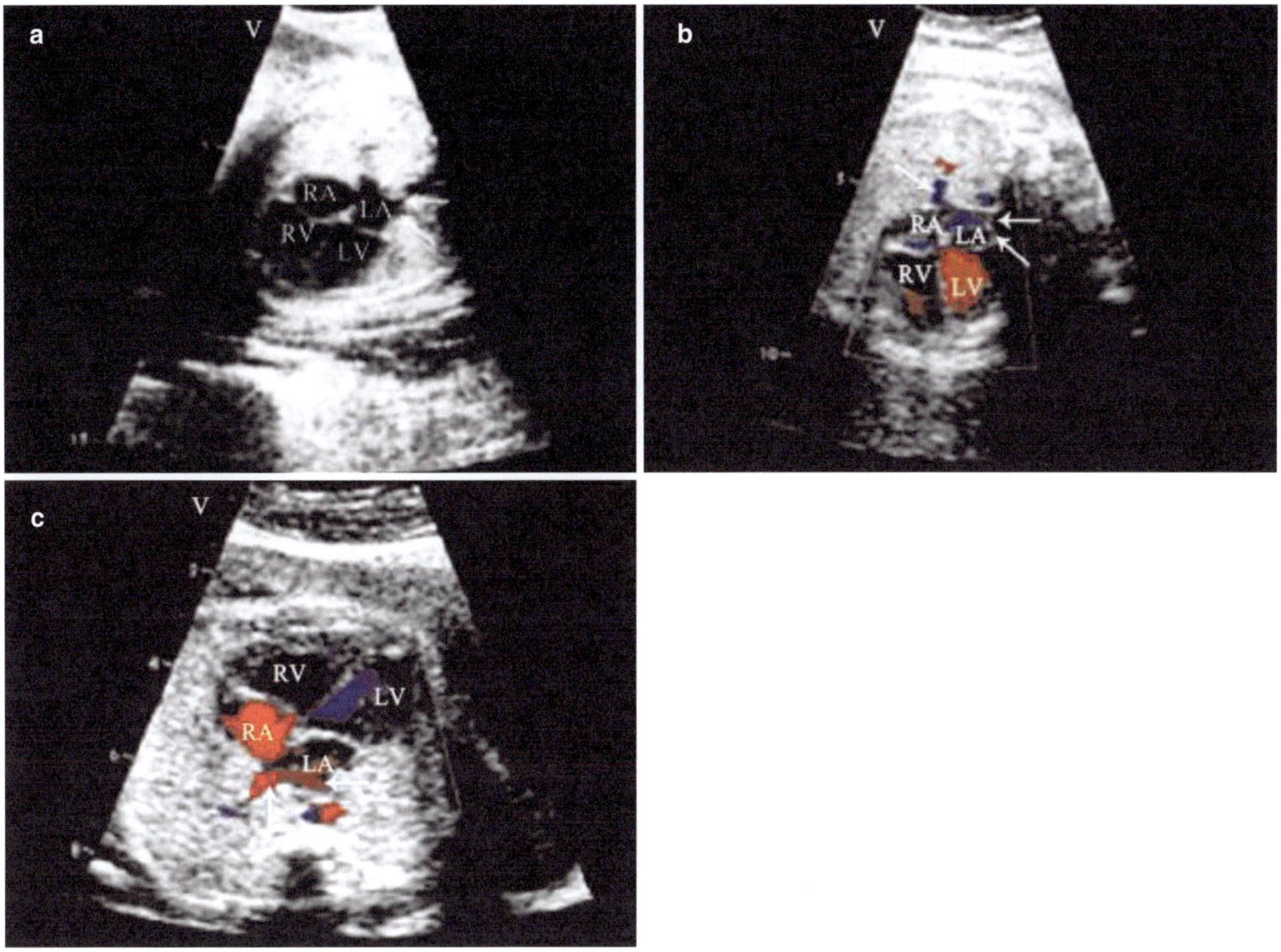

Fig. 4.32 Normal view of the pulmonary vein. (**a**) Three pulmonary veins (arrows) return into the left atrium in the four-chamber view of the normal fetal heart. (**b**) The fetal four-chamber view shows Color flow imaging of pulmonary venous blood flow (arrow) return into the LA. (**c**) Color flow imaging of pulmonary vein blood flows to the LA (arrows show pulmonary veins) in the four-chamber view in a supine position

- Some CHDs cannot be diagnosed by prenatal ultrasonic examination as follows: patent ductus arteriosus and patent foramen ovale.

7. Notice Items in Fetal Echocardiography.

   There are some difficulties and limitations in fetal echocardiography. To avoid unnecessary medical disputes, we should pay attention to the following aspects:

   - Standardize medical behaviors. Performing fetal echocardiography is highly specialized, which requires relevant clinical knowledge of cardiovascular disease, knowledge of basic cardiac anatomy, and the ability to diagnose various heart diseases with ultrasound.
   - The limitations of ultrasonography should be understood sufficiently. During pregnancy, small fetal cardiovascular volume, variable fetal position, maternal obesity, polyhydramnios, and oligohydramnios are important factors that affect the fetal heart examination. Screening is challenging, which requires patience and meticulousness to improve the diagnosis of fetal cardiovascular disease.
   - Due to the ultrasonic biological effect, shorten the examination time as much as possible.
   - You can ask the pregnant woman to lie on the left or right side or to perform appropriate activities, if the fetal position is not suitable or some structures are not well displayed, to obtain a satisfactory image of the fetal heart.
   - For complex fetal CHD, only partial malformation images can be obtained, and make a relevant qualitative diagnosis, which is difficult to further accurate classification.

8. Development of fetal echocardiography

   - New applications of fetal 2-D echocardiography

     In the past decades, with the booming development of minimally invasive surgery in neonates, the

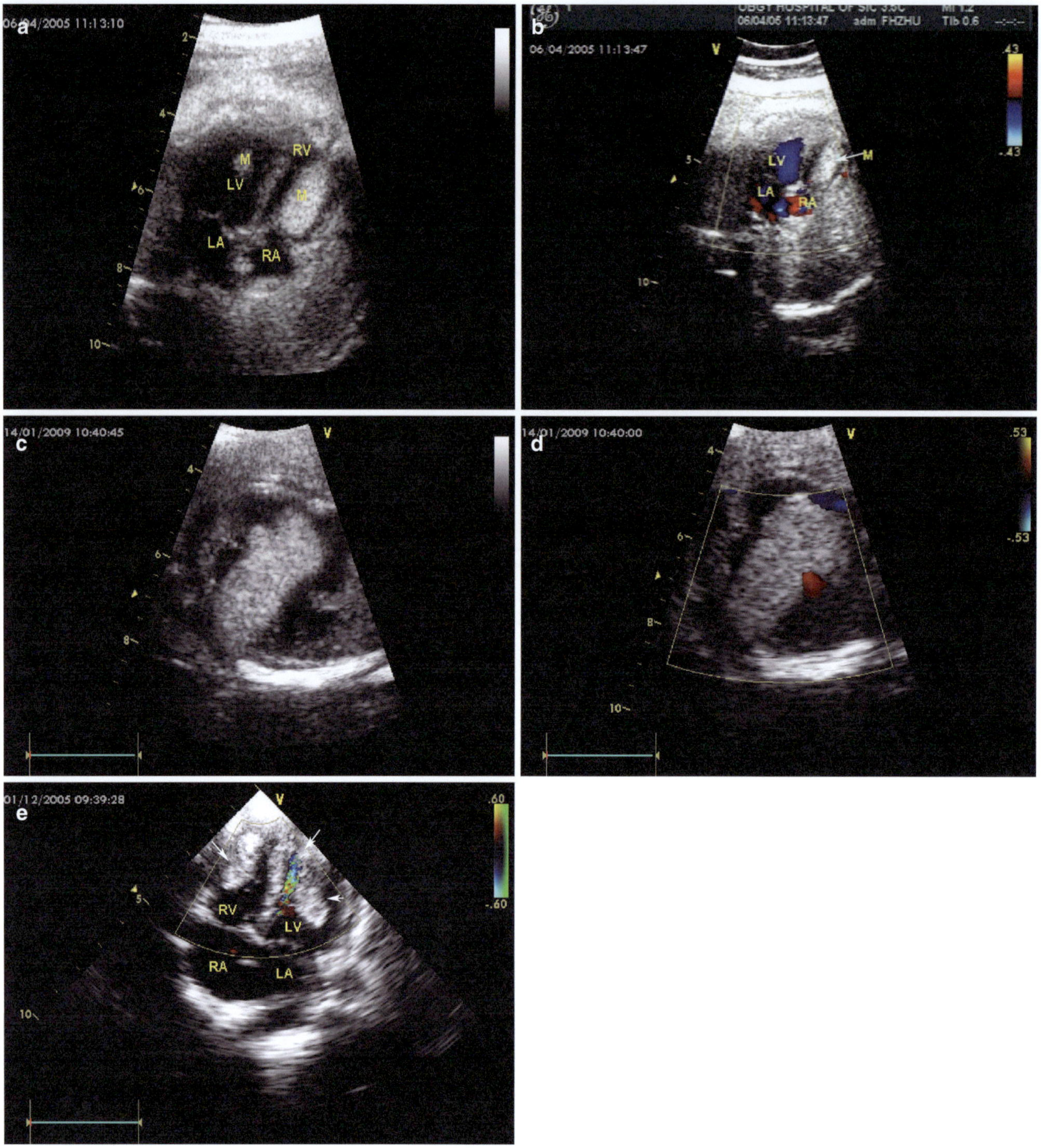

Fig. 4.33 Fetal cardiac tumor. (**a**) The four-chamber view shows hyperechogenic masses in the RV and LV. (**b**) Color flow imaging of the same view shows no obvious obstruction. (**c**) The interventricular septum is thickened and hyperechogenic in the four-chamber view. (**d**) The same view shows poor blood flow of the cavity, indicating cardiac obstruction. (**e**) In the four-chamber view, multiple hyperechogenic masses are observed both in the RV and LV after birth

application of fetal minimally invasive technology is increasing. 2-D sonography, as an advanced interventional guidance technology, plays a vital role in the minimally invasive operation of fetal closed treatment. Some CHD in fetal period, such as valvular stenosis or atresia, may have hemodynamic changes which affect the development of atrium and ventricle. Fetal development will be affected without early intervention, and further operation for correction is needed after birth. At present, large quantities of researchers are exploring various influencing factors of fetal intervention therapy, in order to improve the success rate of treatment.

- New ultrasonic techniques for fetal cardiac examination

  The increasingly widespread application of ultrasound requires the improvement of technology for ultrasonic diagnosis. Therefore, with the development of computer and ultrasound application technology, a variety of new ultrasonic technologies have developed, demonstrating an amazing prospect. Among them, many of the latest technologies can be applied in fetal echocardiography. For example, tissue Doppler technology is used to determine the location and classification of fetal arrhythmia, analyze myocardial activity, and monitor the overall and local functions of the heart. Harmonic imaging technology is used to improve the image quality of the fetal heart, especially that of obese pregnant women.

- The application of fetal 3-D echocardiography

  Since the application of 2-D echocardiography in fetal heart examination, the diagnostic accuracy of prenatal CHD, especially some severe CHD, has remained at a low level. The quality of the images is limited by various objective factors, such as gestational age, fetal position, shadow of the ribs, and maternal abdominal wall thickness. Moreover, qualified images depend on the operator's skills in screening and extensive experience in diagnosing. In the 1970s, with the introduction of 3-D ultrasound in adult transthoracic echocardiography, this technique was also introduced into fetal echocardiography subsequently. Fetal 3-D echocardiography has undergone a process from static to dynamic, from delayed to real time.

  – Spatial-temporal image correlation (STIC)

    STIC realizes two key points in 3-D dynamic imaging technology. One is to collect lots of volume datasets at a certain time of the cardiac cycle, and the other is the electrocardiogram (ECG) gating. STIC is a kind of delayed 3-D imaging technology with fast reconstruction speed and satisfied reconstructed images. STIC has a powerful post-analysis technology in offline analysis software, which has become the study focus in recent years. The following are the applications of 3-D ultrasonography based on STIC for the structural and functional evaluation of the fetal heart.

  – Application of STIC and tomographic ultrasound imaging (tomographic ultrasound imaging, TUI) (TUI-STIC) in the segmental analysis of fetal CHD

    Segmental analysis is often used to describe cardiovascular characteristics of the fetus with CHD. The segmental analysis method includes the analysis of all the views from the fetal abdominal to the ductal arch. TUI-STIC benefits to display the structural lesions of complex CHD vividly, such as visceral ectopic syndrome, complex conotruncal anomalies, etc. TUI imaging mode can be used to display several parallel cardiac plans simultaneously after volume data reconstructed by STIC, which helps to understand fetal cardiac structural abnormalities spatially. D. Paladini et al. performed a TUI-STIC examination on 103 CHD fetuses confirmed by 2-D fetal echocardiography. The research shows that all cases can obtain precise segmental analysis results using TUI-STIC.

  – 3-D cardiac imaging of STIC with surface rendering (STIC-rendering)

    Many planes cannot be displayed by standard views of 2-D fetal echocardiography, such as the lateral view of the atrial septum and ventricular septum, the transverse view of the atrioventricular annulus. STIC-Rendering can render the plane of hole ventricular septum or atrial septal on the screen, enabling observers to view the complete septum from the atrium–atrium and ventricle–ventricle perspectively. The number and motion of atrioventricular valves are vital to atrioventricular connection. The shape of the semilunar valve plays an important role in determining the ventricular arterial connection. However, regular 2-D ultrasound, which can only observe the heart from the long axis: the anterior and posterior view of the atrioventricular valve ring and the plane of the coronary-atrioventricular valve. Whereas, STIC-rendering can display the above views.

  – STIC combined with 2-D B-flow imaging mode (STIC-B flow) for the diagnosis of pulmonary vascular abnormalities

    B-flow imaging is a new imaging technology of coded digital ultrasound, which uses "coded excitation" to enhance signals from weak blood flow and suppress signals from the static tissues.

Because of the simultaneous imaging of blood flow and tissue, the flow in the blood vessel and the anatomic relationship with vessels are displayed intuitively and clearly while performing 2-D scanning. The advantages include higher frequency and spatial resolution, high sensitivity to blood flow signals, and angle-independent, which contribute to an ideal display of fetal pulmonary vessels. In recent years, many scholars have combined B-flow technology with STIC to achieve a 3-D visualization of small vessels in the fetal pulmonary circulation, improving the hemodynamic interpretation and diagnosis of CHD with abnormal pulmonary circulation.

- STIC in cardiac function assessment

  An accurate and reliable cardiac output measurement method is of great significance for evaluating the abnormalities of fetal cardiac structure and function. In the measurement of fetal heart function by 2-D echocardiography, it is relatively reliable to measure the time velocity integral (TVI) by detecting the Doppler spectrum of blood flow in the outflow tract. Measure the inner diameter (D) of the aorta and pulmonary artery, and calculate the stroke volume of LV and RV respectively, using the formula $SV = \pi \times (D/2)^2 \times TVI$. The angle between the sampling line and the blood flow is required less than 20 °, which needs a very suitable fetal position and is very time-consuming. It is a pity that this application has limited clinical value. Recently, researchers collect fetal heart volume data by STIC and have used various powerful post-processing technologies to objectively calculate the fetal cardiac volume and evaluate cardiac function.

- Clinical application of RT-3DE

  Real-time three-dimensional echocardiography (RT-3DE) can collect images in real time and simultaneously display 3-D dynamic cardiac images. RT-3DE contains four display modes: real-time 3-D, color 3-D, full-volume 3-D, and three-plane 3-D. At present, RT-3DE has been widely used in the diagnosis of heart structure and valve disease, measurement of ventricular volume, and cardiac function. At the same time, RT-3DE has developed a new way for the diagnosis of fetal CHD. RT-3DE, as a supplement to 2-D echocardiography, enables prenatal diagnosis of congenital structural and functional abnormalities of the fetus. The volume data obtained by RT-3DE is less affected by fetal movement and fetal respiration in the process of image collection, which reduces the distortion and pseudo-image caused by fetal movement. The clinical application of RT-3DE mainly includes the following aspects: (1) Observe the fetal cardiac anatomical structure, especially some views that are difficult to be displayed by 2-D echocardiography. (2) Display the plane view of the heart and great arteries and complex cardiac malformations visually, such as ASD and VSD, DORV, tricuspid atresia, transposition of the great arteries, permanent arterial trunk, etc. (3) Measure the fetal cardiac volume and evaluate the fetal heart function in a relatively accurate way.

9. Clinical application of 4-D fetal echocardiography

   In recent years, many researchers are devoted to the development of new technologies to improve the prenatal diagnosis rate of CHD. The latest technology applied to fetal cardiac examination is real-time and single cardiac cycle 4D imaging (4D), which can acquire the full volume cardiac images within a cardiac cycle. 4-D echocardiography can visually display the spatial structure of the fetal heart in real time, realizing veritable real-time full-volume cardiac imaging. Compared with traditional full-volume cardiac imaging, 4-D echocardiography can reach 90 × 90 °, with flexible size according to frame frequency and resolution, no longer requires image splicing, electrocardiogram trigger, or breath-holding. 4-D echocardiography starts a new era of four-dimensional cardiac imaging. With the progress of computer technology, these new technologies, which will play a more prominent role in prenatal screening of fetal CHD and eugenics, will inevitably become a necessary complement to 2-D echocardiography.

10. New application of fetal cardiac function evaluation

    A reliable noninvasive assessment of fetal cardiac function is affected by many factors, including small fetal heart volume, unclear display of ventricular intima, difficulty in standardizing fetal cardiovascular structure, orientation, fetal movement, a poor acoustic window of maternal abdominal wall, and irregular geometry of fetal RV. The RV may have geometric changes if there is a fetal arrhythmia accompanied by abnormal heart function. It is challenging to evaluate fetal ventricular function accurately by the conventional evaluating method of adult and child. Abnormal myocardial systolic and diastolic functions coexist in fetal cardiac insufficiency cases, so it is more reasonable to perform a detailed cardiac functional assessment comprehensively.

    Tei index is not affected by ventricular geometry shape, heart rate, and gestational age in the fetus. The measurement of the Tei index is reproducible and straightforward, which is a practical method to evaluate fetal cardiac function. Tei index can evaluate fetal cardiac function reliably, under physiological or pathological conditions. In the case of cardiac insufficiency, Tei index of fetal ventricular cavity increases. Some researches show that the Tei index can evaluate the cardiac function of edema fetus. Tei index measurement is limited by the small volume of the fetal heart in early pregnancy. Moreover, the Tei index detection in the fetal ventricle is difficult, limiting the application of the Tei index in fetal arrhythmia.

Huhta and colleagues developed the cardiovascular profile score (CVPS, Table 4.1), a multivariate scoring system to evaluate cardiovascular function. CVPS helps to predict the outcome of hydrops and guide its treatment. Furthermore, CVPS can be used to evaluate the prenatal intervention of severe congenital cardiovascular malformation. It is also commonly applied to choose the right opportunity for intrauterine treatment and evaluate the efficacy of fetal arrhythmia/heart failure. It is generally considered that intervention should be performed once the CVPS system score decreases. The treatment, according to etiology, can achieve ideal results when the score of CVPS is more than 7 points. If 7 points > CVPS ≥5 points, whether to take treatment measures or not remains controversial. Most of these cases observe the dynamic changes after individual treatment. The perinatal mortality is high, and the treatment is of little significance when the CVPS is less than 5 points. Clinical intervention may inhibit the adaptive protection of the mother and fetus, exposing the mother–fetus complex to a state of high stress, and result in unnecessary complications that threatening the safety of the mother and fetus. CVPS is negatively correlated with the Tei index. Therefore, the combination of CVPS and Tei index in the evaluation of the diagnosis, treatment, and prognosis of fetal cardiac failure will be more instructive in clinical.

4.3 Echocardiography of Fetal Arrhythmia

Fetal cardiac arrhythmia is defined as irregular fetal cardiac rhythm or abnormal fetal heart rate that beyond the normal range when there is no uterine contraction during a routine prenatal examination. Fetal arrhythmias are detected in 1% ~ 2% of all pregnancies. Normal fetal heart rate (FHR) ranges between 120 and 160 beats per minute (bpm), with a regular rhythm. When the FHR is less than 80% of the low normal FHR, there is a sign of fetal bradycardia. And fetal tachycardia is suggested if the FHR is more than 120% of the high normal FHR. Premature contraction is the premature beats of the atria or ventricles. The difference between supraventricular tachycardia and ventricular tachycardia is that the former originates from atrial premature beats and the latter from ventricular premature beats. There is an entirely contractive dissociation of the atria and ventricle in complete heart block cases. The first-degree heart block refers to a prolonged PR interval caused by the delayed atrioventricular conduction. The second-degree atrioventricular block refers to cyclical ventricular block because of intermittent conduction abnormalities, consisting of Mobitz type I and Mobitz type II. Mobitz type I is characterized by the gradually prolonged PR interval and gradually shortening RR interval, following by a heart block. Mobitz type II refers to the cyclical atrioventricular block without progressive prolonged PR interval. Irregular heart rhythm refers to the heart rate ranges within normal limits, while its fastest heart rate is 25–30 more beats per minute than the slowest—serious arrhythmia resulting in fetal heart failure and demise. In the fetus, auscultation can reflect no more than whether the heart rate is regular, failing to define the rhythm characters. It is challenging to acquire fetal ECG by other noninvasive methods. Fortunately, fetal echocardiography can observe the fetal cardiac structure and function in real time, and deter-

Table 4.1 Cardiovascular profile score (CVPS)

Project	2 points	1 point	0 points
Hydrops	None	Ascites, pleural effusion, or pericardial effusion	Edema of skin
Heart area/ chest area	> 0.20 and ≤ 0.35	0.35 ~ 0.50	>0.50 or <0.20
Cardiac function	Normal MV and TV biphasic diastolic filling	Holosystolic tricuspid regurgitation	Holosystolic mitral regurgitation Monophasic filling
Arterial Doppler of umbilical artery	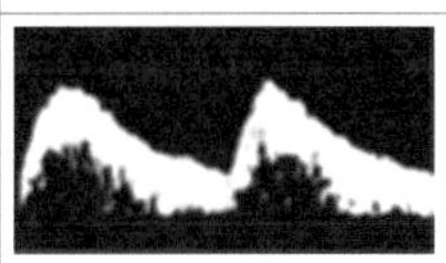	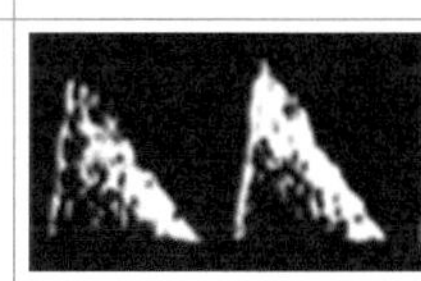	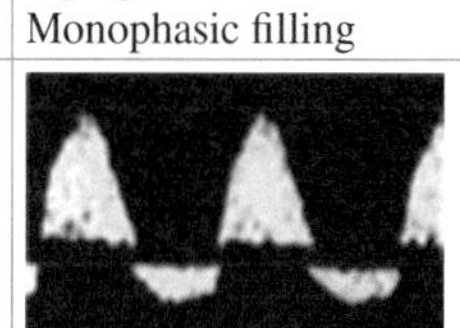
Venous Doppler of umbilical vein and ductus venosus	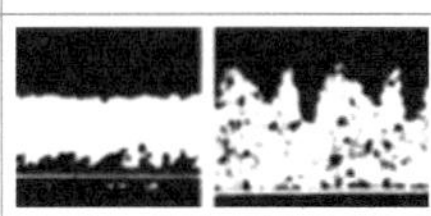	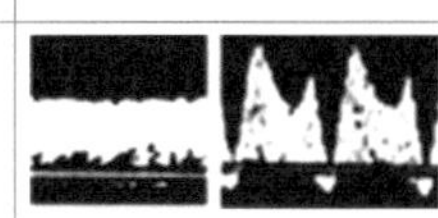	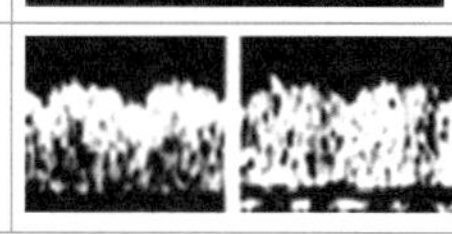

mine the type of fetal arrhythmia, becoming the most valuable method to diagnose fetal arrhythmia.

The diagnosis, classification, and treatment of fetal arrhythmia by fetal echocardiography are based on the electrophysiology and timing analysis of the atria and ventricle. Currently, M-type, spectral Doppler and tissue Doppler imaging (TDI) are used to describe the movement at the atrioventricular level, separately. Although fetal echocardiography is difficult to diagnose complex arrhythmias, it is competent to indicate the prognosis and guide the treatment for its validity and relative accuracy.

1. Echocardiographic assessment of the fetal arrhythmia
   - M-mode echocardiography

     M-mode ultrasound is the most classical and commonly used method to evaluate arrhythmia. By 2-D ultrasound, place the M-mode sampling line across the atrial wall and the ventricular wall to obtain a clear M-mode image. The motion curve of the atrial wall represents atrial systole and diastole, and so does the curve of the atrioventricular valve. The moving curve of the ventricular wall represents ventricular systole and diastole, and so does the curve of the semilunar valve. These motion curves are representations of ECG conduction, intuitively showing the sequence and rhythmic relationship of the atrial and ventricular conduction. Determine the types of fetal arrhythmia by analyzing the corresponding relationship among the motion curves above (Fig. 4.34).
   - Spectral Doppler echocardiography and tissue Doppler echocardiography

     Position the spectral Doppler ultrasound sample volume at different sites of the heart, containing left ventricular inflow - outflow tract area, the adjacent area of SVC and ascending aorta, the adjoining area of IVC and abdominal aorta, and area of pulmonary artery and vein. Atrial rate, ventricular rate, and time interval are calculated according to the blood flow spectrum. Determine the types of arrhythmias depending on the corresponding relationship between the atrial rate and the ventricular rate. The spectral imaging of the inflow and the outflow tract can be obtained when placing the sampling volume at the intersection of the ventricular inflow and the outflow tract. The starting point of the inflow tract spectral A wave represents the beginning of atrial systole, and that of the outflow tract spectrum represents that ventricular diastole starts. According to the above description, we can define specific fetal arrhythmia by analyzing and the corresponding relationship between the systolic and diastolic motion of the atrium and ventricle. Tissue Doppler imaging, reflecting the atrioventricular movement, is acquired when placing tissue Doppler sampling volume in the lateral septum of mitral/tricuspid annular and left/right ventricular wall (Fig. 4.35).
2. Classification of fetal arrhythmia

   Fetal cardiac arrhythmia is defined as irregular fetal cardiac rhythm or abnormal fetal heart rate that outside the normal range when there is no uterine contraction during a routine prenatal examination. When the FHR is less than 80% of the low normal FHR, there is a sign of fetal bradycardia. And fetal tachycardia is suggested if the FHR is more than 120% of the high normal FHR.

   Fetal arrhythmia is generally divided into irregular arrhythmia, tachyarrhythmia, and bradyarrhythmia. Tachyarrhythmia is defined as FHR higher than 200 bpm,

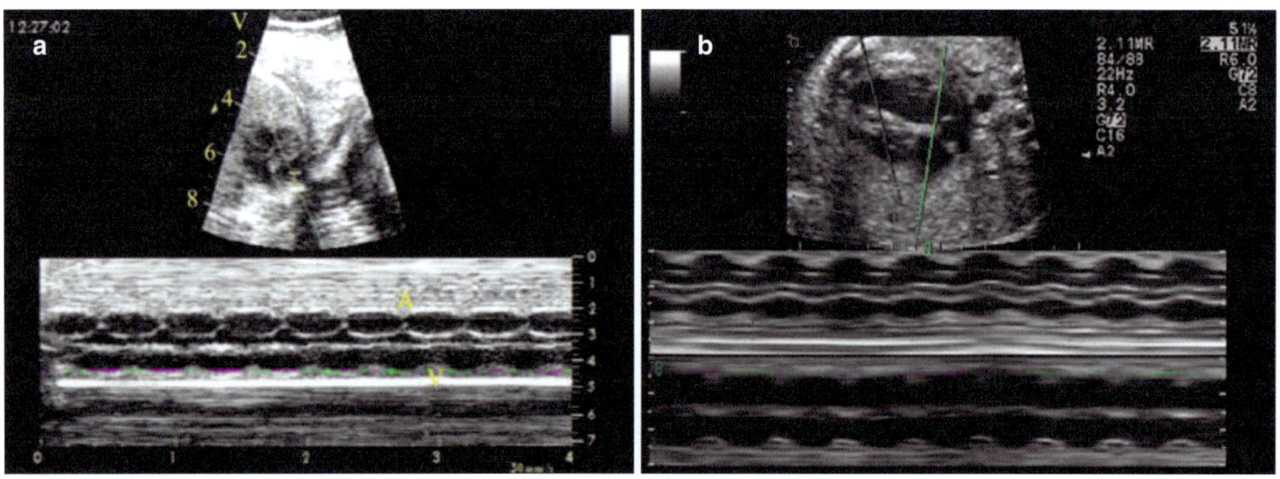

Fig. 4.34 Atrioventricular motion curves of the normal fetal heart. (**a**) The upper curve represents the atrial wall, and the lower one represents the ventricular wall. The lines in the middle are the motion curves of the ventricular septum and the atrioventricular valve. There is a one-to-one correspondence between the motion curve of the atrial wall and the ventricular wall. (**b**) Two sampling lines pass through the atrial wall and the ventricular wall, respectively, and the motion curves of them show a one-to-one correspondence either

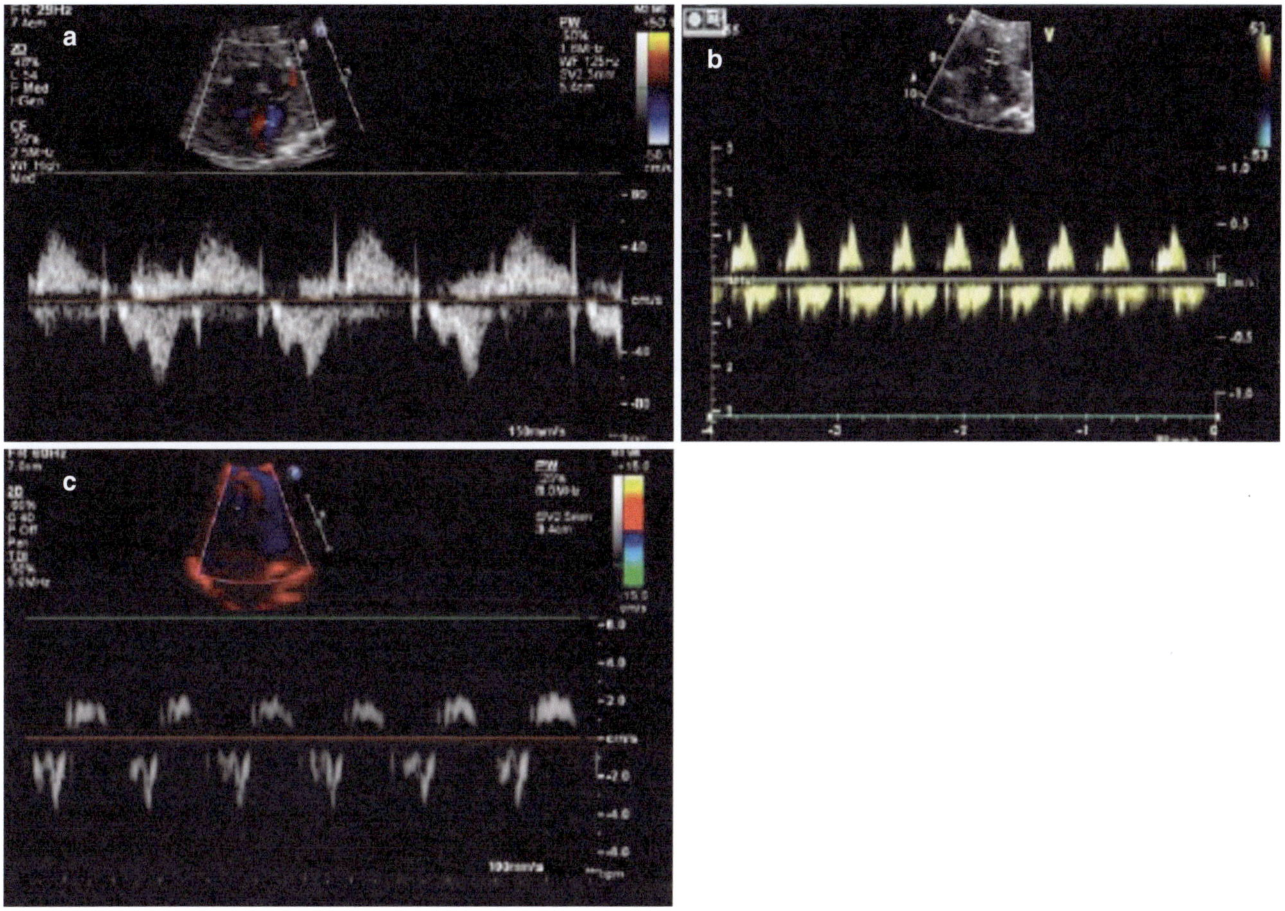

Fig. 4.35 Pulsed Doppler and tissue Doppler echocardiography images. (**a**) It shows A wave, the atrial excitation wave, when the PW samples are placed at the adjacent areas of the inflow and outflow tracts of the left ventricle. (**b**) PW is sampled at PA and PV, showing normal fetal rhythm. (**c**) Tissue Doppler spectrums of ventricular septal movement are obtained by placing sample volume at the lateral ventricular septum of mitral/tricuspid annulus

consisting of sinus tachycardia, supraventricular tachycardia, atrial flutter, and atrial fibrillation. Bradyarrhythmia is characterized by FHR less than 100 bpm, including sinus bradycardia, non-conductive premature beat, and complete heart block. The irregular types include premature atrial contraction, premature ventricular contraction, and tachyarrhythmia with heart block.

3. Echocardiographic characteristics of fetal arrhythmia
   - Irregular arrhythmia

     Irregular rhythm refers to that the heart rate ranges within normal limits, while its fastest heart rate is 25–30 more beats per minute than the slowest. According to the frequency of occurrence, the atrial and ventricular premature contractions that happened in the fetus can be divided into incidental (<5 bpm) and frequent (≥6 bpm) premature contractions.
     – Premature Atrial Contraction

       Premature atrial contraction (PAC): It is a common fetal arrhythmia, which refers to that the atrial contraction is premature, following an incomplete compensatory pause, which can be conducted to the ventricle or blocked. The appearance of a corresponding ventricular movement represents that the PAC has conducted to the ventricle. Conversely, there is no corresponding ventricular motion with a blocked PAC. Both the above two characteristics are shown if the PAC partly conducts to the ventricle (Fig. 4.36).

       M-mode echocardiography shows the premature atrial motion wave with a low amplitude.

       The Doppler echocardiography of PAC shows that wave of the inflow tract blood flow appears in advance, similar to that in M-mode echocardiography. The wave of ventricular ejection will appear if the PAC conducts to the ventricle. In contrast, no wave of ventricular ejection will appear if the PAC is blocked. It is challenging to

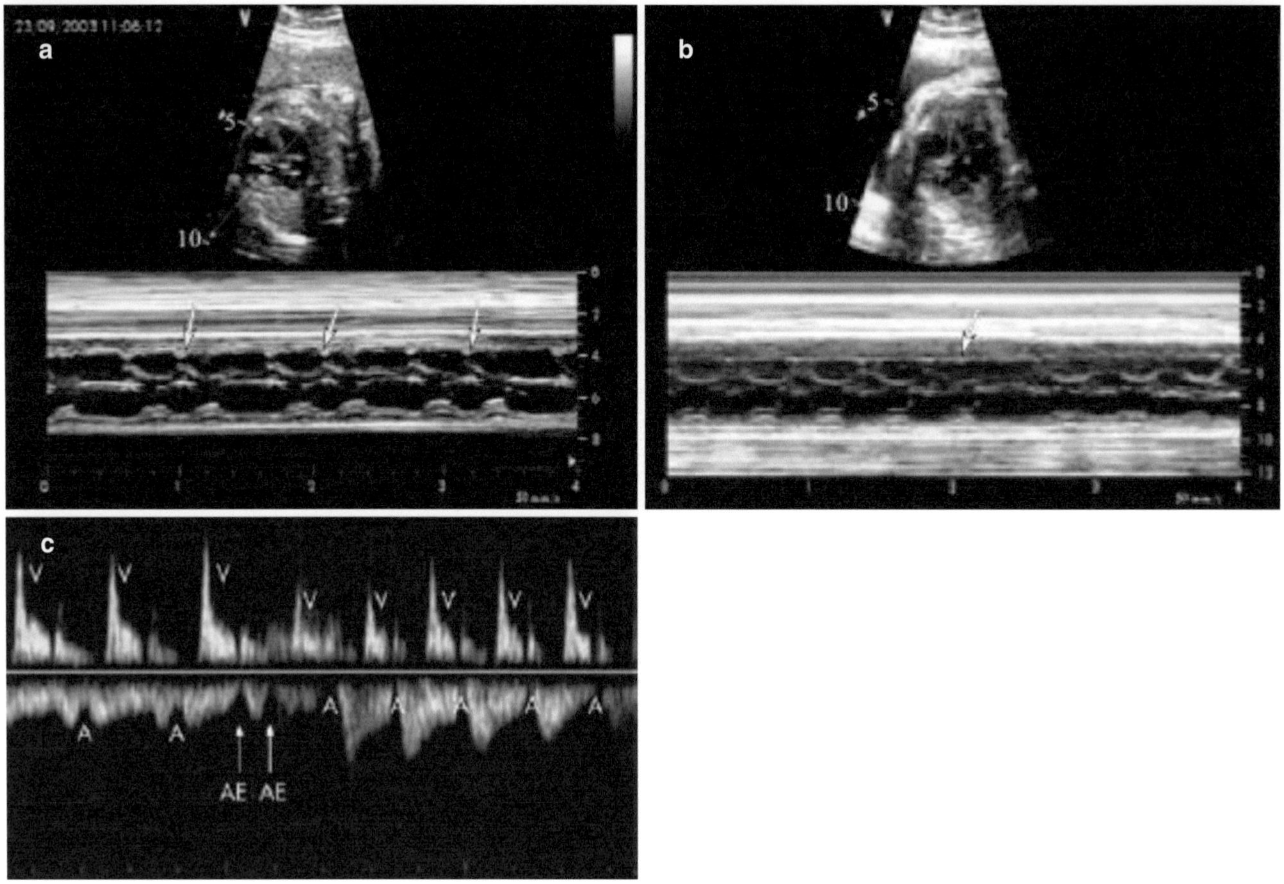

Fig. 4.36 Fetal irregular arrhythmia (Premature Atrial Contraction). (**a**) M-mode ultrasound shows the frequent atrial bigeminy caused by PAC conducted to the ventricle. (**b**) Accidental blocked PAC and the premature contraction of the atrial wall (arrow). (**c**) Spectrum Doppler imaging shows the accidental blocked PAC and the premature contraction of the atrial wall (arrows). (References: Carvalho JS, Prefumo F, Ciardelli V, et al. Evaluation of fetal arrhythmias from simultaneous pulsed wave Doppler in pulmonary artery and vein. Heart, 2007, 93:1448–1453)

show the ventricular outflow tract wave if the atrial contraction is exceptionally in advance.

– Premature ventricular beat

Premature ventricular beat, originating from the ventricle without conducting reverse to the atrium, is uncommon in the fetus. It is characterized by the ventricular contraction premature and long compensative interval, without corresponding atrial contraction.

M-mode echocardiography shows the premature ventricular wave with a low amplitude. There is no corresponding atrial wave in the anterior region. A long interval can be shown in the posterior of the premature ventricular wave, which is longer than that of PAC (Fig. 4.37).

The Doppler echocardiography of premature ventricular beat shows that wave of the outflow tract blood flow appears in advance, without an anterior wave of the inflow tract blood flow, following by a long interval.

- Tachyarrhythmia
  – Sinus tachycardia. The fetal heart rate ranges from 180 to 200 bpm, with a 1:1 ratio of atrial: ventricular rhythm. The movement curves of the atrium and ventricular wall are regular and corresponding.
  – Supraventricular tachycardia. Supraventricular tachycardia (SVT) refers to the fetal heart rate in the 220 to 300 bpm range, with 1:1 atrial: ventricular conduction. The motion curves of the atrial and ventricular wall are corresponding and regular (Fig. 4.38).
  – Ventricular tachycardia. Ventricular tachycardia (VT) refers to the fetal ventricular rate > 200 bpm, the ventricular rate > the atrial rate. The ventricular movement curve is regular, while the atrial curve is regular or irregular.

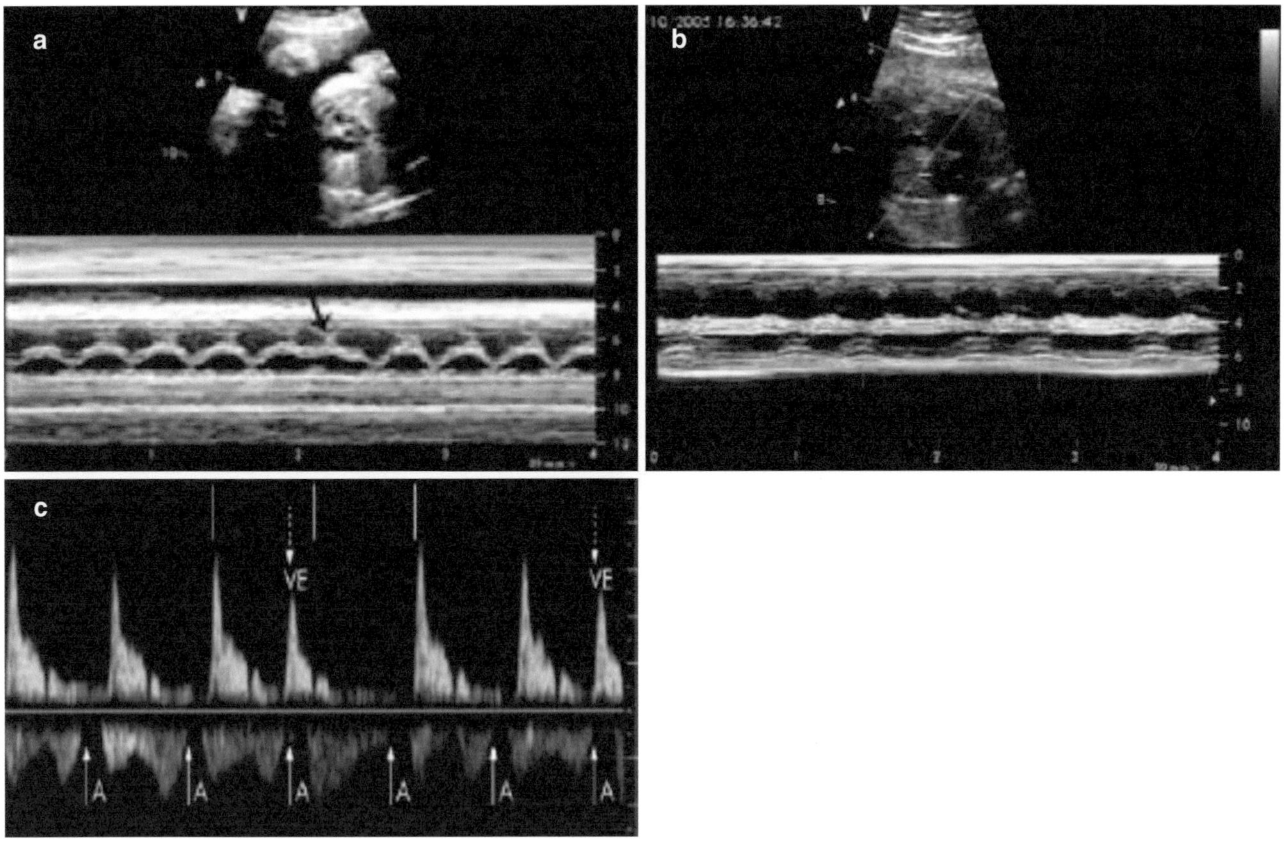

Fig. 4.37 Fetal irregular arrhythmia (Premature ventricular beat). (**a**) In M-mode, the upper curve represents the ventricular wall, and the lower one represents the atrial wall. The line in the middle is the motion curve of the atrioventricular valve. The premature ventricular beat is shown. (**b**) In the M-mode of fetal ventricular bigeminy, the upper curve represents the atrial wall, the lower one represents the ventricular wall, and the middle one is the motion curve of the ventricular septum. The premature ventricular beat is shown. (**c**) The spectrum Doppler shows the ventricular trigeminy in the fetus (References: Carvalho JS, Prefumo F, Ciardelli V, et al. Evaluation of fetal arrhythmias from simultaneous pulsed wave Doppler in pulmonary artery and vein. Heart, 2007, 93:1448–1453)

  - Atrial flutter. Atrial flutter (AF) is defined as the fetal atrial rate in the 300–500 bpm range, faster than the rate of the ventricle. The movement curve of the atrial wall is regular, and that of the ventricular wall is irregular (Fig. 4.39).
  - Atrial fibrillation. Fetal atrial fibrillation refers to fetal atrial rate > 400–500 bpm, atrial rate > ventricular rate. Curves of the atrial wall and the ventricular wall are irregular (Fig. 4.40). Incessant fetal tachyarrhythmia can lead to fetal heart failure, hydrops, and even fetal demise.
- Bradyarrhythmia
  - Sinus bradycardia. Fetal sinus bradycardia refers to a fetal heart rate of 100 bpm or less, with synchronized atrial and ventricular rate. Motion curves of the atrial and ventricular walls are corresponding, regular (Fig. 4.41).
  - Heart block. Normally, the distance between the beginning of the atrial wave and that of the ventricular wave in M-mode ultrasound or the A-V interval in spectrum Doppler is within 150 ms. The heart block can be determined by estimating the A-V interval by M-mode or spectral Doppler ultrasound (Fig. 4.42).

    First-degree heart block refers to the PR interval is longer than 150 ms. All the atrial contractions are conducted to the ventricle (Fig. 4.43).

    Second-degree heart block

- Mobitz type I is characterized by the progressive lengthening of the A-V interval in spectrum Doppler, following by a heart block (short-long-long-drop) (Fig. 4.44).
- Mobitz type II refers to the regular A-V interval under spectrum Doppler, with cyclical atrioventricular block. No progressive prolonging PR interval is detected (Fig. 4.45).
- Third-degree atrioventricular block, also known as a complete atrioventricular block (CAVB), is character-

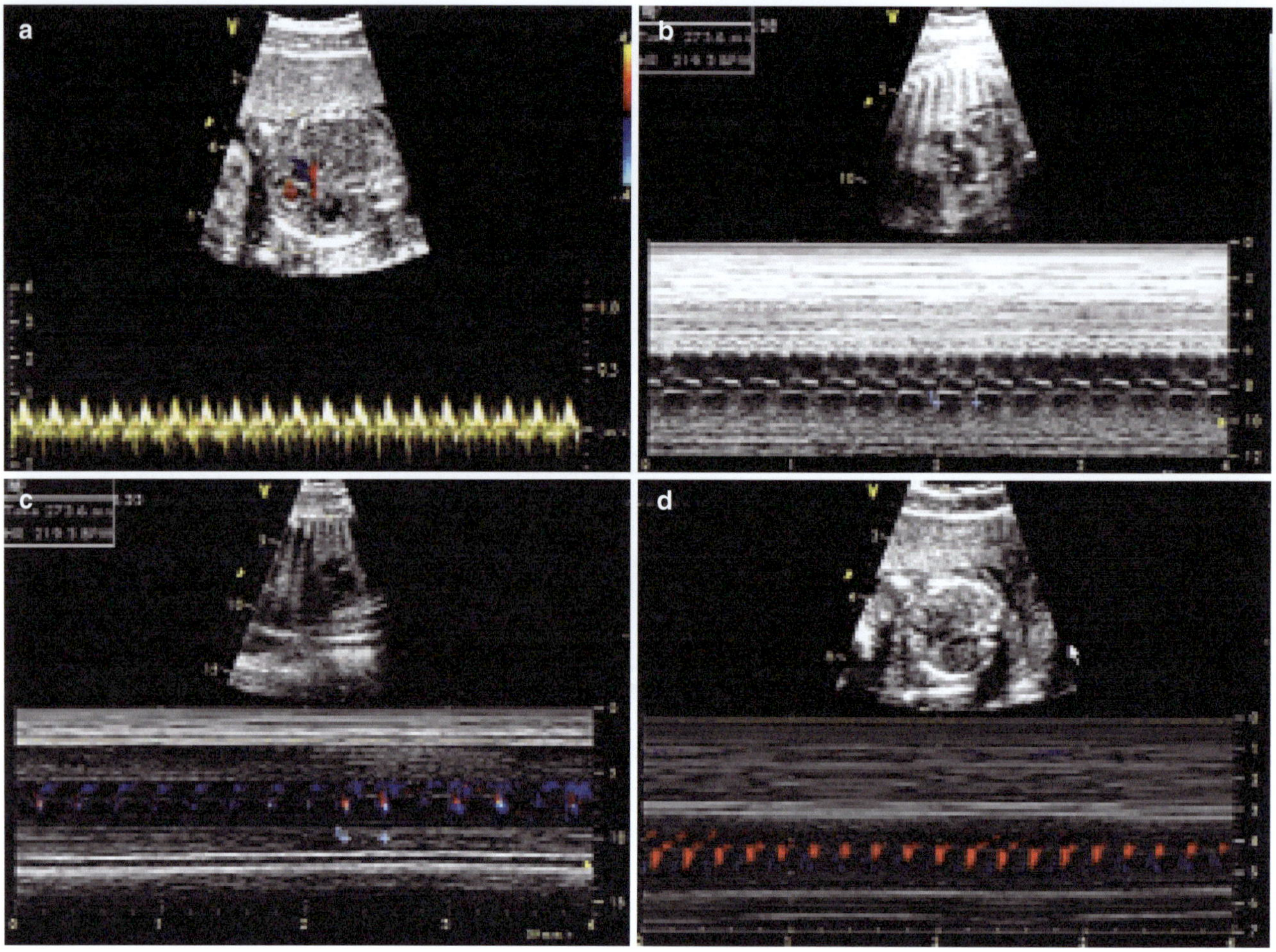

Fig. 4.38 Supraventricular tachycardia. (**a**) Doppler of supraventricular tachycardia. (**b**) M-mode ultrasound of fetal supraventricular tachycardia. (**c**, **d**) M-mode color ultrasound in fetal supraventricular tachycardia

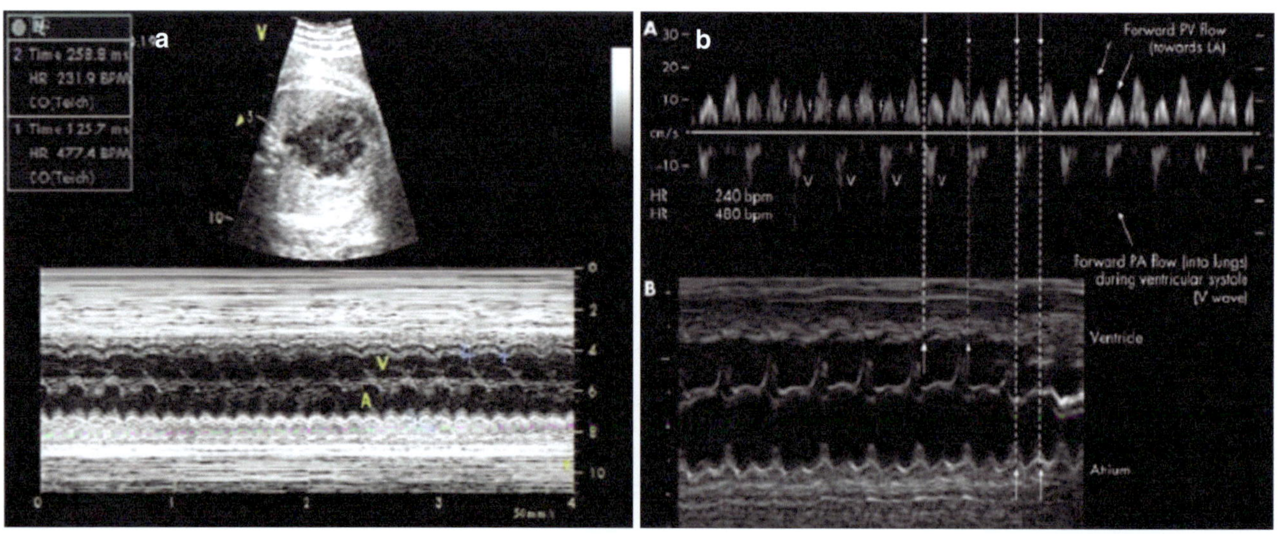

Fig. 4.39 Fetal atrial flutter. (**a**) M-mode ultrasound shows fetal atrial flutter with a 2:1 atrioventricular conduction, atrial rate > ventricular rate. (**b**) It shows pulsed wave Doppler (PWD) recording of pulmonary vessels (A) and M mode (B) of the same fetus with atrial flutter and 2:1 atrioventricular block, simultaneously. The vertical dashed line shows the corresponding atrial and ventricular activity both in the PWD and M mode. (References: Carvalho JS, Prefumo F, Ciardelli V, et al. Evaluation of fetal arrhythmias from simultaneous pulsed wave Doppler in pulmonary artery and vein. Heart, 2007, 93:1448–1453)

ized by the fetal ventricular rate less than 80 bpm, atrial rate >ventricular rate, and atrial and ventricular dissociation (Fig. 4.46).

- Notices in screening fetal arrhythmia.

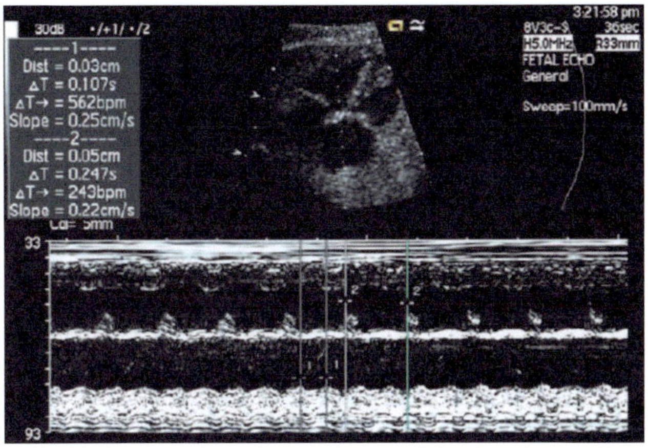

Fig. 4.40 M-mode echocardiography of fetal atrial fibrillation, atrial rate > ventricular rate

  - When detecting fetal arrhythmia, M-mode echocardiography should simultaneously record the motion curve of the atrial wall and the ventricular wall, and calculate the atrial rate and ventricular rate, respectively. Define the type of arrhythmia according to the corresponding relationship between atrial and ventricular rate and between atrial and ventricular contraction.
  - In Doppler echocardiography, place the sampling volume at the intersection of the ventricular inflow and outflow tract to obtain the spectral imaging of the inflow and outflow tract, analyze, and determine the type of arrhythmia.
  - The diagnosis of first- to second-degree heart block is based on the atrial and ventricular dissociation. Besides, it depends on the PR interval by recording the spectrum of the right pulmonary artery and right superior pulmonary vein simultaneously, or the spectrum of SVC and ascending aorta simultaneously. These methods help to make a correct diagnosis of fetal first- to second-degree atrio-

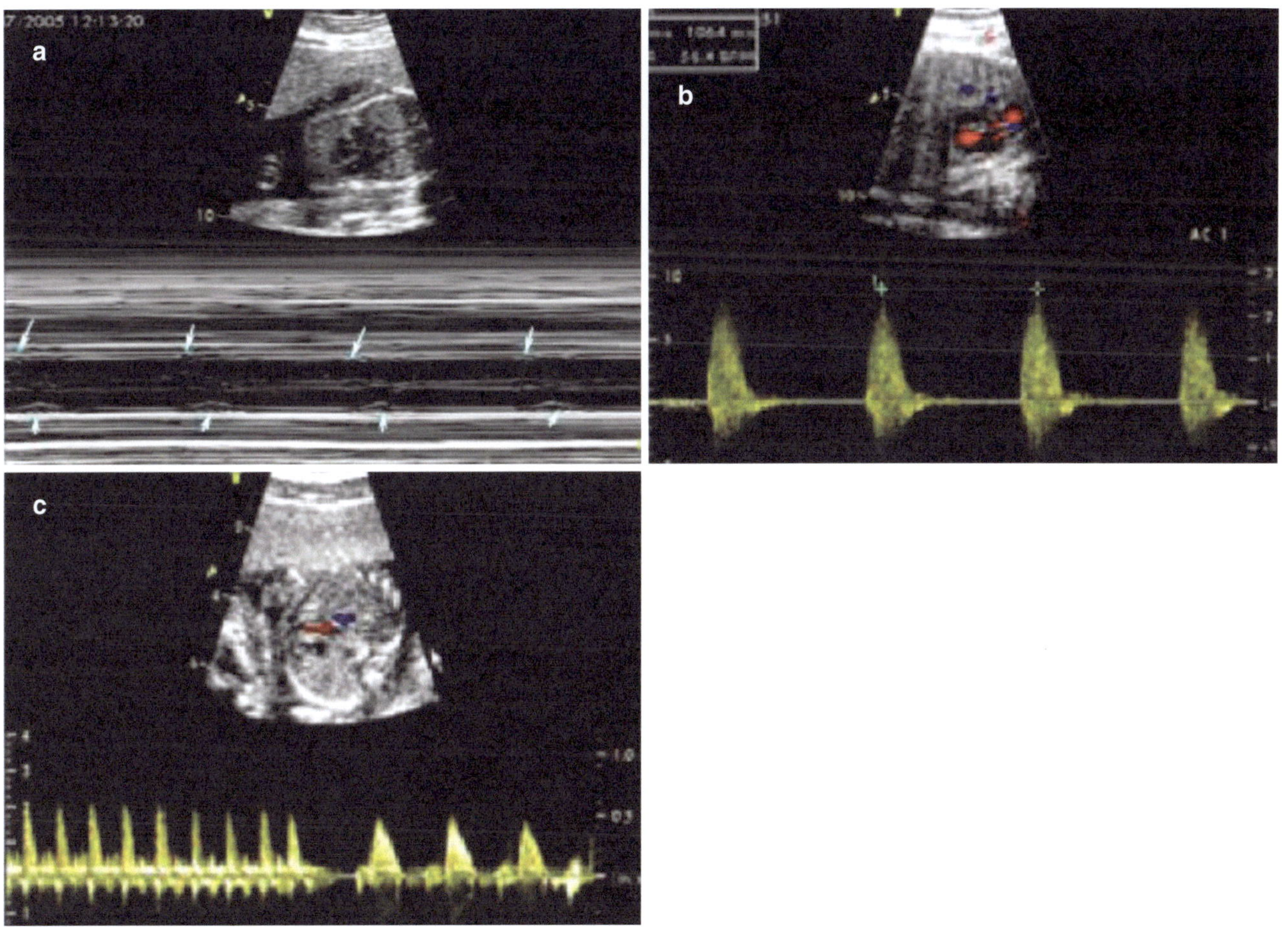

Fig. 4.41 Fetal sinus bradycardia. (**a**) M-mode ultrasound shows fetal bradycardia. (**b**) Spectrum Doppler ultrasound shows fetal bradycardia. (**c**) Spectrum Doppler ultrasound shows fetal tachycardia changing into bradycardia, with alternating fast and slow heart rate

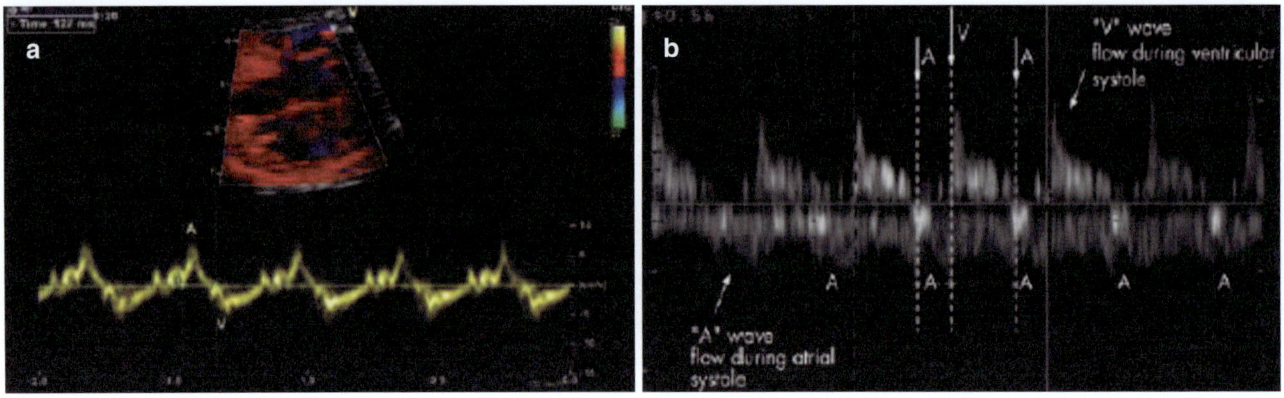

Fig. 4.42 Evaluation of the PR interval (A-V interval in the figure) by the method of simultaneous spectrum Doppler A-V interval (**a**) and recording the spectrum of pulmonary artery and vein (**b**). References: Carvalho JS, Prefumo F, Ciardelli V, et al. Evaluation of fetal arrhythmias from simultaneous pulsed wave Doppler in pulmonary artery and vein. Hear, 2007, 93:1448–1453

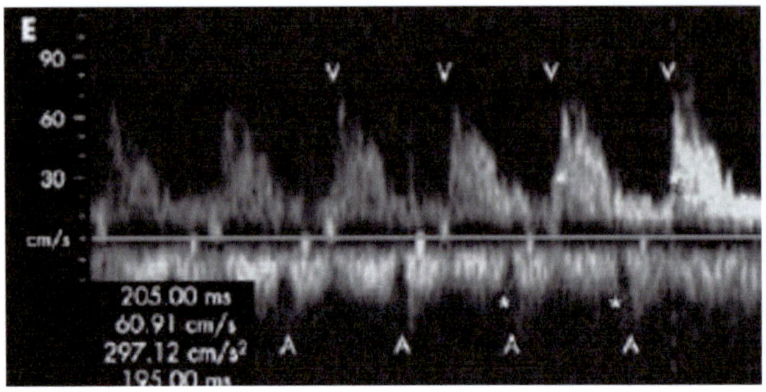

Fig. 4.43 Spectrum Doppler of first-degree heart block shows AV interval > 150 ms. References from: Carvalho JS, Prefumo F, Ciardelli V, et al. Evaluation of fetal arrhythmias from simultaneous pulsed wave Doppler in pulmonary artery and vein. Heart, 2007, 93:1448–1453

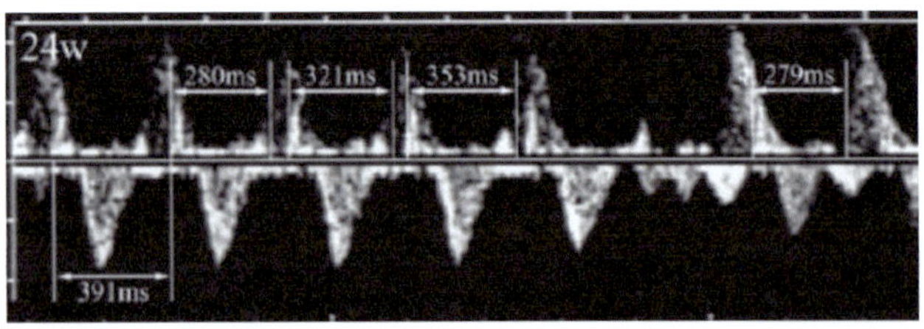

Fig. 4.44 Second-degree heart block, type I. This simultaneous SVC/AA Doppler recording shows the venous waves are below the zero-velocity line and the aortic waves above the line. A tall "A" wave is superimposed on the aortic wave. The progressive lengthening of the AV time intervals from 280 to 353 ms leads to a complete block, observed in a classical Luciani–Wenckebach phenomenon. It should be noted that the A-A interval remains constant at 391 ms. (References: Fouron JC. Fetal arrhythmias: the Saint-Justine hospital experience. Prenat Diagn, 2004, 24:1068–1080.)

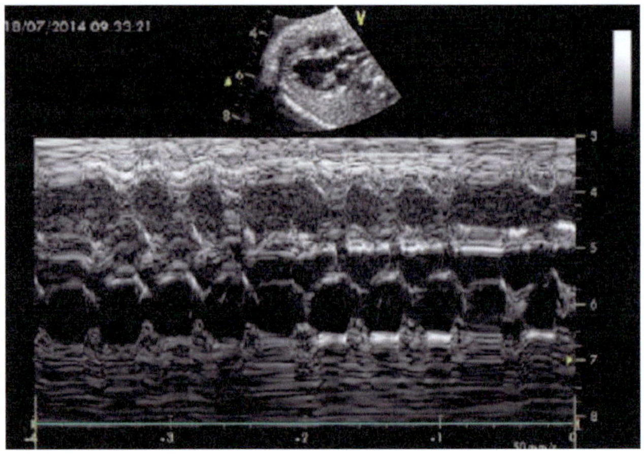

Fig. 4.45 The second-degree heart block, type II. In M-mode, the upper curve represents the ventricular wall, and the lower one represents the atrial wall. The line in the middle is the motion curve of the ventricular septum and the atrioventricular valve. The atrial wave beats regularly, and the ventricular wave stops once after three pulsations, indicating a cyclical atrioventricular block

ventricular block or dominant preexcitation syndrome.

– It is transient when the arrhythmia duration <10 min. Premature more than 10 bpm is defined as frequent premature. The transient bradycardia, tachycardia, and occasional premature are normal variations, which are kinds of immature functional changes. They may repeatedly occur in heart development and then disappear. No particular treatment is needed.

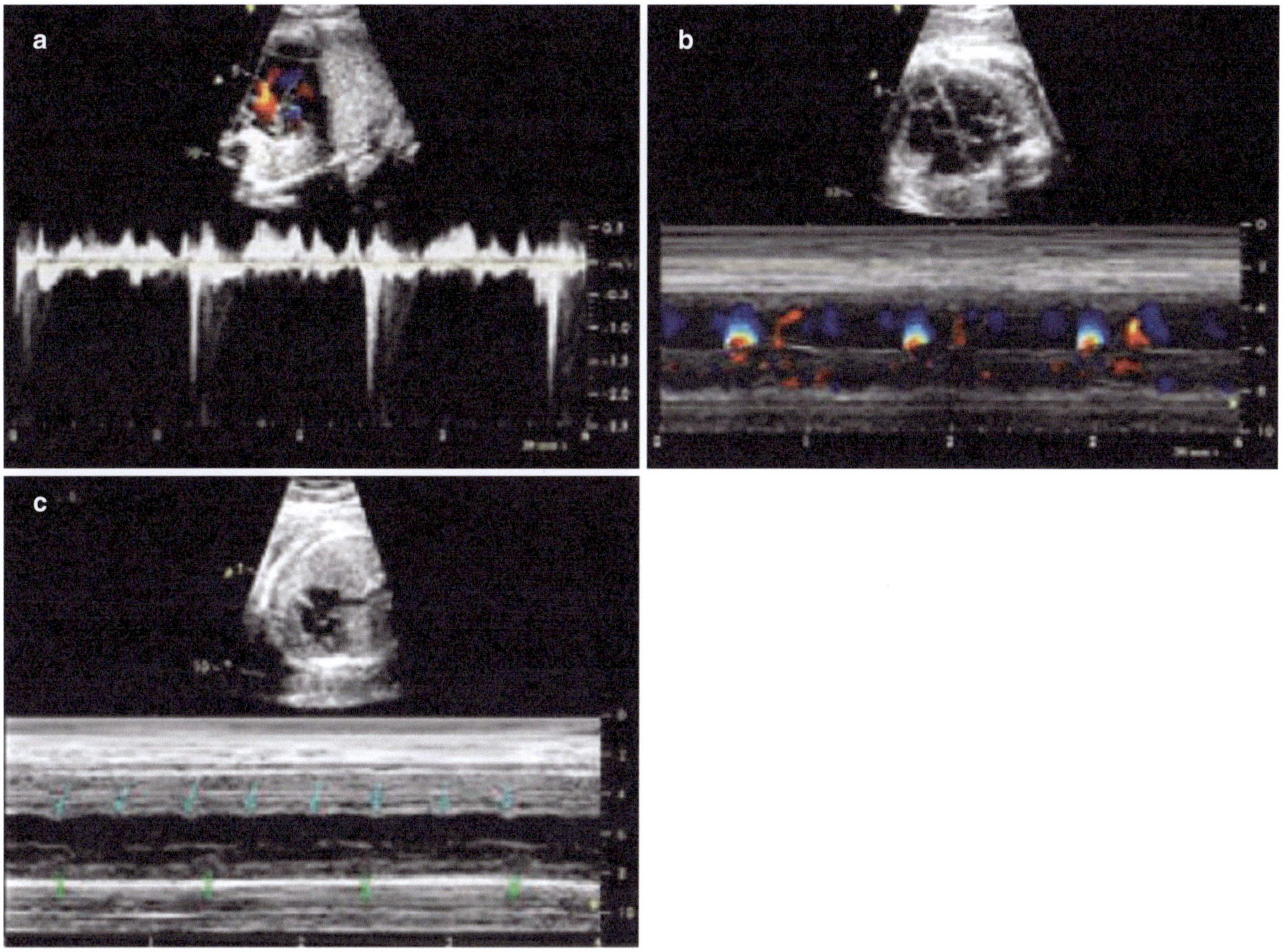

Fig. 4.46 Bradyarrhythmia. (**a**) Spectral Doppler ultrasound shows that the atrial and ventricular dissociation without dependence. (**b**) M-mode color ultrasound shows that the movement curves dissociation of the atrial and ventricular wall, without correlation. Picture a and picture b are from the same fetus, suggesting CAVB. (**c**) The separation of the atrial and ventricular motion curves, uncorrelated and independent

– The type of arrhythmia varies with pregnancy, so does the severity of arrhythmia. The earliest diagnosis time of fetal arrhythmia is about 16 weeks, while the best diagnosis time is 18–22 weeks. For the early detection of fetal pathological arrhythmia, fetal heart auscultation should be carried out carefully in the middle of pregnancy, especially in the 16–20 weeks. These actions contribute to further clinical diagnosis, avoiding the delay of optimal diagnosis and treatment.

Suggested Reading

1. Carvalho JS, Prefumo F, Ciardelli V, et al. Evaluation of fetal arrhythmias from simultaneous pulsed wave doppler in pulmonary artery and vein. Heart. 2007;93:1448–53.
2. Fouron JC. Fetal arrhythmias: the saint-Justine hospital experience. Prenat Diagn. 2004;24:1068–80.
3. Hofstaetter C, Hansmann M, Sturla H. Eik-nes, et al. A cardiovascular profile score in the surveillance of fetal hydrops. J Maternal-Fetal Neonatal Med. July 2006;19(7):407–13.

Application of Diagnostic Ultrasound in Gynecology

5

Taizhu Yang, Ying Tang, Min He, Hong Xu, and Yu Tian

5.1 Ultrasonic Diagnosis of Uterine Leiomyomas

(I) Basic Concepts

- Uterine leiomyomas, commonly referred to as fibroid or myoma, are composed of amounts of smooth muscle and fibrous tissue, and the etiology is due to uterine smooth muscle cell proliferation. It is the most common benign tumor in the female reproductive system, the incidence accounting for 4–11% and 70–80% occurrence in women between 30 and 50 years old.
- Almost 80% of the uterine leiomyomas are multiple according to the pathoanatomy, sometimes even more than one hundred. Fibroids are commonly classified into two subgroups by location: corpus and cervical, of which the former accounts for about 90%. The corpus leiomyomas are classified as intramural, subserosal, submucosal, and broad ligament leiomyomas. These tumors are usually multiple and various types of leiomyomas can coexist in one uterus.
- The appearance of leiomyomas may be various which may be according to the replacement of various degenerative tissues as abnormal blood supply. The degeneration is classified into hyaline, myxoid, cystic, calcific, red, necrosis, fatty, infection, and malignant degeneration. Special types, such as cellular leiomyoma, atypical leiomyoma, mitotically active leiomyoma, and intravenous leiomyoma, are also listed here.
- The clinical manifestations are mainly related to the location and size of uterine leiomyoma. The most common symptoms include menstrual cycle changing, abdominal mass, and compression symptoms. The majority of patients complain of abnormal uterine bleeding, heavy menstrual bleeding and shortened menstrual cycle. Bowel dysfunction and bladder symptoms such as urinary frequency and urgency may be present by large fibroids.
- During physical examination, we can find an enlarged, solid uterus with an irregular contour which is consistent with fibroids. In addition, submucosal fibroids may prolapse to the endometrial cavity, cervix, or vagina.
- Ultrasonography is particularly helpful to assess the location, size, and number of myomas. Transvaginal ultrasonography provides superior resolution for fibroids smaller than 2 cm in diameter. However, ultrasonic attenuation is usually accompanied by large fibroids, and it is recommended to choose low-frequency probe and increase the gain.

(II) Ultrasonic diagnosis

- Enlarged or irregular-shaped uterine can be caused by multiple leiomyomas. The size and shape of the uterine are normal when accompanied by a single small intramural leiomyoma. In cases of submucosal leiomyoma or multiple leiomyomas, the uterine shape is abnormal with distorted endometrium (Figs. 5.1, 5.2, and 5.3).
- Leiomyomas may have variable appearances because of the different portions of smooth muscle and fibrous tissue. The leiomyomas can represent hypoechoic, hyperechoic, isoechoic, or punctate echo, with a typical linear shadowing effect (also known as swirling echo, Figs. 5.4, 5.5, and 5.6).
- Leiomyomas are easy to be diagnosed and measured by ultrasonography. Most represent a spherical mass, with hypoechoic or lightly hyperechoic pseudocapsule (Fig. 5.7).

This chapter was translated by **Linlin Ma**, Department of Obstetrics and Gynecology, Beijing Hospital, National Center of Gerontology, Beijing, China

T. Yang (✉) · Y. Tang · M. He · H. Xu · Y. Tian
Department of Ultrasonography, West China Second University Hospital, Sichuan University, Chengdu, China

T. Yang, H. Luo (eds.), *Practical Ultrasonography in Obstetrics and Gynecology*,
https://doi.org/10.1007/978-981-16-4477-1_5

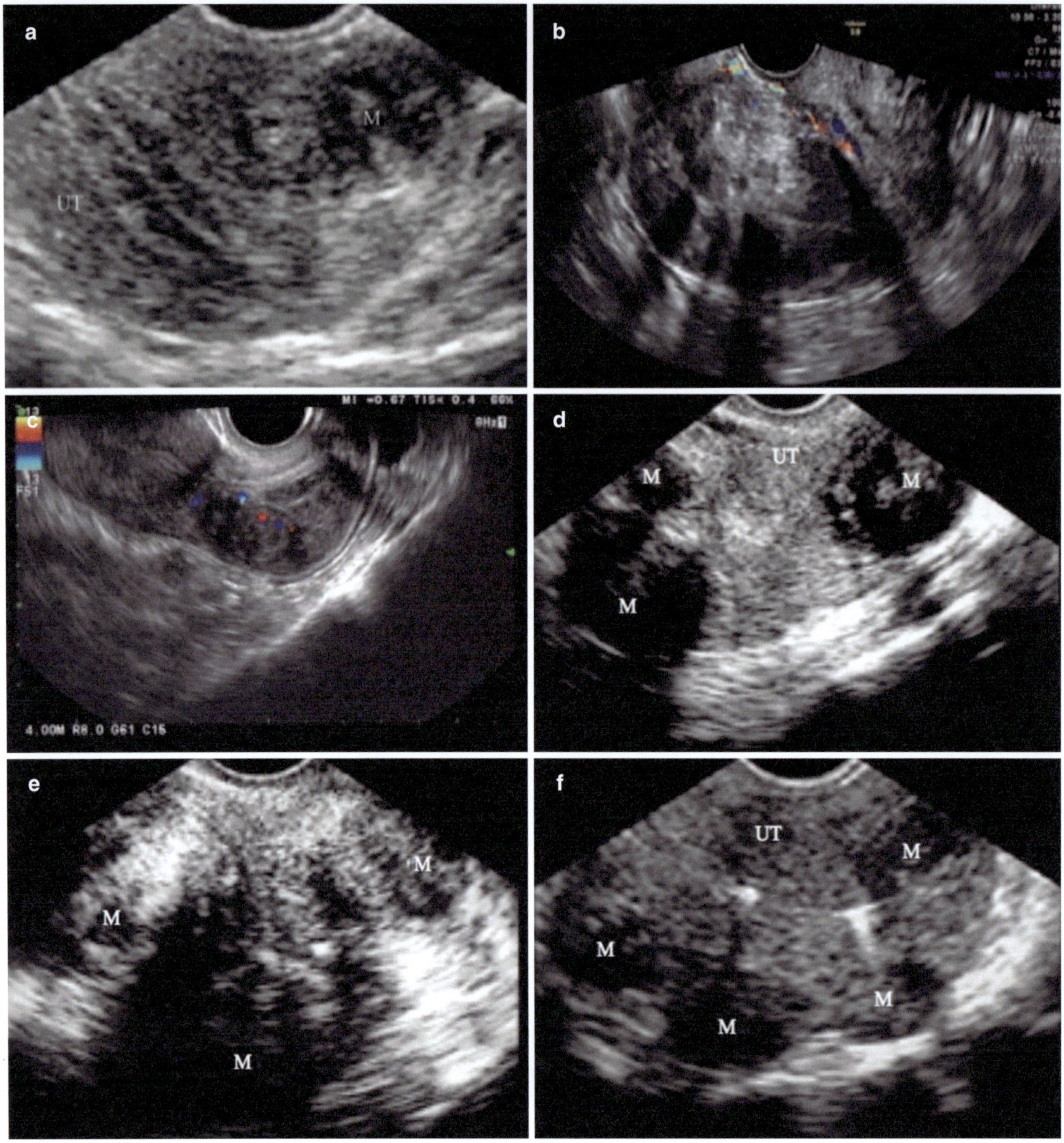

Fig. 5.1 Leiomyoma (I). (**a**) A well-defined uterus with an intramural leiomyoma. (**b**) Subserosal leiomyoma. (**c**) Cervical leiomyoma. (**d-f**) Abnormal-shaped uterus with multiple subserosal and intramural leiomyomas

- Color Doppler flow imaging shows a circular or semicircular blood flow around the leiomyomas (Fig. 5.8).
- Uterine leiomyomas occasionally undergo various forms of degeneration. The ultrasonic changes include the disappearance of normal swirling structure, hypoechoic mass, irregular cystic area in the mass, and hyperechoic area accompanied by attenuated acoustic shadowing within or around the mass. Degenerated leiomyoma is more common in pregnancy and postpartum, and often manifests as hypoechoic mass. In addition, calcification of leiomyoma usually occurs in postmenopausal women (Figs. 5.9 and 5.10).

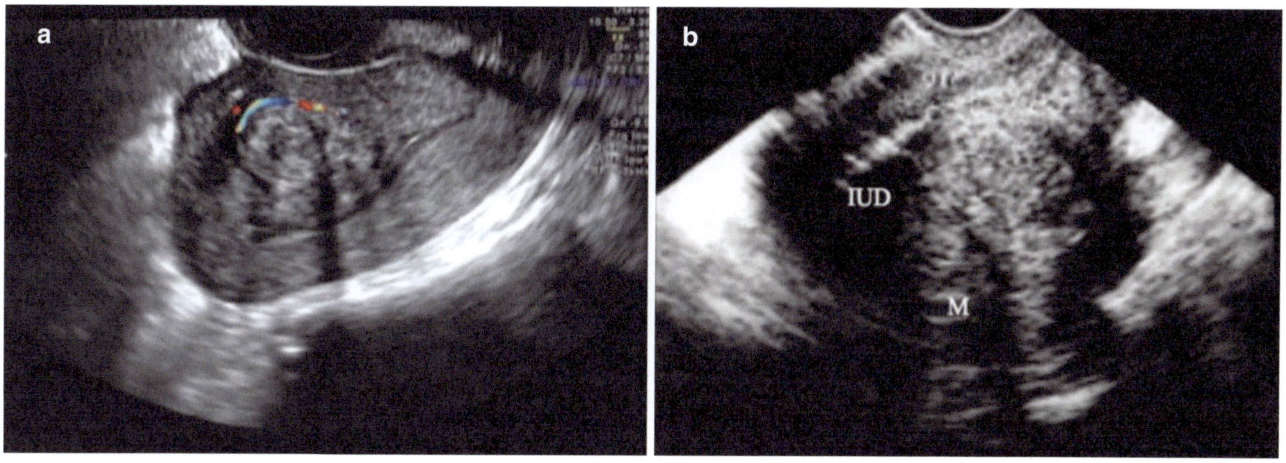

Fig. 5.2 Leiomyoma (II). (**a**) Backward and distorted endometrium caused by a fibroid in the anterior wall of the uterus. (**b**) Forward and distorted endometrium caused by a fibroid in the posterior wall of the uterus

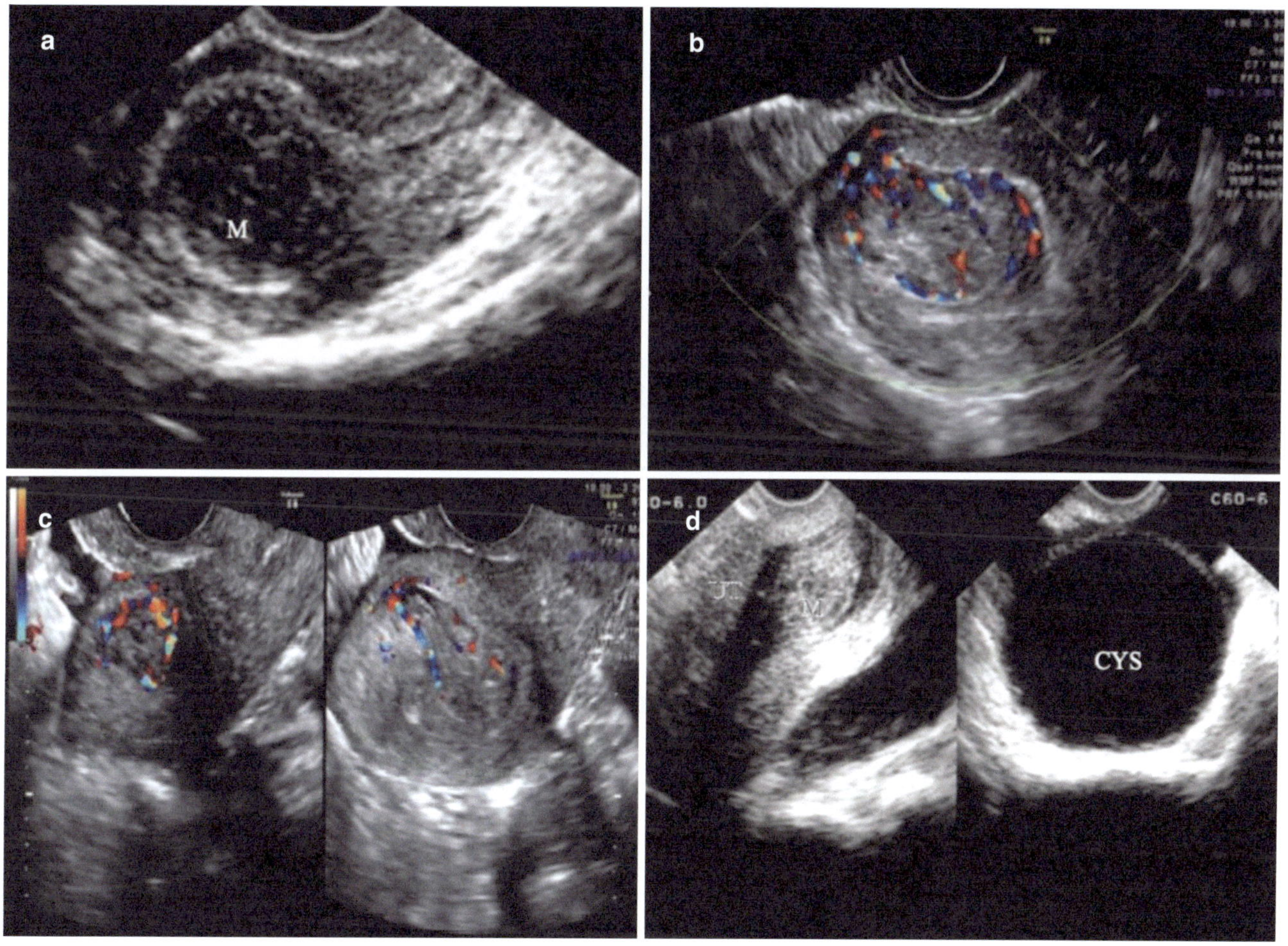

Fig. 5.3 Leiomyoma (III). (**a**) A submucosal leiomyoma, surrounded by the endometrium. (**b**) An intramural leiomyoma in the anterior wall, partially protruding into the uterine cavity. (**c**) A submucosal leiomyoma. (**d**) A submucosal leiomyoma that prolapsed into the cervical canal, with an adnexa cyst

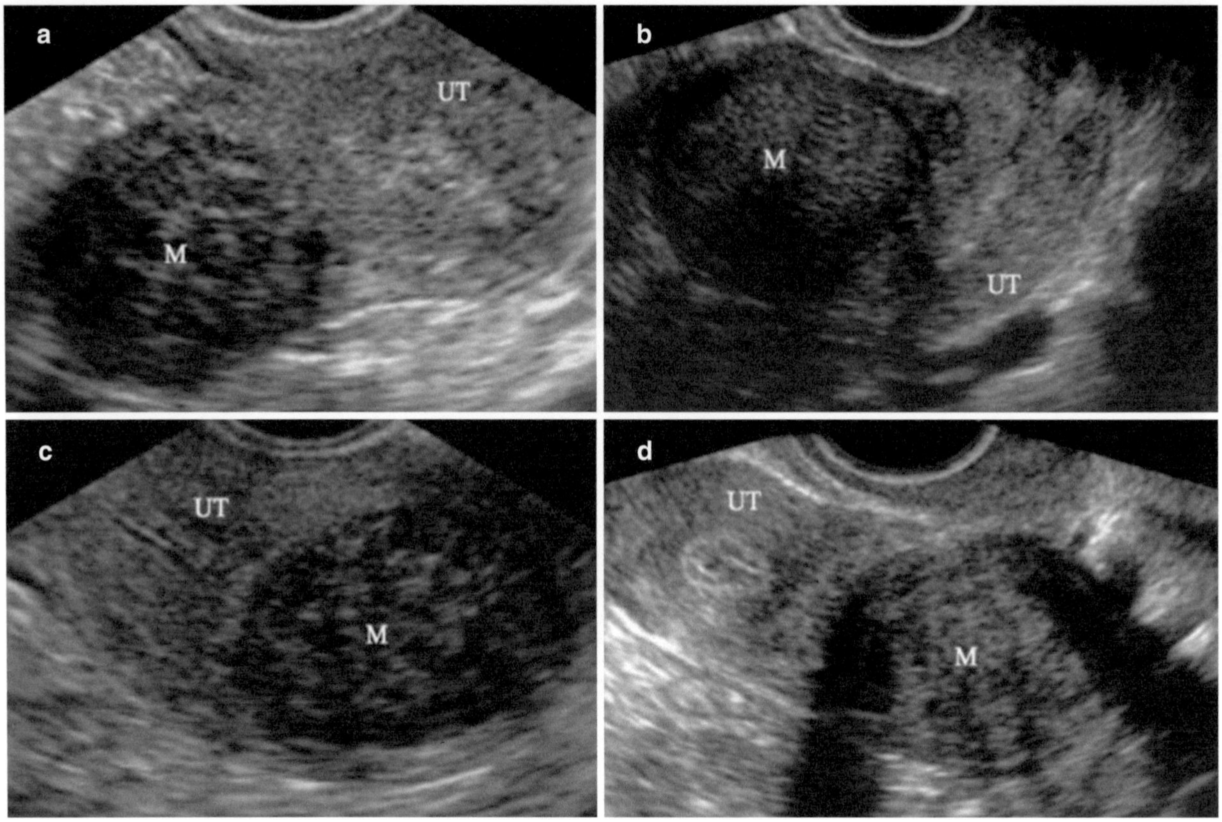

Fig. 5.4 Leiomyoma (IV). (**a**-**c**) Hypoechoic leiomyomas shown by sonogram. (**d**) Leiomyoma with bilateral attenuation

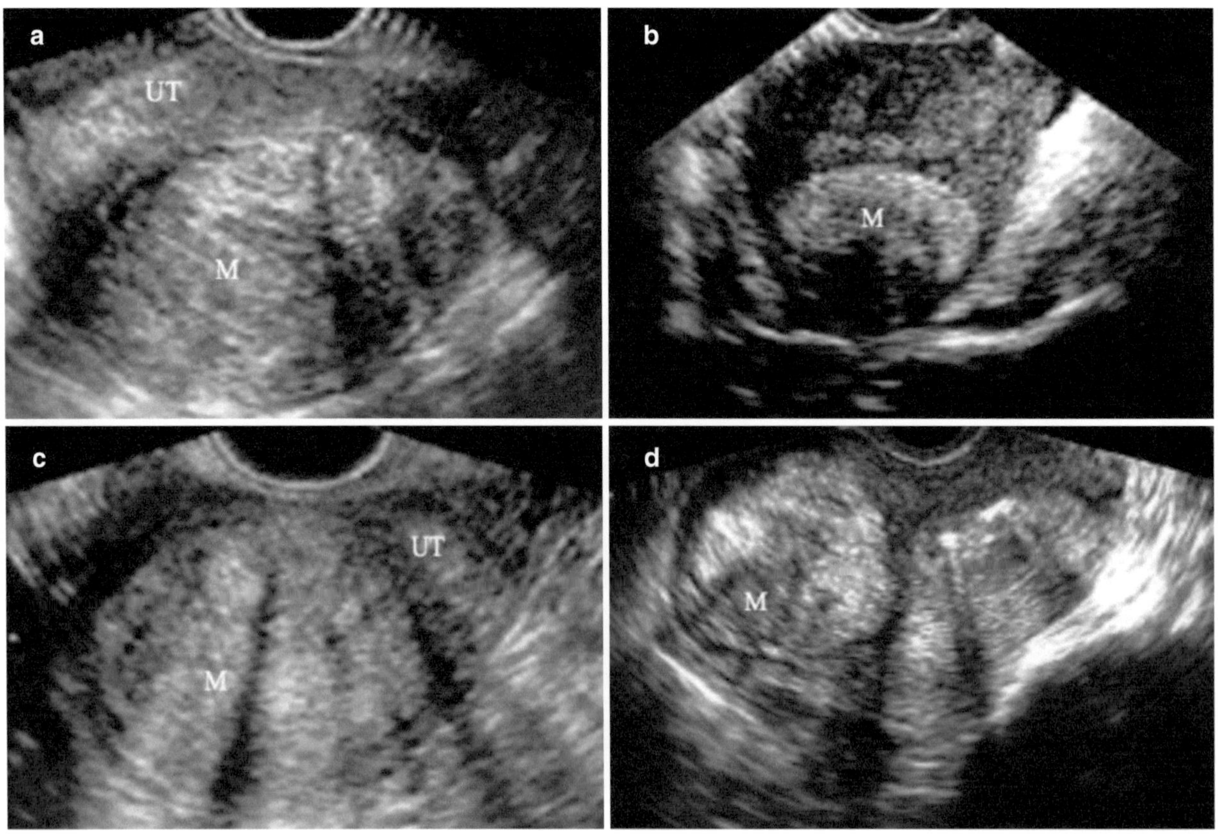

Fig. 5.5 Leiomyoma (V). (**a**-**d**) Hyperechoic leiomyomas

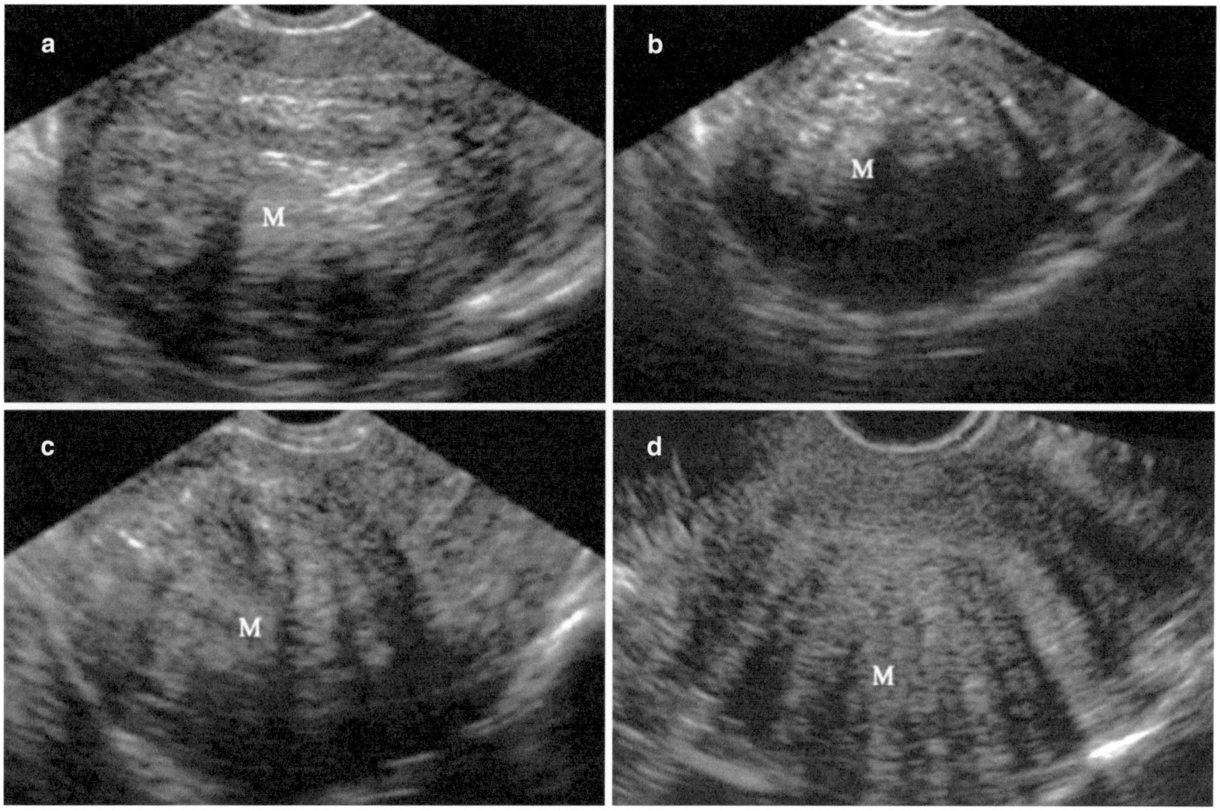

Fig. 5.6 Leiomyoma (VI). (**a**, **b**) Fibroids shown as granophyric hyperechoic. (**c**, **d**) Fibroids with typical linear shadowing effect

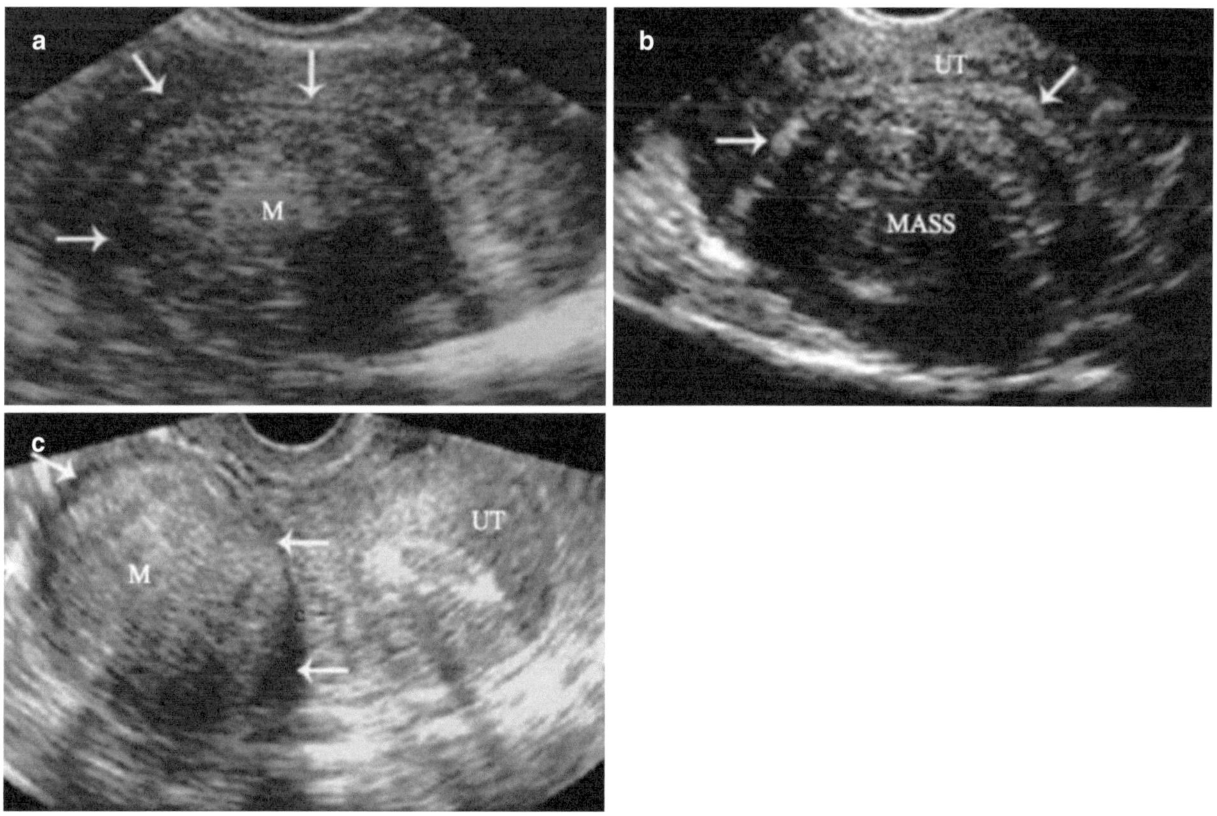

Fig. 5.7 Leiomyoma (VII). (**a-c**) Leiomyomas with hyperechoic or hypoechoic pseudocapsule (arrow)

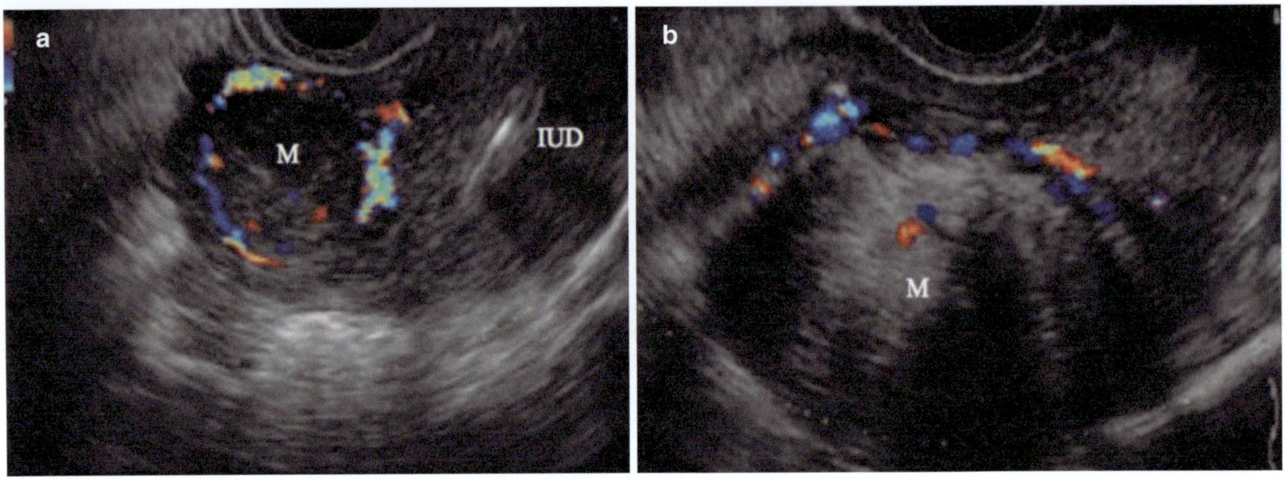

Fig. 5.8 Leiomyoma (VIII). (**a**, **b**) The image of circular or semicircular flow around the fibroid shown by color Doppler

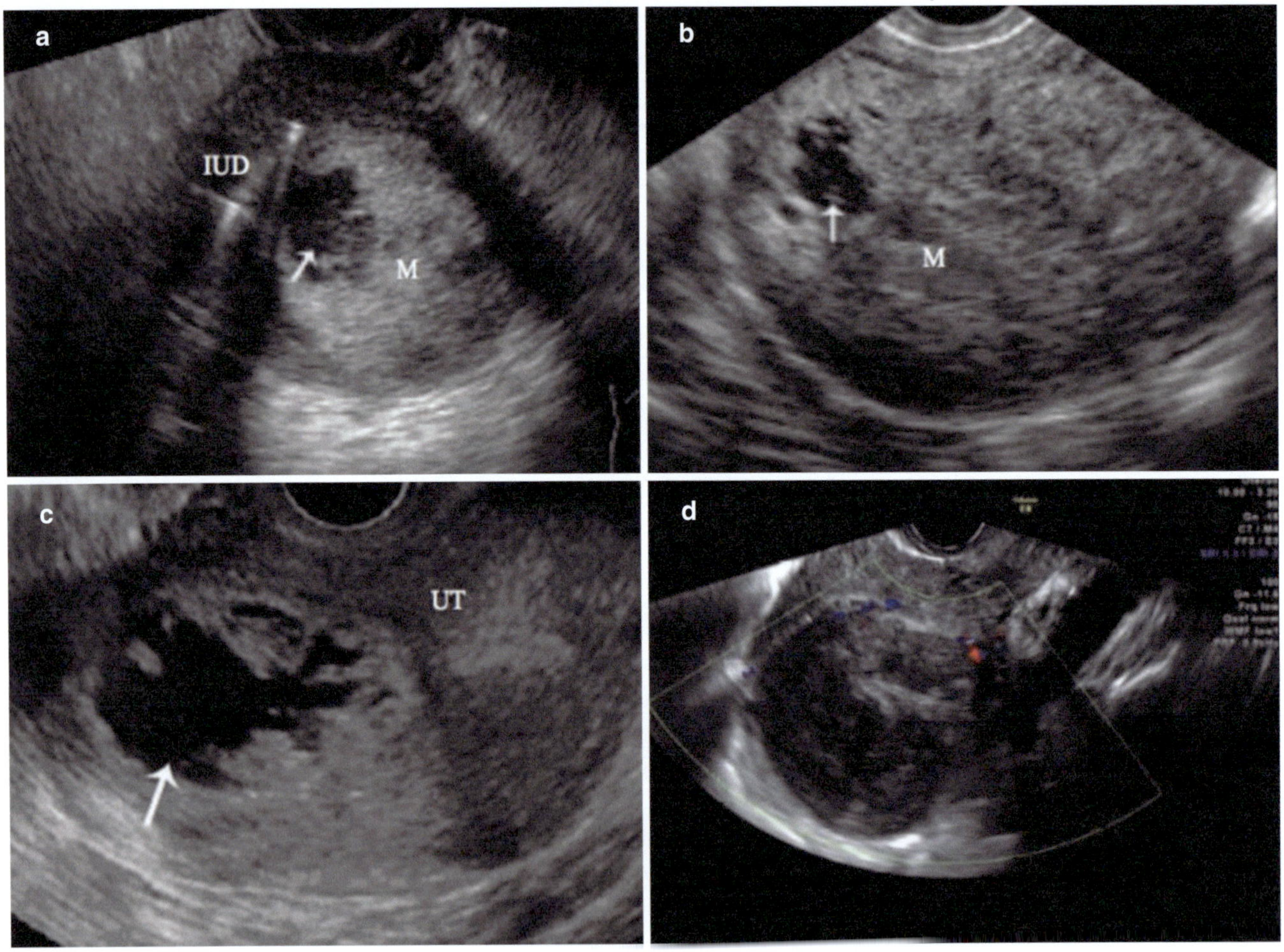

Fig. 5.9 Degenerated leiomyoma. (**a-d**) Different degrees of hydropic degeneration of the fibroids. Sonogram shows the heterogeneous leiomyoma with irregular fluid areas (arrow)

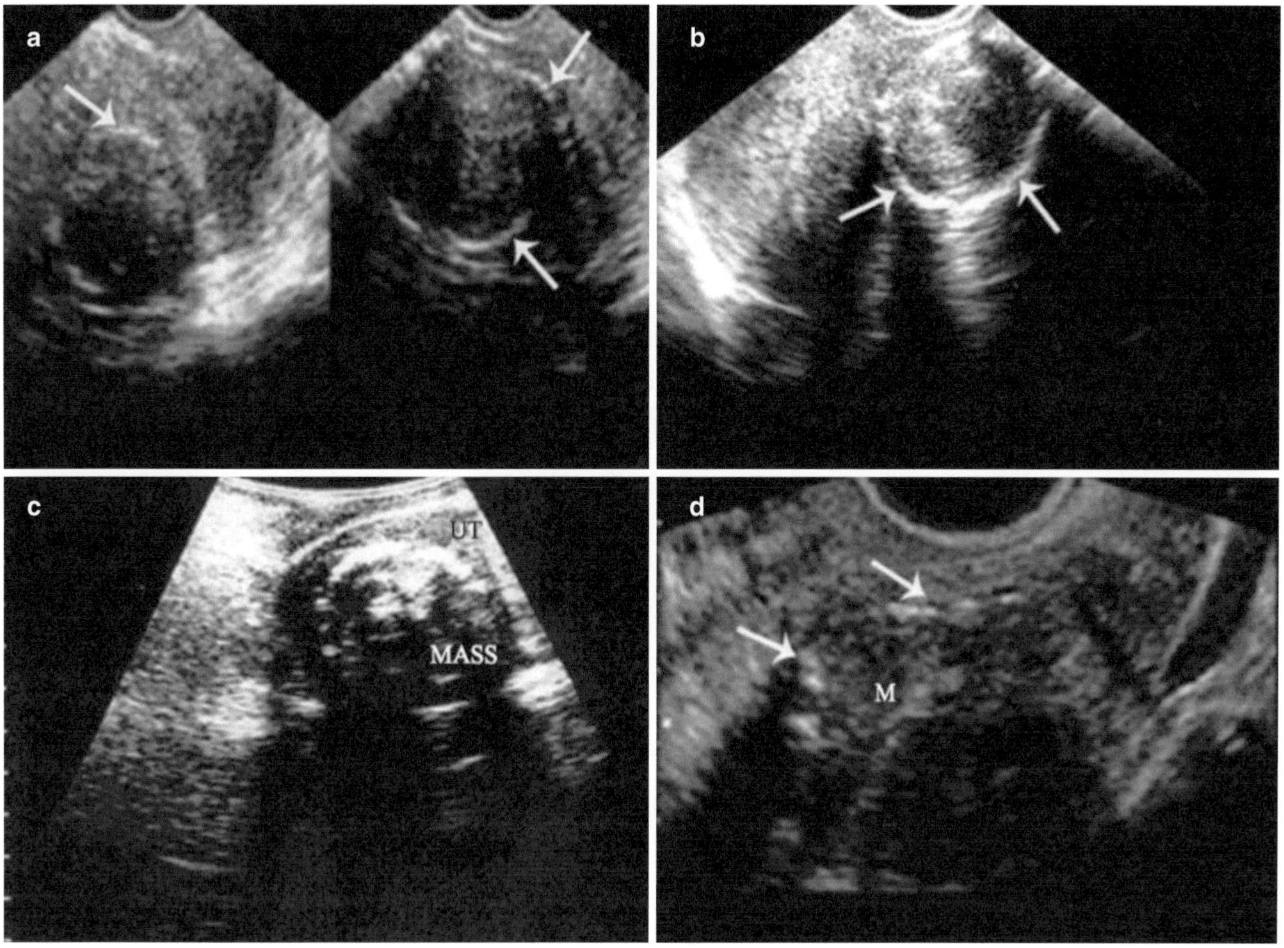

Fig. 5.10 Calcified leiomyoma. (**a**, **b**) Leiomyoma with peripheral calcification. (**c**, **d**) Hyperechoic plaque accompanied by attenuated shadowing within the mass shown by sonogram. Arrow shows the calcification

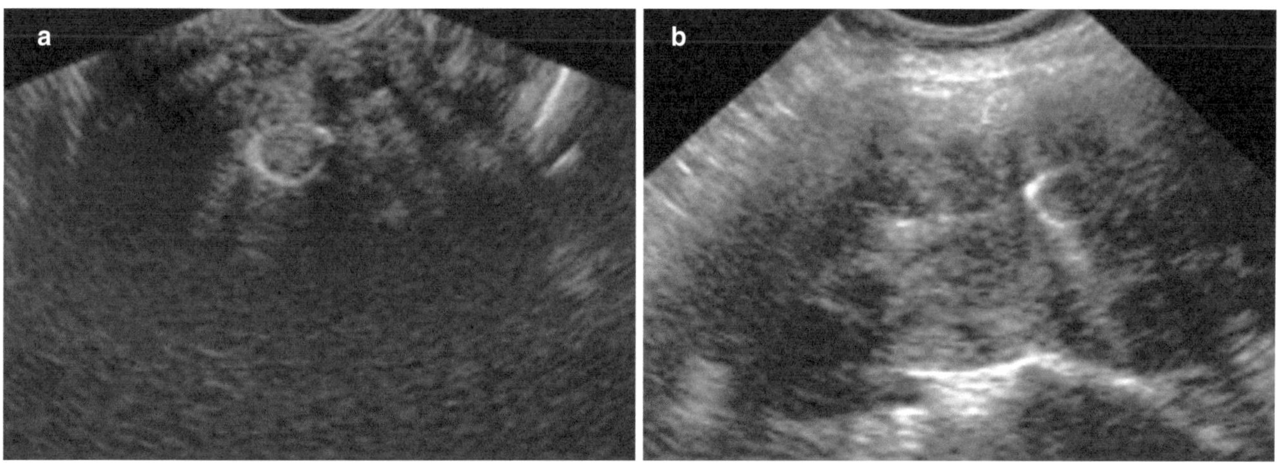

Fig. 5.11 Leiomyoma (IX). (**a**) Only use the TVS fails to show the whole fibroid. (**b**) TAS shows the outline of the fibroid

(III) Special tips

- A relatively full bladder is important for transabdominal ultrasonography. Transvaginal sonography alone may fail to show the entire fibroids larger than 8 ~ 10 cm in diameter, and the combination scanning of TAS with TVS is recommended (Fig. 5.11).
- Subserosal leiomyoma with long peduncle or broad ligament leiomyoma may be misdiagnosed as ovar-

ian mass. Pay attention to the relationship between the leiomyoma and the ovary (Fig. 5.12).
- Cystic degenerated leiomyoma should be distinguished from adnexa cyst and pregnant sac (Fig. 5.13).
- The leiomyoma should be distinguished from adenomyosis, uterine hypertrophy, endometrial polyp, adnexa mass, and uterine malformation, etc. (Fig. 5.14, 5.15, 5.16, 5.17, and 5.18).

(IV) Typical cases
See Figs. 5.19 and 5.20.

5.2 Sonographic Features of Adenomyosis

(I) Basic concepts
Adenomyosis is characterized by the endometrial glands and stroma are present in the myometrium, which is combined with a proliferation of smooth muscles and fibrous tissues. The etiologies are commonly reported as chronic endometritis and trauma in the myometrium which is secondary to multiple gravidity and deliveries. Adenomyosis was called internal endometriosis previously.

Adenomyosis commonly occurs in 30–50 years old multipara and 50% of the patients coexists with leiomyoma. Adenomyosis may coexist with pelvic and other organic endometriosis, also known as external endometriosis.

Adenomyosis affects the myometrium diffusely and shows as an enlarged global uterus. The diffuse or focal lesions in the myometrium are clarified and the lesions often locate in the posterior myometrium. It leads to more thickened posterior myometrium than the anterior. The ultrasonic display of focal adenomyosis, sometimes called adenomyoma, is similar to leiomyoma. While the former shows indistinct demarcate, island glands and stroma are visible in the myometrium under a microscope.

The symptoms of adenomyosis are characterized by progressive dysmenorrhea, menometrorrhagia, meno-

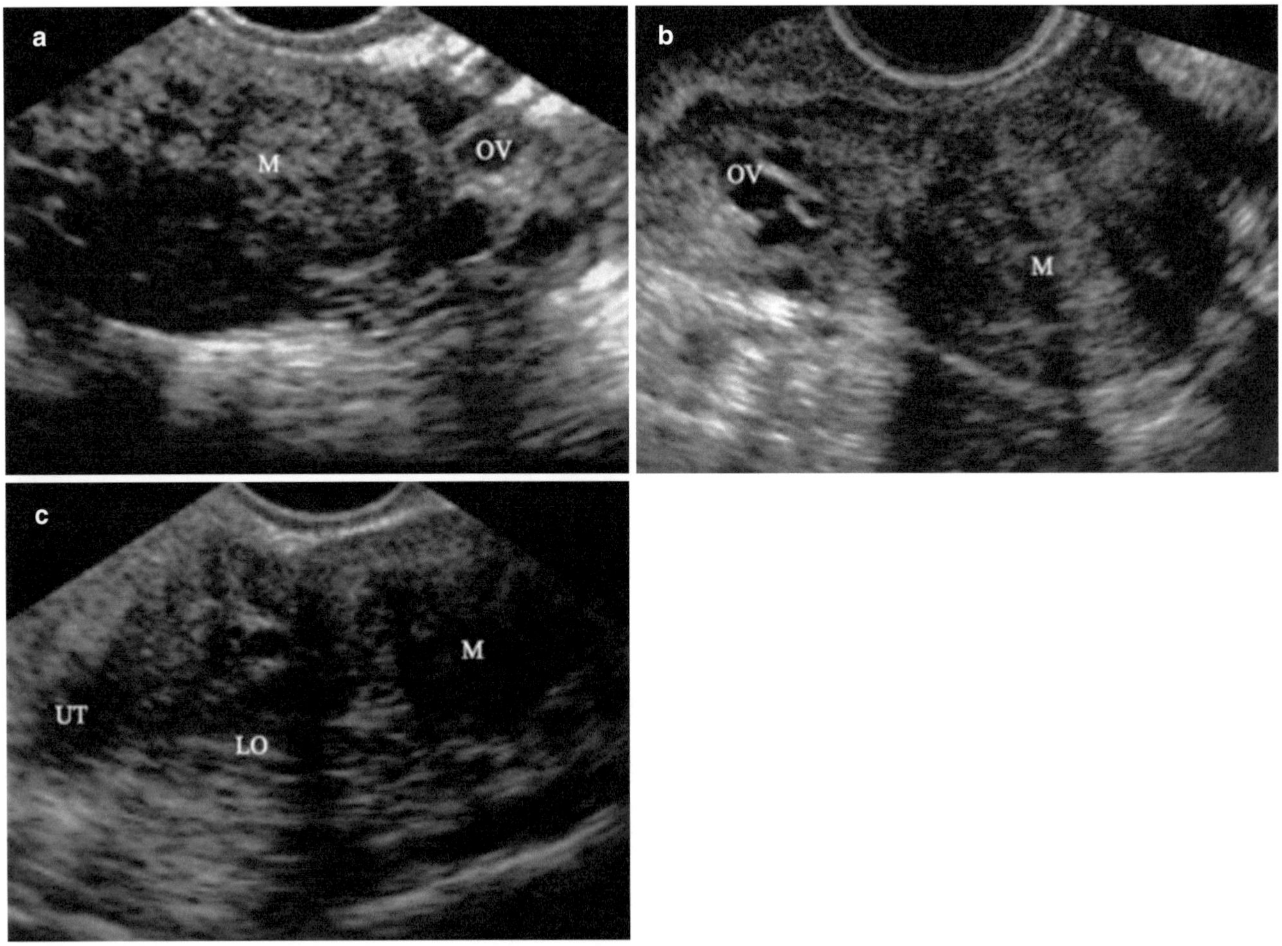

Fig. 5.12 Leiomyoma (X). (**a**, **b**) Sonogram shows the subserosal fibroid in the annex area and ipsilateral ovary. (**c**) Sonogram shows the fibroid within the broad ligament, with a certain distance from the uterus. The ipsilateral ovary is visible

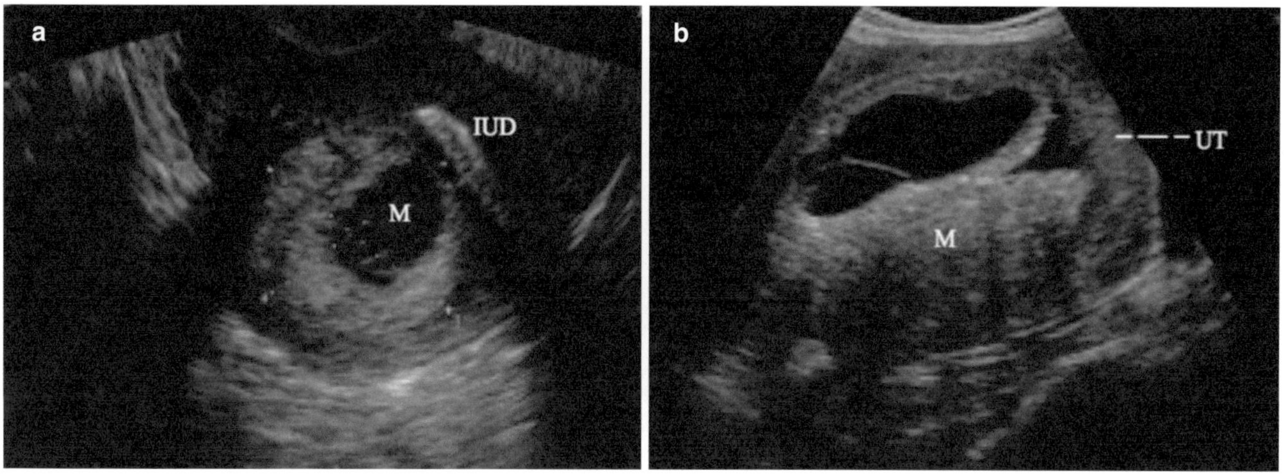

Fig. 5.13 Differential diagnosis of cystic leiomyoma and cyst. (**a**) Cystic spaces locate in the myometrium. (**b**) Cystic spaces locate outside the uterus

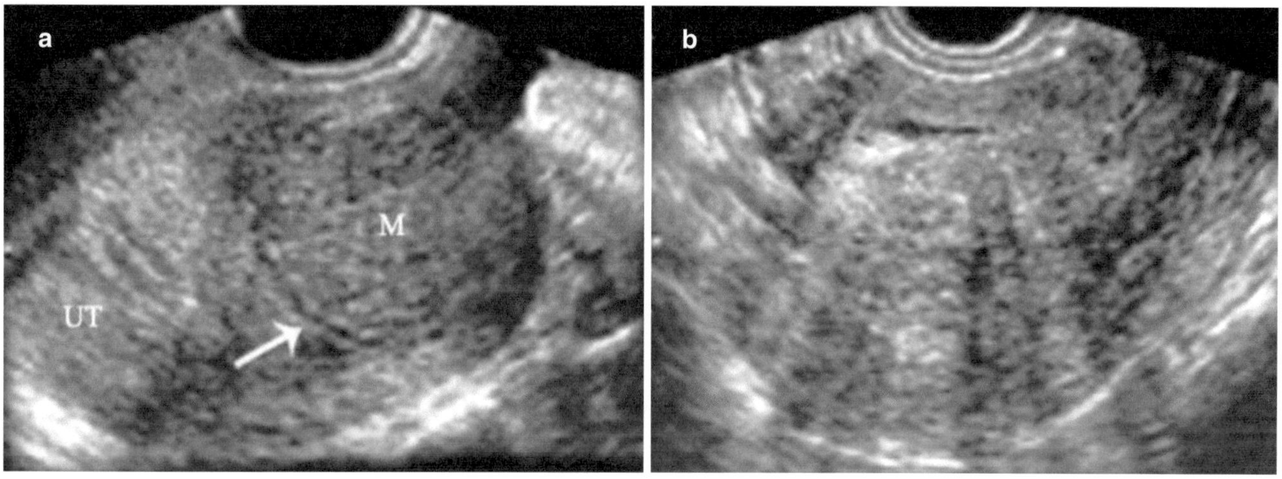

Fig. 5.14 Differential diagnosis of leiomyoma and adenomyosis. (**a**) Sonogram shows the leiomyoma with surrounding pseudocapsule. (**b**) Sonogram shows the adenomyosis lesion with an indistinct boundary in the posterior wall of the uterus

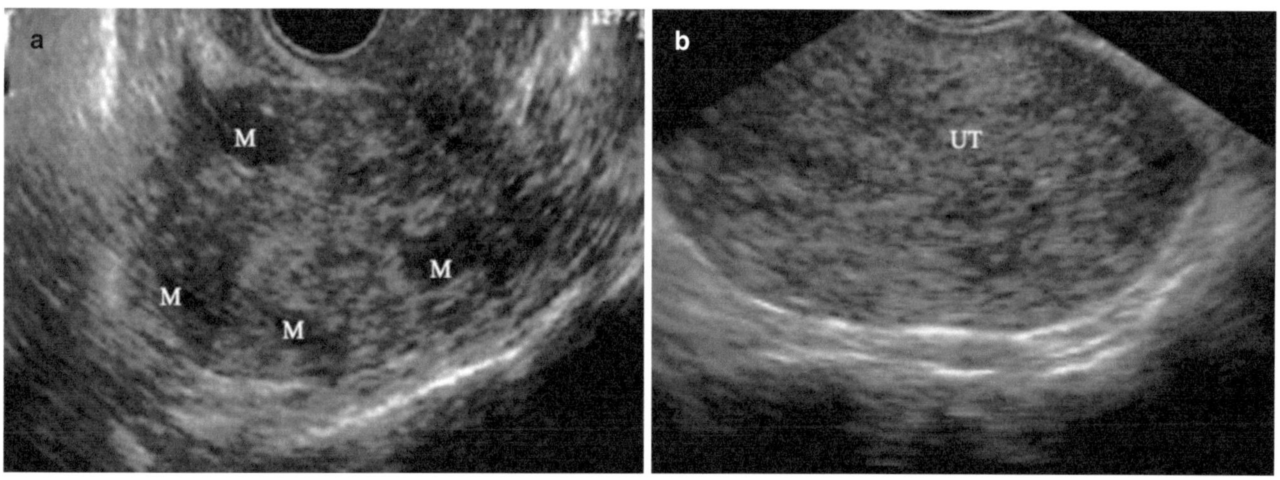

Fig. 5.15 Differential diagnosis of leiomyoma and uterine hypertrophy. (**a**) Small fibroids with boundary in a normal-shaped uterus. (**b**) Sonogram shows the enlarged uterus in a normal shape, without intramural lesion

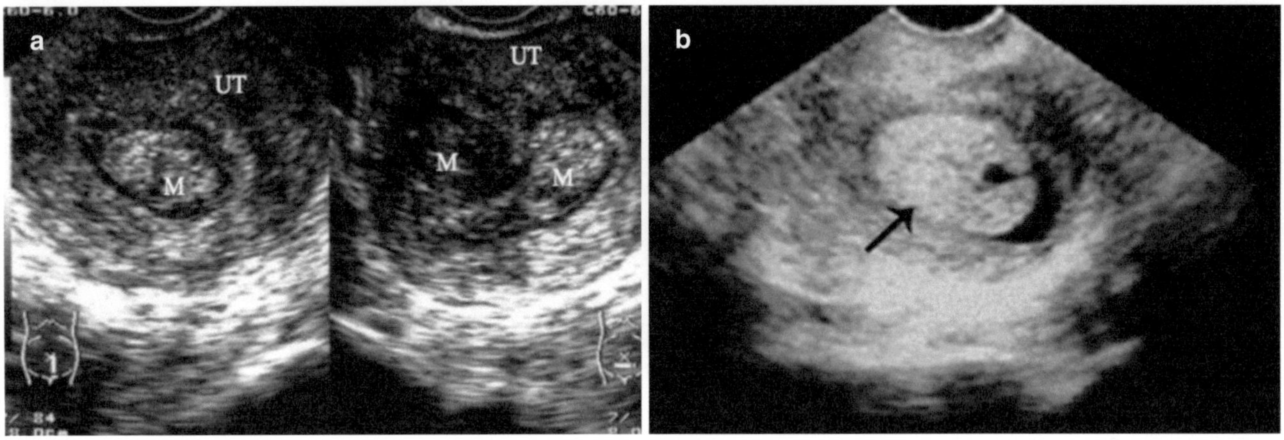

Fig. 5.16 Differential diagnosis of leiomyoma and endometrial polyp. (**a**) Hypoechoic submucosal fibroid. (**b**) A well-defined hyperechoic polyp (arrow) with the fluid area

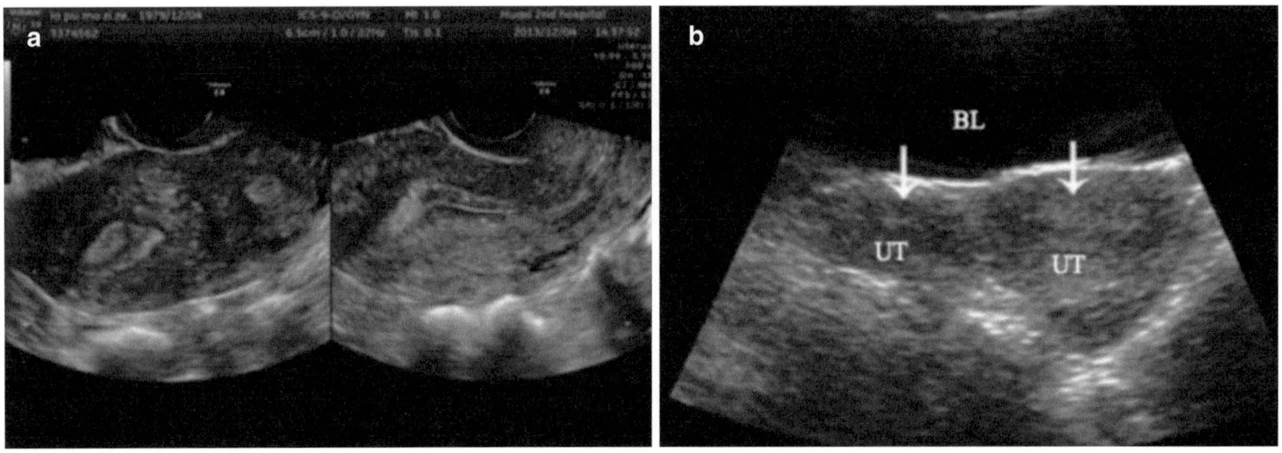

Fig. 5.17 Differential diagnosis of leiomyoma and the rudimentary horn of uterus. (**a**) TAS shows a round fibroid close to the uterus. (**b**) TAS demonstrates a rudimentary uterus with endometrium (arrow)

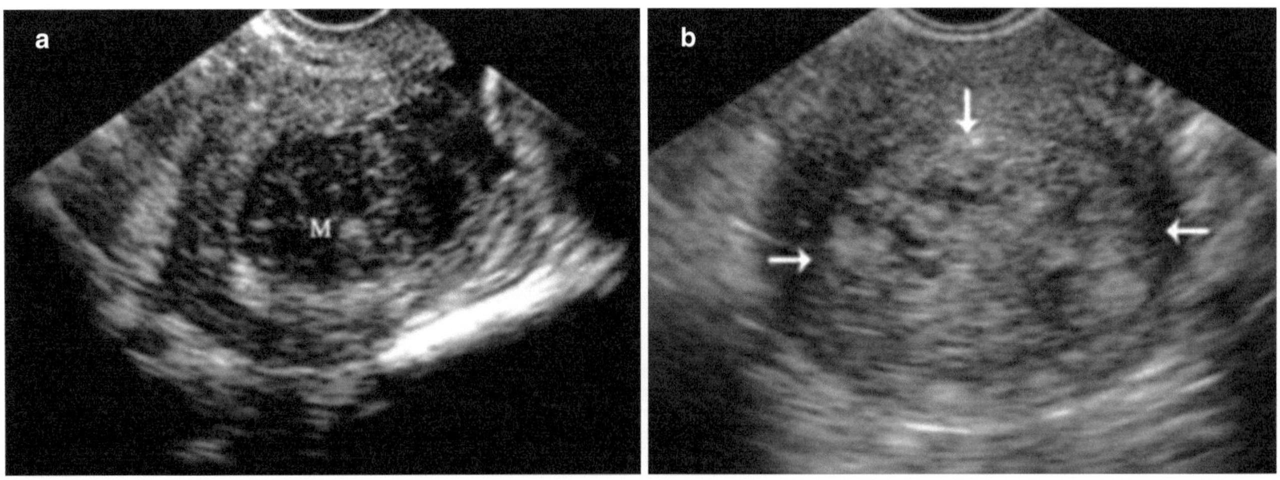

Fig. 5.18 Differential diagnosis of leiomyoma and intrauterine remainder. (**a**) A hypoechoic subserosal fibroid with a distinct boundary. (**b**) Seven days after a drug-induced abortion. Sonogram shows a heterogeneous hyperechoic mass in the uterus of a patient with vaginal bleeding. The arrow indicates the intrauterine residual

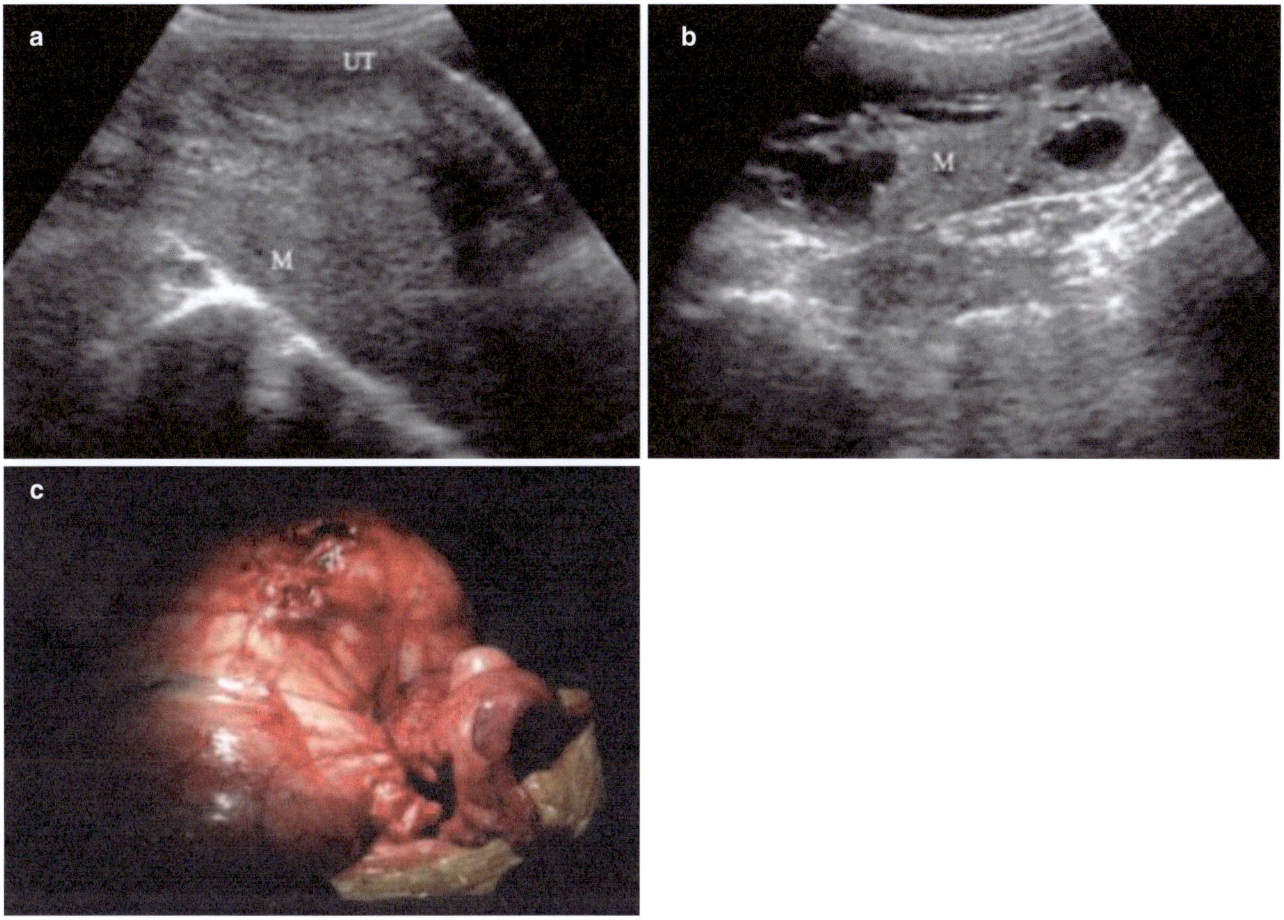

Fig. 5.19 A 41-year-old patient presents with a palpable mass in the abdomen, with normal menstruation. (**a**, **b**) The ultrasonography shows a normal-appearing uterus and a mixed mass at the right posterior to the uterus with solid and cystic heterogeneous. As there are irregular fluid areas in the mass, it is suspected as an ovarian tumor. (**c**) Gross specimen from operation shows a fibroid located in the posterior of the uterine isthmus. The pathological diagnosis is leiomyoma with extensive degeneration

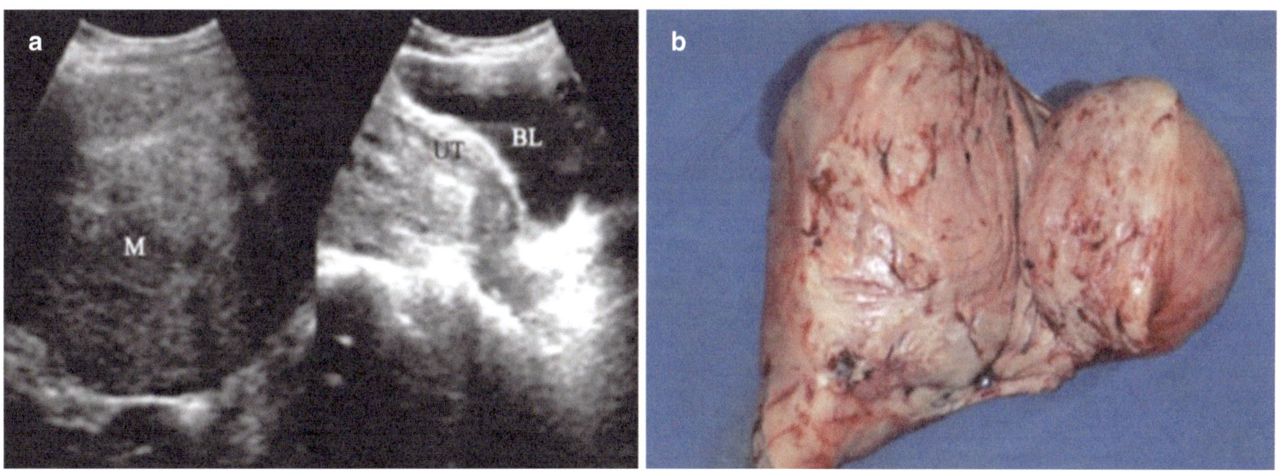

Fig. 5.20 A 30-year-old patient complains of pain for 1 month. (**a**) Ultrasonography shows a normal uterus with an intrauterine device. A huge solid mass is shown in the pelvic and is suspected as a solid ovarian tumor. The operation confirms that it is a leiomyoma in the left broad ligament. (**b**) Gross specimen. The pathological diagnosis is leiomyoma with myxoid degeneration

staxis, and even infertility. Some patients are asymptomatic. A diffusely enlarged and solid uterus can be palpable, accompanied with tenderness sometimes.

(II) Sonographic features

- Sonogram shows a diffused enlarged uterus in a normal shape or globular shape. In general, the uterus shows a longer length, width, and anteroposterior diameter (Fig. 5.21).
- Most patients with adenomyosis represent a thickened posterior myometrium and the endometrium is distorted forward or backward (Fig. 5.22).
- Thickened myometrium usually represents hyperechoic. The ultrasonic display of focal adenomyosis is similar to leiomyoma but shows an indistinct border with peripheral myometrium (Fig. 5.23).
- Sporadic and irregular tiny fluid areas are visible in the lesion during the menstrual period, which disappears after menstruation (Fig. 5.24).
- The image of diffuse adenomyosis shows that the whole myometrium is thickened, and diffusely enhanced echo. The location of the endometrium is normal (Fig. 5.25).
- Color Doppler shows that the blood flow is sporadic and stellate distributed in the focus of adenomyosis (Fig. 5.26).

(III) Special tips

- The ultrasound images of adenomyosis and hysteromyoma are extremely similar. Except to consider the clinical manifestations, we should pay more attention to the boundary of the lesion and surrounding muscle.
- Transvaginal ultrasonic scanning is recommended to identify the lesion boundary and endometrium in multipara patients (Fig. 5.27).

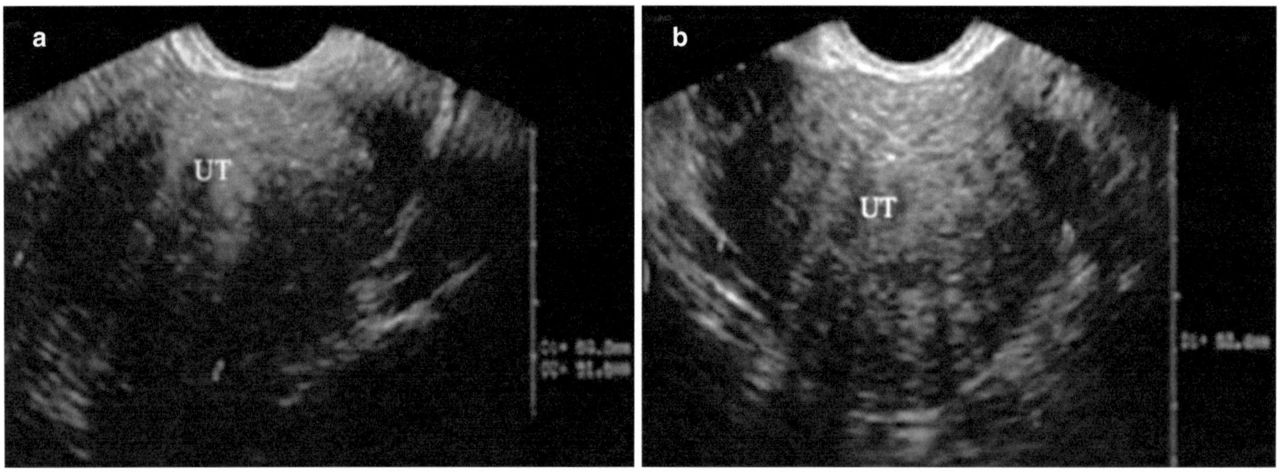

Fig. 5.21 Adenomyosis (I). (**a**) Sagittal TVS shows the enlarged uterine with elongated length and anteroposterior diameter. (**b**) Transverse TVS shows the increased width

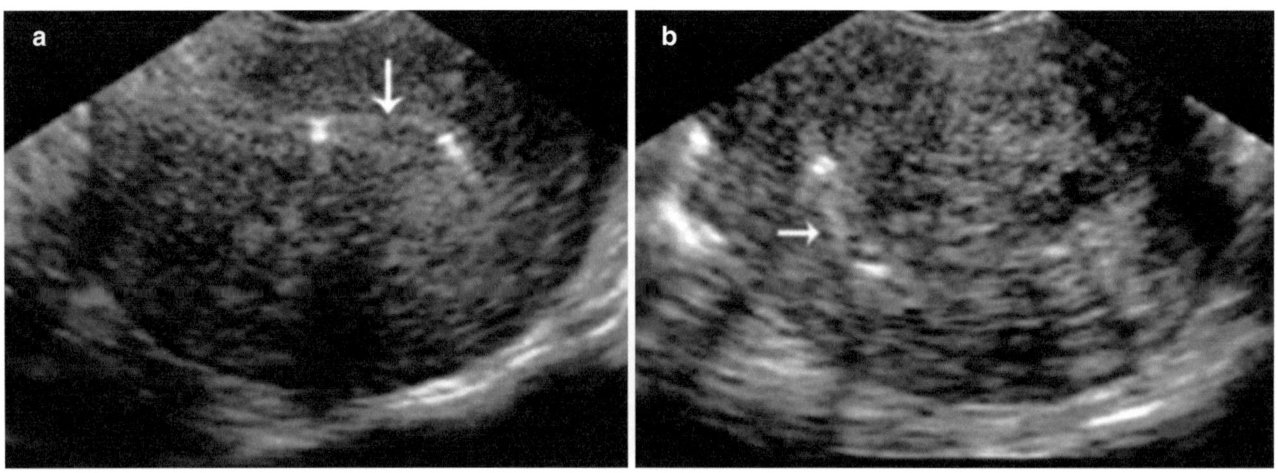

Fig. 5.22 Adenomyosis (II). (**a**) Sonogram shows the thickened anterior myometrium and backward distorted endometrium (arrow). (**b**) Sonogram shows the thickened posterior myometrium and distorted endometrium (arrow)

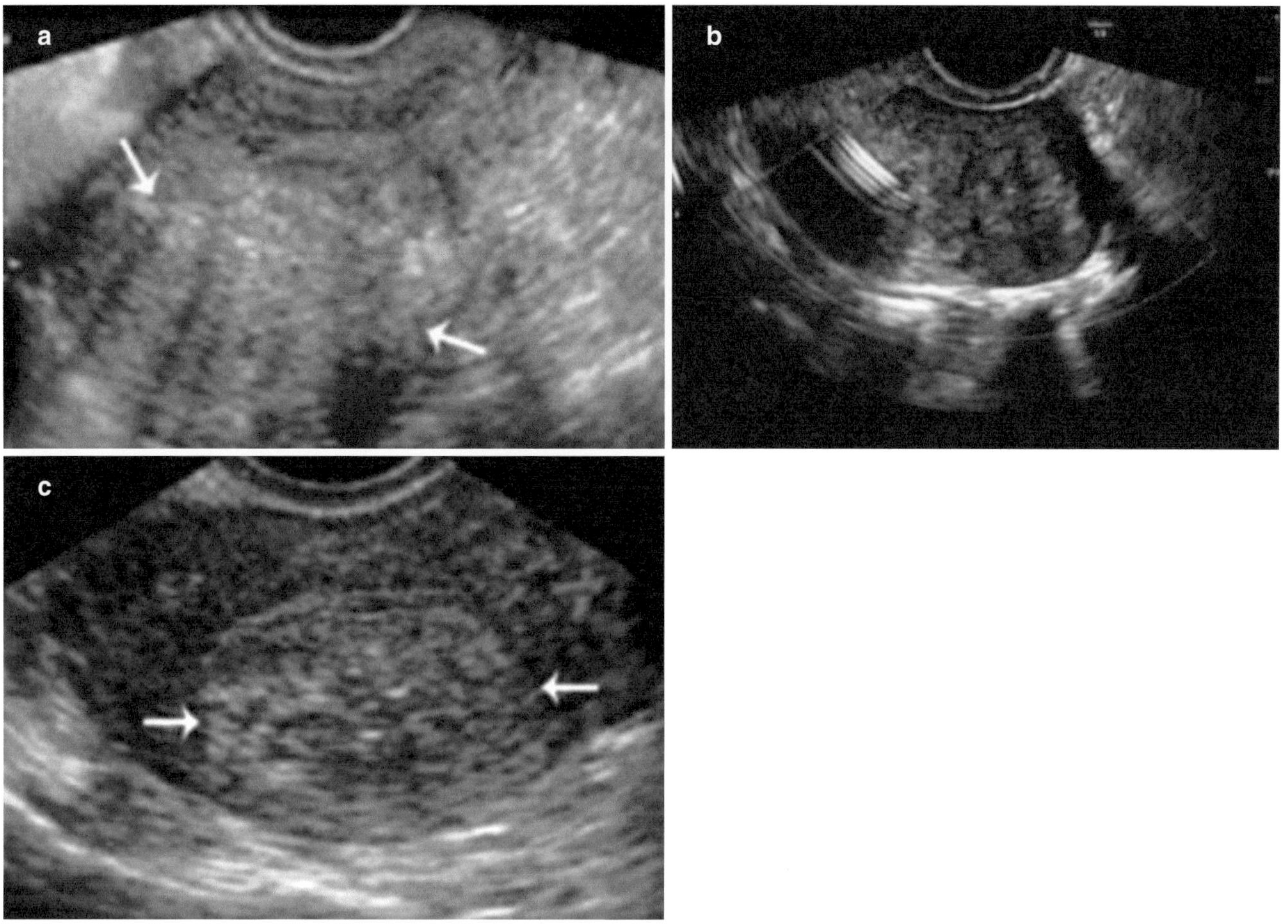

Fig. 5.23 Adenomyosis (III). (**a-c**) Adenomyosis affects the anterior and posterior myometrium. The lesion is hyperechoic (arrow), which is similar to leiomyoma but without obvious peripheral pseudocapsule

5.3 Ultrasonic Diagnosis of Endometrial Carcinoma

(I) Basic concepts

Endometrial carcinoma, one of the three common malignant reproductive tumors in females, accounts for 20–30% of the malignant reproductive tumors in females. The incidence is related to race and region. According to recent statistical data, the incidence of endometrial carcinoma increases, which is most prevalent in patients aged 58–61.

The exact cause of endometrial carcinoma remains unclear. The high-risk factors include long-term and continuous endometrial stimulation by exogenous or endogenous estrogen, endometrial hyperplasia, obesity, hypertension, diabetes, unmarried, nulliparous, delayed menopause, genetic factors, etc.

The pathological findings of endometrial carcinoma are mainly divided into the diffuse type and localized type. Most of the lesions of localized type locate in the fundus of the uterus, especially near the uterine cornu. In the early stages, the endometrium shows a rough surface, the lesions are superficial and small without a mass. Sometimes, a pathological section could probably not find an obvious carcinoma lesion, which might be due to the previous diagnostic curettage or multiple curettages. Diffuse endometrial carcinoma involves a wide range of endometrium or multifocal lesions. Localized carcinoma shows polypoid or cauliflower-like growth in the uterine cavity. The common cell types of endometrial carcinoma include endometrioid adenocarcinoma (accounting for 70–80% of endometrial carcinoma), adenocarcinoma with squamous epithelial differentiation, special types such as serous papillary carcinoma and clear cell carcinoma, etc. The typical metastasis of endometrial carcinoma involves myometrial invasion, lymphatic invasion, vascular invasion, and advanced hematogenous metastasis, etc.

The typical clinical symptoms are intermittent or persistent postmenopausal vaginal bleeding. Premenopausal patients usually complain of increased menstrual volume, prolonged menstrual period, or

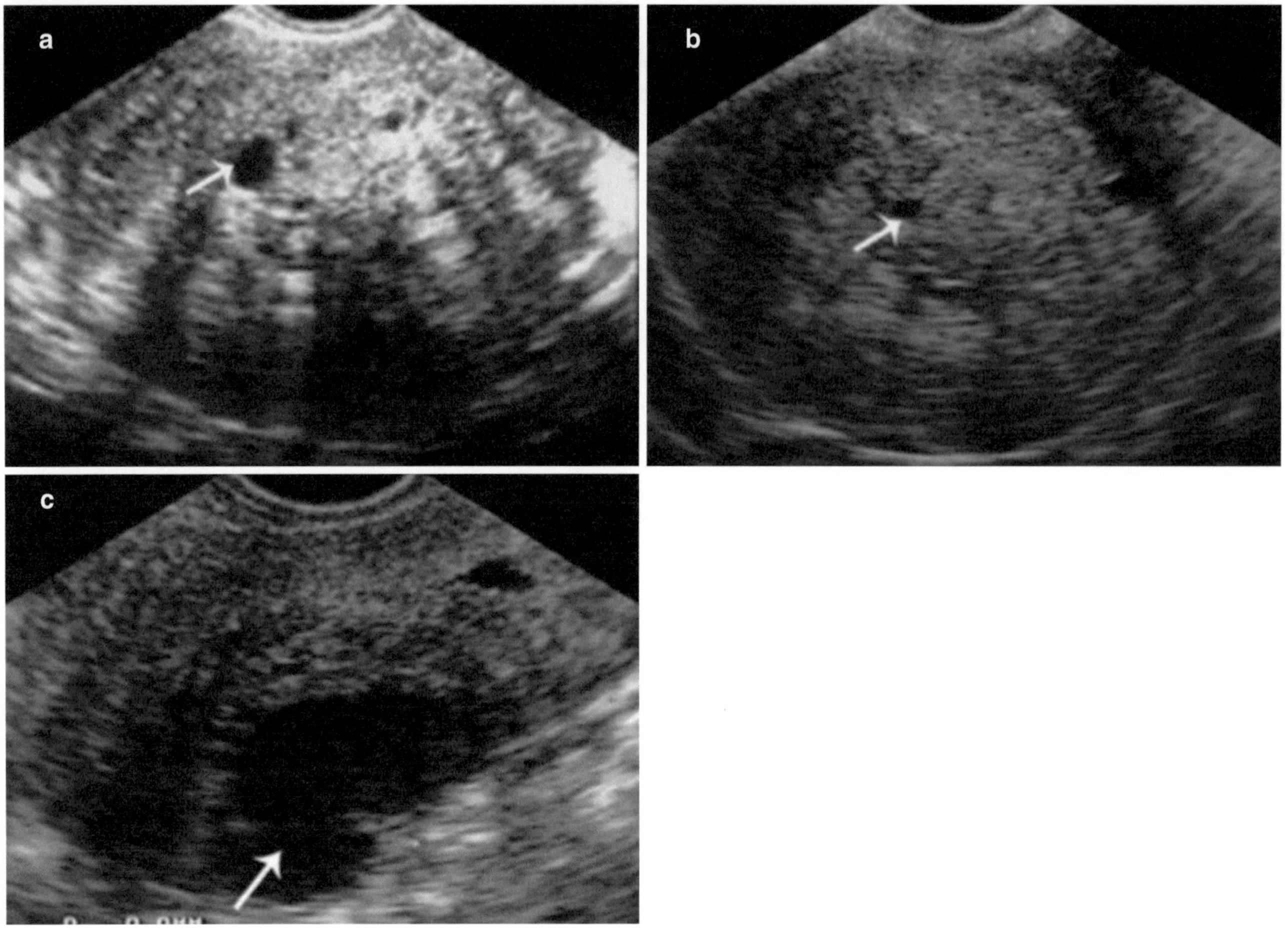

Fig. 5.24 Adenomyosis (IV). (**a-c**) Irregular tiny fluid areas (arrow) are visible, especially during the menstrual period

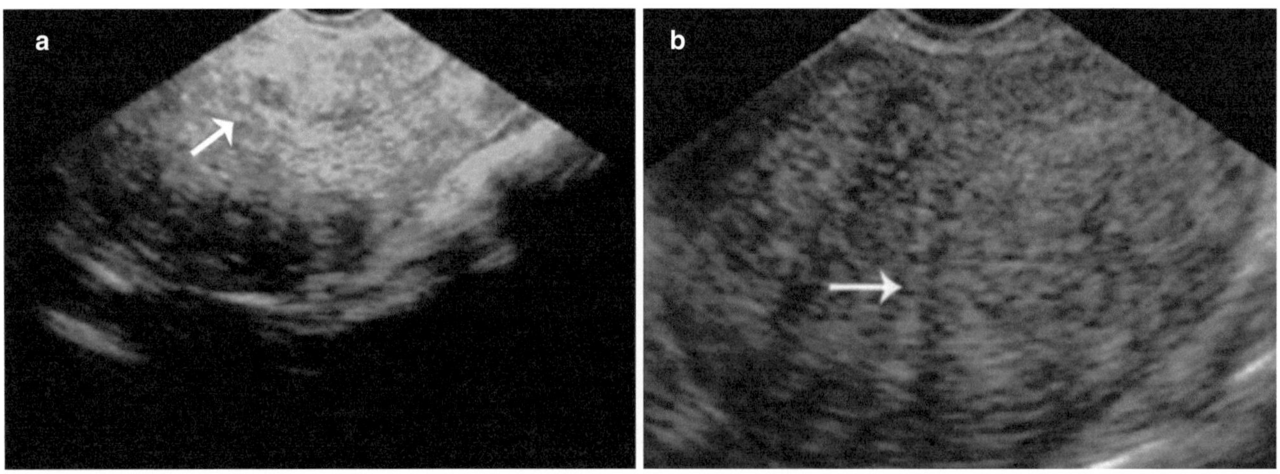

Fig. 5.25 Adenomyosis (V). (**a-b**) Diffuse lesions of adenomyosis and normal endometrium (arrow) are shown

intermenstrual bleeding. Some patients manifest with vaginal discharge, while bloody and pyometra discharge with the strong stench in advanced patients. The cervical invasion of tumor may lead to obstruction of the cervical canal, resulting in hematocele or pyometra in the uterine cavity and manifesting lower abdominal pain. In the late stages, it may cause pain in the lower abdomen and lumbosacral region which is related to the tumor invasion of surrounding tissue or compression of the mass.

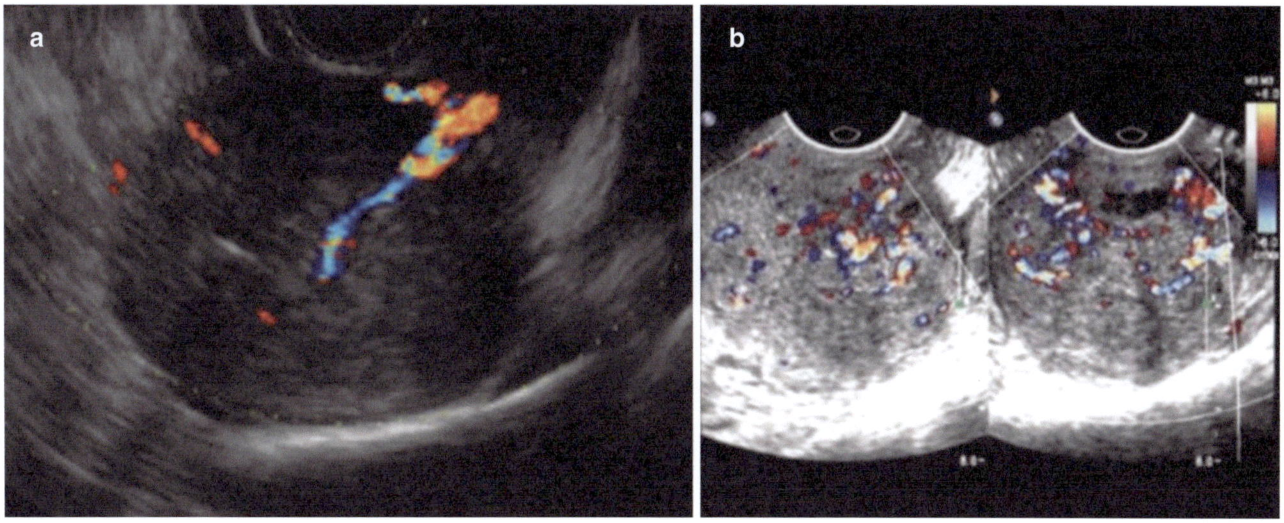

Fig. 5.26 Adenomyosis (VI). (**a-b**) The blood flow in the focus of adenomyosis is sporadic and stellate distributed by Color Doppler

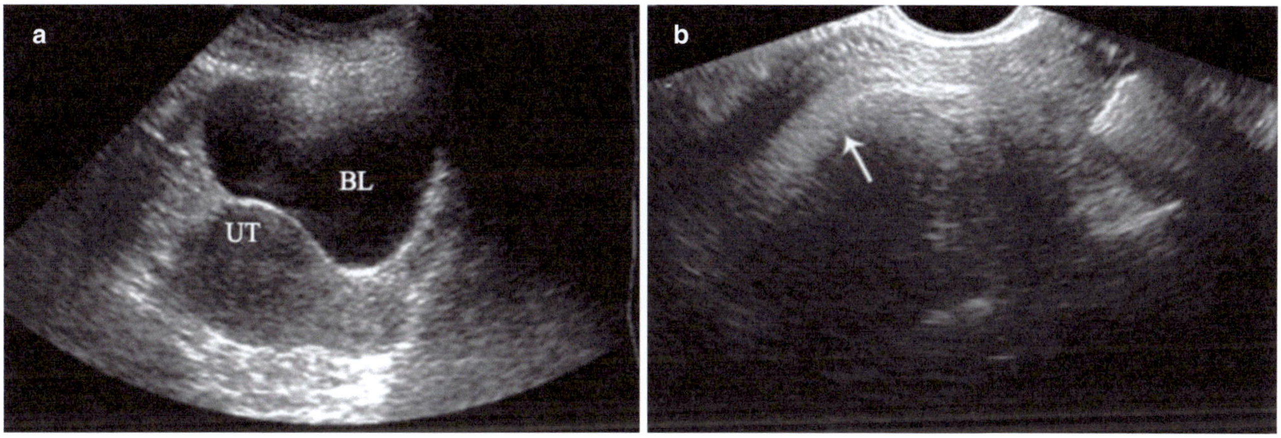

Fig. 5.27 Adenomyosis (VII). (**a**) Transabdominal scanning fails to show the features of adenomyosis. (**b**) The shape of the uterus and adenomyosis lesions can be clearly shown by transvaginal scanning

In the early stages, most patients do not have any obvious systemic symptoms or signs. The enlarged and softened uterus could be palpated. Irregular nodular masses around or beside the uterus could be found in advanced patients.

The diagnosis of endometrial carcinoma is based on the pathological results of curettage.

(II) Ultrasonic diagnosis

- In the early stages of endometrial carcinoma, doctors could not find obvious endometrial morphologic changes by ultrasonographic image. Some patients with endometrial carcinoma only show slightly thickened endometrium or fluid in the uterine cavity (Fig. 5.28).
- Sonographic image finds enlarged uterus in patients with advanced stages of endometrial carcinoma. The enlarged uterus is especially found in patients with original atrophic after menopause. The single layer of endometrium may be thicker than 0.5 cm, with an irregular solid mass in the uterine cavity in some cases (Fig. 5.29).
- When the infiltration is involved into the myometrium, the endometrial-like echo extends to the myometrium. Endometrial carcinoma may also obstruct the cervical canal, resulting in irregular hyperechoic findings in the cervical canal (Fig. 5.30).
- An ultrasonographic image shows fluid, hematometra, and pyometra in the endometrial cavity, due to the obstruction of the cervix (Fig. 5.31).

(III) Special tips

- For postmenopausal women with the single layer of endometrial thickness $\geq$ 0.4 cm, or unevenly thickened, or space-occupying lesions; or premenopausal women with menstrual disorder accompanied by menometrorrhagia, it is advisable to carry out the diagnostic dilatation and curettage as soon as possible (Fig. 5.32, 5.33, 5.34, and 5.35).

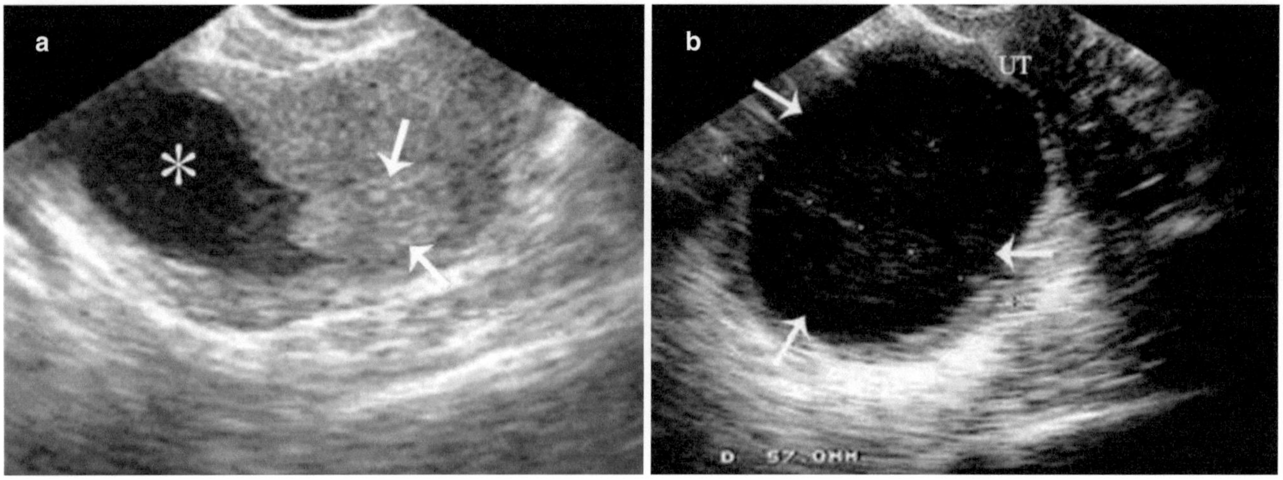

Fig. 5.28 Endometrial carcinoma (I). (**a**) A 57-year-old patient represented with irregular vaginal bleeding for 1 month. A solid mass (arrow), 2.0 cm in diameter, and fluid (shown with "*") are shown in the uterine cavity. (**b**) A 63-year-old postmenopausal patient, menopause for 13 years, presents mild vaginal bleeding. Sonogram shows the fluid area (arrow) in the uterine cavity, with a diameter of 5.7 cm

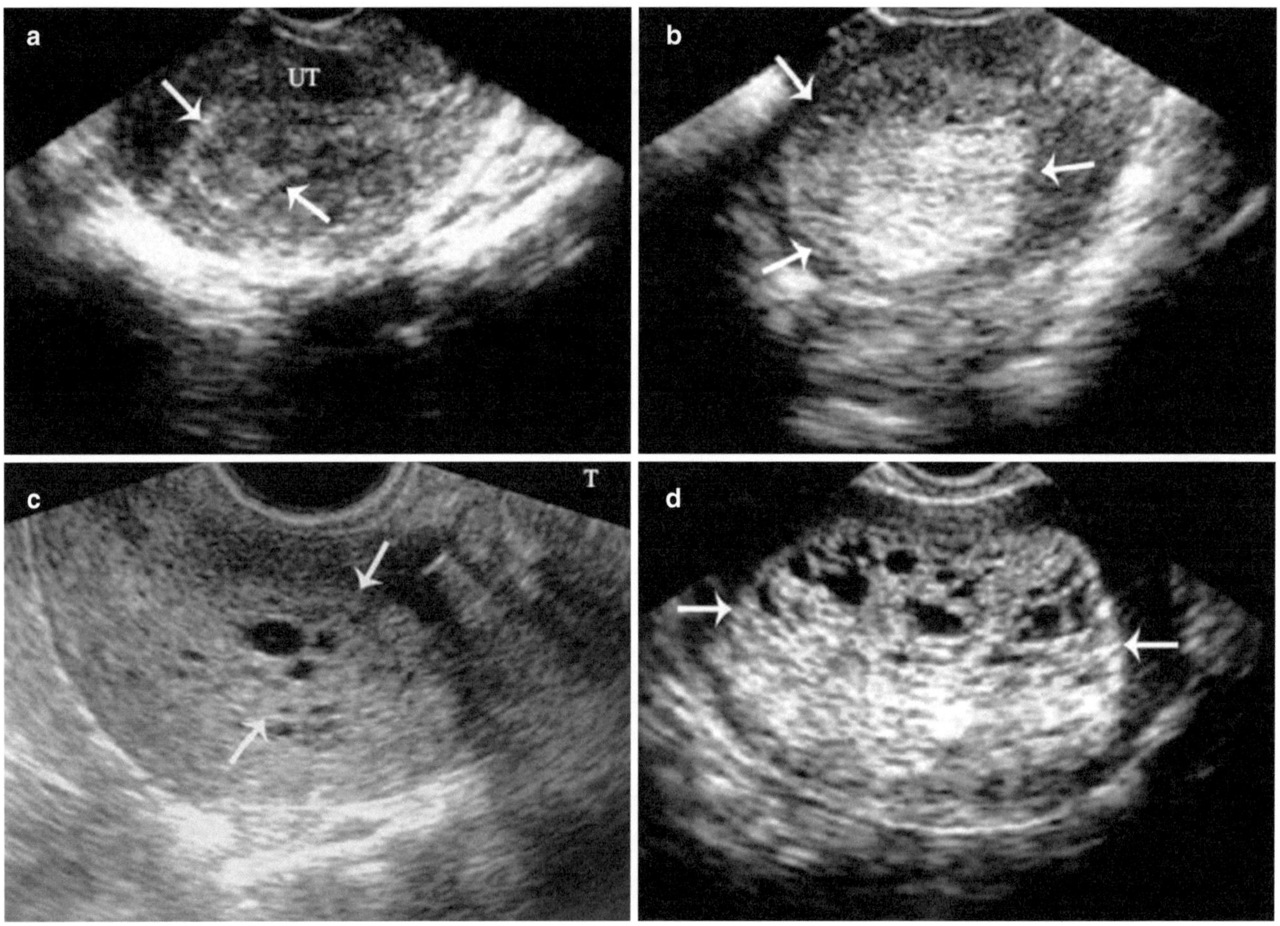

Fig. 5.29 Endometrial carcinoma (II). (**a**) A 44-year-old patient with a history of menstrual disorder for half a year. Sonogram represents a thickened endometrium and heterogeneous echo. (**b**) A woman with a postmenopausal period of 10 years. Sonogram shows an enlarged uterus with thickened hyperechoic endometrium. (**c**) A woman with a postmenopausal period of 6 years, represented with mild vaginal bleeding. The ultrasonogram shows the thickened heterogeneous endometrium, with multiple cystic changes. (**d**) Ultrasonographic findings showed the thickened, heterogeneous, and mass-like endometrium, with fluid area in it (arrow)

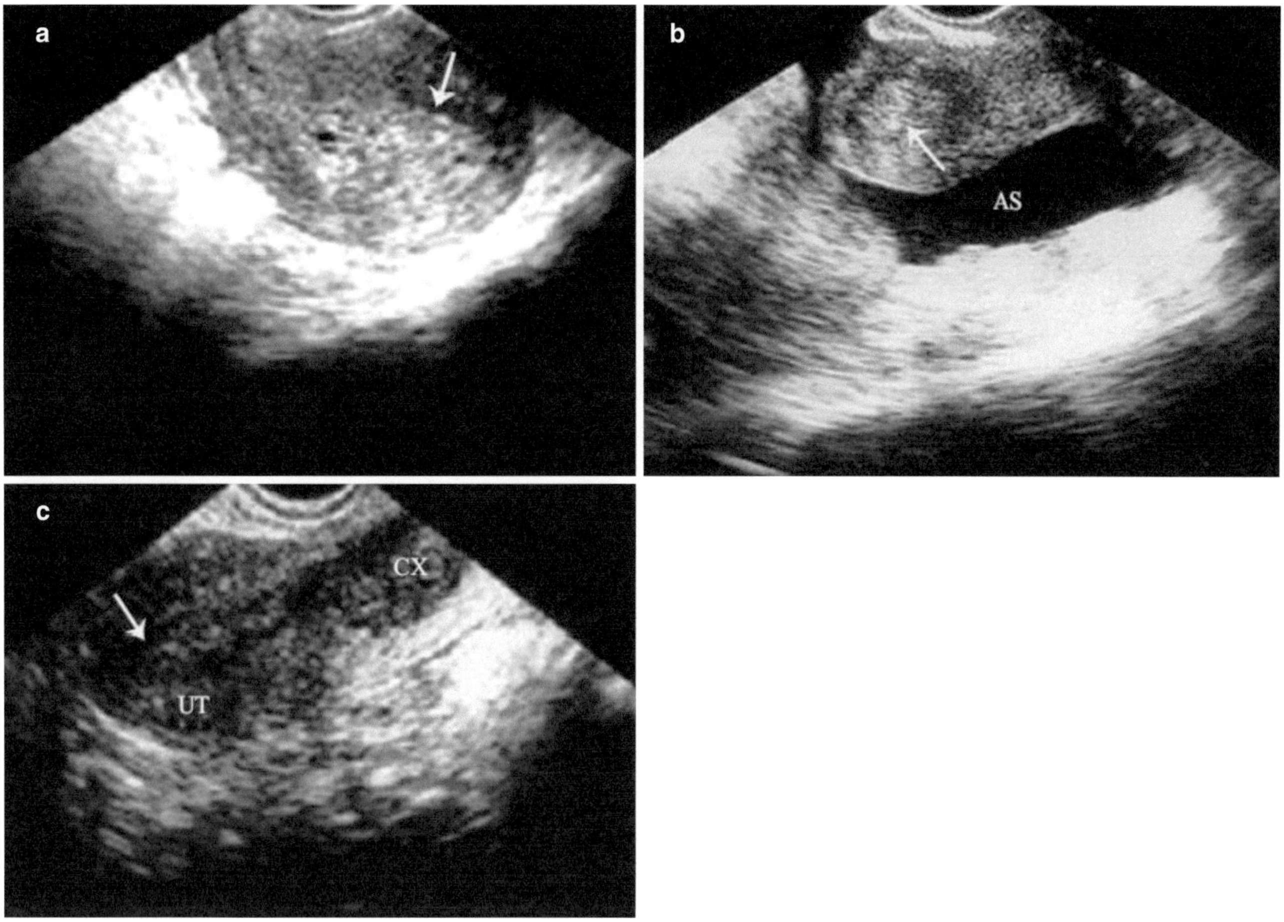

Fig. 5.30 Endometrial carcinoma (III). (**a**) Sonogram shows the thickened endometrium and the "nibbling like" endometrial invasion. (**b**) A 61-year-old patient complained of vaginal bleeding for half a year. Ultrasonographic images show the thickened hyperechoic endometrium with ascites around the uterus. (**c**) A patient with endometrial and cervical adenocarcinoma. Sonogram shows the hypoechoic mass in the uterine cavity and posterior wall of the cervix (arrow)

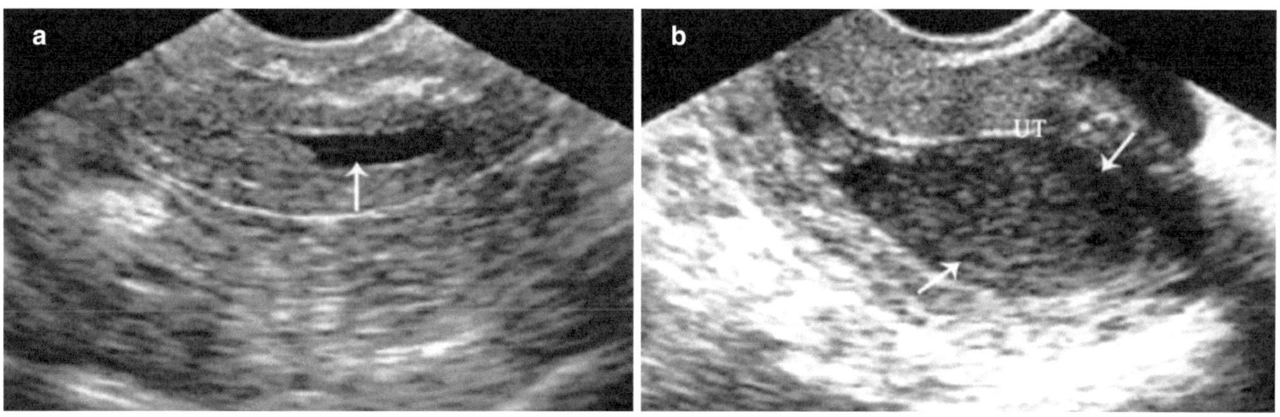

Fig. 5.31 Endometrial carcinoma (IV). (**a**) A 65-year-old patient, with a postmenopausal period of 10 years, represented mild vaginal bleeding. Ultrasonographic image shows a small amount of fluid in the uterine cavity and a hyperechoic mass in the anterior wall of myometrium, with a diameter of nearly1.5 cm. (**b**) A patient with a postmenopausal period of 6 years, accompanied by hypertension and diabetes mellitus, represented with vaginal spotting for one month. Ultrasonographic images show the fluid area with a diameter of 3.0 cm and tiny dot-like echoes (arrow) in the uterine cavity

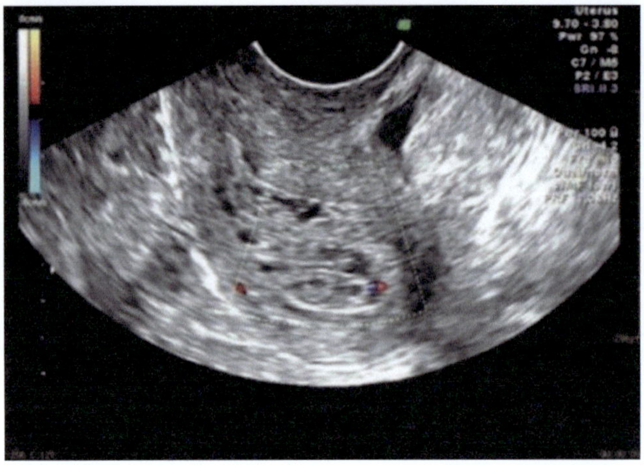

Fig. 5.32 Endometrial hyperplasia. A woman with a postmenopausal period of 4 years represented no vaginal bleeding. Conventional ultrasonic examination shows thickened endometrium with vesicular echoes. The subsequent curettage identified the diagnosis of endometrial hyperplasia

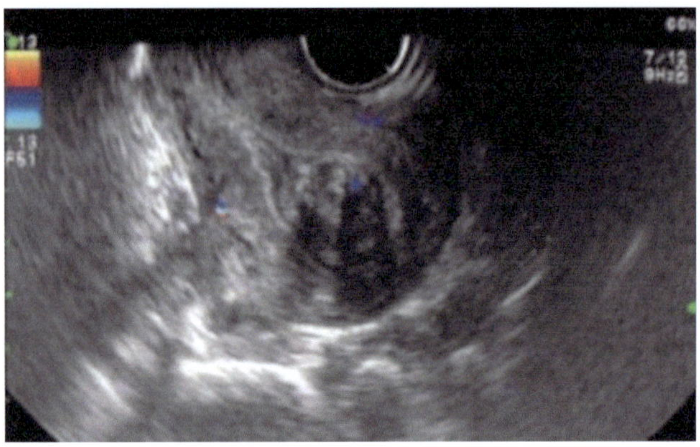

Fig. 5.33 Submucous myoma. A 48-year-old patient with menorrhagia for 2 years. Sonogram shows a solid mass with a diameter of nearly 2.5 cm in the uterine cavity. Submucous myoma is confirmed after an operation

- Endometrial carcinoma should be distinguished from endometrial hyperplasia, submucous myoma, endometrial polyp, senile endometritis, uterine effusion, and functional uterine bleeding.

(IV) Classic cases

- A reproductive woman represented with irregular vaginal bleeding for 3 months. Ultrasonography shows a space-occupying mass in the uterine cavity, which is suspected residue, and endometrial carcinoma is confirmed by pathological examination after curettage (Fig. 5.36).
- An elderly woman, with no vaginal bleeding, represented an obvious fluid area in the uterine cavity, without thickened endometrium. The uterine effusion and endometrial carcinoma were confirmed by diagnostic dilation and curettage (Fig. 5.37).

5.4 Ultrasonic Diagnosis of Benign Endometrial Lesion

(I) Basic concept

Endometrial polyp is a common tumor-like lesion, which is composed of local hyperplasia of endometrial glands and stroma. Endometrial polyps with pedicles grow into the uterine cavity. Some of the pedicels are relatively long, even protruding to the internal cervical os. It can occur at any age, especially in women aged 50–60 years.

Histologically, endometrial polyp has smooth surface, sometimes complaint as hemorrhage, necrosis and ulceration when accompanied by infection. It can be single, multiple, or diffuse lesions with different shapes and ranges from millimeters to centimeters. Pathologically, it can be divided into functional,

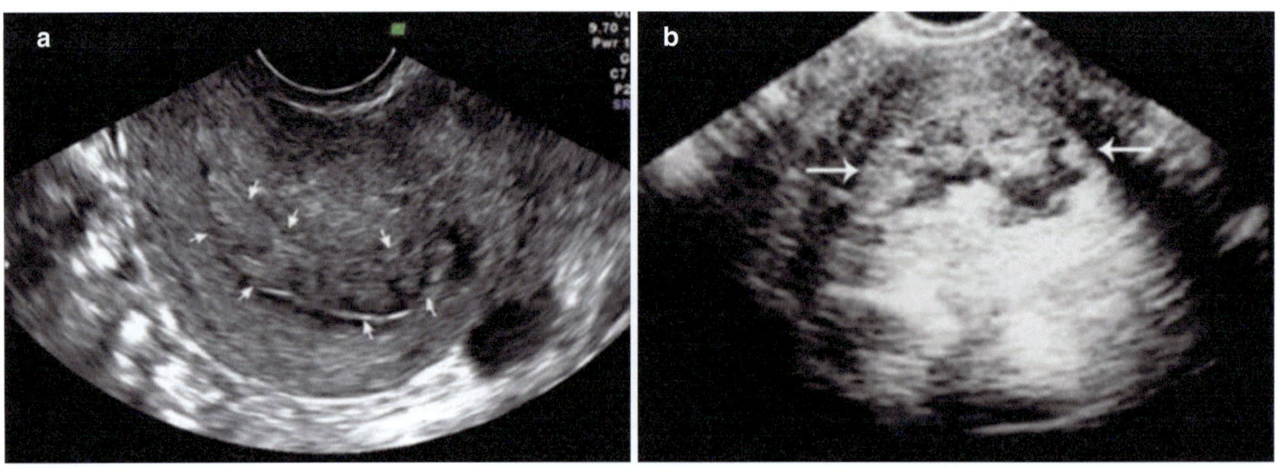

Fig. 5.34 Endometrial polyp. A 29-year-old patient represented with menstrual disorder and infertility. Ultrasonography shows an enlarged uterus and heterogeneous echoes with a diameter of nearly 6.0 cm in the uterine cavity. Multiple polyps are diagnosed after curettage (arrow)

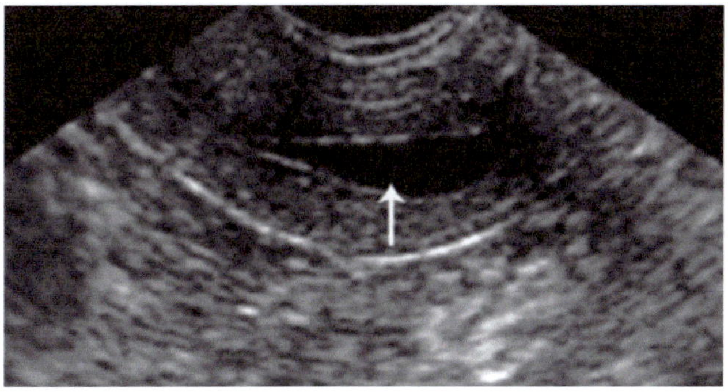

Fig. 5.35 Uterine effusion. A woman with a postmenopausal period of 3 years represented with abnormal vaginal discharge. Sonogram shows the atrophied uterus, the clear fluid in the uterine cavity (1.6 cm in diameter), and the smooth inner wall of the uterus (arrow)

nonfunctional, adenomyomatous, and postmenopausal endometrial polyps. The pedicles are different in thickness and length.

The typical clinical manifestation is menometrorrhagia or spotting bleeding. A single small polyp can be asymptomatic.

(II) Ultrasonic diagnosis

- The uterus is normal or slightly enlarged, without morphology change.
- Space-occupying lesion is visible in the uterine cavity, with discontinued or distorted endometrium. Most of them are hyperechoic, round, or punctate, attached to the inner wall of the uterine cavity, and well-defined with the endometrium (Figs. 5.38 and 5.39).

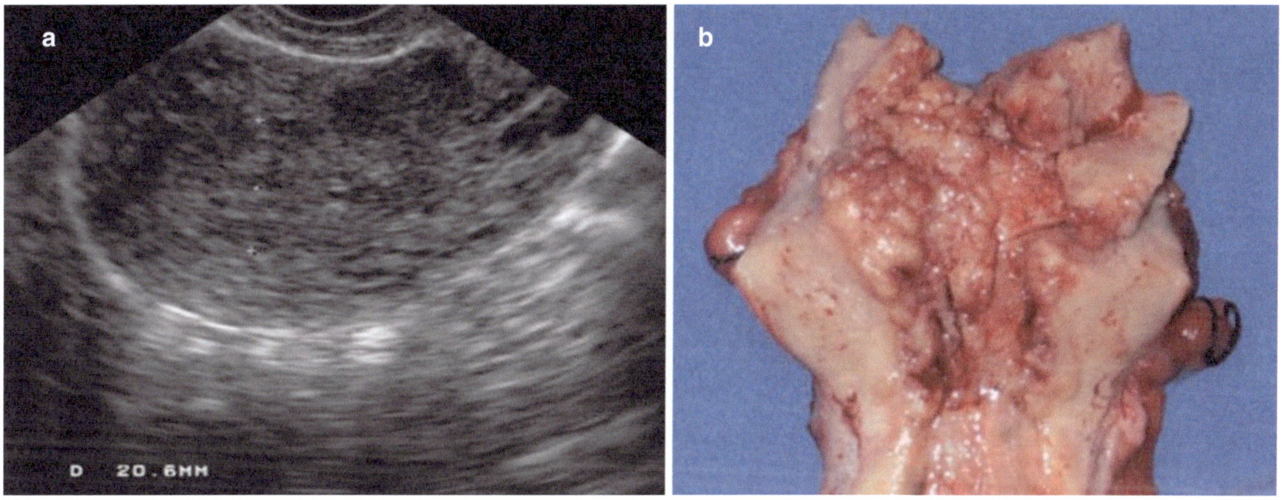

Fig. 5.36 Endometrial carcinoma (V). A 38-year-old patient represented irregular vaginal bleeding for 3 months. (**a**) Ultrasonography showed a space-occupying mass in uterine cavity, which was suspected residue. (**b**) Gross specimen. Endometrial carcinoma was diagnosed after an operation, with a confirmed pathological diagnosis of moderately and highly differentiated endometrial adenocarcinoma

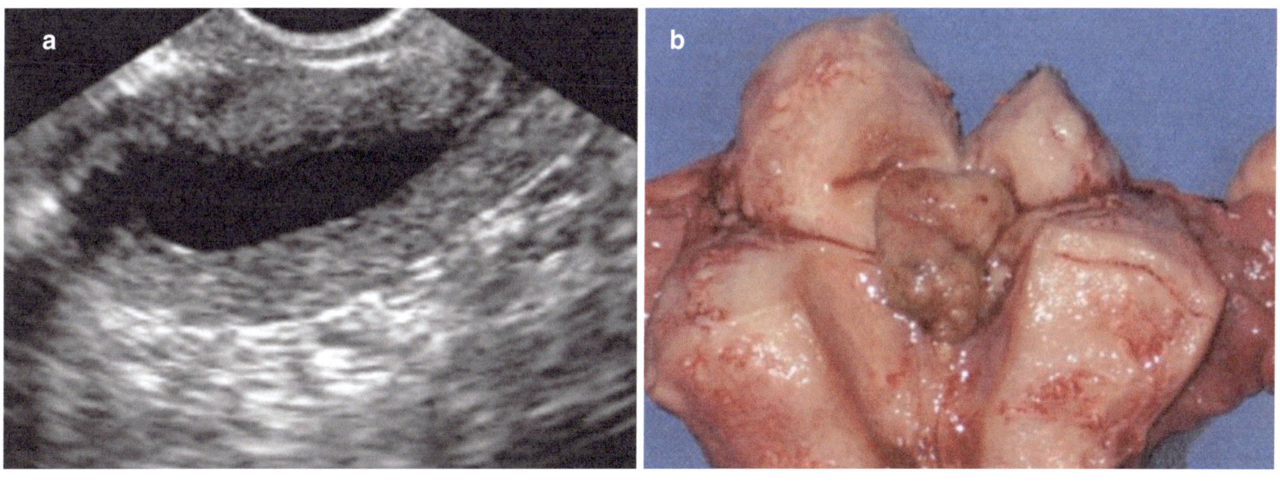

Fig. 5.37 Endometrial carcinoma (VI). A 57-year-old patient with a postmenopausal period of 9 years represented vaginal bleeding for 5 days. (**a**) Ultrasonography shows the fluid in the uterine cavity and a slightly hyperechoic mass with a diameter of 2.0 cm at the fundus. Endometrial carcinoma was diagnosed by subsequent curettage. (**b**) Gross specimens after the operation

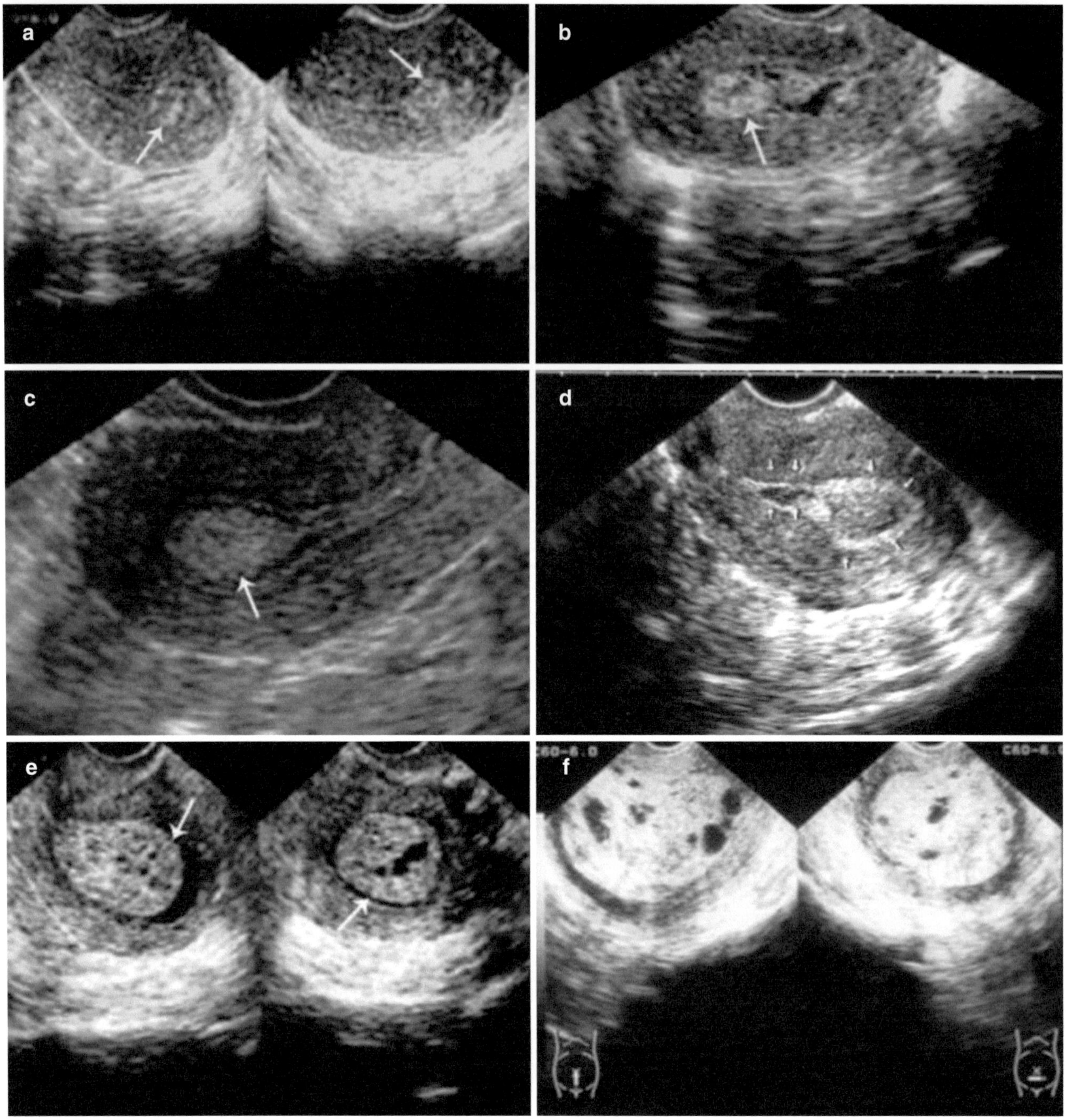

Fig. 5.38 Endometrial polyps (I). (**a-d**) Sonogram shows the space-occupying lesions and the discontinued endometrial line. (**e**) A 61-year-old patient with a postmenopausal period of 10 years represented a little amount of vaginal bleeding. Sagittal and transverse TVS shows a slightly hyperechoic lesion with a diameter of about 2.0 cm in the uterine cavity, with multiple small cysts in it. (**f**) A 66-year-old patient with a postmenopausal period of 13 years. Sagittal and transverse TVS shows an intrauterine space-occupying hyperechoic lesion with a diameter of about 3.5 cm. Multiple small cysts are visible in the lesion (arrow)

(III) Special tips

- Transvaginal ultrasound is recommended to show the morphology of the endometrium. Ultrasound images show abnormally thickened endometrium in the cases of diffuse heterogeneity polyps. Sonohysterography is helpful to distinguish between the endometrial polyps and endometrial thickening.
- Endometrial polyps should be differentiated from endometrial hyperplasia, submucous myoma, endometrial carcinoma, and intrauterine residue (Figs. 5.40, 5.41, 5.42, 5.43, 5.44 and 5.45).

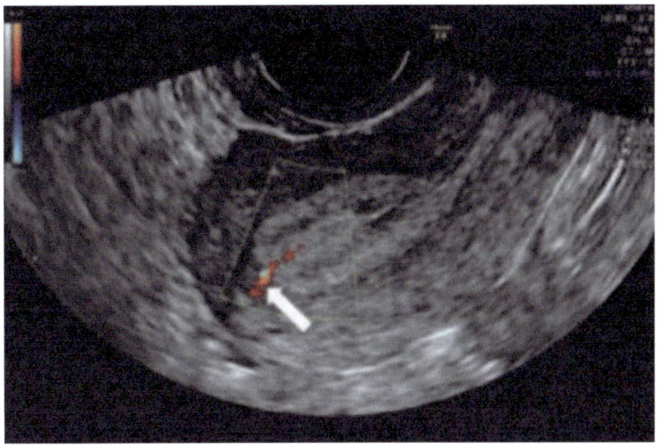

Fig. 5.39 Color Doppler shows the blood vessels supplying the endometrial polyp (arrow)

5.5 Ultrasonic Diagnosis of Cervical Lesions

(I) Basic concepts

- The cervix, a part of the uterus, is mainly composed of fibrous connective tissue and a small amount of smooth muscle cells. It is cylindrical and 2.5–3.0 cm in length. The cervical canal locates in the center, and the inner membrane of the canal can secret alkaline mucus. Cervix has many defense functions, but it is vulnerable to be injured by childbirth and uterine cavity operation, leading to chronic cervicitis, which is the most common disease in gynecology.

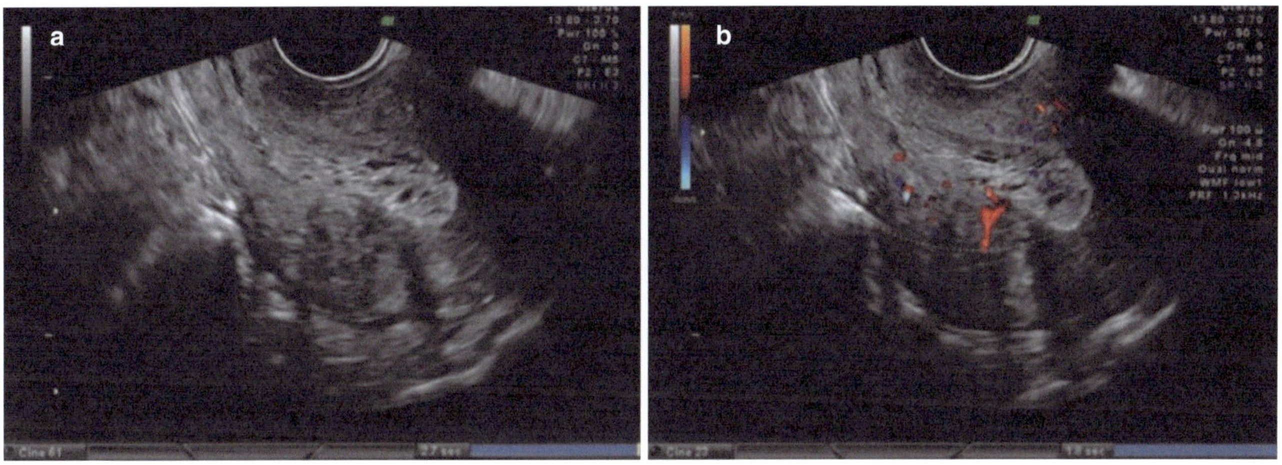

Fig. 5.40 Endometrial hyperplasia. Ultrasound images show thickened endometrium with multiple small cysts (**a**. two-dimension, **b**. Color Doppler flow image). Endometrial hyperplasia is confirmed by pathological examination after diagnostic D&C

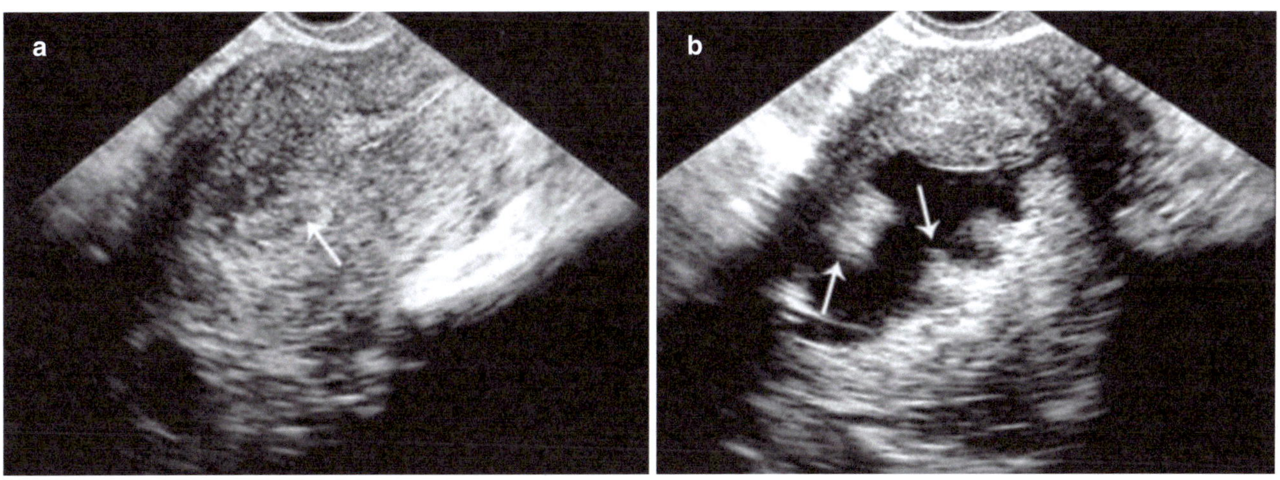

Fig. 5.41 Endometrial polyps (II). A 45-year-old patient with a history of menstrual disorder for 1+ year received an ultrasonic examination. (**a**) Sagittal view of TVS shows heterogenous thickened endometrium. (**b**) Multiple polyps are shown protruding into the fluid in the uterine cavity after saline infusion (arrow)

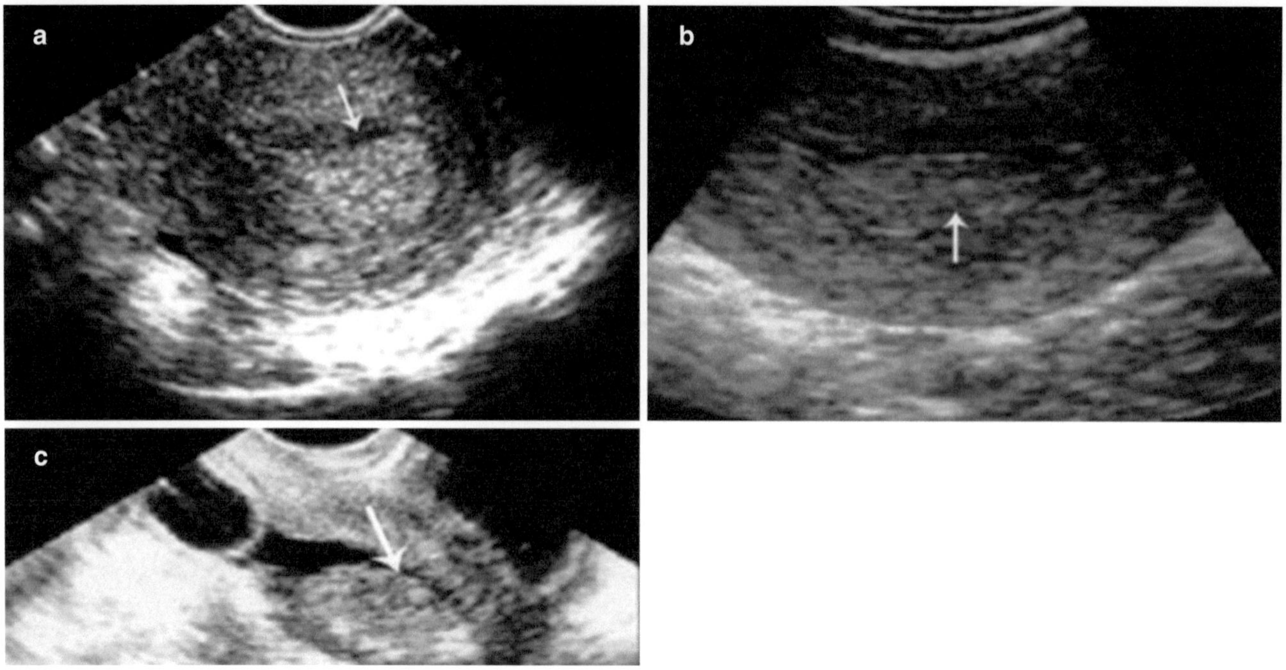

Fig. 5.42 Identification of endometrial polyp and intrauterine residue. (**a**) The space-occupying lesion was shown in the uterine cavity and the endometrium discontinued; (**b**) Sagittal view of TVS shows the thickened endometrium. (**c**) Sonogram shows a hyperechoic mass with a diameter of about 3.0 cm floating in uterine fluid after saline infusion (arrow)

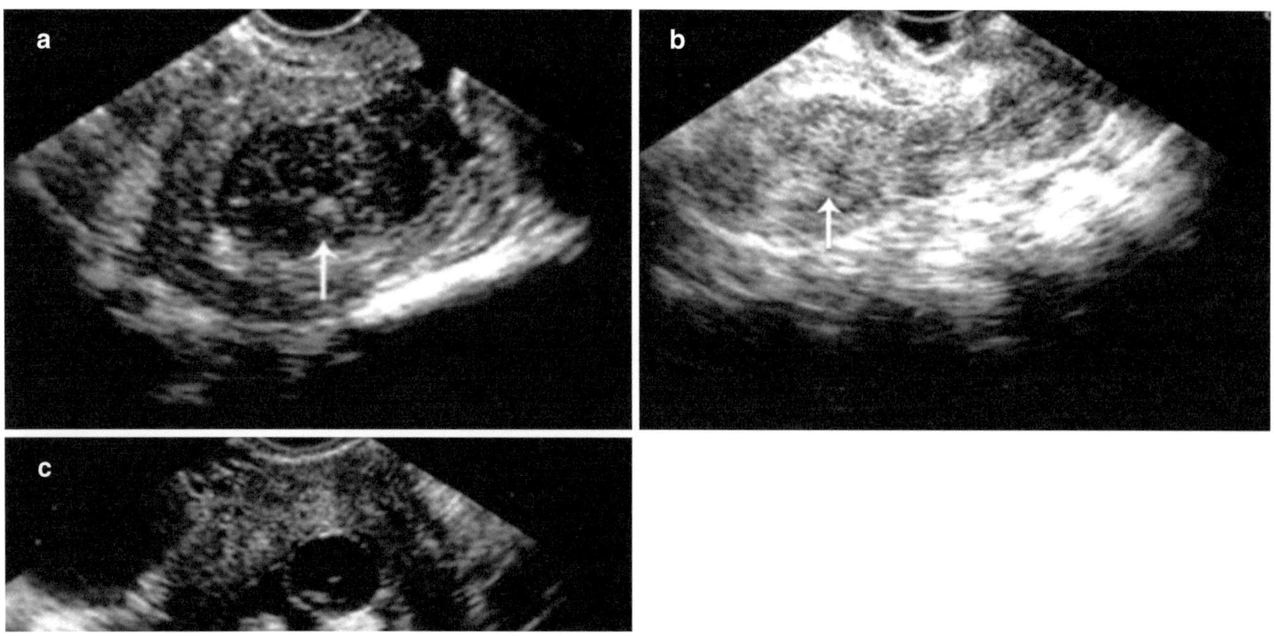

Fig. 5.43 Identification of submucous myoma and endometrial polyp. (**a**) A patient complained of excessive volume of menses with blood clots for 2+ years. Sonogram shows a hypoechoic mass, 2.4 cm in diameter with a well-defined boundary, in the uterine cavity. (**b**) A patient diagnosed with primary infertility represented menstrual disorder for 3 years. Sonogram shows the thickened endometrium. (**c**) Multiple hyperechoic masses are shown in the uterine cavity after saline infusion (arrow)

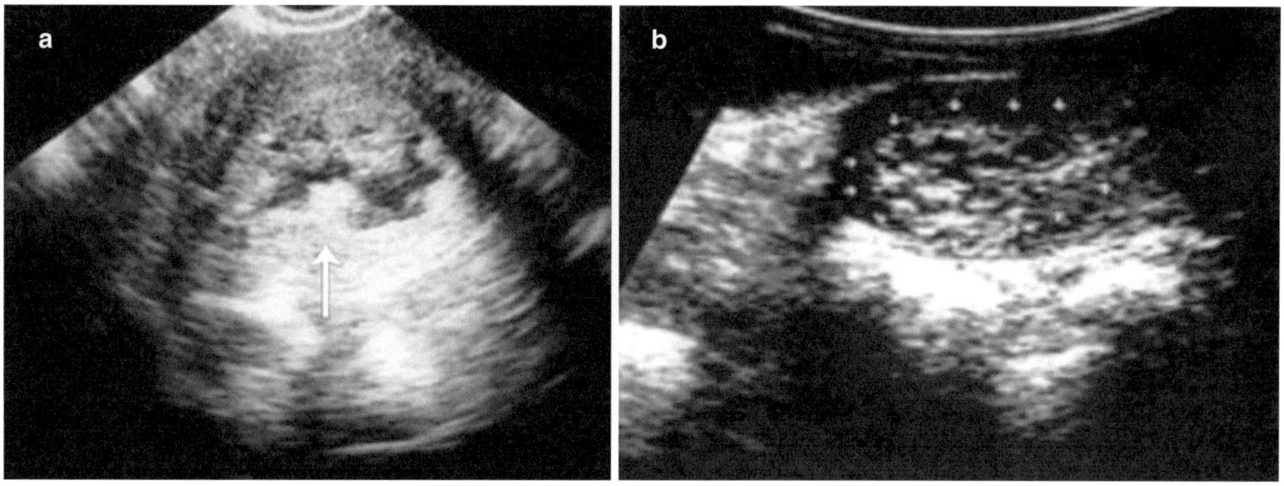

Fig. 5.44 The differential diagnosis of endometrial polyp and tuberculosis. (**a**) A 37-year-old patient represented menstrual disorder with an excessive volume of menses for 2 years. Ultrasonography shows multiple irregular, heterogeneous hyperechoic masses in the uterine cavity; (**b**) A 24-year-old patient with a history of tuberculosis and secondary amenorrhea for 7 years. Heterogeneous hyperechoic mass is shown in the uterine cavity, which is suspected as endometrial tuberculosis (arrow)

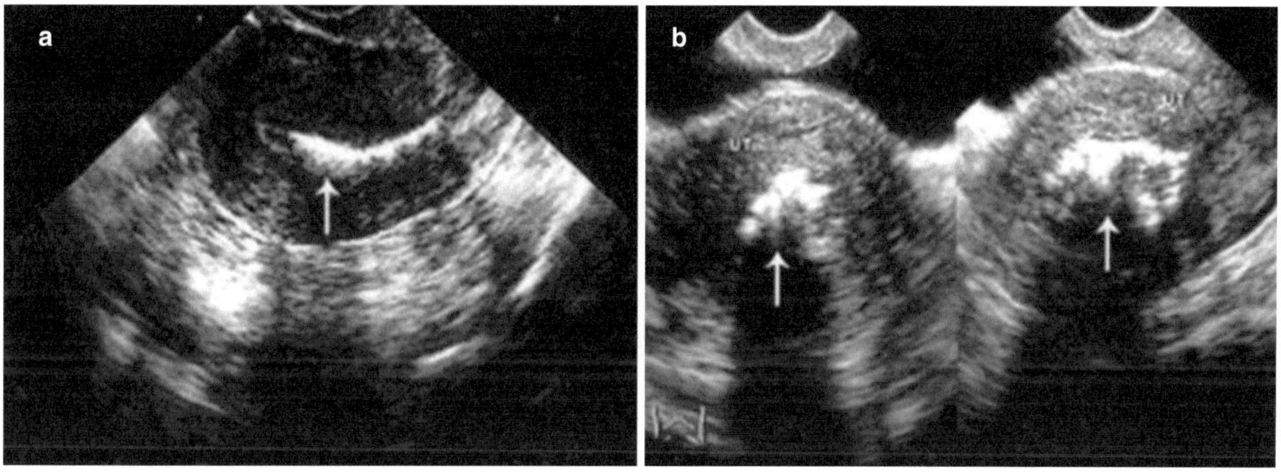

Fig. 5.45 Other endometrial lesions. (**a**) A 32-year-old patient complained of secondary amenorrhea for 7 years after induced abortion. Strip-like hyperechoic tissue with an attenuated shadow is found in the uterine cavity, which is identified as residual calcification and intrauterine adhesions. (**b**) Hypomenorrhea for 3 years after induced abortion. Sonogram shows irregular hyperechoic tissue with acoustic shadow, indicating calcification (arrow)

- Due to the special characteristics of cervical anatomy and histology, the formation of the squamous columnar junction is highly sensitive to the stimulations caused by some carcinogenic factors. Cervical cell dysplasia, disordered cell arrangement, abnormal cells, and increased mitosis may exist and lead to invasive cervical cancer eventually.
- Cervical cancer is the most common malignant tumor of the reproductive tract, with a high incidence in 35–39-year-old and 60–64-year-old women. The exact cause is not completely understood. Recently, human papillomavirus (HPV) infection, especially persistent high-risk HPV infection, is considered to be the main cause of cervical precancerous lesions and cervical cancer. Other related risk factors include early childbirth, multipara, high-risk male partners, and immune suppression.
- Common histological types include squamous cell carcinoma, adenocarcinoma, squamous adenocarcinoma, spinous adenocarcinoma, clear cell carcinoma, and undifferentiated carcinoma. According to the differentiation level, cervical cancer is divided into high differentiated, moderately differentiated, and poorly differentiated carcinoma. According to the different development stages, cervical carcinoma is divided into carcinoma in situ, early invasive carcinoma, and late invasive carcinoma.

- Exogenic type, endogenic type, ulcerative type, and endocervical type are common cervical squamous cell carcinoma, which accounts for 80–85% of all cervical carcinoma. Cervical adenocarcinoma accounts for about 15%. The main metastasis of cervical cancer is direct invasion and lymphatic metastasis.
- In general, there are not any obvious clinical symptoms and signs are shown in the early stage of cervical cancer. Once manifestations are present, usually shown as vaginal bleeding and abnormal vaginal discharge. Symptoms such as frequent urination, urgent urination, constipation, edema and pain of lower limbs, and even systemic cachexia can be complained in the late-stage patients with lesions spreading to pelvic connective tissue. In advanced-stage patients, cervical cauliflower mass can be seen protruding to the vagina during the pelvic examination, with a bleeding tendency. In the endocervical types, the cervix is hypertrophic and firm, with smooth surface or superficial ulcer, cervical canal is enlarged, and depressed ulcers are visible in advanced-stage patients. Thickened and nodular parametrial tissues can be palpated in the gynecological examination, even invaded into the pelvic wall, forming a frozen pelvis.
- The main clinical symptoms of chronic cervicitis are increased vaginal discharge, hemorrhagic leucorrhea, and postcoital bleeding. When the inflammation involves other adjacent organs or spreads to the pelvis, lumbosacral pain and lower abdominal pain may occur.
- The pathological changes of chronic cervicitis include cervical erosion, cervical polyp, cervical mucositis, cervical Nabothian's cyst and cervical hypertrophy, etc.

(II) Ultrasonic diagnosis

- The main ultrasonic manifestations of chronic cervicitis, including cervical Nabothian's cyst, cervical hypertrophy, and cervical polyp.
- The enlarged cervix with multiple anechoic cysts (Fig. 5.46).

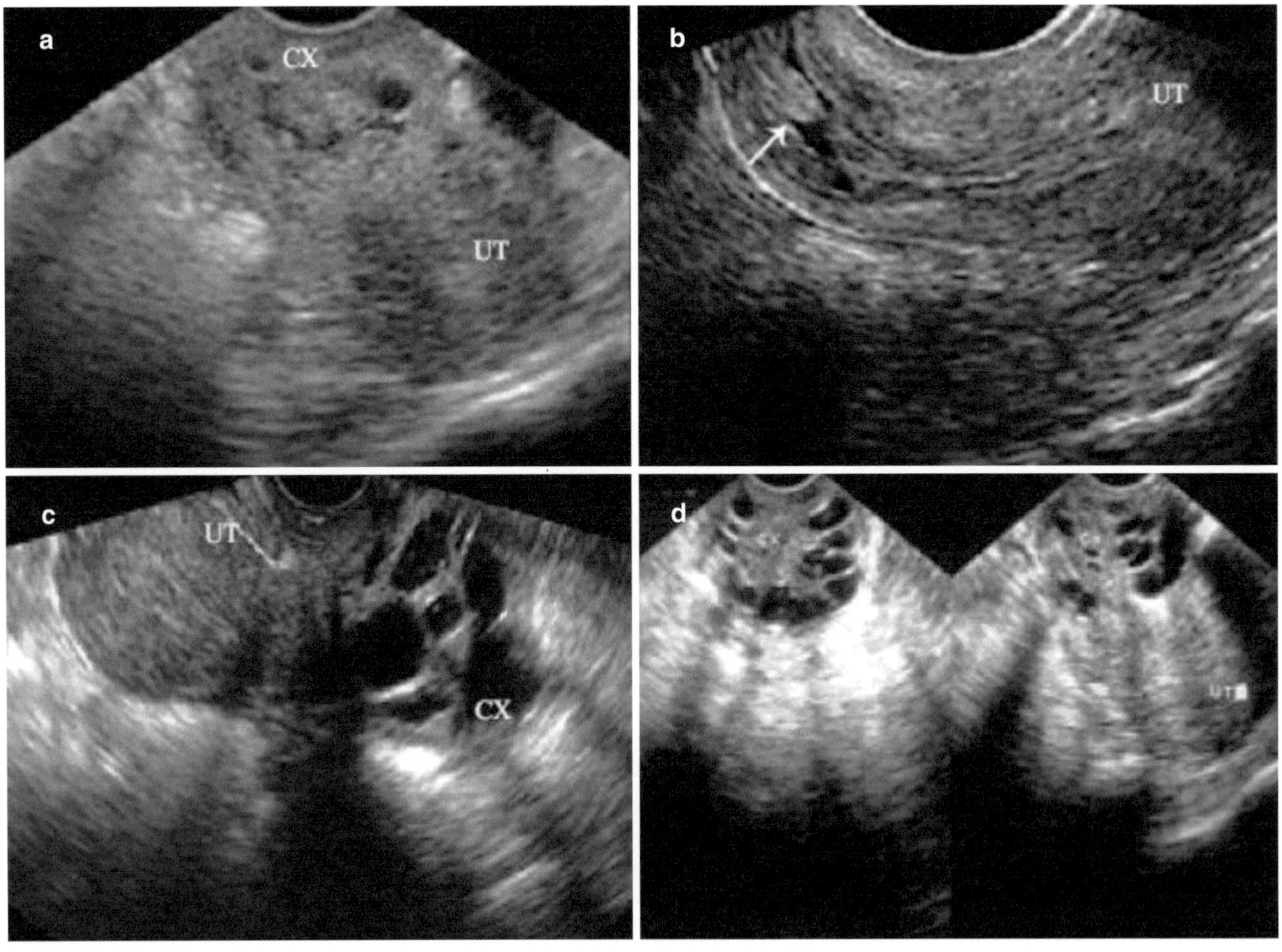

Fig. 5.46 chronic cervicitis. (**a**) Hypertrophy of cervix with Nabothian's cysts. (**b**) Polyp in the cervical canal (arrow). (**c**, **d**) cervical hypertrophy with Nabothian's cysts

- Ultrasonic images of cervical cancer.
  - No obvious ultrasonic findings are shown in the early stage of cervical cancer. When the lesion grows to a certain size and protrudes to the external os or appears as a mass, the ultrasonic image shows an enlarged cervix with a diameter of more than 3 cm. The morphology of the endocervical membrane is abnormal or disappeared (Figs. 5.47 and 5.48).
  - A heterogeneous, hypoechoic, or hyperechoic, irregular mass can be shown in the cervix. When the tumor infiltrates the bladder and parametrium, the ultrasonic images show an unsmooth bladder wall and irregular hypoechoic tissue around the uterus (Fig. 5.49).
  - Color Doppler shows abundant blood flow in cervical cancer (Fig. 5.50).

(III) Special tips

- Cervical cancer should be differentiated from cervical pregnancy in women of reproductive age. Serum hCG level should be tested (Fig. 5.51).
- Cervical cancer should be differentiated from cervical myoma (Fig. 5.52).

5.6 Ultrasonic Diagnosis of Uterine Sarcoma

(I) Basic concepts

Uterine sarcoma, which is rare, is the most malignant tumor of the female genital system. Leiomyosarcoma accounts for about 0.64% of the smooth muscle tumors of the uterus, and 45–75% of the leiomyosarcoma. Leiomyosarcoma generates from

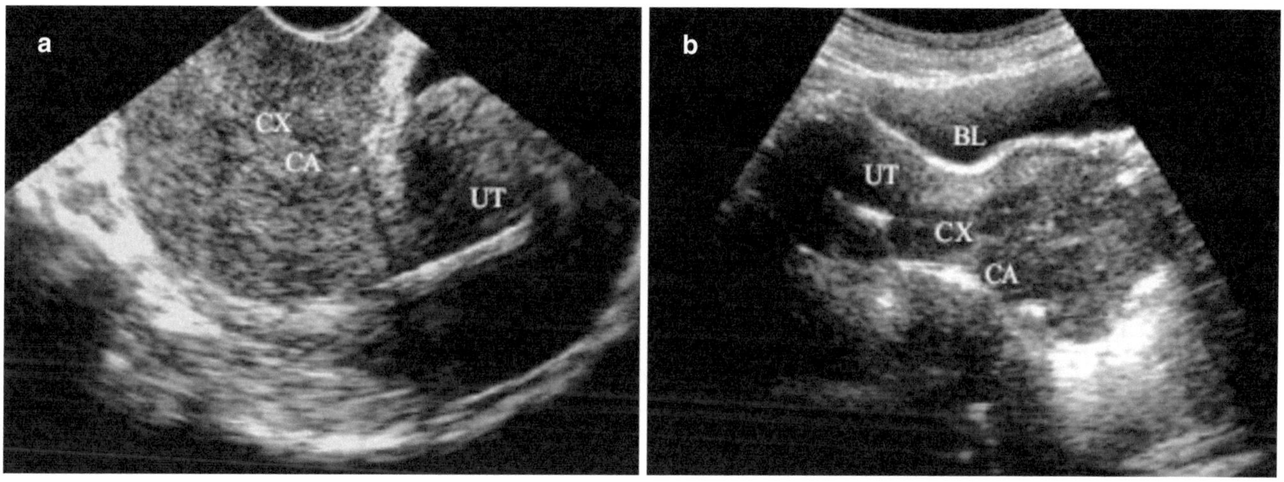

Fig. 5.47 Cervical cancer (I). (**a**) Sagittal view of TVS shows a larger cervical diameter compared with the uterine anteroposterior dimension, and the cervix is hypoechoic. (**b**) Transabdominal ultrasonography shows a larger cervical diameter compared with the uterine anteroposterior dimension, and the cervical canal is disappeared, accompanied by the abnormal cervical morphology

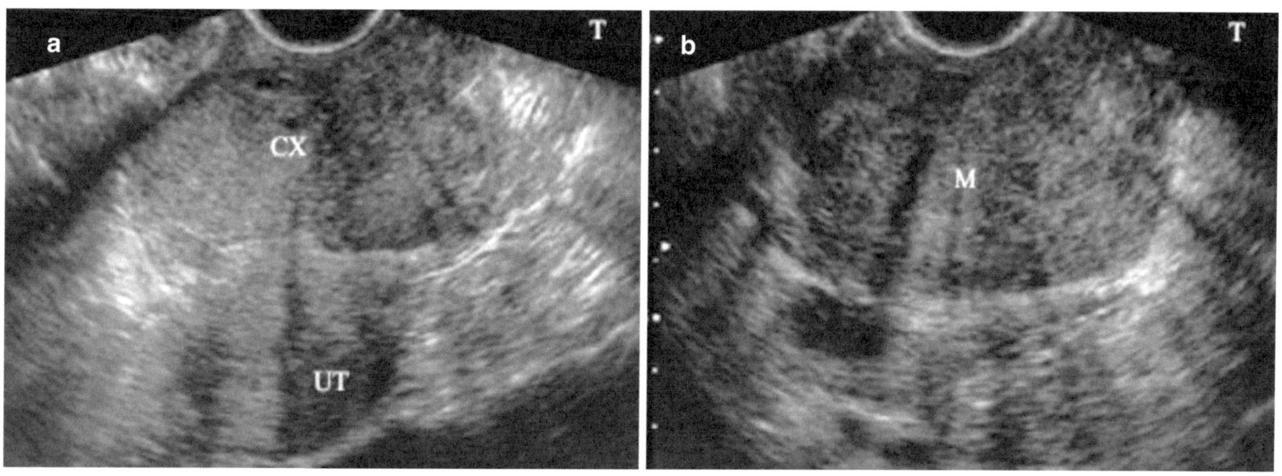

Fig. 5.48 Cervical cancer (II). A 59-year-old patient with a postmenopausal period of 7 years represented vaginal bleeding for 3 months. (**a**) Ultrasonic images show atrophic corpus, abnormal cervical morphology, and an irregular mass with a diameter of about 7.0 cm. (**b**) Transverse images show the mass of the same patient

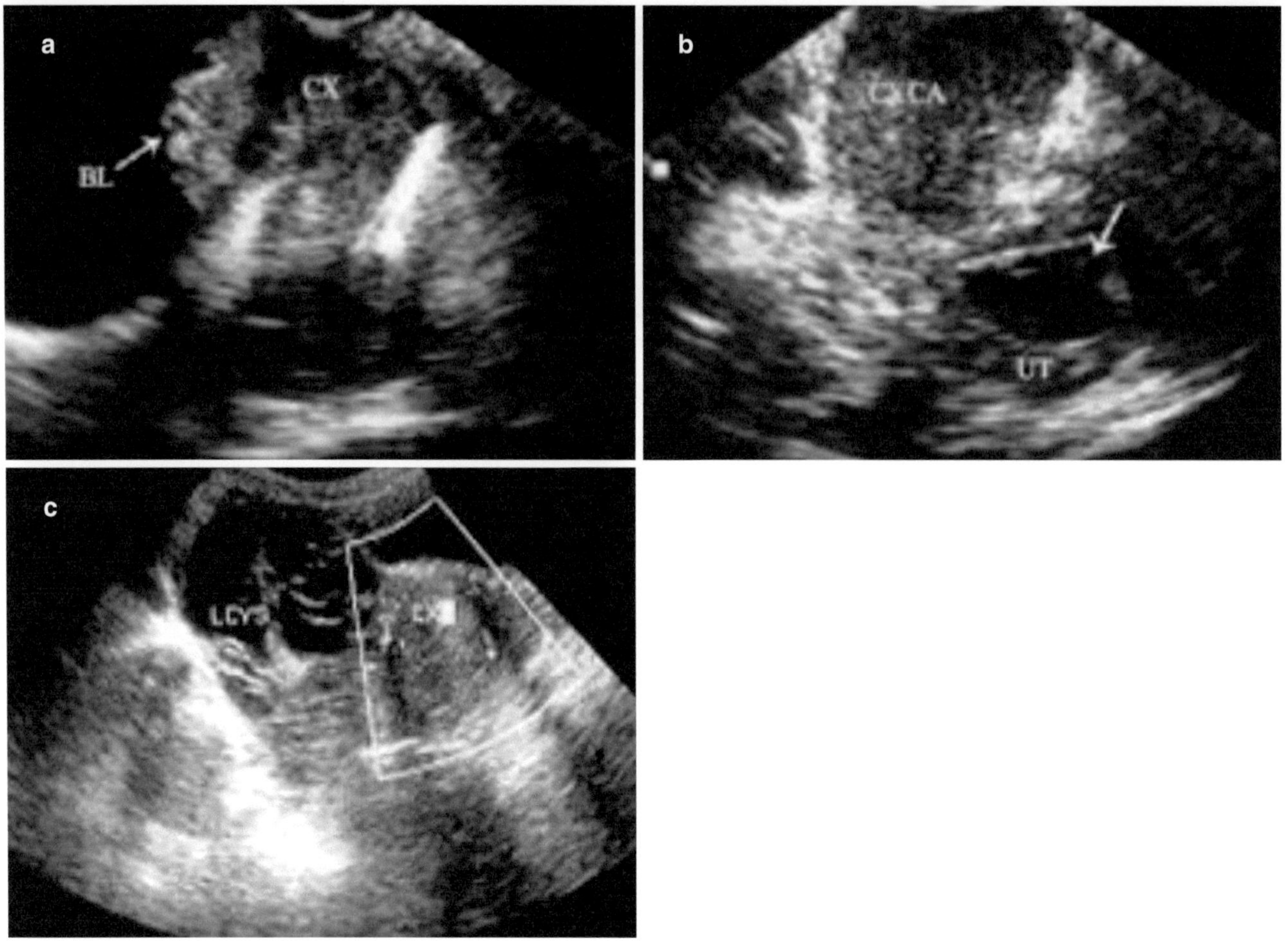

Fig. 5.49 Cervical cancer infiltration. (**a**) Sonogram shows the enlarged cervix with abnormal shape, and the mass infiltrated into the bladder wall (arrow). (**b**) Sonogram shows the enlarged cervix without the normal cervical canal, obstructed internal os, and uterine effusion (arrow). (**c**) Sonogram shows the irregular parametrial cystic lesion, indicating parametrial invasion

the myometrium or the connective tissue in the myometrium. Uterine sarcomas are susceptible in perimenopausal women but also can occur in young women.

According to the different original tissues, sarcomas are mainly divided into the following types: (1) Leiomyosarcoma of the uterus, which arises from the myometrium or the smooth muscle fibers of the uterine vascular wall, or from the malignant transformation of uterine fibroids. (2) Endometrial stromal sarcoma, which is derived from endometrial stromal cells and divided into low-grade and high-grade malignant stromal sarcoma. (3) Malignant mixed müllerian disease, also known as carcinosarcoma, arises from residual embryonic cells or interstitial cells metaplasia.

The main clinical symptom is vaginal bleeding, which is characterized by an excessive volume of menses, irregular bleeding, or postmenopausal bleeding. The amount of the blood varies from bloody leucorrhea to purulent discharge with a peculiar smell. Some patients have no obvious symptoms and are diagnosed as palpable abdominal mass. Advanced patients may represent anemia, cachexia, lower abdominal pain, backache, and so on. Gynecological examination revealed an enlarged, irregular, and soft uterus, even occupying the whole pelvic cavity.

(II) Ultrasonic diagnosis

- Ultrasonic scanning shows the myoma grows rapidly within a short time, with obvious attenuation, and it is difficult to recognize the three-layer structure of the uterus (Fig. 5.53).
- A large solid mass is visible in the pelvic cavity, while the uterus is pressed to the side. Normal uterine morphology fails to be shown in some cases (Fig. 5.54).
- Ultrasonography shows heterogeneous or disordered echo in large myomas.

(III) Special tips

- When a patient with a history of uterine fibroids represents rapidly fibroids enlargement within a short

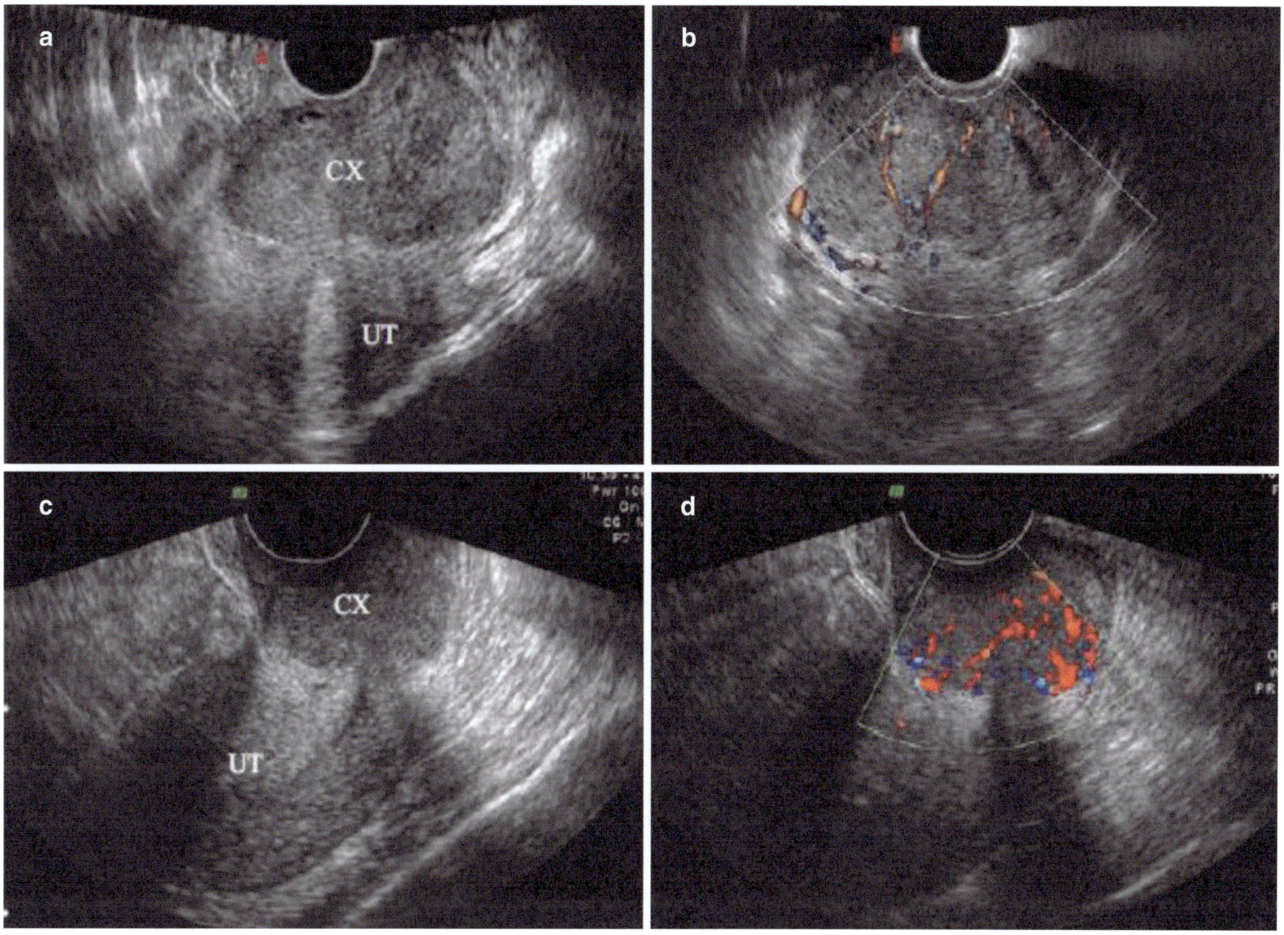

Fig. 5.50 The blood flow of cervical sarcoma and cervical cancer. A 51-year-old patient represented recurrent vaginal bleeding four times. (**a**) Sonogram shows the abnormal cervix morphology, absent endocervical endometrium, with the cervical diameter larger than the corpus. (**b**) In the same patient, color Doppler shows abundant blood flow in the cervical tumor. Pathological diagnosis of cervical sarcoma is confirmed. (**c**) A 67-year-old patient represented with irregular vaginal bleeding history for half a year. Sagittal view of TVS shows an obvious enlargement of the cervix. (**d**) Sagittal view of the same patient. Abundant blood flow is shown in the cervical lesions by color Doppler. Cancer cells are found on the cervical smear and cervical carcinoma is diagnosed by operation and pathological examination

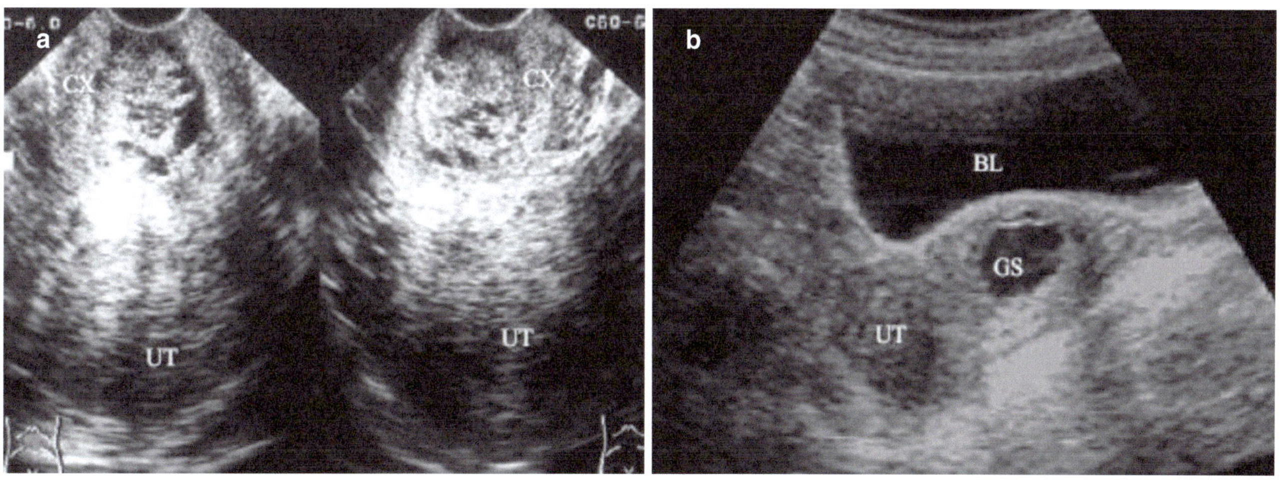

Fig. 5.51 The differentiation of cervical cancer and cervical pregnancy. (**a**) A cervical cancer patient shows an abnormal cervix with an enlarged diameter and hCG is negative. (**b**) The cervix is "barrel-like" enlarged, with gestational sac or heterogeneous hyperechoic tissue in the cervical canal, and hCG is positive

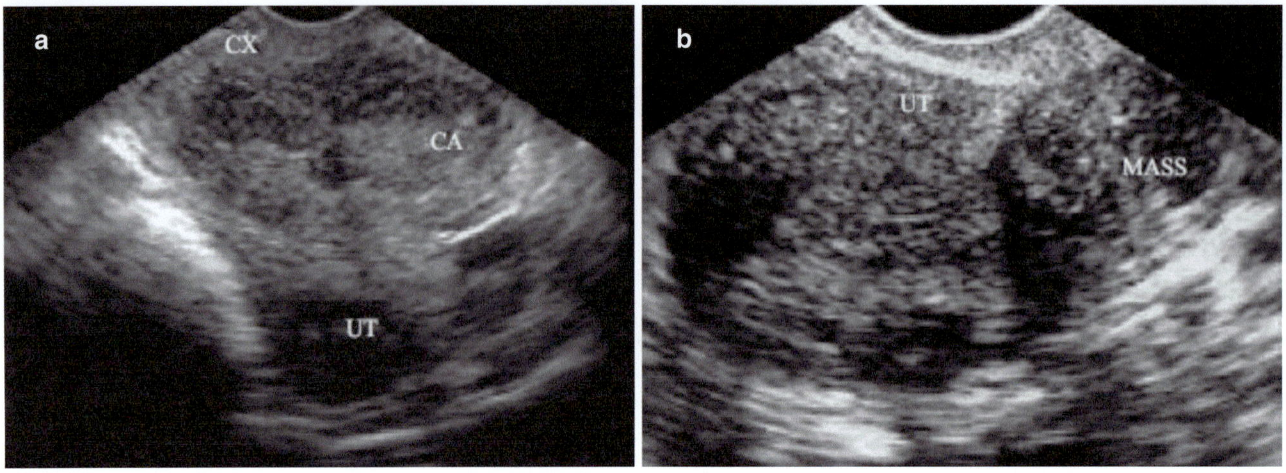

Fig. 5.52 The differentiation of cervical cancer and cervical myoma. (**a**) A cervical cancer patient. Sonogram shows the larger cervical diameter compared with the corpus, abnormal cervical morphology, and irregular and heterogeneous mass. (**b**) Cervical leiomyoma, which is mostly located in the posterior labium of the cervix, is usually well-defined, and the endocervical endometrium is visible by altering the scanning angle

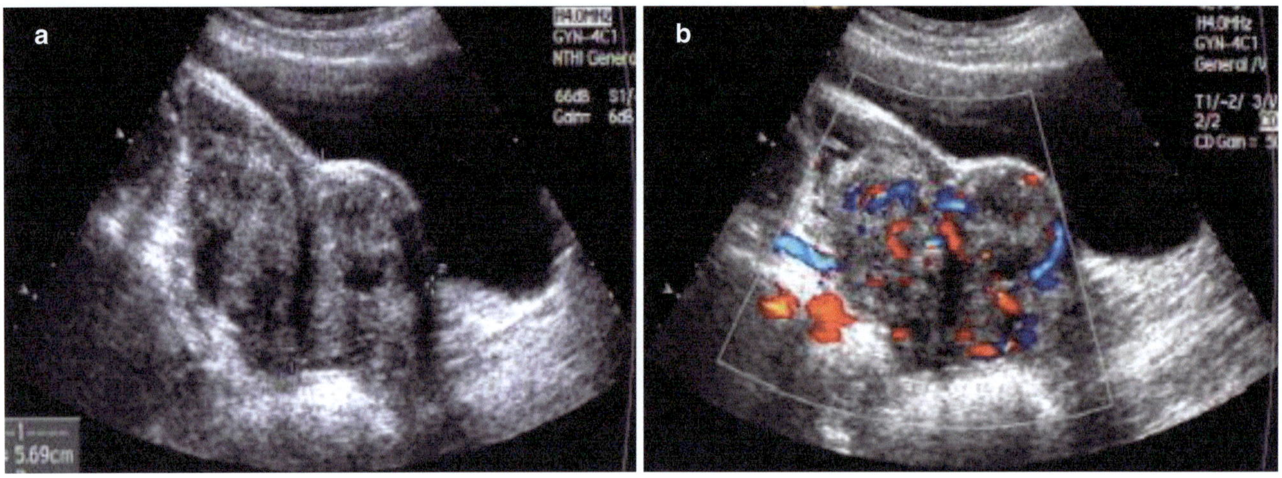

Fig. 5.53 Uterine sarcoma. A 17-year-old female patient recurred with fibroids 1 year after myomectomy. (**a**) 2-D TAS shows multiple hypoechoic masses conglobated together in the myometrium of the right lower segment area and subserosal area, with the size of about 5.7 cm × 8.1 cm × 7.8 cm. The other one is located in the right anterior area of myometrium with the size of 2.2 cm × 2.9 cm × 2.9 cm. (**b**) Abundant blood flow signals are shown in the masses and peripheral area. Pathology confirmed the diagnosis of uterine leiomyosarcoma

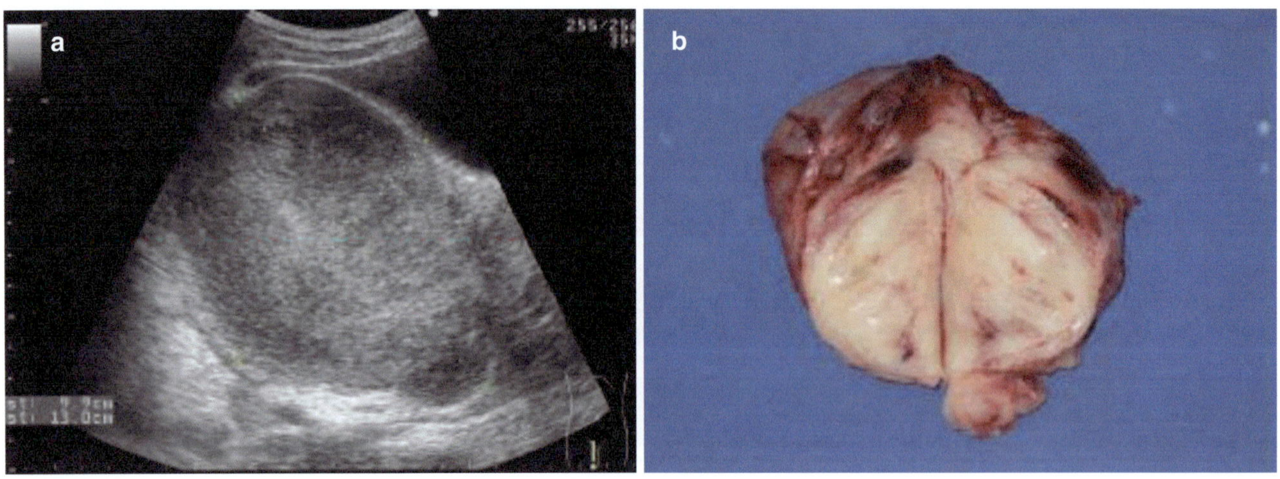

Fig. 5.54 Pelvic sarcoma. An 18-year-old patient experienced left lower abdominal pain for 1 month. Ultrasound image shows a mass in the pelvic cavity. (**a**) TAS shows a solid mass in the pelvic cavity, which is measured comparably to the uterus of 16 gestational weeks. The uterus is challenging to be recognized. (**b**) The gross specimen. Pathological diagnosis is embryonal rhabdomyosarcoma

time, it should be a concern for the clinicians. The characteristics of the uterine echo and the three-layer structure should be identified during ultrasonic scanning.

- Sarcomas should be distinguished from huge benign uterine fibroids and ovarian tumors. Women of childbearing age should be paid more attention to bilateral ovaries.

5.7 Ultrasonic Diagnosis of Abnormal Development of Female Reproductive Organs

(I) Basic concepts

- At the third to fourth gestational weeks, primordial germ cells appear in the yolk-sac endoderm. At the fourth to fifth week, a genitourinary crista is formed. At the fourth to sixth week, primordial germ cells migrate to genitourinary crista to form primordial gonad. At the eighth week, primordial gonad differentiates into the ovary.
- After the gonads develop into ovaries, the mesonephric tube on the lateral side of the urogenital ridge degenerates. The head segments of the accessory mesonephric tubes on both sides form two fallopian tubes, and the middle and tail segments on both sides combine to form the uterus and the upper segment of the vagina. At the early stage of syncopation, there is still a septum, which divides the syncopation into two chambers. The septum disappears at the end of 12 weeks and becomes a single lumen. The caudal end of the accessory mesonephric duct is connected with the urogenital sinus, meanwhile, it divides and proliferates to form the vagina cavity.
- The abnormalities caused by the obstruction of normal duct formation of female reproductive organs include hymen atresia, vagina transverse, vagina mediastinum, congenital vagina atresia, and cervical atresia, etc. The abnormal uterine development caused by the hypoplasia or fusion obstacle of accessory mesonephric duct derivative includes a congenital absence of uterus, primordial uterus, uterine dysplasia (immature uterus), unicornuate uterus, uterus duplex, and uterus bicornis, saddle form uterus, mediastinal uterus, etc.
- The clinical manifestations of female congenital malformation are as follows:
  - No menarche after puberty accompanied by periodic lower abdominal pain may experience following diseases, such as imperforate hymen, vaginal septum (diaphragm or oblique septum), partial atresia of the vagina and congenital cervical atresia, etc.
  - No menarche after puberty should be distinguished from the following situations, such as ametria, primordial uterus, and immature uterus, etc.
  - Patients with dyspareunia after marriage, recurrent abortions, premature delivery or infertility, should be examined to exclude the following conditions, such as the congenital absence of vagina, ametria, vaginal septum, vagina atresia, unicornuate uterus, uterus bicornis, and uterus septus, etc.

(II) Ultrasonic diagnosis

- Congenital absence of uterus is also called ametria. No uterus is visible by both TVS and TAS behind the bladder. Relatively smaller ovaries can be detected on both sides of the pelvic cavity in most patients. Congenital absence of uterus is often combined with congenital absence of vagina, resulting in the absence of vaginal gas line (Fig. 5.55).

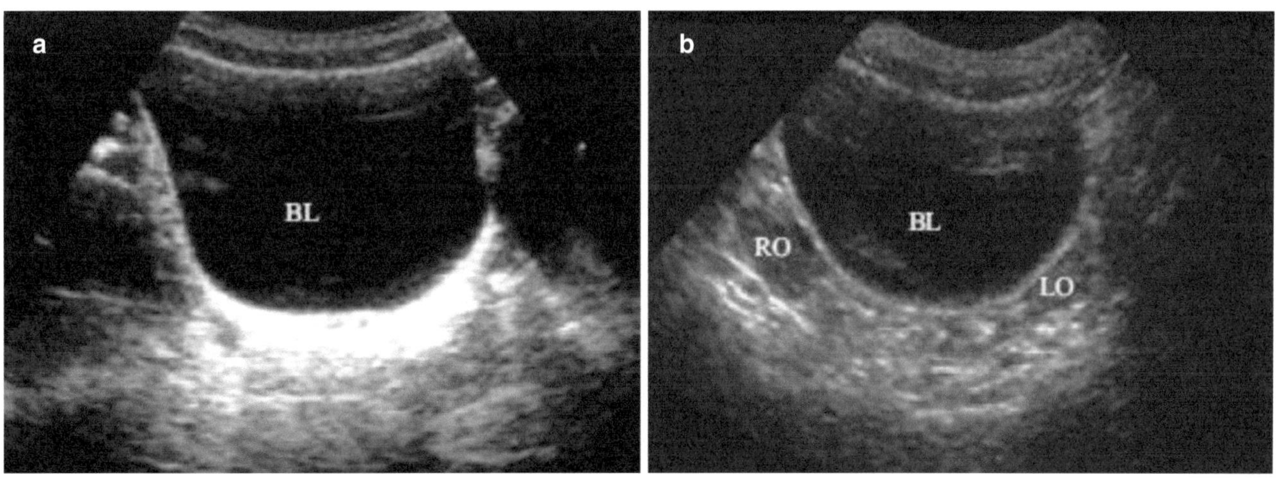

Fig. 5.55 Congenital absence of uterus. (**a**) TAS. No uterus is visible behind the filled bladder. (**b**) Bilateral ovaries are shown by TAS

- Rudimentary uterus. Transabdominal or transvaginal ultrasonic images show only a small cord-like hyperechoic mass behind the filled bladder. No normal uterine morphology or endometrium is shown. Ovaries can be found on both sides of the pelvic cavity in some patients (Fig. 5.56).
- Hypoplasia of uterus (infantile uterus). The uterus is shown in the pelvic cavity with a shorter anteroposterior dimension, length, and width compared to normal uterus. The anteroposterior dimension is less than 2 cm. The endometrium is unclear or in a thin line shape (Fig. 5.57).
- Uterus didephys. Ultrasonography shows two separate uterus and two separate uterine cavities. When the transabdominal ultrasonic examination is used, it should be transversely scanned from the fundus to the cervix and vagina, or from the vagina to the cervix and fundus. On the transverse view, the fundus shows like a butterfly. When moving down the probe to the uterine body, the transverse diameter of the uterine body is wider than normal. Then the two cervical canals and vaginal gas lines can be displayed when the probe is a slant to the posterior pubis. In the longitudinal scanning, place the probe on the lower abdomen and move slowly to the opposite side, two separate uteruses are displayed in turn (Figs. 5.58 and 5.59).
- Uterus bicornis or arcuate uterus. Transabdominal transverse scanning shows two uterine horns similar to the shape of sheep's horn in the level of the fundus, accompanied by a separate uterine cavity. The lower segment of the uterine and cervix usually represents normal. When the probe is moved to scan the uterine body longitudinally, two uterus images may be shown, while only one cervix and vagina can be found. When the uterus

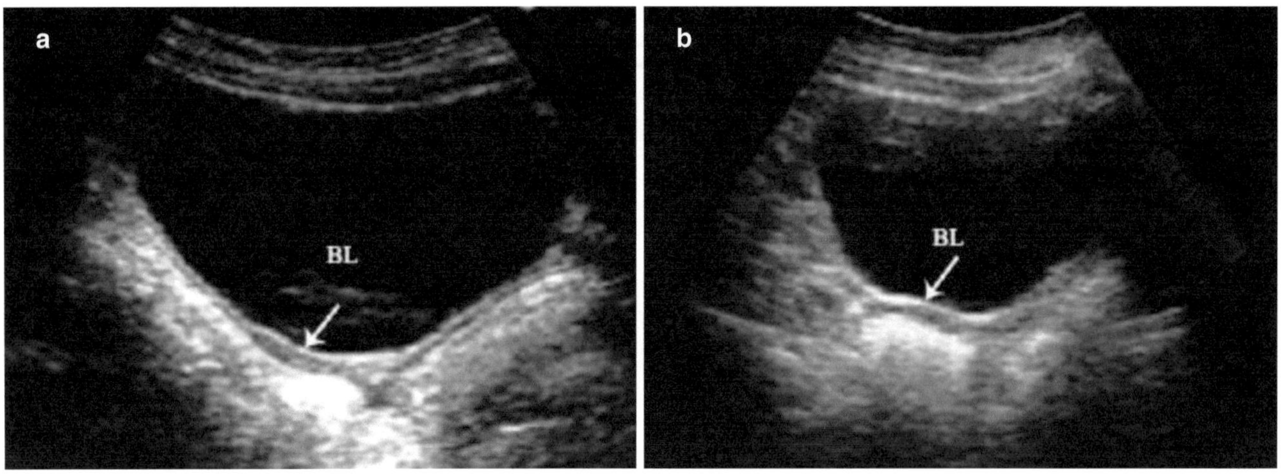

Fig. 5.56 Rudimentary uterus. (**a**) TAS shows a cord-like hyperechoic mass in the pelvic cavity. No uterus and endometrium are shown. (**b**) TAS shows no ovary. Primordial uterus is shown by the arrow

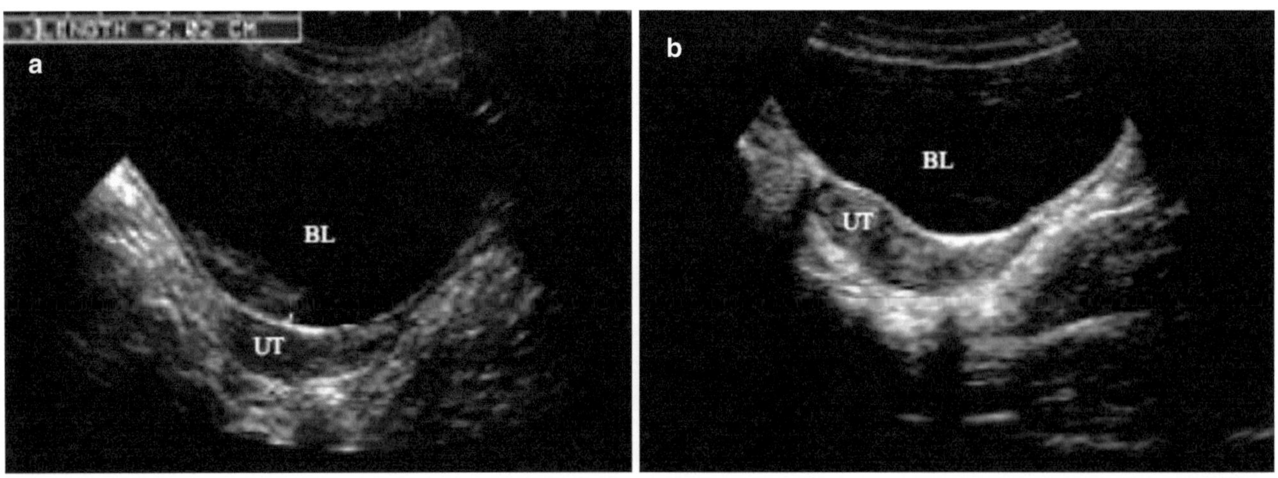

Fig. 5.57 Hypoplasia of uterus. (**a**) A 21-year-old patient represented with no menarche. TAS shows the anteroposterior dimension of uterus is 1.8 cm, without endometrium shown. (**b**) A 19-year-old patient represented oligomenorrhea and hypomenorrhea. The size of the uterus is 2.2 cm × 4.4 cm × 2.0 cm and the endometrial is extremely thin

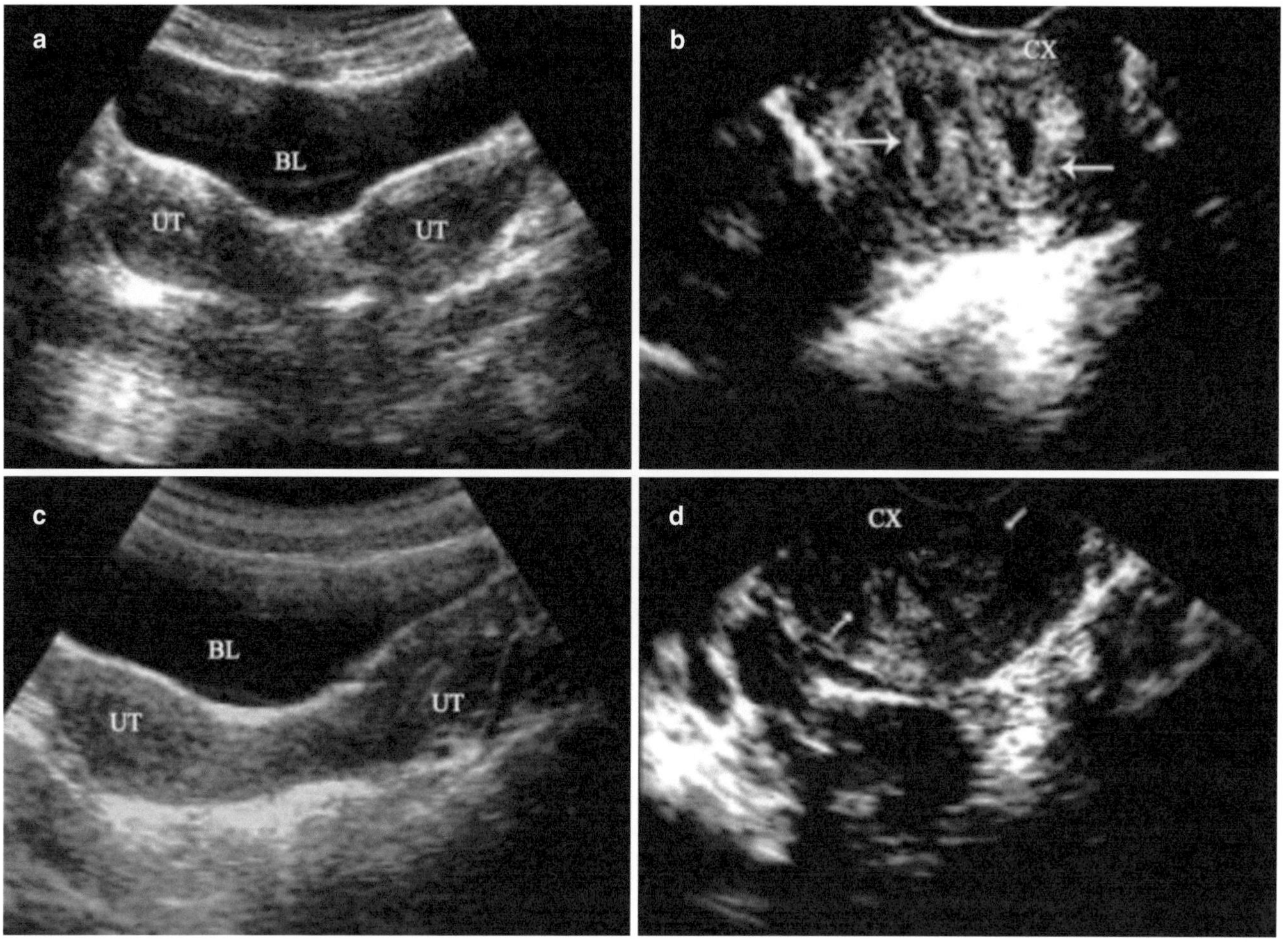

Fig. 5.58 Uterus didephys. (**a**, **b**) TAS shows two separate uteruses with separate endometrium by transverse scanning. TVS shows two cervical canals. (**c**, **d**) TAS shows similar results with a and b

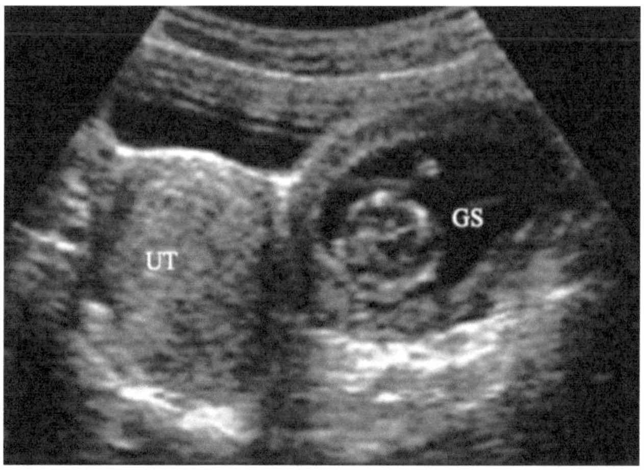

Fig. 5.59 Uterus didephys with pregnancy. TAS shows gestational sac in left uterus with an enlarged right uterus and thickened endometrium

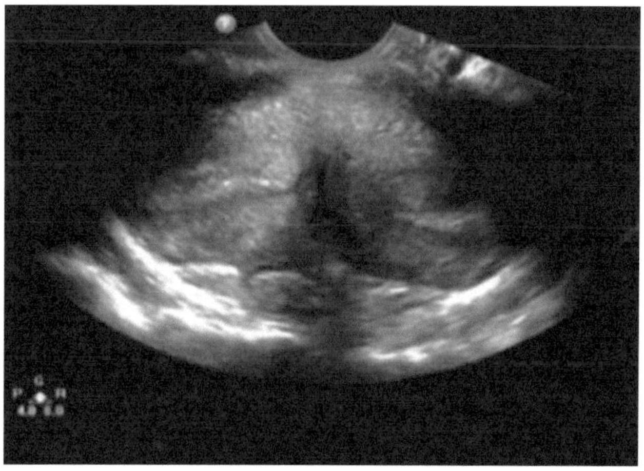

Fig. 5.60 Uterus bicornis. TVS shows the separate endometrium on the left and right side in a similar shape of a Chinese character "八" in the uterine cavity. The myometrium of the fundus is depressed into the cavity

bicornis shows a concave uterine fundus on transverse section, it is also called arcuate uterus (Fig. 5.60).

- Uterus septus. No obvious changes can be found in the contour and morphology of the uterus. The transverse images show the wider fundus with a larger transverse diameter than normal. The uterine cavity shows similarly with the shape of the Chinese character "八" or the English letter "Y." Two separate endometriums are visible from the fundus to the cervix in the complete septate uterus, from left to right or from anterior to posterior. Partial uterus septus is characterized by the attenuated septal echo between endometrium, as the septum does not extend from the fundus to the cervix (Figs. 5.61 and 5.62).

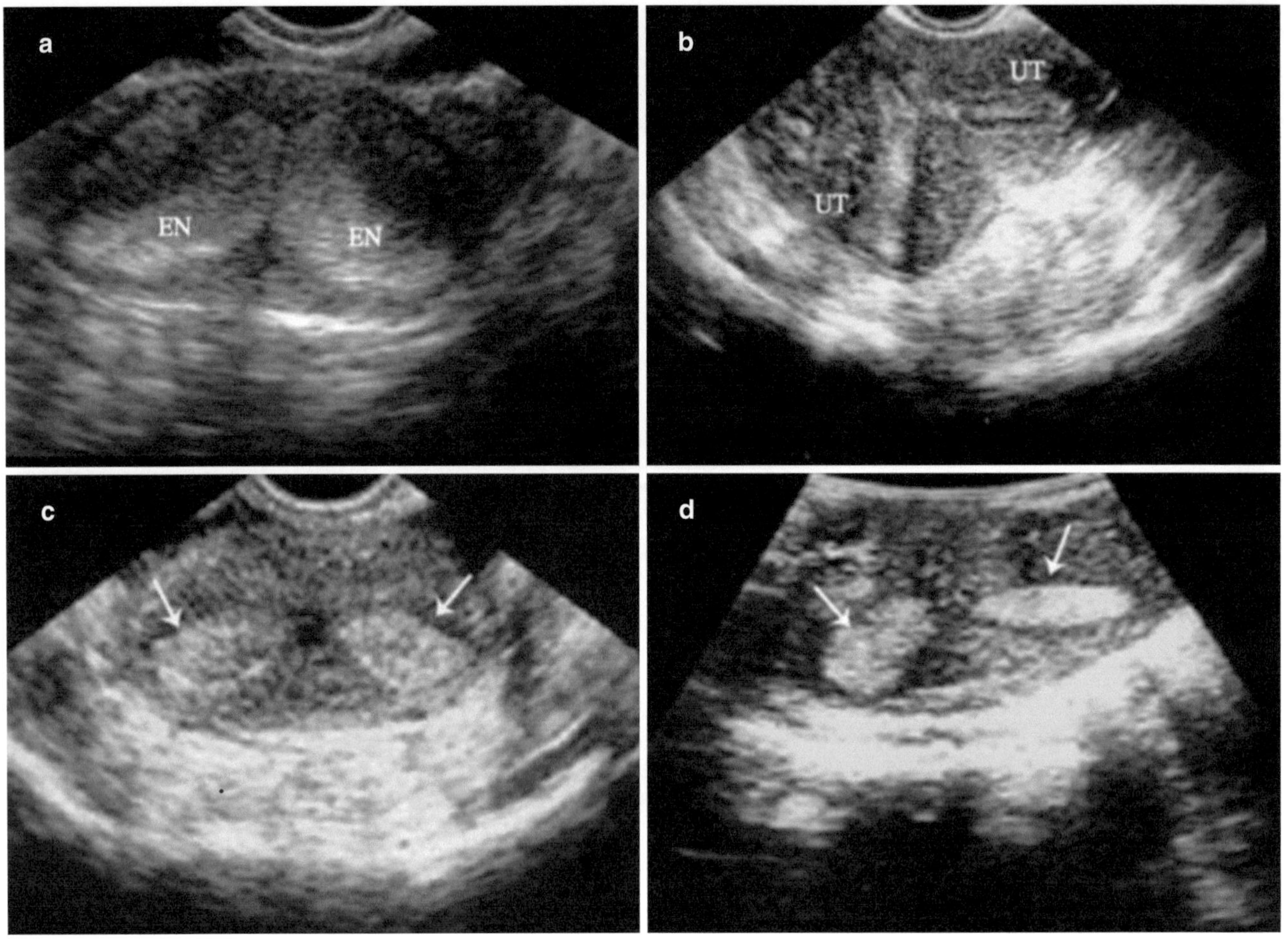

Fig. 5.61 Septate uterus. (**a**) Complete septate uterus is shown on the coronal plane. (**b**) The endometrium is shown as the shape of letter "Y" on the coronal view. (**c**) The transverse image of the uterus shows the typical endometrial morphology similar to "cat's eye" (arrow). (**d**) The transverse view of the uterus showed the endometrium in the shape of the Chinese word "八" (arrow)

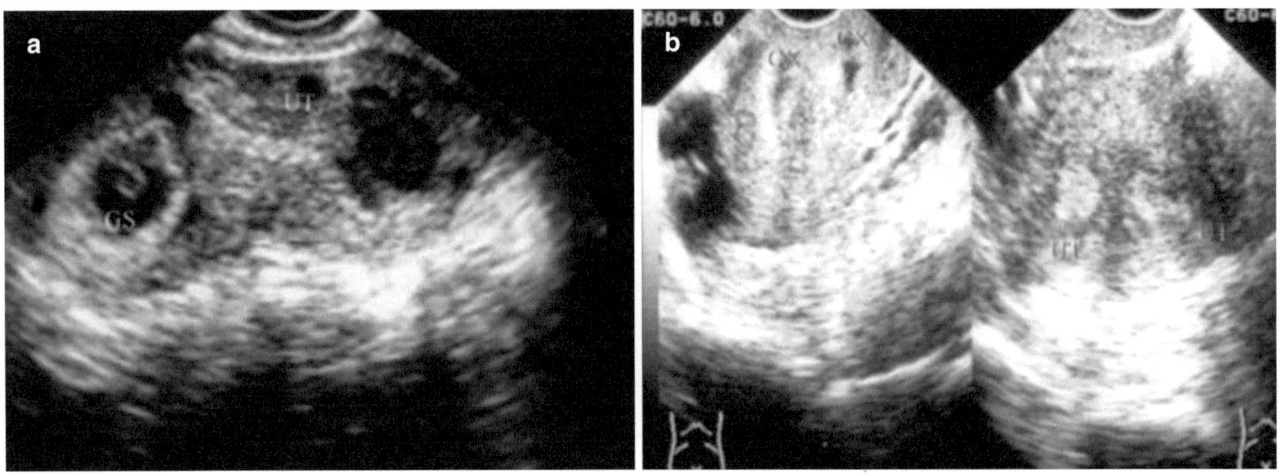

Fig. 5.62 Septate uterus with pregnancy. (**a**) Septate uterus with early pregnancy in the right cavity. (**b**) Transvaginal ultrasonography shows only one uterine body and two endometriums from the fundus to the cervix

- Rudimentary horn of uterus. A normal uterus can be seen in the pelvis with a solid mass on either side of the uterus. The echo of mass is similar to the non-pregnant uterus, without endometrium. It is easy to be confused with subserosal myoma. A small amount of fluid may be found in some rudimentary uterus. When pregnancy occurs in the rudimentary horn, the diagnosis of rudimentary horn of uterus may be considered (Fig. 5.63).
- Congenital imperforate hymen. Sonogram shows the normal uterus, saccular or oval dilatation from cervix to the vagina, with weak or enhanced echo inside. Some patients combined with uterine cavity dilatation and cervix dilatation (Fig. 5.64).
- Atrasia of vagina or vaginal septum. Sonogram shows the normal uterus, dilatated uterine cavity or cervix, and vaginal dilatation above the vaginal septum or oblique septum. Patients with a relatively longer history of the disease may accompany dilation of bilateral fallopian tube or bilateral adnexal masses, with retention of menses inside (Fig. 5.65).

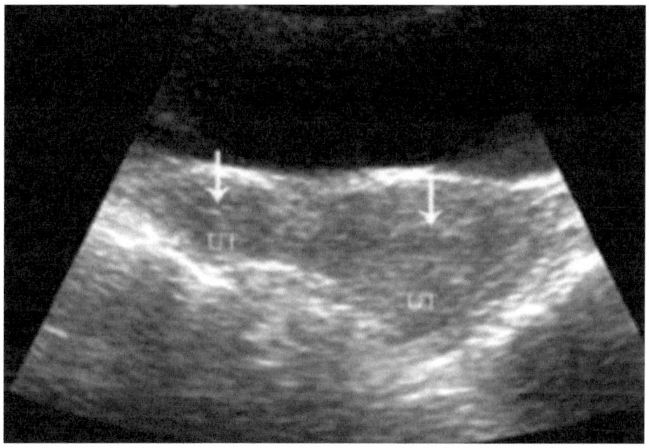

Fig. 5.63 Rudimentary horn of uterus. TAS shows a normal uterus in the pelvis and a solid mass located on its right side with endometrial echo

(III) Special tips

- There are many different types of female congenital genital malformation. Various scanning methods are recommended. TAS is utilized to show the position and structure of the uterus for further diagnosis of the uterus didephys, uterus bicornis, and septate uterus. The endometrial echo is an important sign to identify uterine malformation.
- Attention should be paid to differentiate bicornate uterus and rudimentary horn uterus from subserosal myoma and ovarian mass.
- Female congenital genital malformation may be combined with malformation of urinary system, such as the absence of kidney, ectopic kidney, etc. (Fig. 5.66).
- When it is difficult to identify the malformation of uterus by two-dimensional ultrasound, sonographic hysterography can be performed to show the endometrium and uterine cavity more clearly (Fig. 5.67).

5.8 Ultrasonic Diagnosis of Ovarian Masses in Pelvic Cavity

The ovary is an important reproductive organ in the female pelvic cavity. The ovary is small while the ovarian histoembryology, anatomy, and endocrine function are extremely complex. The type, morphology, and nature of the ovarian mass are various. The traditional diagnostic method of ovarian masses is pelvic bimanual examination. The examiners evaluate the ovarian size, shape, and texture by hand, which

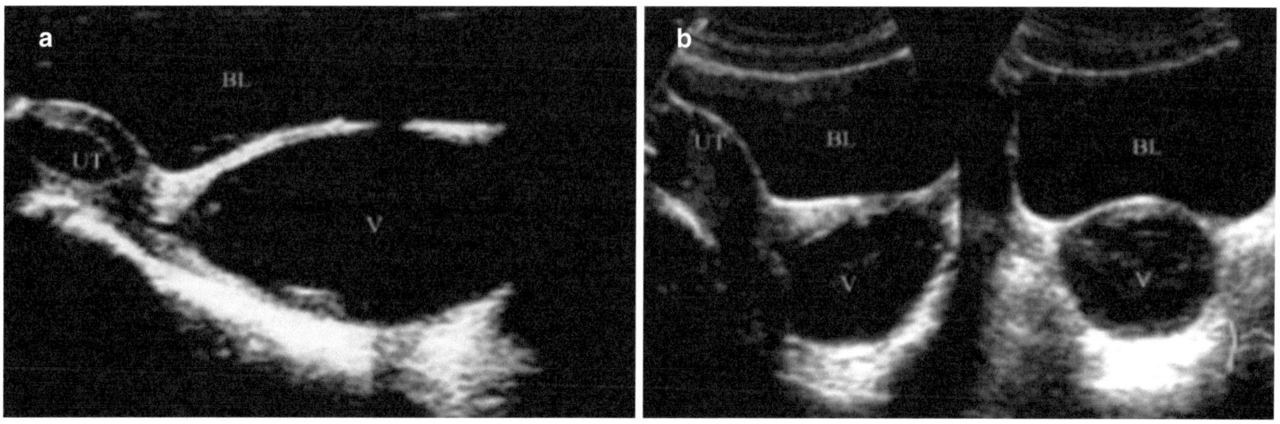

Fig. 5.64 Congenital imperforate hymen. (**a**) A 14-year-old patient represented periodic lower abdominal pain for 4 months. TAS shows a normal uterus with fluid area in the uterine cavity, and cystic dilatation from the lower cervix to the vagina. (**b**) An 11-year-old patient represented periodic pain in the lower abdomen for half a year. TAS shows normal uterus and cystic dilatation of the vagina with tiny and weak echo inside

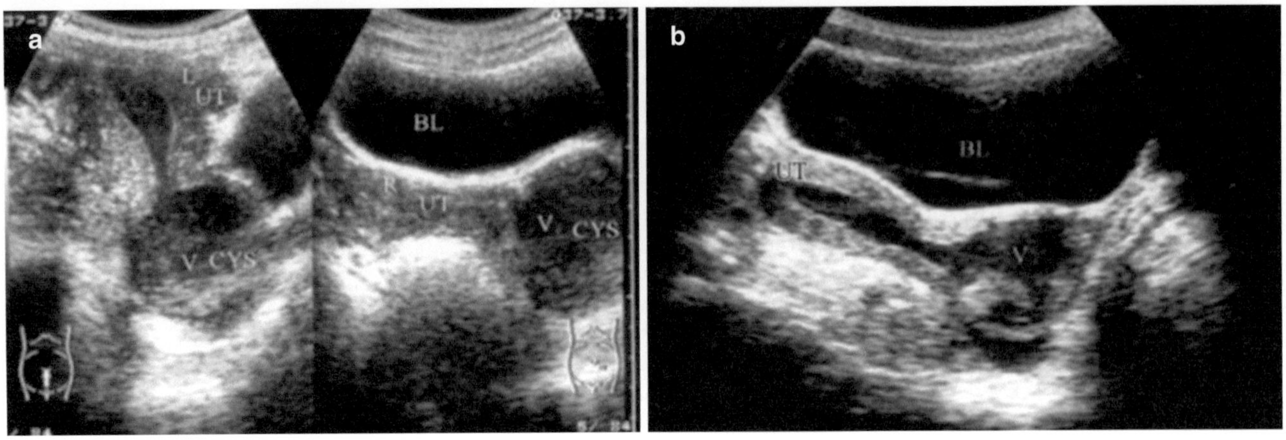

Fig. 5.65 Atrasia of vagina (**a**) A 15-year-old patient had menstruation for 2 years with dysmenorrhea. TAS shows two uteruses, with hematometra in the right uterine cavity and vagina. The fluid area in the uterine cavity is connected with the vagina. The left uterus is slightly smaller than the right one, with normal morphology. Uterus didephys with atresia of the right vagina is confirmed by operation. (**b**) A 14-year-old patient represented with secondary amenorrhea and periodic lower abdominal pain for 1+ years. Sagittal TAS shows intrauterine hematometra connected with the fluid area in the middle and upper segments of the vagina. Adhesion and atresia of lower segment of vagina are diagnosed after operation

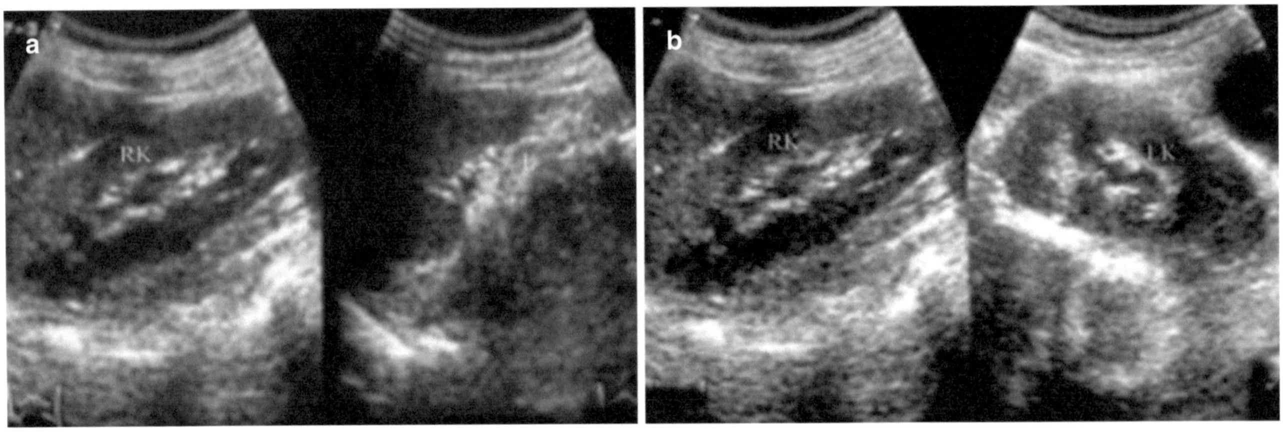

Fig. 5.66 The absence of kidney (**a**) and ectopic kidney (**b**) A 28-year-old patient represented with primary amenorrhea. Ultrasonography shows no uterus and ovary, with absent left kidney and normal right kidney. (**b**) No uterus or ovary is shown in the pelvis, and the left kidney is found in pelvic cavity

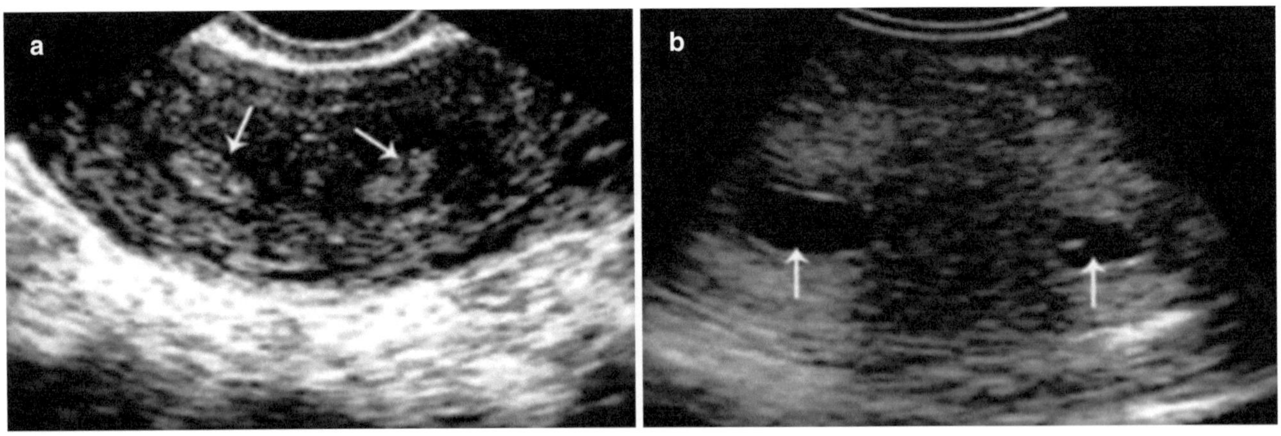

Fig. 5.67 Sonographic hysterography. (**a**) Transverse scanning shows "cat's eye sign" of endometrium in septate uterus before hysterography. (**b**) Hysterography with saline shows the relationship between the uterine cavity and septum

is difficult to detect early masses. When the masses can be palpable by bimanual examination, most patients are already in the middle and late stage of the tumor. In recent years, with the rapid development of imaging technology, CT and MRI can clearly show the mass less than 5 mm, lymph node metastasis, and ascites. However, due to the high price, it is limited to screen early ovarian masses. The serum markers for the diagnosis of ovarian cancer (CA125, AFP) are one of the screening tools for ovarian cancer, while the screening sensitivity needs to be improved.

Recently, the application of ultrasonography in the diagnosis of ovarian diseases has shown obvious advantages. Transvaginal ultrasound scanning is especially well which can clearly show the physical properties and size of ovarian masses and provide valuable information for the clinician. Transvaginal Color Doppler ultrasonography is used in the diagnosis of ovarian tumors, which can obtain clear two-dimensional images. Moreover, it is helpful for the diagnosis and differentiation of benign and malignant ovarian masses by measurement of blood flow signals and the vascular resistance index. Due to the different characteristics of ovarian masses, the ultrasonic images are complex and diverse. Meanwhile, a given disease may be shown as different images and different diseases may be revealed as similar images. As a result, it is relatively difficult to determine the type of ovarian masses by ultrasound. According to the ultrasonic characteristics and clinical and pathological changes, the ultrasonic diagnosis of ovarian masses will be discussed in this section, including non-tumor cyst and ovarian tumor.

I. Non-tumor cysts
- Basic concepts

  Most of the non-neoplastic cysts are retention cysts due to functional changes of the ovaries, mostly appeared in women of childbearing age. They are often associated with menstrual cycle, pregnancy, and endocrine disorders, and sometimes be related to iatrogenic medication. Most of these cysts can be absorbed by their own.

  The volume of ovarian non-neoplastic cyst is generally small, with a diameter of 3–5 cm. Most of them have no clinical symptoms, while some of them can cause uterine functional bleeding, or irregular vaginal bleeding, menstrual disorders and so on. If the cyst ruptures or twists, acute abdominal pain can occur suddenly. Ovarian non-neoplastic cysts include follicular cysts, luteal cysts, luteinized cysts, parovarian cysts, polycystic ovaries, fallopian tube-ovarian cysts, simple cysts, and ovarian endometriotic cysts, etc.
- Ultrasonic diagnosis
  - Follicular cysts

    Mature follicles fail to rupture, ovulate, or atresia during menstrual cycles, and then the follicular fluid accumulates in the follicle cavity leading to cysts formation in females.

    The diameter of the follicular cyst is generally less than 5.0 cm, round-shaped with thin-wall, well-circumscribed, and the fluid in the cyst is clear. Unilateral cyst is more common and most of them can vanish on their own during routine observation (Fig. 5.68).
  - Corpus luteum cyst.

    The disordered blood and lymphatic supply of the corpus luteum from the ovary, or the formation of the hematoma in the corpus luteum, leads to the accumulation of clear fluid in the corpus luteum and results in cysts. This kind of cyst mostly belongs to the physiological lesion. Some of them are accompanied by delayed menstruation. The cysts will disappear naturally after menstrual onset. Similar corpus luteum cyst may also occur in early pregnancy disappear during the second trimester.

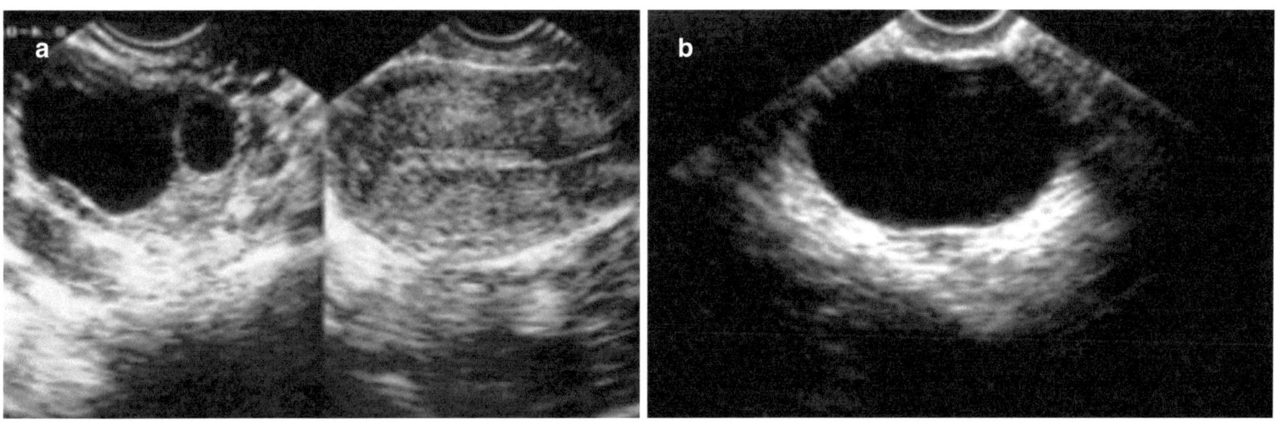

Fig. 5.68 Follicular cysts. (**a**) Sonogram shows a cyst, 2.6 cm in diameter, with clear fluid and thin wall. (**b**) Sonogram shows a cyst, 4.0 cm in diameter, with clear fluid and thin wall. The cyst absorbed naturally during routine observation

The corpus luteum cyst is mostly isolated with a translucent wall. It is usually glossy in appearance, mostly monolocular and round-shaped, with a diameter less than 5.0 cm. Color Doppler ultrasound shows abundant blood flow inside (Fig. 5.69).

– Theca-lutein cyst

Theca-lutein cyst refers to the luteinization of theca cells on the wall of the follicular cyst, which is related to gonadal hormones from the placental, dysfunction of hypothalamic–pituitary–gonadal axis, application of ovulation induction drugs, and other factors. Theca-lutein cyst is more common in patients diagnosed as hydatidiform mole, with an incidence of 35–50%.

Bilateral theca-lutein cysts are more common, with a diameter of 20 cm or more, while some tiny ones can only be diagnosed under the microscope. The serum β-hCG level in patients with trophoblastic disease is significantly higher than in normal pregnancy. The masses are shown as multilocular cysts with uneven surfaces and thin septa. A clear liquid is visible in the cysts, with good acoustic transmission. The theca-lutein cysts can disappear after the primary disease is cured (Fig. 5.70).

– Polycystic ovary, POC

The basic pathological change of polycystic ovary is homogeneously enlarged bilateral or unilateral ovaries, which is 2–3 times larger than normal with a smooth surface and thick capsule. The membrane of the ovary is thickened and the cortex is widened. Multiple follicles less than 1.0 cm usually locate peripherally along the envelope as "pearl strings"

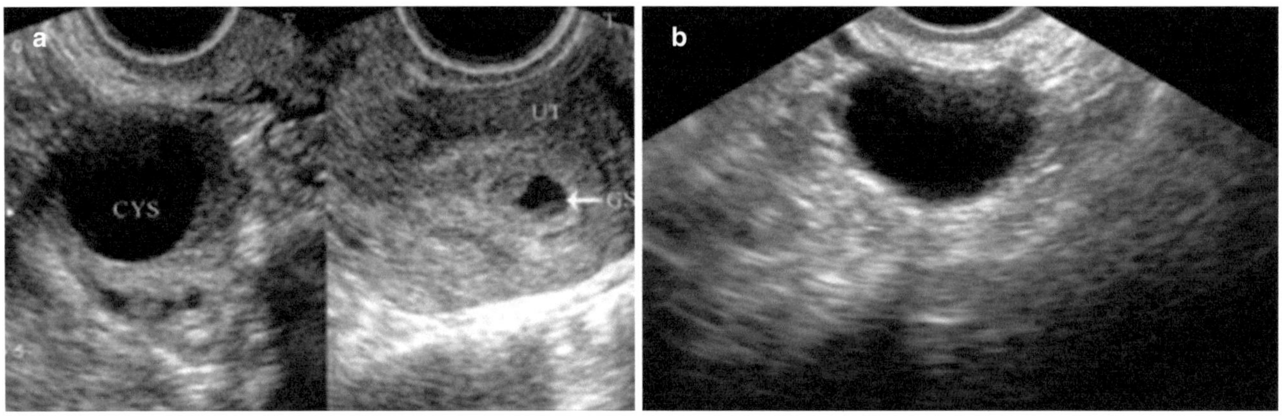

Fig. 5.69 Corpus luteum cyst. (**a**) On the 42nd day of pregnancy, ultrasonography shows intrauterine gestational sac and embryo. A mass with a diameter of about 3.0 cm is found in the right ovary, and the cystic fluid is clear. (**b**) On the patient's 35th day of amenorrhea, hCG is negative. Ultrasound scanning shows normal uterus without an intrauterine gestational sac. A mass with a diameter of about 3.0 cm is found in the left ovary, with clear cystic fluid. The cyst disappeared after menstrual onset

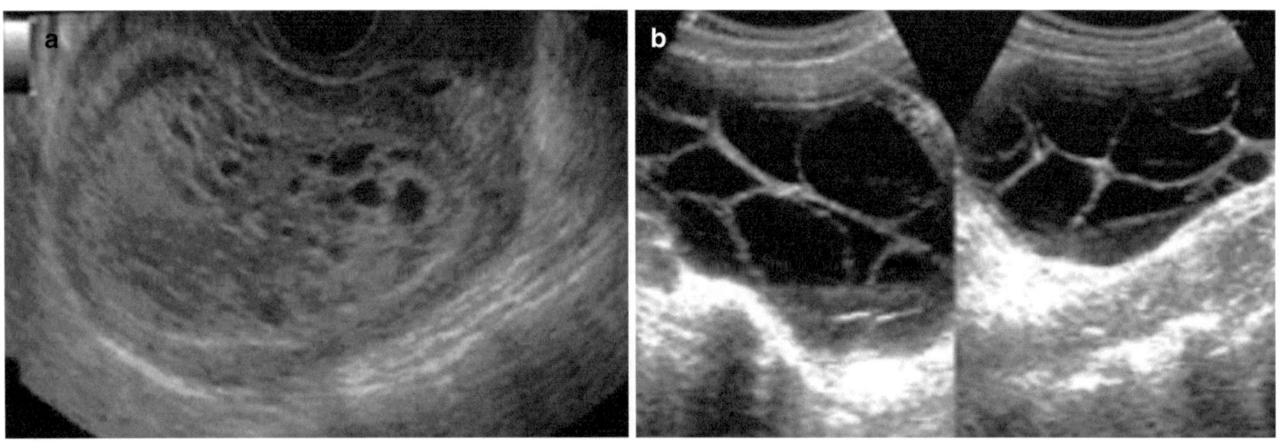

Fig. 5.70 Theca-lutein cyst. (**a**) The uterine cavity represents "honeycomb-like" echo in a patient with hydatidiform mole. (**b**) Bilateral theca-lutein cysts are shown in the same patient and then disappeared after the hydatidiform mole is cured.

sign. Microscopical images show fibrosis of the cortical surface with fewer cells and there is little mature follicle formation and ovulation. PCO is more common in women of adolescence and childbearing age. The ultrasonic images show the increased volume of bilateral ovaries, occasionally unilateral. The capsule is hyperechoic and thickened with multiple follicles less than 1.0 cm located peripherally along the cortex. They are in wheel-shaped or in net-like morphology. More than ten follicles can be seen on a single section with no mature follicle and no ovulation observed routinely. The ovarian medulla is acoustically enhanced. The ovaries are usually enlarged with multilocular cystoid alteration after the application of ovulation induction drugs (Fig. 5.71).

– Simple ovarian cyst.

  Ovarian simple cysts are usually monolocular, originated from follicular cysts or serous monolocular cysts which is usually not accompany by clinical manifestation. Pathologic examination cannot determine the origin of the cysts. Most of simple ovarian cysts are unilateral and monolocular, regular round or oval shaped, with clear boundary, thin capsule, and clear fluid inside. Generally, it is rare to vanish naturally (Fig. 5.72).

– Ovarian endometriotic cyst.

  Ovarian endometriotic cyst is one of the most common lesions in external endometriosis. About 80% of the patients are involved in unilateral ovary and 50% of the patients are involved in bilateral ovaries. In the early stage

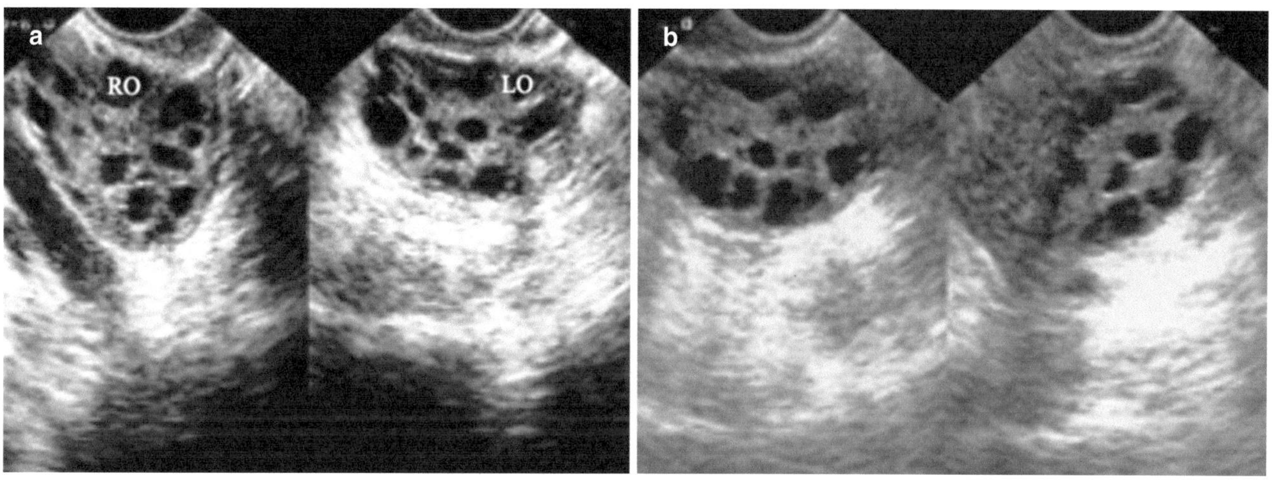

Fig. 5.71 Polycystic ovary. (**a**, **b**) Multiple follicles are shown in wheel-shaped bilateral ovaries; more than ten follicles can be seen on a single section. The ovarian medulla is acoustic enhanced and polycystic changed as a result of medication

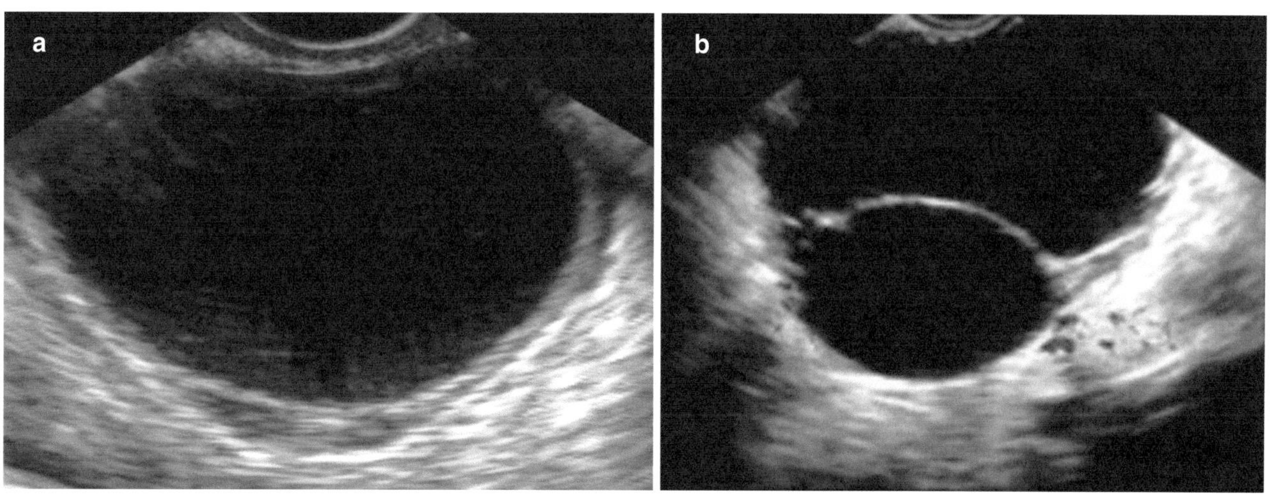

Fig. 5.72 Simple ovarian cyst. (**a**) Sonogram shows a monolocular cyst in the pelvis, with thin capsule, clear boundary, and clear fluid inside. (**b**) Sonogram shows a multilocular cyst with a thin capsule and clear fluid inside

of the lesion, small purple-brown spots or vesicles can be seen on the surface and in the cortex of the ovary. With the development of the disease, a single cyst or multiple cysts can be seen on the ovary, filled with dark brown, viscous and old blood, like chocolate, also known as "chocolate cyst" clinically.

Most patients represent dysmenorrhea and persistent pain in the lower abdomen. Progressive dysmenorrhea is usually aggravated year by year with the development of local lesions. The degree of pain is not necessarily related to the size of the lesions. About 20% of the patients do not have any obvious clinical symptoms. A few patients may have menstrual disorders. Forty percent of the patients accompany by infertility which is also a common cause of infertility.

Ultrasonic scanning shows round, oval, or irregular cysts on bilateral or rear of the uterus in the pelvic cavity. The capsules of the cysts are thick with an unsmooth surface. Larger cysts are usually pressed by surrounding organs or adhered to the surrounding organs. The boundary is not clearly shown.

The ultrasonic image of chocolate cyst varies according to the duration of lesion. The different echoes in the cysts include slightly hyperechoic uniform and dense spots, complex hyperechoic and weak echo, or anechoic clear liquid.

The diameter of a chocolate cyst is about 5 ~ 6 cm, and unilateral cyst is more common. The cyst may have fissures or even ruptures which may cause exuding or spreading of the cystic fluid into the pelvic cavity. And it results in adhesion between the ovary and adjacent organs. At this time, the contour of the cyst alters or even disappears (Figs. 5.73 and 5.74).

- Special tips
  - Most of the non-tumor cystic masses on the ovary are caused by the change of an ovarian function. They are usually small in size and vanish by themselves without clinical management. But its morphology is often confused with tumor cyst.
  - TVS is very helpful to detect small lesions of an endometriotic cyst. However, it is easy to be misdiagnosed with other tumors due to the variety of sonograms of a chocolate cyst.

II. Ovarian tumors

- Basic concepts
  - The ovary is a small and complex organ, which has the most tumor types. Ovarian tumor is a common tumor of gynecologic malignancies, including benign, borderline, and malignant tumor. Cystic tumors are common and most of them are benign. Solid tumors are relatively rare. Exception for primary malignant ovarian tumors, metastasis from other organs is common, too.
  - Various types of ovarian malignant tumors have various pathological characteristics. The common pathological characteristics are the disorder of cell structure and arrangement, hemorrhage, and necrosis in the tumor. According to the histologic classification of ovarian tumors formulated by the World Health Organization (WHO), they are generally divided into epithelial tumors (50–70%), sex cord stromal tumors (about 5%), germ cell tumors (20–40%) and metastatic tumors (5–10%).
  - Ovarian cancer is one of the three common tumors of the female reproductive system, which accounts for about 15% of gynecological cancer, only lower than cervical cancer. It can occur at any age with the peak age of 45–64 years old. The survival rate is about 25–30%. The pathogenesis of ovarian cancer is mainly related to heredity, family history, environmental factors, and endocrine factors. 20–25% of patients with ovarian cancer have a family history.
  - Primary ovarian cancer can be divided into two categories: epithelial cancer and nonepithelial cancer. Metastatic tumors may metastasize from the primary malignancies of any other organs. Common metastatic tumors are common from breast, stomach, intestine, reproductive urinary tract, and other organs. The main metastasis methods are intraperitoneal implantation and lymphatic metastasis, followed by diaphragm metastasis.
  - Benign ovarian tumors are mostly asymptomatic clinically. They are often found occasionally in the routine gynecological examination. The tumors are moderately enlarged, which causes abdominal distention or palpablation. Spherical masses can be palpable unilateral or bilateral adnexal areas, either cystic or solid, indicating smooth and movability by gynecological examination. The tumors can grow big enough to occupy the full pelvis, even to the abdominal cavity. And compression symptoms may occur, such as frequent urination, constipation, difficulty in breathing and cardiopalmus, etc. Abdominal distention without shifting dullness can be found. Once the clinical symptoms of ovarian cancer appear, most patients are in advanced stages. If the tumor invades or compresses the nerves, it may cause abdominal pain, backache, lower limb pain, and anemia in the late stage.

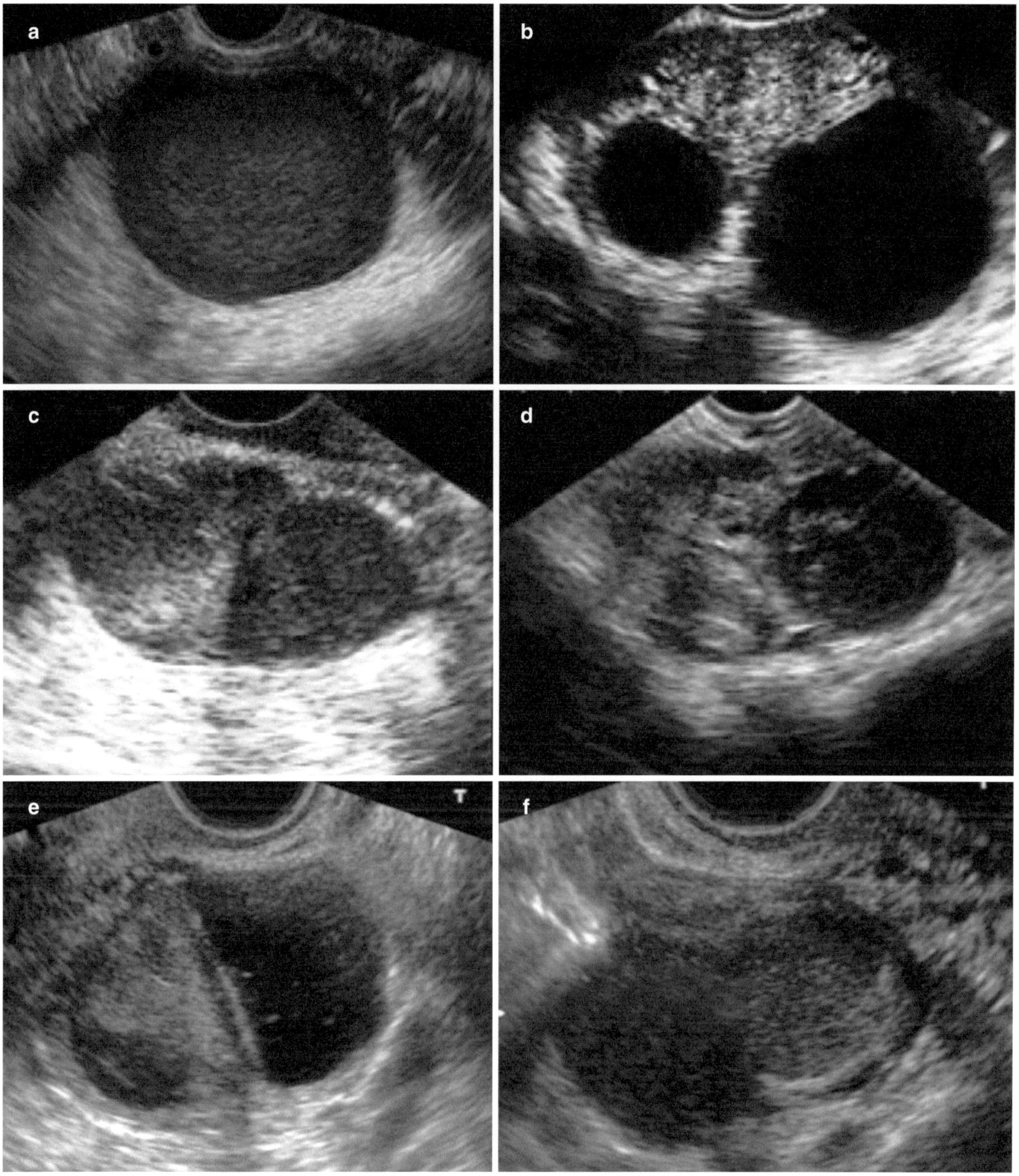

Fig. 5.73 Ovarian endometriotic cyst (chocolate cysts). (**a**) The cyst is shown full of homogeneous and hypoechoic dots. (**b**) Bilateral chocolate cysts. (**c-f**) The chocolate cyst is filled with heterogeneous and complex echoes in an irregular shape

- The ovary locates in the deep pelvis, which makes it difficult to be palpable. Nowadays, reliable methods are not available for the early detection and diagnosis of ovarian tumors. Ultrasonography is a convenient and reliable noninvasive method for early detection of pelvic masses, which enables the possible early detection of ovarian tumors.

- Ultrasonic diagnosis
  - The diagnosis of an ovarian tumor can be made by its characteristics of morphology and echo.

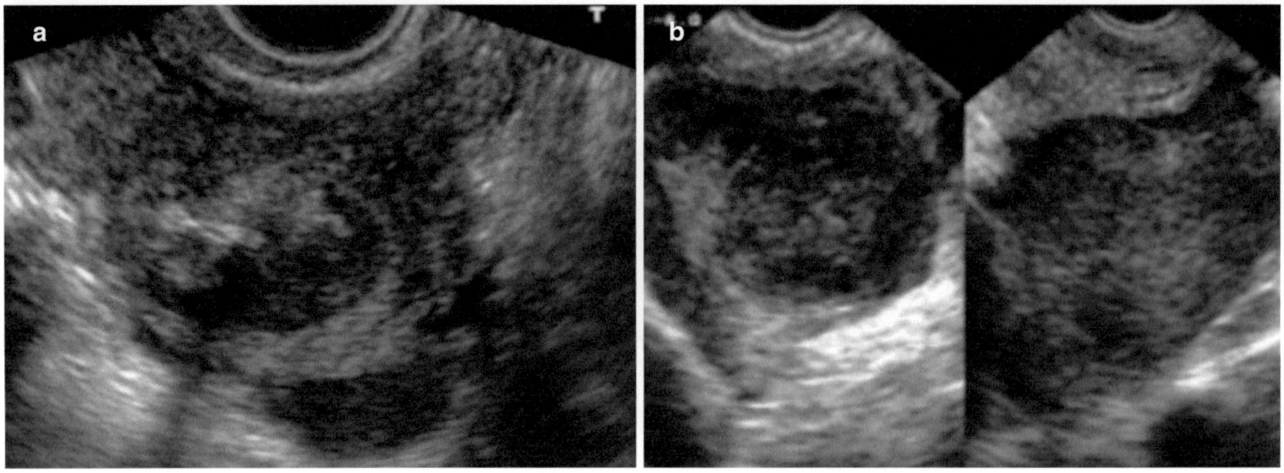

Fig. 5.74 Ruptured ovarian endometriotic cyst. (**a**) A 36-year-old patient represented abdominal pain for 3 hours with a history of dysmenorrhea. Emergency ultrasonography shows an irregular and heterogeneous hypoechoic mass in the left adnexa area, without an obvious cyst wall. (**b**) A patient represented pain in the lower abdomen for 2 days with a history of "chocolate cyst." Sonogram shows irregular hypoechoic in bilateral adnexa area without clear boundary. The free fluid area in the pelvis is about 3.0 cm

Transvaginal ultrasound and color Doppler flow examination provide referable information for the primary judgment of ovarian tumor.

- The sonographic images of ovarian cystic tumors are mostly unilateral or bilateral spherical or spheroid masses. Anechoic dark area can be seen in the cyst, unilocular or plurilocular. The septum of benign multilocular cysts is thin, without blood flow in the septum. Occasionally, the inner wall of some cystic tumors is uneven, or papillary solid hyperechoic protrusions are visible (Fig. 5.75).
- The ultrasonic image of solid ovarian tumor mostly shows unilateral and moderately enlarged mass, with an unclear wall. The tumor is a homogeneous or heterogeneous solid mass, and calcification with an acoustic shadow is visible.
- Solid tumors include ovarian fibroma, Boehner's tumor, ovarian endometrial cancer, ovarian clear cell cancer, endodermal sinus cancer, dysgerminoma of the ovary, granular cell tumor, and theca cell tumor, etc. There are many kinds of solid tumors, without specific sonographic images, which should be confirmed by pathological examination (Fig. 5.76).
- The ultrasound images of ovarian mixed tumors show the fluid, fibrous, and fatty structures inside the tumors. Fluid area, hypoechoic, hyperechoic, or attenuated echo is visible in the tumor, which is characterized by a disordered echo. The most common type of ovarian mixed tumor is ovarian teratoma, most of which have specific manifestations on the sonogram. Cystic teratomas appear variably ranging from completely anechoic to completely hyperechoic. The common images include dough sign, hair-clot sign, fat fluid level sign, and star-flower sign, etc. (Figs. 5.77, 5.78, 5.79, 5.80, and 5.81).
- The size of ovarian malignant tumors varies, unilateral or bilateral. The shape is mostly irregular, spherical, or oval with an unsmooth surface. The capsules are unevenly thickened, incompletely or unclearly displayed. Complex and disordered echoes are commonly seen inside the masses. The multilocular masses are more common, with a dense and thick septum. Blood flow may be seen on the septum. Ascites are visible in the pelvic and abdominal cavity (Fig. 5.82, 5.83, 5.84, and 5.85).

- Special tips
  - Ovarian tumors are complex and the ultrasonic images lack specific signs. Some different kinds of tumors may have similar images and a certain tumor may have different images. The diagnosis should be confirmed in combination with the clinical manifestations, medical history, and related auxiliary examination.
  - In the ultrasonic examination of pelvic ovarian tumors, the first step is to determine the position of the uterus, in order to identify the relationship between the tumor and the uterus and to exclude the diseases of the uterus. According to ultrasonic characteristics of the tumor, benign or malignant mass was presumptive diagnosed. Once uneven or disordered mass with ascites is found in the pelvis, a related auxiliary examination should be considered to exclude malignant neoplasia.

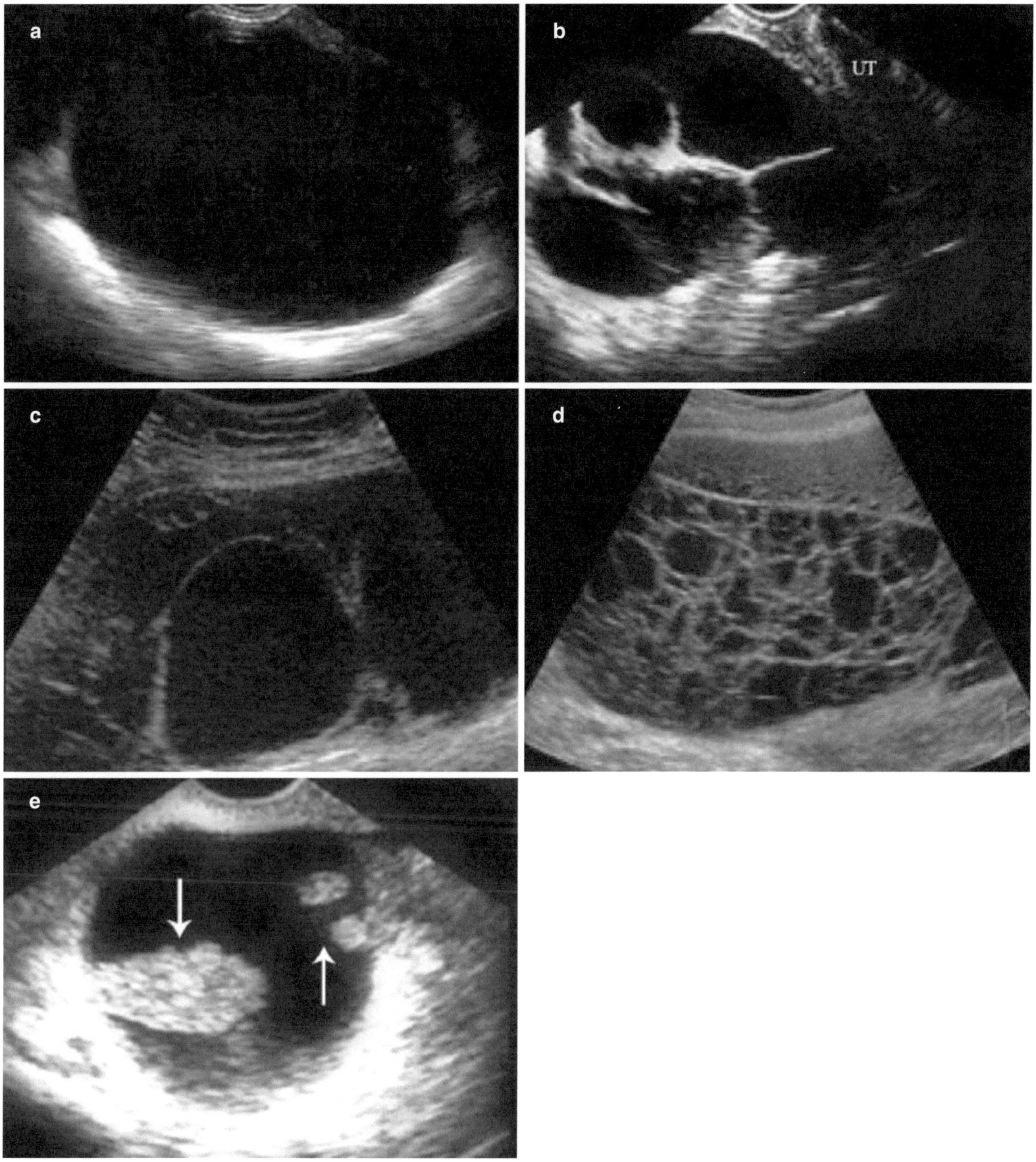

Fig. 5.75 Ovarian cystic tumor. (**a**) The cyst is unilocular, with clear fluid and clear boundary. (**b**, **c**) Septal cyst with clear fluid and clear septum; (**d**) An ovarian hemorrhagic cyst with a reticular septum, which disappeared after 3 months. (**e**) Solid echonic protuberance grows into the inner wall of the cyst

- Solid ovarian mass should be differentiated from intramural and subserosal myoma. Cystic mass should be differentiated from a cystic change of uterine myoma. Large cyst should be differentiated from massive ascites.

III. Ultrasound diagnosis of other masses in pelvic cavity
- Inflammatary mass
  - Basic concepts
  - The infection of female internal genitalia are related to postpartum or abortion, uterine cavity

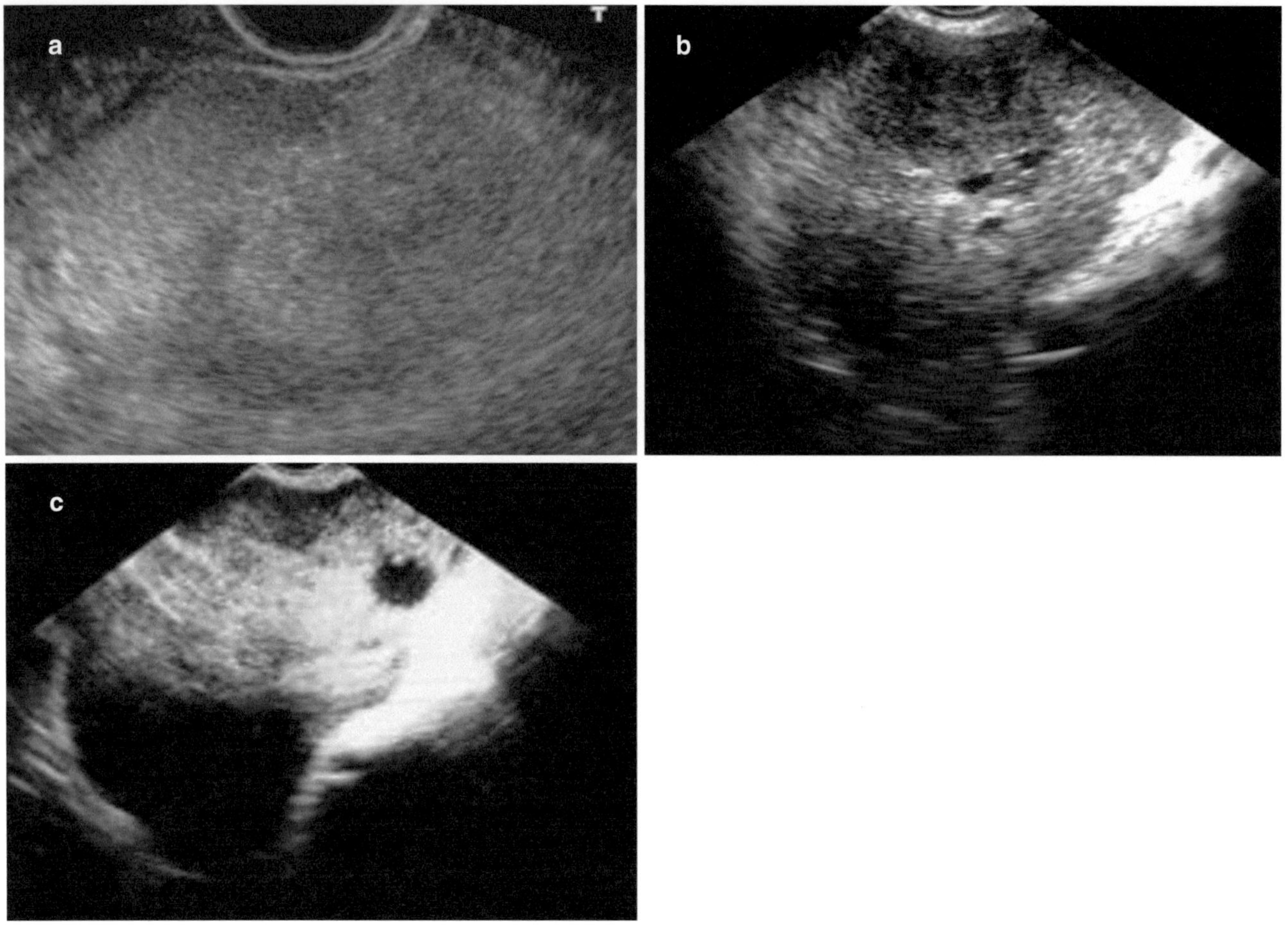

Fig. 5.76 Ovarian solid tumor. (**a**) Sonogram shows a homogenic solid mass in the pelvic cavity, with similar echoic characteristics to uterine fibroma. Ovarian fibroma is confirmed by operation. (**b**, **c**) A 21-year-old patient represented with an abdominal mass. The ultrasonography revealed an irregular solid mass in the pelvic cavity, 9.0 cm in diameter, with a small amount of fluid area in the mass. It is diagnosed as an endodermal sinus tumor by the operation and pathology

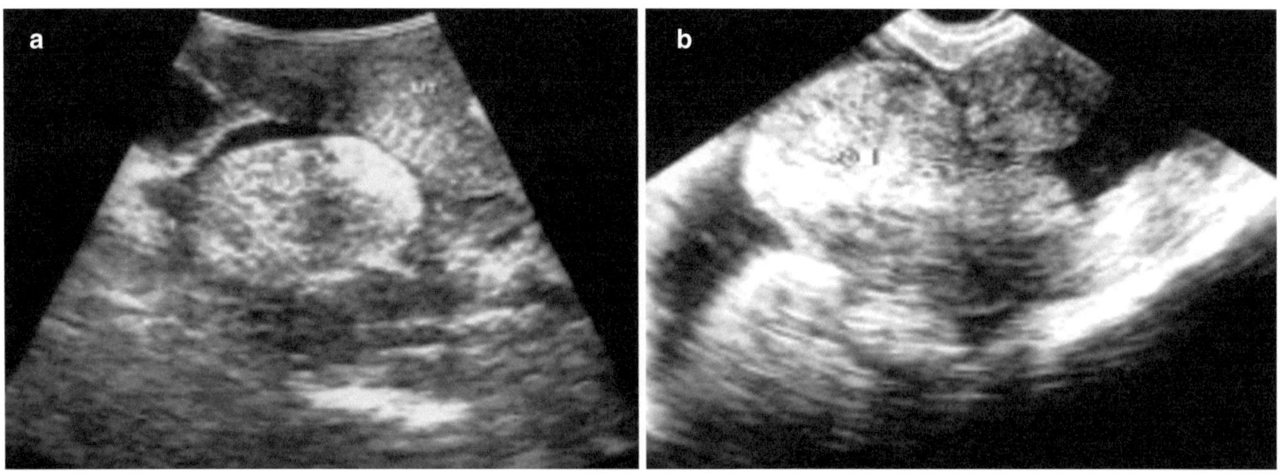

Fig. 5.77 Ovarian teratoma (I). (**a**, **b**) Ultrasonic images show hyperechoic dough sign

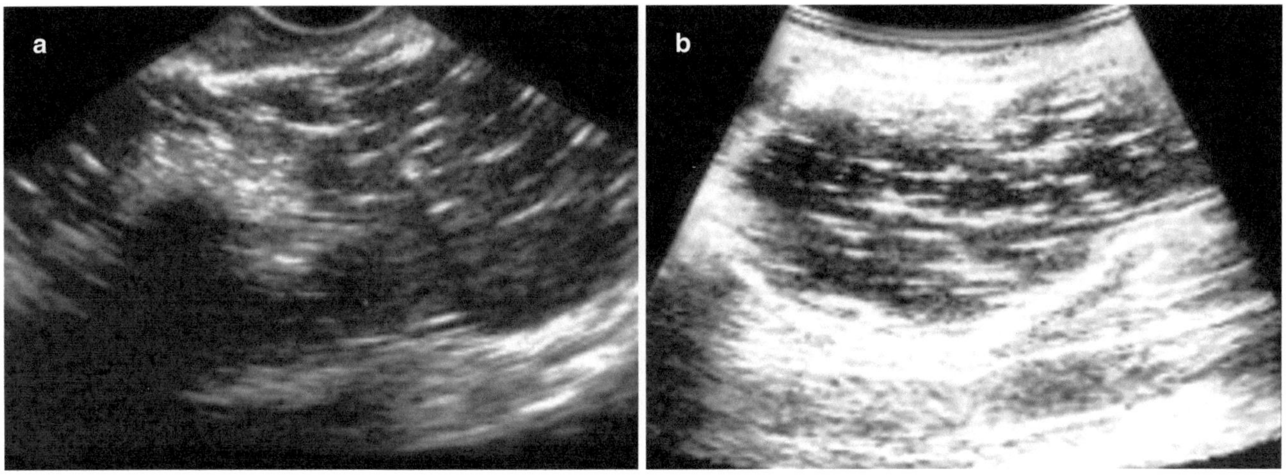

Fig. 5.78 Ovarian teratoma (II). (**a**, **b**) Ultrasonography shows cystic mass, with sporadic or multiple hyperechoic lines floating inside, like "starflower"

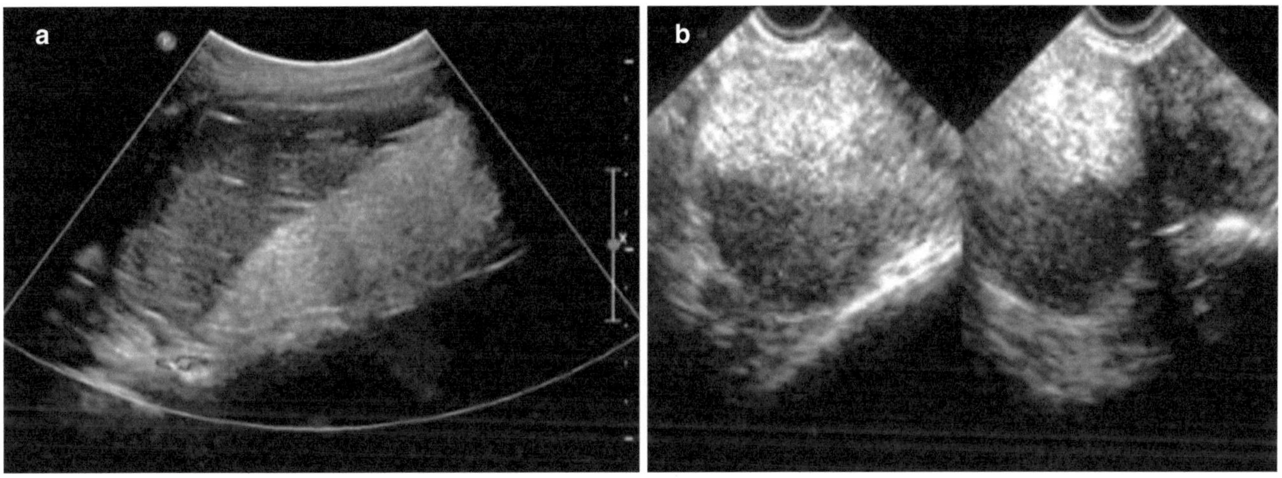

Fig. 5.79 Ovarian teratoma (III). (**a**, **b**) Ultrasound image shows the mass with fat-fluid level. The hyperechoic fatty tissue located in the upper part

operation, menstrual period infection with sexually transmitted diseases, and directly spreading from inflammation of adjacent organs, which can cause infection of the pelvic internal genitalia and surrounding connective tissue as well as pelvic peritoneum.

- The pelvic inflammatory diseases include acute endometritis and myometritis, acute salpingoophoritis, pyosalpinx, tubo-ovarian abscess, acute parametritis, acute pelvic peritonitis, and sepsis.
- The clinical manifestations include lower abdominal pain, some severe patients may present with chills, high fever, headache, and anorexia. Increased volume and menotaxis may occur in the period, while increased leucorrhea may occur non-menstrual period. Vaginal hyperemia and purulent secretion from the cervix can be seen in gynecological examination and inflammatory mass can be palpable in the pelvis. The mass may be fluctuant and tender. Total number of leukocytes and proportion of the neutrophils can be increased obviously.
- Ultrasonic diagnosis

  Endometritis and acute myometriitis: (i). Endometrium is swollen, thickened, and hypoechoic (Fig. 5.86). (ii). Myometritis shows a slightly enlarged uterus, attenuated echo, and obvious tenderness (Fig. 5.87).

  Acute and chronic salpingoophoritis (also known as adnexitis): (1) Adnexitis is characterized by unilateral or bilateral adnexal masses, with a diameter of 4–6 cm in general. The ovary is slightly enlarged and hypoechoic, surrounded by a fluid area (Figs. 5.88 and 5.89). (2) The adnexal mass is cystic or septate cystic, with

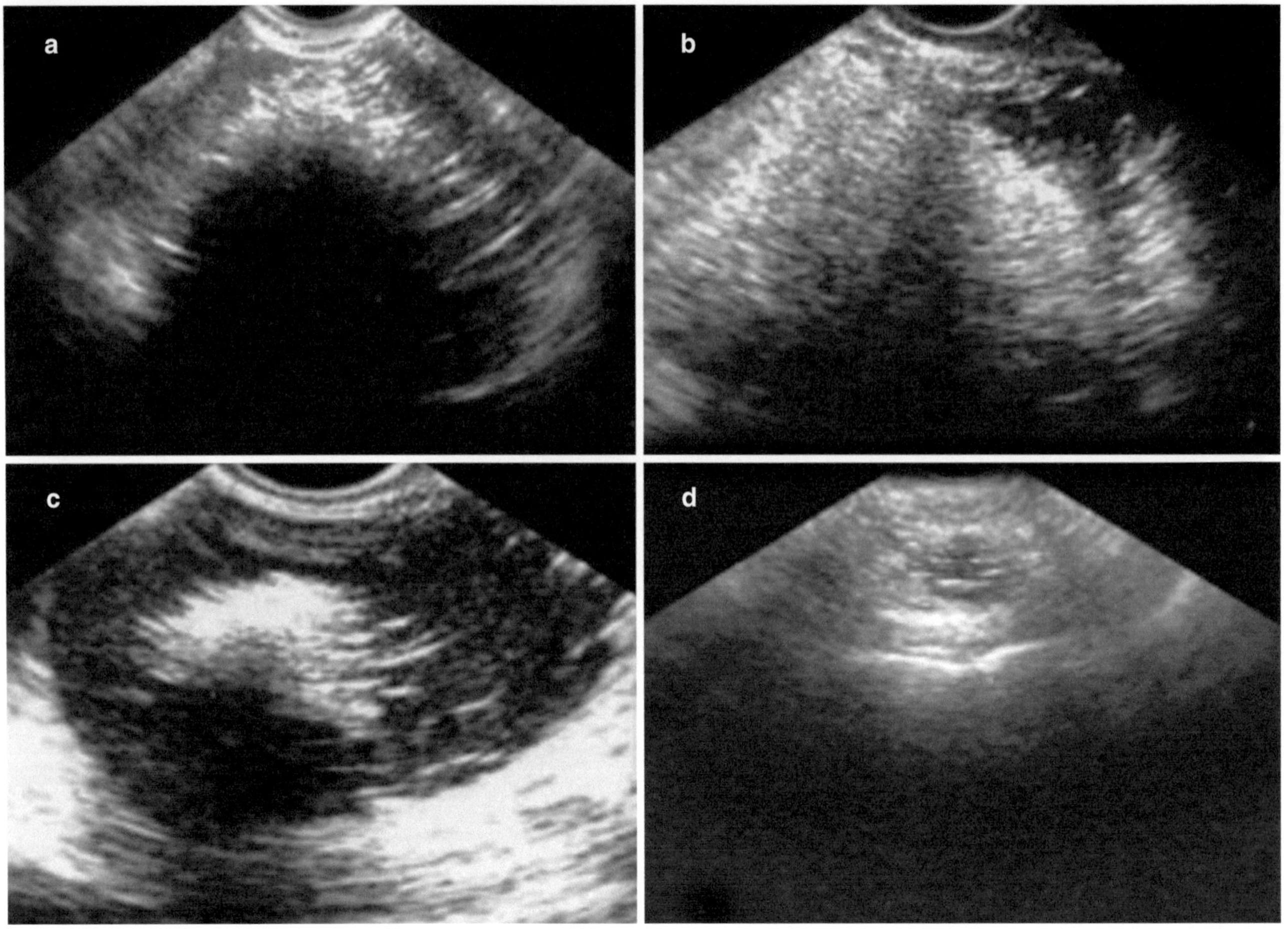

Fig. 5.80 Ovarian teratoma (IV). (**a-d**) Ultrasonography shows an inhomogeneous mass with some hypoechoic areas. Hyperecho is often accompanied by attenuation shadow, resulting in unclear boundary

flocculent or reticular echo inside. The wall is thickened and rough. The fallopian tube can be found thickened with tenderness (Fig. 5.90).

Pyosalpinx and tube-ovarian abscess: Unilateral or bilateral cystic masses are shown with tiny echoes or flocculent hyperechoic material inside. Masses, with unclear boundary, are adhered to both sides and posterior uterus with an obscure margin of ovary and fallopian tube. Pyosalpinx shows flaky weak echoes, and severe tenderness when touching (Figs. 5.91 and 5.92).

- Ultrasonic diagnosis of masses after pelvic surgery
  - Basic concepts

    Hysterectomy or subtotal hysterectomy is carried out because of uterine diseases or ovarian tumors, and unilateral or bilateral ovaries remain. Anatomical relationships of the pelvic organs change after extensive procedures for malignant tumors. The recurrence of the tumor or inflammation and endocrine disorders may also occur. All the situations above may result in masses in the pelvis.

    Ultrasonography has been a common method in following up for postoperative patients. The vaginal stump, masses in the pelvis, ascites, and effusion between intestines should be observed when scanning.
  - Ultrasonic diagnosis

    Recurrence of myoma after operation. It usually occurs in the uterine body or the residual cervix, and the mass represents solid echoes of different sizes (Fig. 5.93).

    Recurrence of ovarian or uterine malignancies. Heterogeneous or homogeneous solid mass can be found in pelvis, may be accompanied by ascites (Figs. 5.94 and 5.95).

    Lymphocyst after tumor surgery: Most lymphocysts locate in bilateral ilium fossa or the posterior part of the pelvic cavity, presenting cystic echoes and clear boundary. Most of the lymphocysts are less than 5 cm (Fig. 5.96).

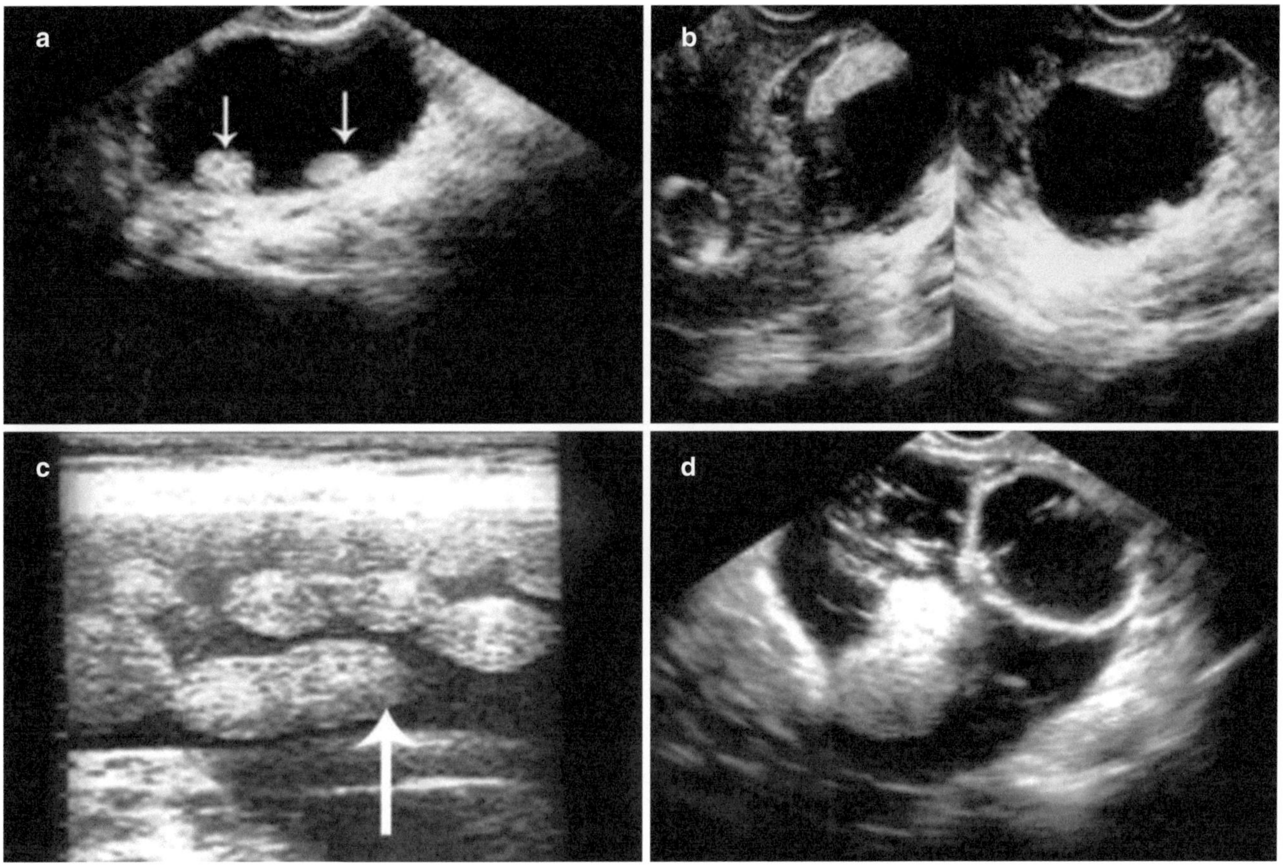

Fig. 5.81 Ovarian teratoma (V). (**a**, **b**) The mass is mainly cystic, with solid nodule protruding into the cystic cavity on the inner wall of the cyst. (**c**) A 52-year-old patient represented abdominal enlargement for half a year. Sonogram shows a huge cystic mass with multiple mobile spherical echogenic structures floating in the cystic fluid. A giant mature teratoma is confirmed by operation. (**d**) A complex echogenic cystic mass with septum

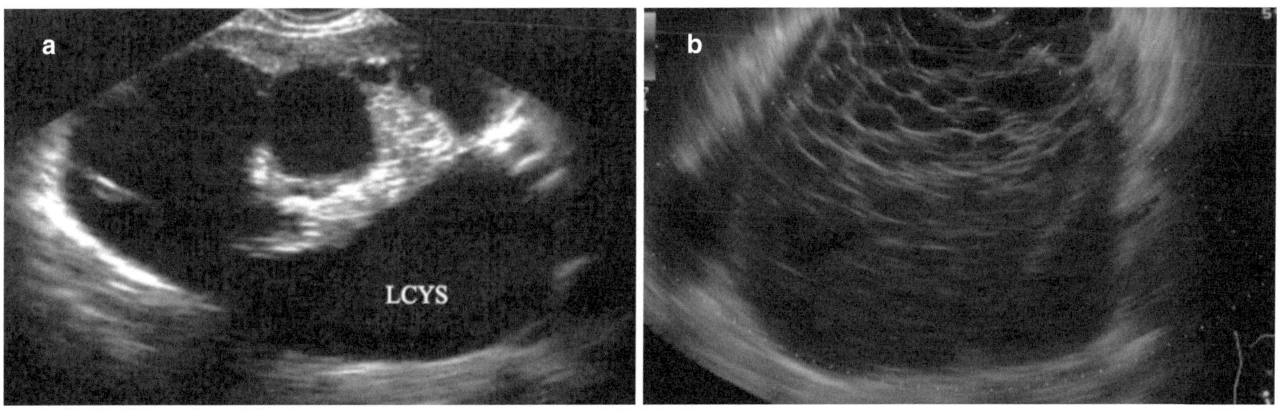

Fig. 5.82 Ovarian malignant tumors (I). (**a**) Ultrasonic images show a septal cystic mass with thick septum, and pathological diagnosis is serous cystadenocarcinoma. (**b**) Ultrasonography shows cystic mass with a dense septum in the pelvis, and pathological diagnosis of serous cystadenocarcinoma is confirmed

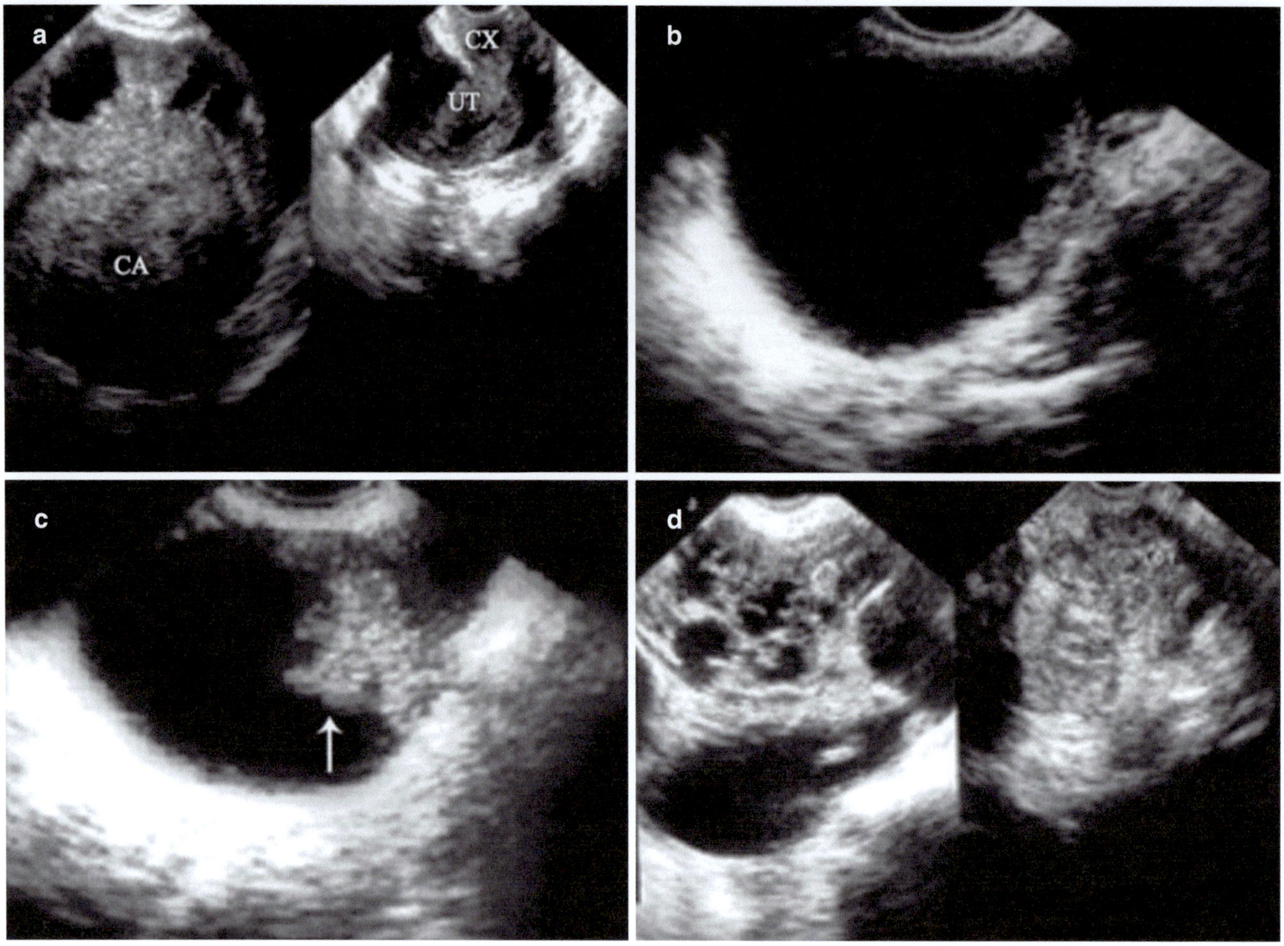

Fig. 5.83 Ovarian malignant tumors (II). (**a**) A 68-year-old patient with a postmenopausal period of 18 years. The ultrasonic images show an atrophic uterus. A cystic domained mixtured echogenic mass with a diameter of 10.0 cm is shown in the right adnexa area, accompanied by ascites. (**b**, **c**) Ultrasonic shows irregular solid echoes on the inner wall of the cystic mass, protruding into the cystic cavity. (**d**) Sonogram shows an irregular and heterogeneous mixed mass in the bilateral adnexa areas, without an obvious capsule

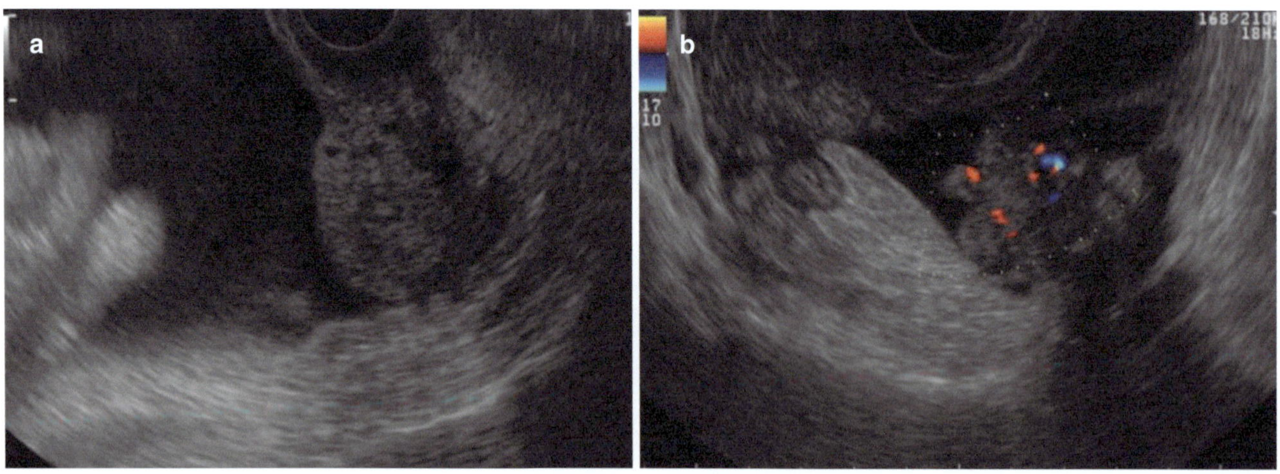

Fig. 5.84 Ovarian malignant tumors (III). (**a**, **b**) A 62-year-old patient with a postmenopausal period of 8 years, represented with abdominal distention. Ultrasonography reveals a large amount of ascites in pelvic and abdominal cavity with an atrophic uterine, with an irregular solid mass measured 4.0 cm × 3.7 cm × 3.2 cm in the right adnexa area. Color Doppler shows inside blood flow

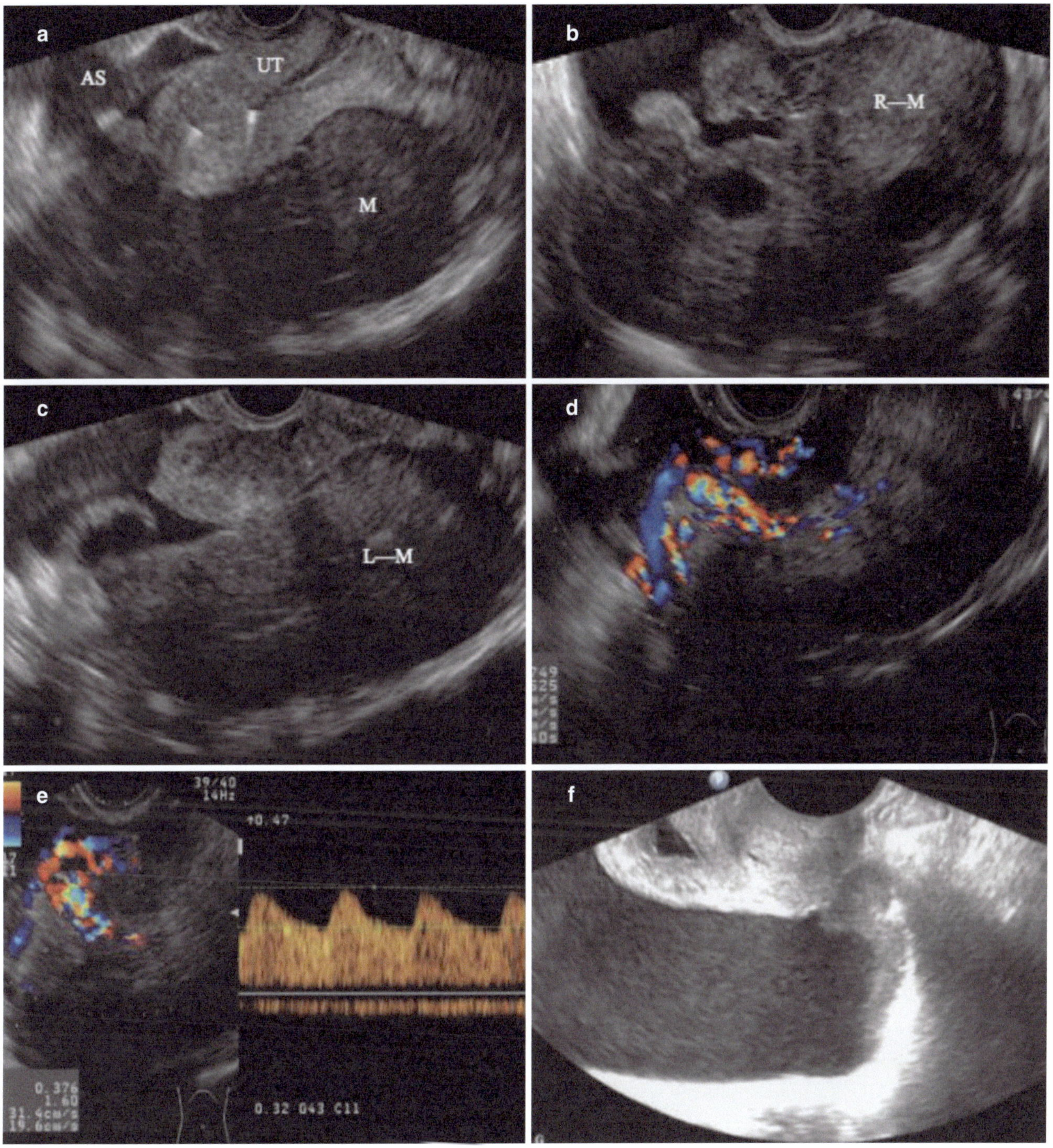

Fig. 5.85 Ovarian malignant tumors (IV). A 29-year-old patient represented abdominal distension for 3 months 1+ years after the operation of gastric cancer. (**a**) Ultrasonic scanning shows a normal-sized uterus with an intrauterine device, and a large amount of unclear ascites in the pelvic and abdominal cavity. (**b**, **c**) Irregular solid masses are found in bilateral adnexa areas, with a small fluid sonolucent area. (**d**, **e**) Color Doppler shows rich blood flow in bilateral masses, with RI = 0.37. (**f**) Uneven thickened pelvic peritoneum is shown

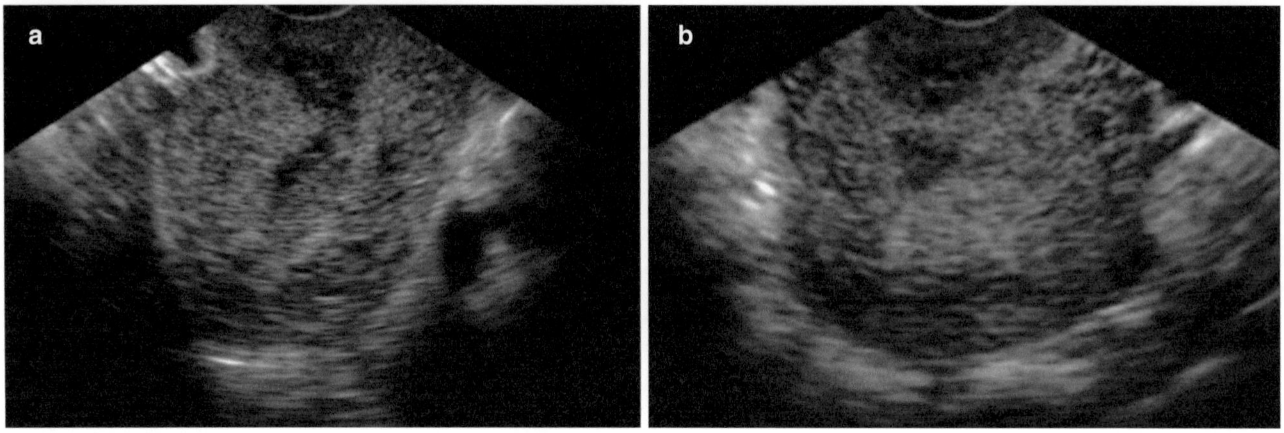

Fig. 5.86 Endometritis. (**a**, **b**) Ultrasonography shows a slightly enlarged uterus, hypoechoic, and thickened endometrium

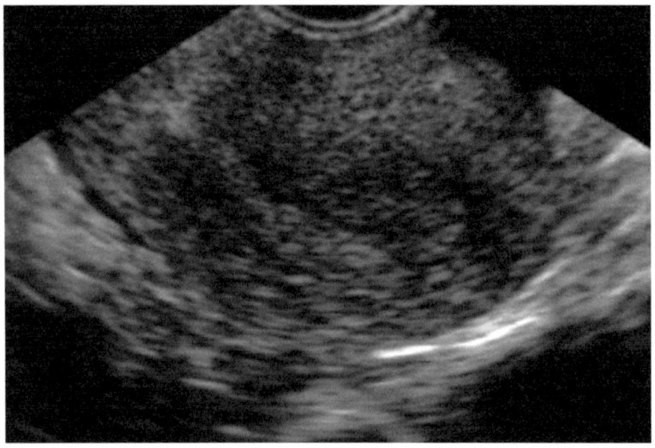

Fig. 5.87 Myometritis. Ultrasonic images show a slightly enlarged uterus, attenuated echo, and obvious tenderness

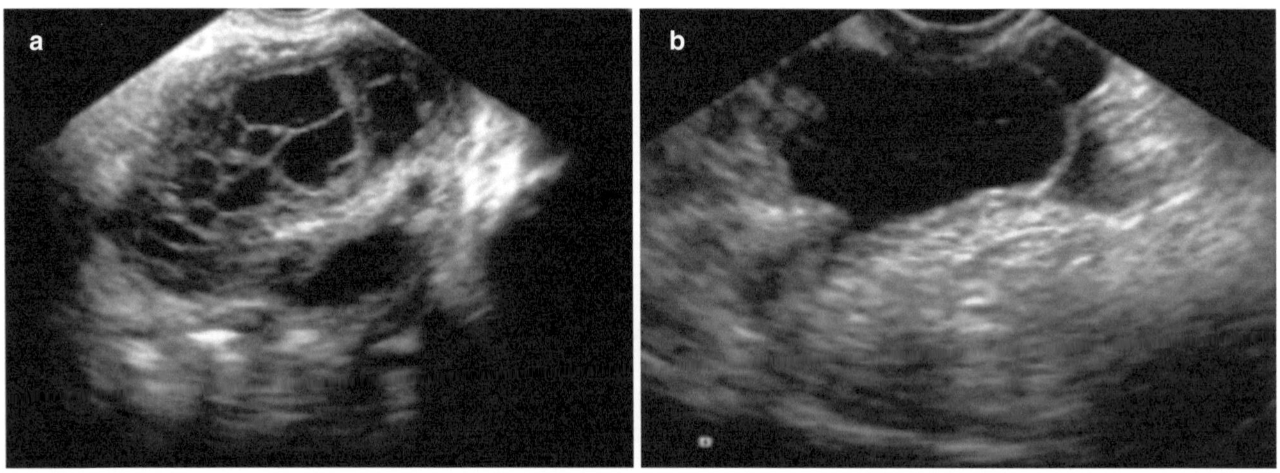

Fig. 5.88 Adnexal inflammatory mass (I). (**a**, **b**) Ultrasonography shows the right adnexal septate cystic mass with irregular shape and abdominal pain. (**a**) Reexamination of the same patient shows the mass significantly reduced after 1 month of treatment. (**b**, **c**, **d**) Ultrasonic image shows strip and flocculent echo in bilateral adnexal cystic masses with thick and rough boundary. (**c**) Reexamination of the same patient shows shrunk cystic masses after 3-month treatment

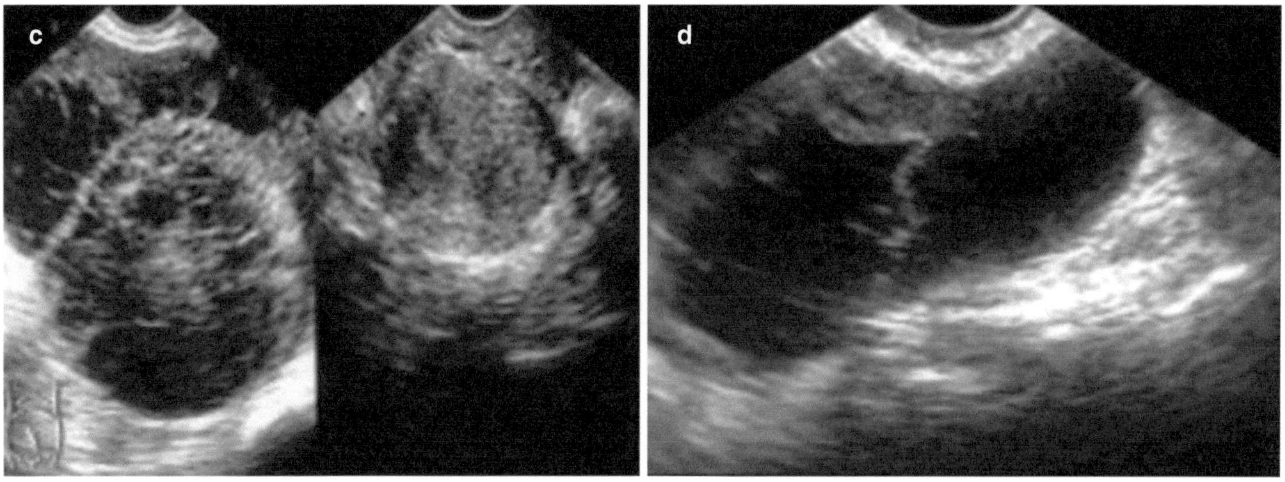

Fig. 5.88 (continued)

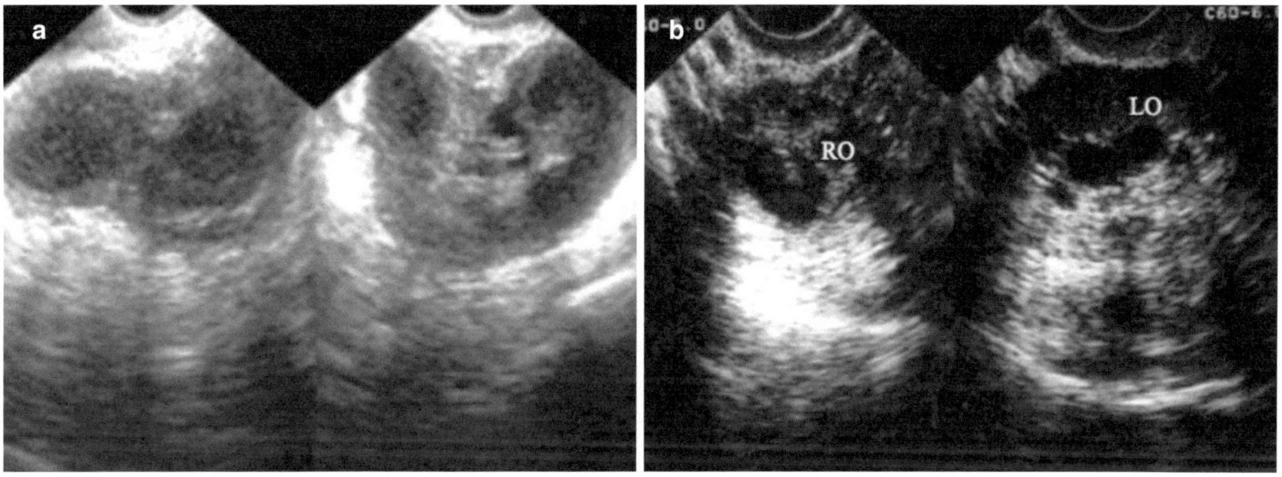

Fig. 5.89 Adnexal inflammatory mass (II). (**a**) A 24-year-old patient represented lower abdominal pain for 1 week after contraceptive operation. The ultrasonic scanning shows a bilateral adnexal hypoechoic mass with obvious tenderness. (**b**) The mass disappeared after treatment of the same patient

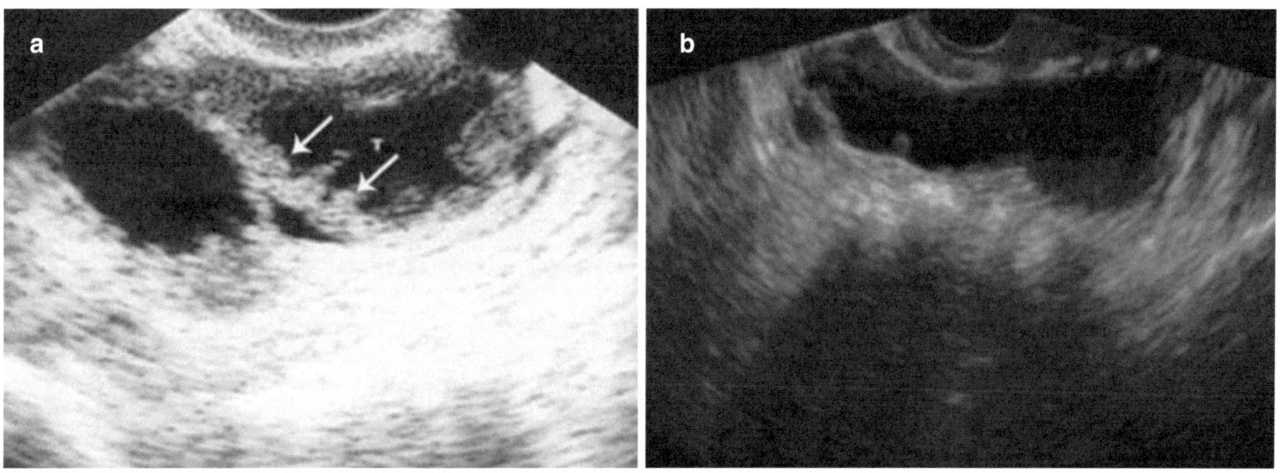

Fig. 5.90 Hydrosalpinx. (**a**, **b**) The coronal images show the dilated and swollen fallopian tube, filled with liquid. The half-fold structure on the tube wall is visible

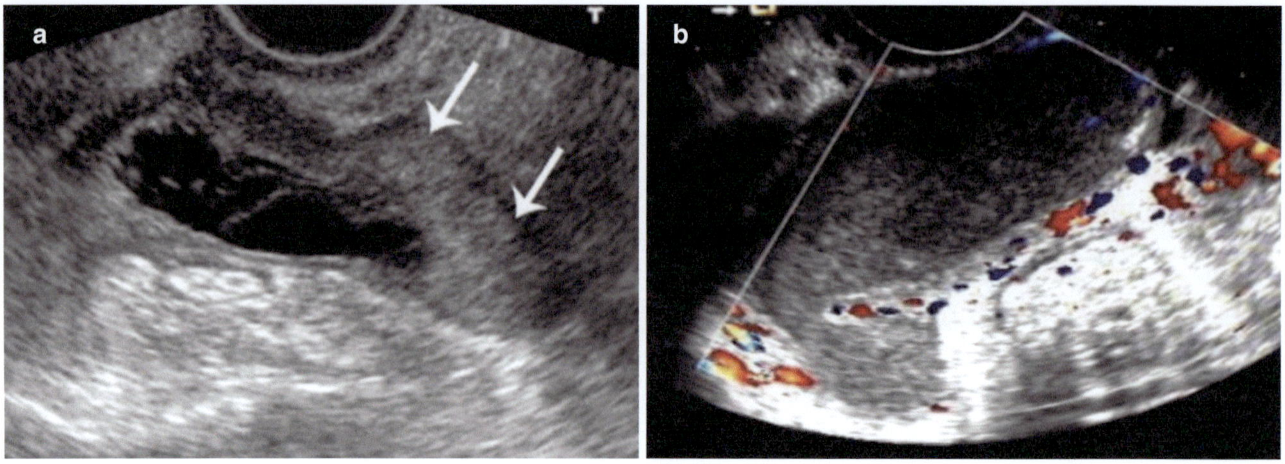

Fig. 5.91 Pyosalpinx. (**a**) A 53-year-old patient represented lower quadrant pain for 10+ days, accompanied with conscious of fever and chills. The coronal image of the left fallopian tube shows dilated fallopian tube with a liquid area and flocculent echoes inside. (**b**) A 33-year-old patient represented with lower abdominal pain for 1+ month. The coronal scanning of the left fallopian tube shows "flask-like" change with hypoechoic materials inside. Both patients recovered after the salpingectomy

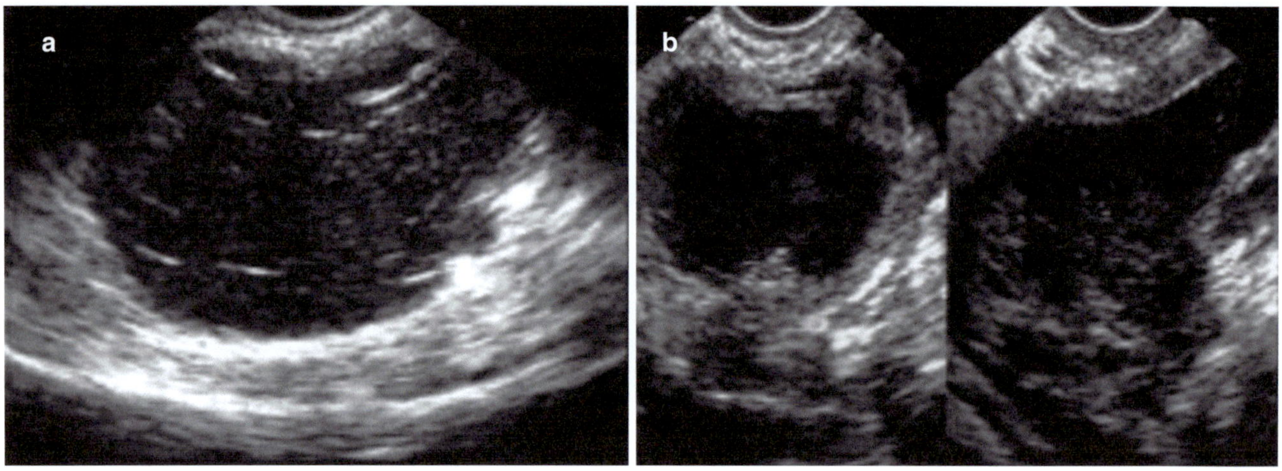

Fig. 5.92 Pelvic abscess. (**a**) A 34-year-old patient represented lower abdominal pain half a year after an operation because of pelvic abscess. The ultrasonography shows a hypoechoic mass located in the posterior and right of the uterus, 8.0 cm in diameter, with tiny and short linear echoes inside. (**b**) A 42-year-old patient represented lower abdomen pain and fever for 1+ month. The ultrasonic scanning shows irregular weak echo mass in bilateral adnexal areas and an abscess is proved by operation

Inflammatory mass. Sonogram shows the irregular cystic mass in the adnexa area, with separated or reticular echoes. The fluid in the mass is not clear. The patient has tenderness and the mass can shrink or disappear after treatment.

Pelvic encapsulated effusion after operation. Sonogram shows irregular mass filled with fluid, with weak tiny echoes or linear septum inside (Fig. 5.97).

Ovary preservation. Ovary can be found in pelvic cavity. Non-tumor cysts or tumor may occur in the residual ovary (Fig. 5.98).

– Special tips

With the widespread use and improvement of ultrasonic technology, it has been widely used in the field of gynecology. Ultrasonography can detect various pelvic masses at an early stage, which has been a routine method for pelvic examination.

Inflammatory mass is the most common one in the female pelvis, and it is also a common disease of gynecology. No special signs could be found by ultrasonography, thus more attention should be paid to differentiate it from other ovarian masses. It is vital to undertake routine ultrasonic follow-up, combined with the clinical history and treatment.

Due to the anatomical changes after pelvic surgery, we should pay attention to the reserved reproductive organs and their positions. Note the recurrence or metastasis in patients with malignant tumor histories.

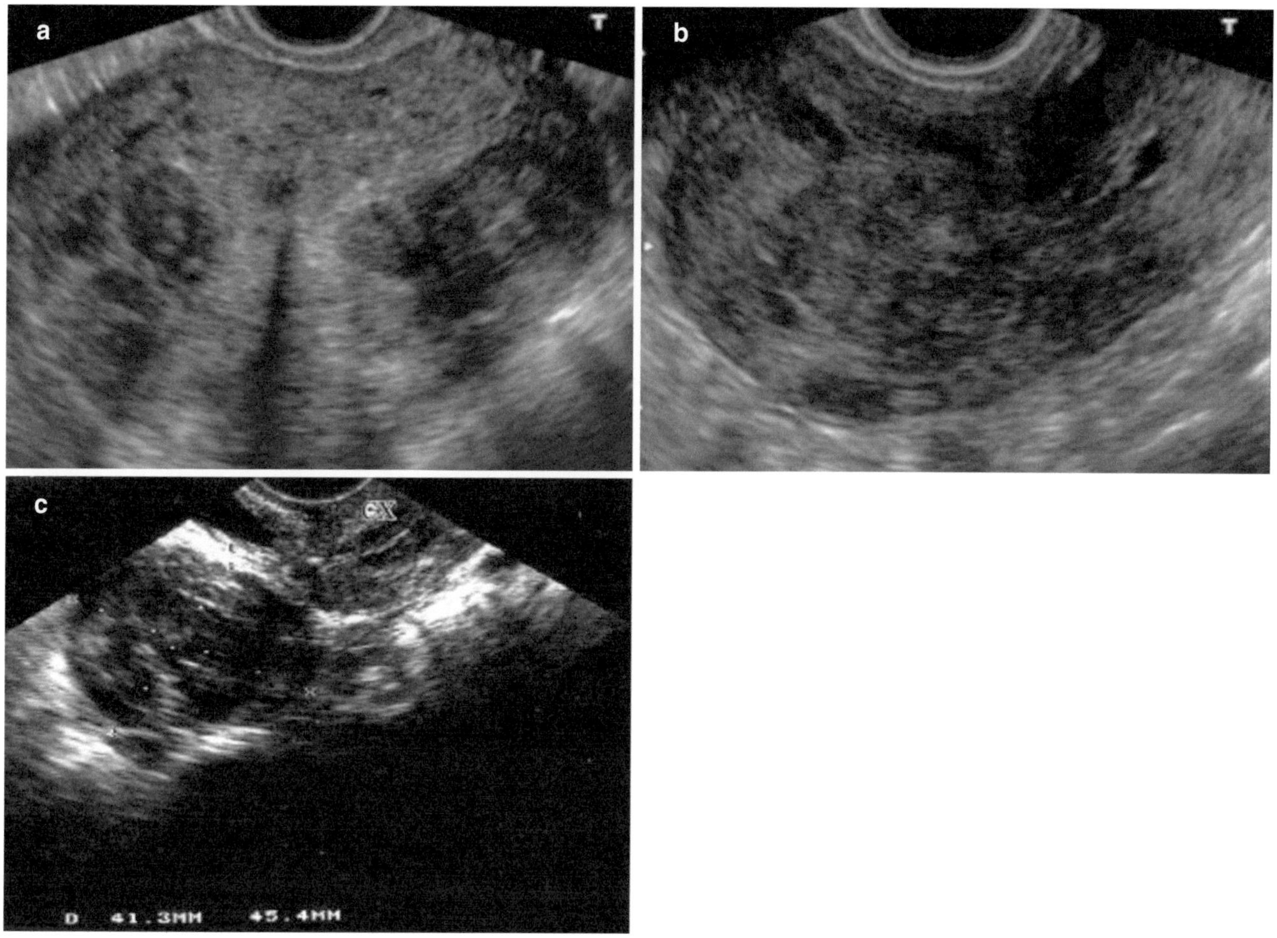

Fig. 5.93 Recurrence of myoma after operation. (**a**, **b**) Myomectomy was carried out before. Ultrasonic reexamination shows in homogeneous myometrium, with multiple small myomas. (**c**) Subtotal hysterectomy was carried out because of myoma 5 years before. Routine ultrasonic following up shows a myoma on the top of the residual cervix

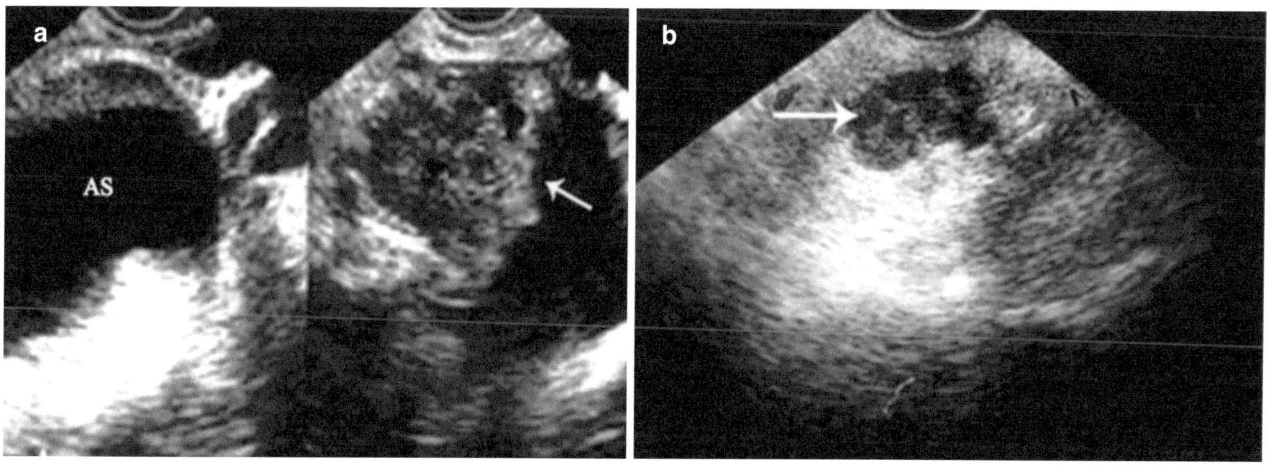

Fig. 5.94 Recurrence of ovarian cancer. (**a**) A patient is followed up by ultrasonography for 1 year after the operation of ovarian cancer. Heterogeneous and irregular hypoechoic solid mass is visible in the pelvis, with a diameter of about 5.0 cm, accompanied by ascites in the intestines. (**b**) A patient undergoes ultrasonography 2 years after the operation for ovarian cancer. Hypoechoic solid mass is found in the pelvis with a diameter of 2.6 cm, and the serum CA125 is significantly increased

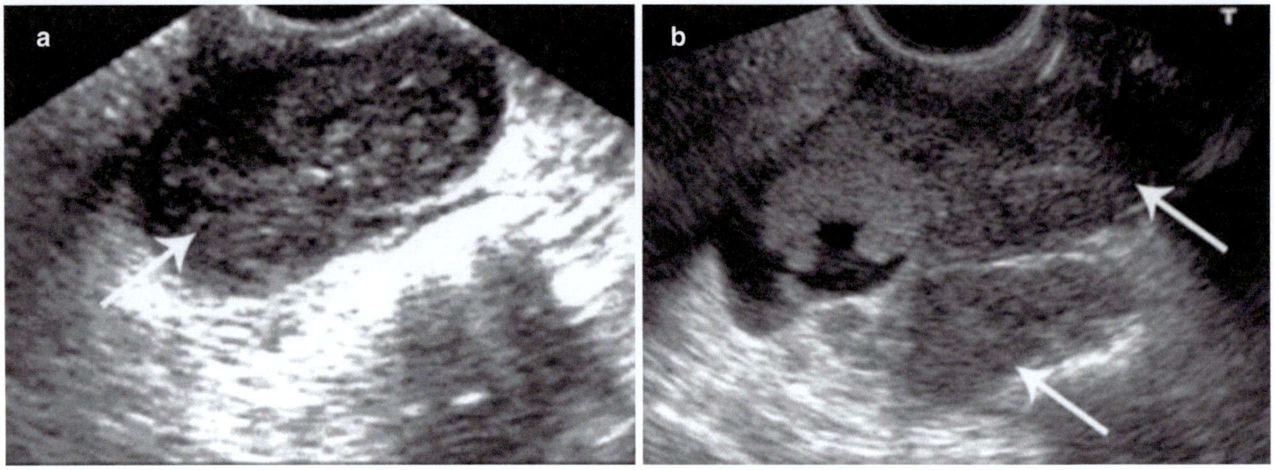

Fig. 5.95 Recurrence of uterine leiomyosarcoma. (**a**, **b**) The patient underwent a hysterectomy for leiomyosarcoma half a year before. Multiple hypoechoic masses are detected in the pelvic and abdominal cavity by ultrasonography

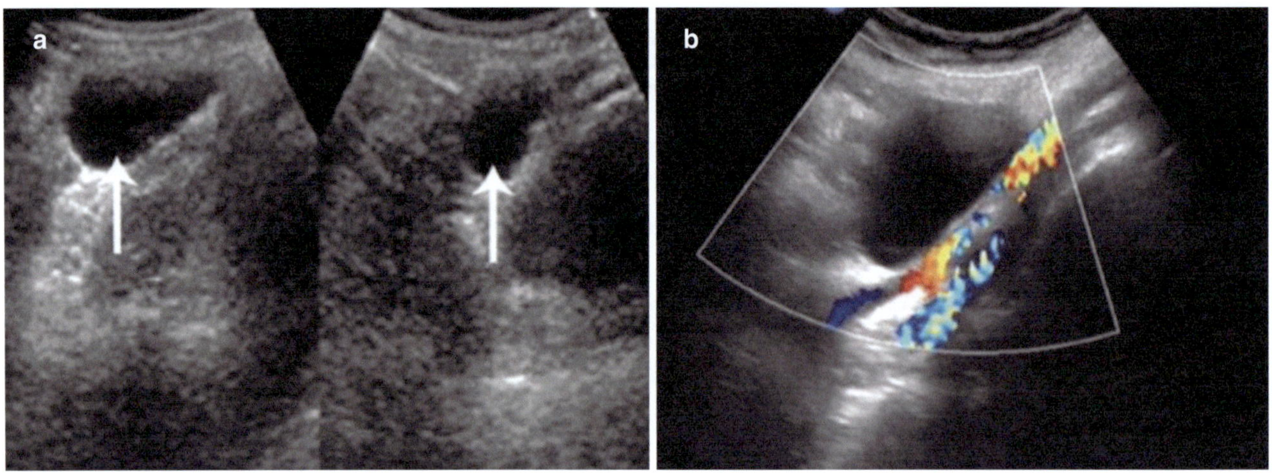

Fig. 5.96 Lymphocyst after tumor surgery. (**a**) Four months after the operation of cervical cancer, the patient represented lower abdominal pain. Ultrasonic scanning shows cystic echoes in bilateral ilium fossa, with a diameter of 2.5 cm and 1.8 cm, respectively. (**b**) TAS shows a cystic mass with a diameter of 4.7 cm in the right ilium fossa, with a thin wall and clear fluid inside

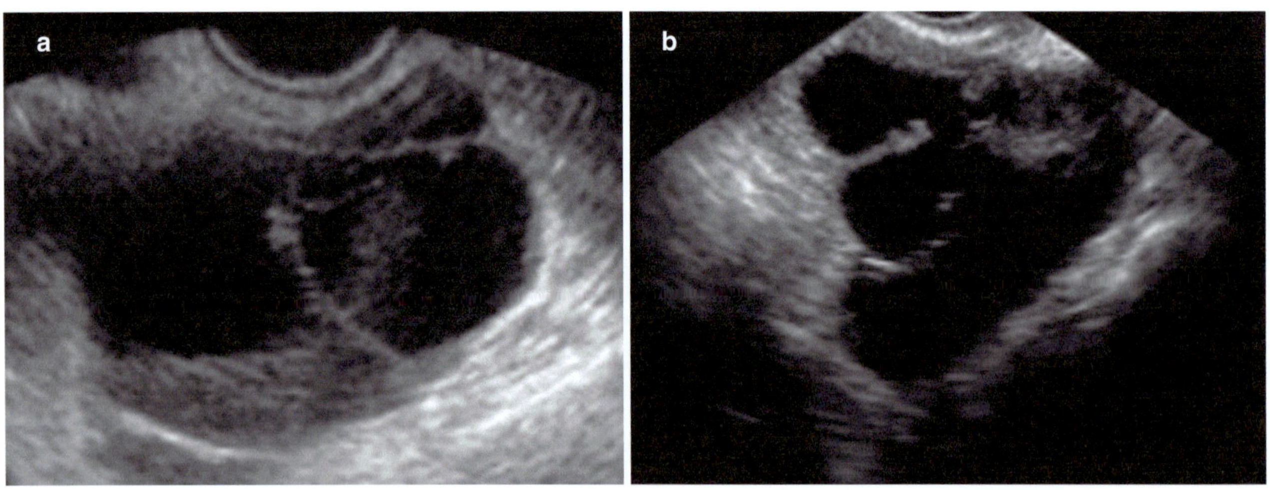

Fig. 5.97 Pelvic encapsulated effusion. (**a**–**d**) Sonogram shows an irregular fluid lesion in the pelvis of a patient after hysterectomy. Septum is visible inside, and some patients may have lower abdominal pain

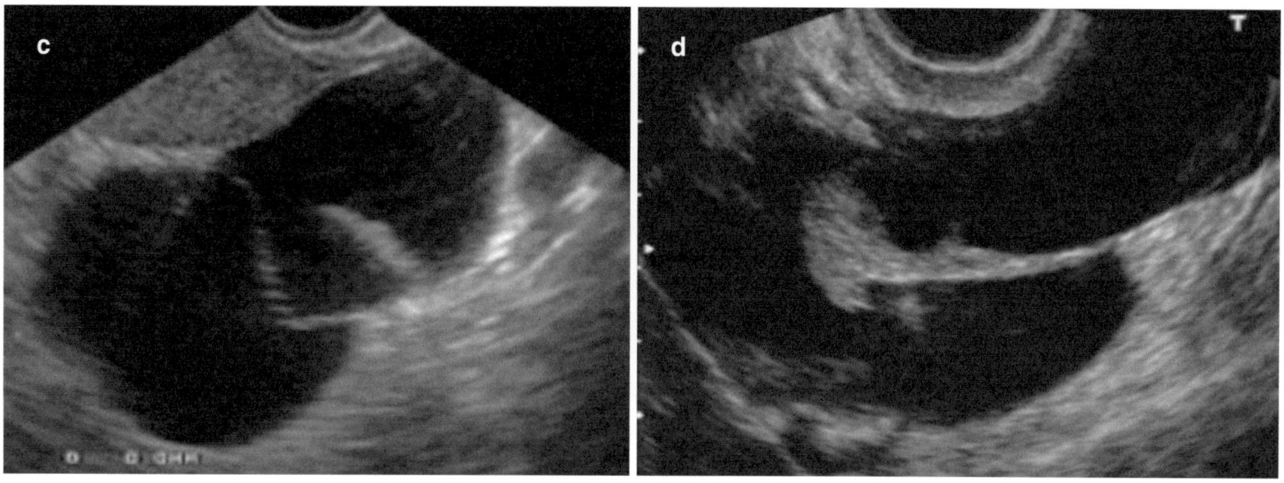

Fig. 5.97 (continued)

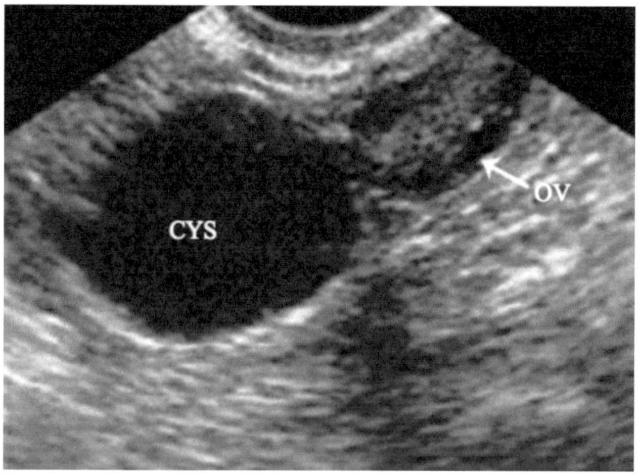

Fig. 5.98 Mesosalpinx cyst. The cyst locates next to the ovary, with a diameter of less than 5.0 cm. The size and shape of the ovary are normal, and the patient has no symptoms.

Suggested Reading

1. Van T, Van D. Ultrasound diagnosis of endometriosis and adenomyosis: state of the art. Best Pract Res Clin Obstet Gynaecol. 2018;8(16–24):16–24.
2. Andres MP, Borrelli GM, Ribeiro J, et al. Transvaginal ultrasound for the diagnosis of Adenomyosis: systematic review and meta-analysis. J Minim Invasive Gynecol. 2017;25(2):635–40.
3. Chen J, Chen W, Zhang L, et al. Safety of ultrasound-guided ultrasound ablation for uterine fibroids and Adenomyosis: a review of 9988 cases[J]. Ultrason Sonochem. 2015;27:671–6.
4. Brindha D, Kandaswamy A, Lakshmideepika C. Digital image analysis of uterine ultrasound for classification of uterine Myoma and Adenomyoma. J Med Imaging & Health Informatics. 2015;5(8):1603–6.
5. Perrot D, Fernandez H, Levaillant JM, et al. Quality assessment of pelvic ultrasound for uterine myoma according to the CNGOF guidelines[J]. J Gynecol Obstetrics Human Reproduction. 2017;S2468784717300326
6. Rizzo S, Femia M, Buscarino V, et al. Endometrial cancer: an overview of novelties in treatment and related imaging key points for local staging. Cancer Imaging. 2018 Dec 04;18(1):45.
7. Lin MY, Dobrotwir A, McNally O, et al. Role of imaging in the routine management of endometrial cancer. Int J Gynaecol Obstet. 2018 Oct;143(Suppl 2):109–17.
8. Hefler L, Lafleur J, Kickmaier S, et al. Risk of endometrial cancer in asymptomatic postmenopausal patients with thickened endometrium: data from the FAME-Endo study: an observational register study. Arch Gynecol Obstet. 2018;298(4):813–20.
9. Skaznik-Wikiel ME, Jelovsek JE, et al. Accuracy of endometrial thickness in detecting benign endometrial pathology in postmenopausal women. Menopause. 2010;17(1):104–8.
10. Cogendez E, Eken MK, Bakal N, et al. The role of transvaginal power Doppler ultrasound in the differential diagnosis of benign intrauterine focal lesions. J Med Ultrason (2001). 2015 Oct;42(4):533–40.
11. Wong M, Crnobrnja B, Liberale V, et al. The natural history of endometrial polyps. Hum Reprod. 2017;32(2):340–5.
12. Bittencourt CA, Dos Santos SR, Bernardo WM, et al. Accuracy of saline contrast sonohysterography in detection of endometrial polyps and submucosal leiomyomas in women of reproductive age with abnormal uterine bleeding: systematic review and meta-analysis. Ultrasound Obstet Gynecol. 2017 Jul;50(1):32–9.
13. Sahdev A. Cervical tumors. Semin Ultrasound CT MR. 2010 Oct;31(5):399–413.
14. Comparetto C, Borruto F. Cervical cancer screening: a never-ending developing program. World J Clin Cases. 2015 Jul 16;3(7):614–24.
15. Park GE, Rha SE. Ultrasonographic findings of low-grade endometrial stromal sarcoma of the uterus with a focus on cystic degeneration. Ultrasonography. 2016 Apr;35(2):124–30.
16. Alcázar JL. Extragenital endometrial stromal sarcoma arising in endometriosis. Gynecol Obstet Invest. 2012;73(4):265–71.
17. Lin LH. Is Doppler ultrasound useful for evaluating gestational trophoblastic disease? Clinics (Sao Paulo). 2015 Dec;70(12):810–5.
18. Asmar FTC. Uterine artery Doppler flow velocimetry parameters for predicting gestational trophoblastic neoplasia after complete hydatidiform mole, a prospective cohort study. Clinics (Sao Paulo). 2017 May;72(5):284–8.
19. Antonini F, Laterza L, Fuccio L, Macarri G. Gastric metastasis from ovarian adenocarcinoma presenting as a subepithelial tumor and diagnosed by endoscopic ultrasound-guided tissue acquisition. World J Gastrointest Oncol. 2017 Nov 15;9(11):452–6.

20. Hong LUO, Tai-zhu YANG, Fan YANG, et al. The value of transvaginal color Doppler ultrasonography in the diagnosis of endometrial polyps. West China Med J. 2011;26(3):410–2.
21. Jiao CHEN, Tai-zhu YANG, Fan YANG, et al. Ultrasonic manifestations of uterine endometrial stromal sarcoma. Chin J Imaging Technol. 2014;30(4):600–2.
22. Xin CHEN, Bo ZHANG, Tai-zhu YANG, et al. Research on the diagnostic value of ultrasonography in examining oblique vaginal septum syndrome. West China Med J. 2011;26(11):1684–6.

Ultrasonography in Female Infertility and Contraceptive Operation

6

Hong Luo and Houqing Pang

6.1 Ultrasonography in the Diagnosis and Treatment of Female Infertility

I. The application of ultrasonography in the diagnosis of female infertility
  - Basic conceptions
  - Infertility, a disease of the reproductive system, is defined as the failure to achieve a clinical pregnancy after 12 months or more of regular unprotected sexual intercourse. The causes include ovulation disorders and congenital genital malformation. In this section, we will talk about infertility caused by ovulation disorders, which is common in polycystic ovary syndrome (PCOS), ovarian hyperstimulation syndrome, luteinized unruptured follicle syndrome, premature ovarian failure, congenital ovarian insufficiency, and bilateral ovarian tumors.
  - Common clinical methods for monitoring ovulation include: basal body temperature, alteration of cervical mucus, the blood level of estrogen and progesterone in vivo.
  - Ultrasonography can continually monitor the periodic variation of ovary and measure the size of follicle to judge whether follicles are growing to mature follicle and then ovulate. Continual ultrasonography monitor can discover some peculiar condition, in which the ovarian morphology is inconsistent with the level of hormone.
  - Ultrasonic diagnosis
    - Ultrasound monitor of normal ovarian period

      To monitor follicle, the ultrasound examination should start on the fifth day of menstruation period to measure the size of ovary and count the number of the follicle.

      From the eighth to 12th day of menstruation period, it is the key point to monitor the growth of follicles every day or every other day and find the primary follicle with a diameter of 1–1.5 cm. The preovulatory phase is defined as the 11th to 13th day of menstruation period, and during this phase the diameter of follicle is up to 1.5–1.7 cm, which is called dominant follicle.

      The 13th and 14th day of menstruation period is called ovulatory phase, during which the diameter of follicle is up to 1.8 cm which is called a mature follicle; the range of volume is 2.5–2.8 ml and the range of diameter is 1.7–2.4 cm. Mature follicle is located on the surface of ovary and protrudes from it, round or oval, with high tension, clear cyst fluid, and thin and clear inner wall. Sometimes germ hillock is located by the side of follicle, meaning that the ovulation will happen in 36 hours. The average growth speed of follicle is 2–4 mm per day, and 5 hours before ovulation the follicle grows 7 mm.

      When the level of hormone is up to some extent, the mature follicle rupture to ovulate and then follicle fluid flow to Douglas pouch. After ovulation, the wall of follicle sac collapses and its outline gets fuzzy. The formed blood body shows slighter weak echo. Five to seven days after ovulation, the blood body is transferred to corpus luteum with spotty echo or latticed echo in it, and CDFI shows surrounding blood flow. When the next menstruation is coming, the corpus luteum disappears and a new period will start (Fig. 6.1).

This chapter was translated by **Feiran Liu**, Department of Obstetrics and Gynecology, Beijing Shijitan Hospital, Bejing, China

H. Luo (✉) · H. Pang
Department of Ultrasonography, West China Second University Hospital, Sichuan University, Chengdu, China

T. Yang, H. Luo (eds.), *Practical Ultrasonography in Obstetrics and Gynecology*,
https://doi.org/10.1007/978-981-16-4477-1_6

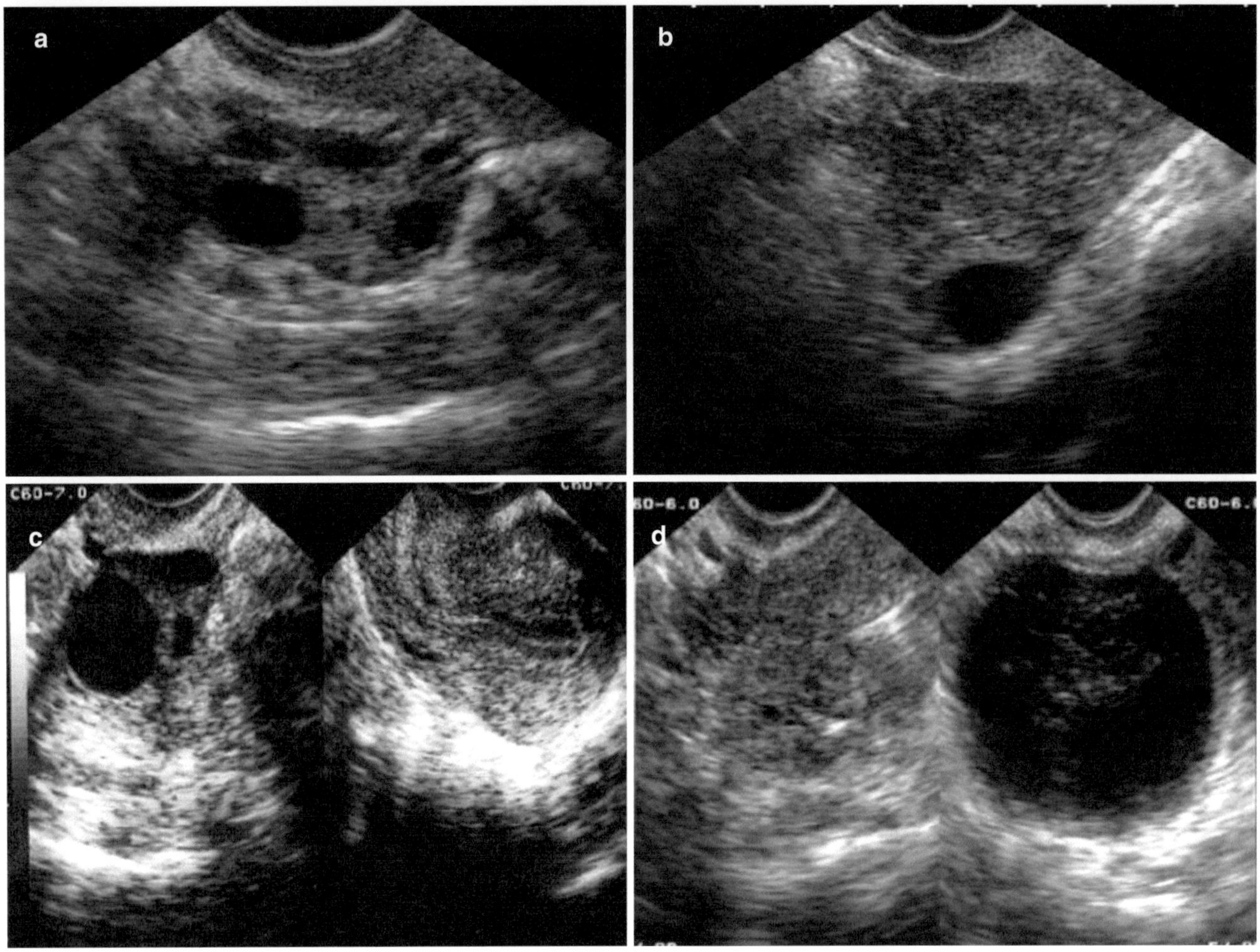

Fig. 6.1 Period of the ovary. (**a**) The fifth day of menstruation period, it shows multiple early follicles in various sizes. (**b**) Dominant follicle. (**c**) Mature follicle. (**d**) Corpus luteum

- Polycystic ovaries

  The ovary is enlarged, mostly bilaterally. The echo of membrane of ovary enhanced and thickened, showing a clear boundary with the surrounding tissue.

  More than 10 follicles can be seen in one sonographic section, with the range of diameter of 2–10 mm, and the majority is no more than 6 mm. Follicles arrange in a wheels-like shape under the ovarian membrane, surrounding the ovary, or all the follicles in ovary are little follicles. The ovarian medulla is enlarged and echo enhanced. Because of anovulation, no typical mature follicle and sign of ovulation can be monitored in continual ultrasound examination (Fig. 6.2).
- Follicles agenesis

  In both of the ovaries, the diameter of cyst is no more than 9 mm. Under continual monitoring, the follicle shows no sign of growing up during the ovarian period (Fig. 6.3).
- Small follicular cycle

  During the continual monitoring through the ovarian period, the average growth speed and the average size of the follicle are significantly lower than normal.

  The diameter of preovulatory follicle is no more than 15 mm with irregular shape and low tension (Fig. 6.4).
- Large follicular cycle

  During ovarian cycle, ovulation happens when the diameter of follicle is more than 30 mm. The egg cell is overripe and cannot be easily fertilized (Fig. 6.5).
- luteinized unruptured follicle

  During the continual monitor, the mature follicle continues to grow up with a thickening follicle wall, and the diameter of follicle can be more than 40 mm.

  The reticular cystic occupation in the ovary will disappear until the next menstruation. (Fig. 6.6).

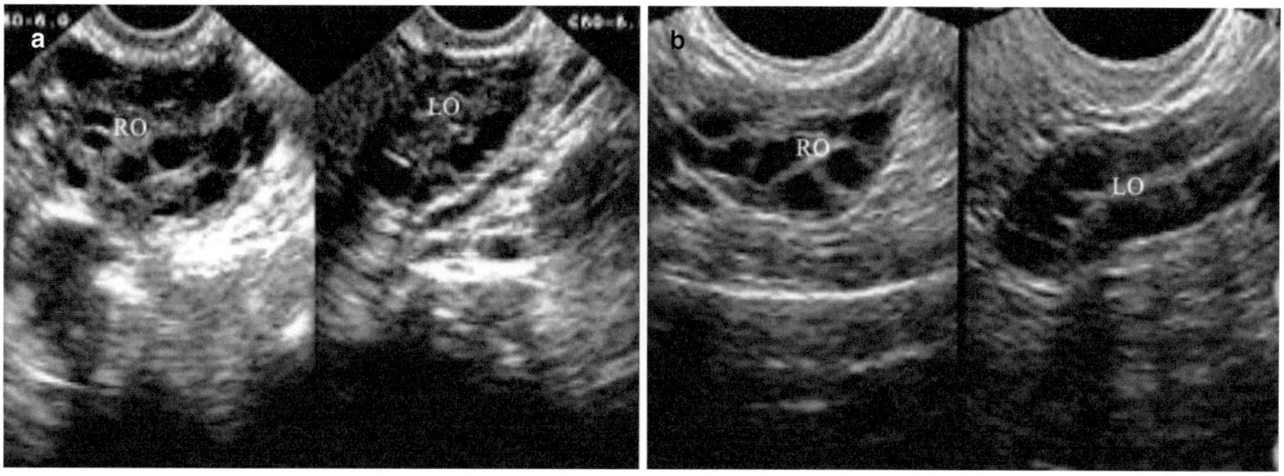

Fig. 6.2 Polycystic ovaries. (**a**) 22-years old, amenorrhea for 2 years with polytrichia. The transvaginal ultrasound shows bilateral enlarged ovaries, and there are more than 10 follicles with diameter no more than 10 mm. (**b**) 27-years-old, infertility. Sonogram shows polycystic ovaries

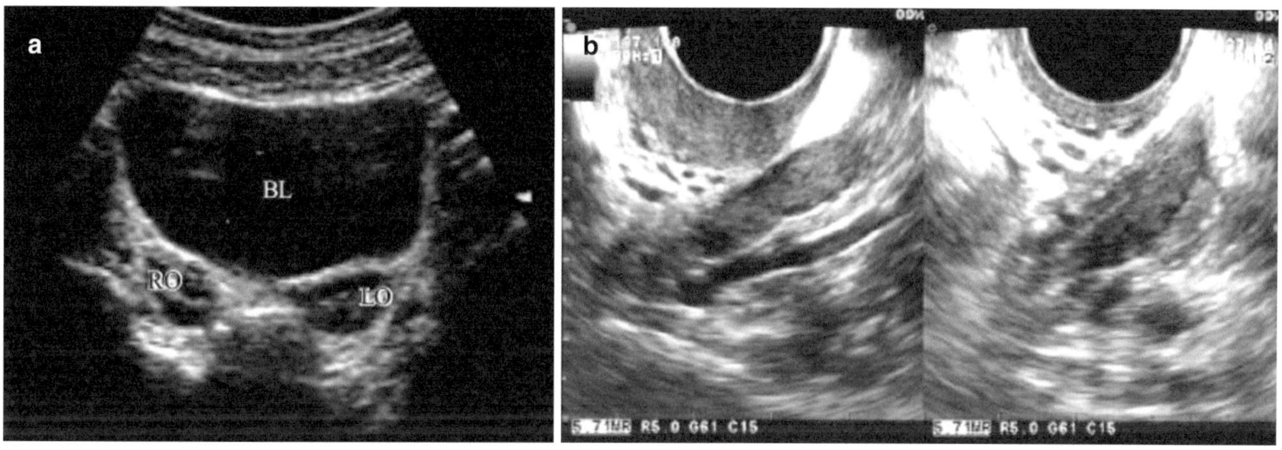

Fig. 6.3 Follicles agenesis. (**a**) During the monitoring through the ovarian period, no follicle is developed. (**b**) 32-years-old, premature ovarian failure. Sonogram shows no follicle in the atrophied ovary

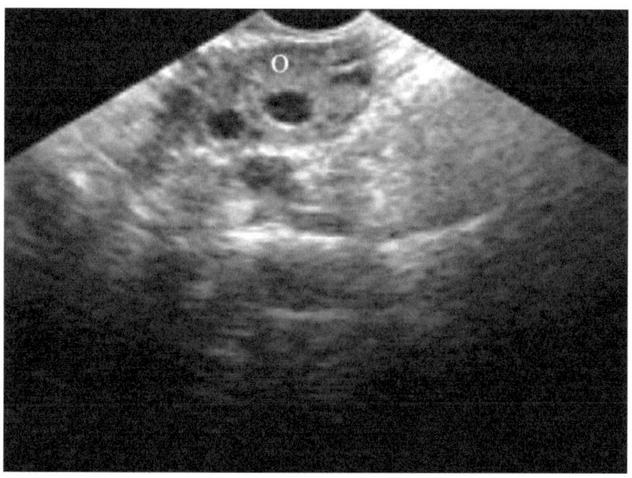

Fig. 6.4 Small follicular cycle. The diameter of follicle is only 15 mm in ovulatory period and disappeared after one day

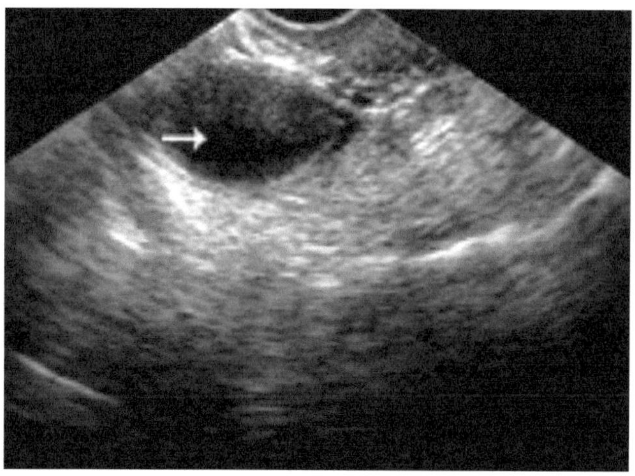

Fig. 6.5 Large follicular cycle. The diameter of follicle in ovulatory period is more than 30 mm

- Ovarian hyperstimulation syndrome (OHSS)

  The bilateral ovaries are significantly enlarged with a thin-wall multilocular cyst, which is 20–60 mm in diameter, with weak spotty echo in it.

  It may combine with hydrothorax and ascites (Fig. 6.7).

- Special tips
  - Ultrasonography can clearly show the number, size, tension, shape, the mature of follicle, estimate ovulation and corpus luteum formation.
  - The growth speed of follicle is much more important than the absolute value of the follicle size in the process of the prediction of ovulation.
  - In general, the follicle with a diameter of more than 17 mm is able to be fertilized.

II. The application of ultrasonography in assisted reproduction

- Ultrasound monitor of endometrium
  - Endometrium is the place where fertilized egg implants. Ultrasound examination can continually monitor the thickness and morphological alteration of the endometrium during menstruation period.
  - In the early stage of hyperplasia, the endometrium shows a thin hyperechoic line with a thickness of less than 5 mm (Fig. 6.8).
  - The thickness of endometrium increases to 10 mm during the upcoming ovulation.
  - During the late stage of hyperplasia and the early stage of secretory phase, the endometrium with characterized lip-shape or ring-shape triple line layer is suitable for the implantation of fertilized egg.
  - As literature reported, during ovulation, endometrium characterized with triple-line sign, the thickness of which is more than 8 mm, is more suitable to be implanted by artificial embryo. However, if the endometrium is hyperechoic and more than 16 mm or less than 8 mm in thickness, the possibility of pregnancy decreases significantly. If the endometrium is no more than 6 mm in thickness, it is not suitable to be implanted (Figs. 6.9 and 6.10).
  - During the treatment of artificial cycle and assisted-reproduction treatment of IVF-ET, ultrasound examination is vital to monitor the morphology, thickness, and echo of endometrium to ensure the prediction of pregnancy and the treatment of artificial cycle.
  - Monitor the blood flow of the endometrium during the mid-luteal phase after ovulation to evaluate the endometrial receptivity (Fig. 6.11).
- Ultrasound monitor of induced ovulation cycle
  - Ultrasound examination can help to monitor the development of follicle, evaluate the therapeutic effect, prevent OHSS, and guide clinical medication in the process of induced ovulation.
  - Patients diagnosed with anovulatory infertility should undertake ultrasound examination to exclude ovarian cyst or polycystic ovaries before treatment.
  - During medication treatment of induced ovulation, the number of ovaries increases and the diameter of ovaries can reach 8–10 mm. More than one dominant primary follicle can be discovered. The diameter of the primary follicle can reach 18–25 mm, indicating that the follicles get mature (Fig. 6.12).
  - Continually monitor the size of follicle with short interval to direct the medication of induced fertilization both in duration and dosage during the process of ovulation induced by medicine.
  - Ultrasound monitor can direct the usage of medicine in the process of induced ovulation to promote rupture and ovulation of follicle at a suitable time.
- Application of color Doppler ultrasound in the monitor of follicle
  - Observe the distribution of uterine arteries and ovarian vessels, the blood flow velocity, and blood flow resistance to evaluate the function of the corpus luteum and the development of follicles.
  - Oyesanya found that the existence of blood flow of follicle is significantly related to the collection of egg cells. Mature follicle with flow blood signals under ultrasound could be collected with egg cells of high quality. On the opposite, immature follicle, without blood flow signals under ultrasound, cannot be easily collected with egg cells (Fig. 6.13).
  - As mentioned in paper, the value of PI reaches the lowest on the 9 days after blood peak of LH, indicating good function of corpus luteum and good

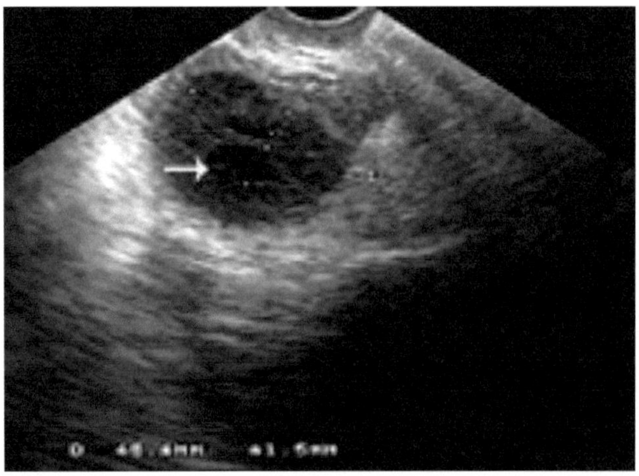

Fig. 6.6 Luteinized follicle. The cyst has thick wall and septum inside. During continual observation, the cyst is disappeared after menstruation

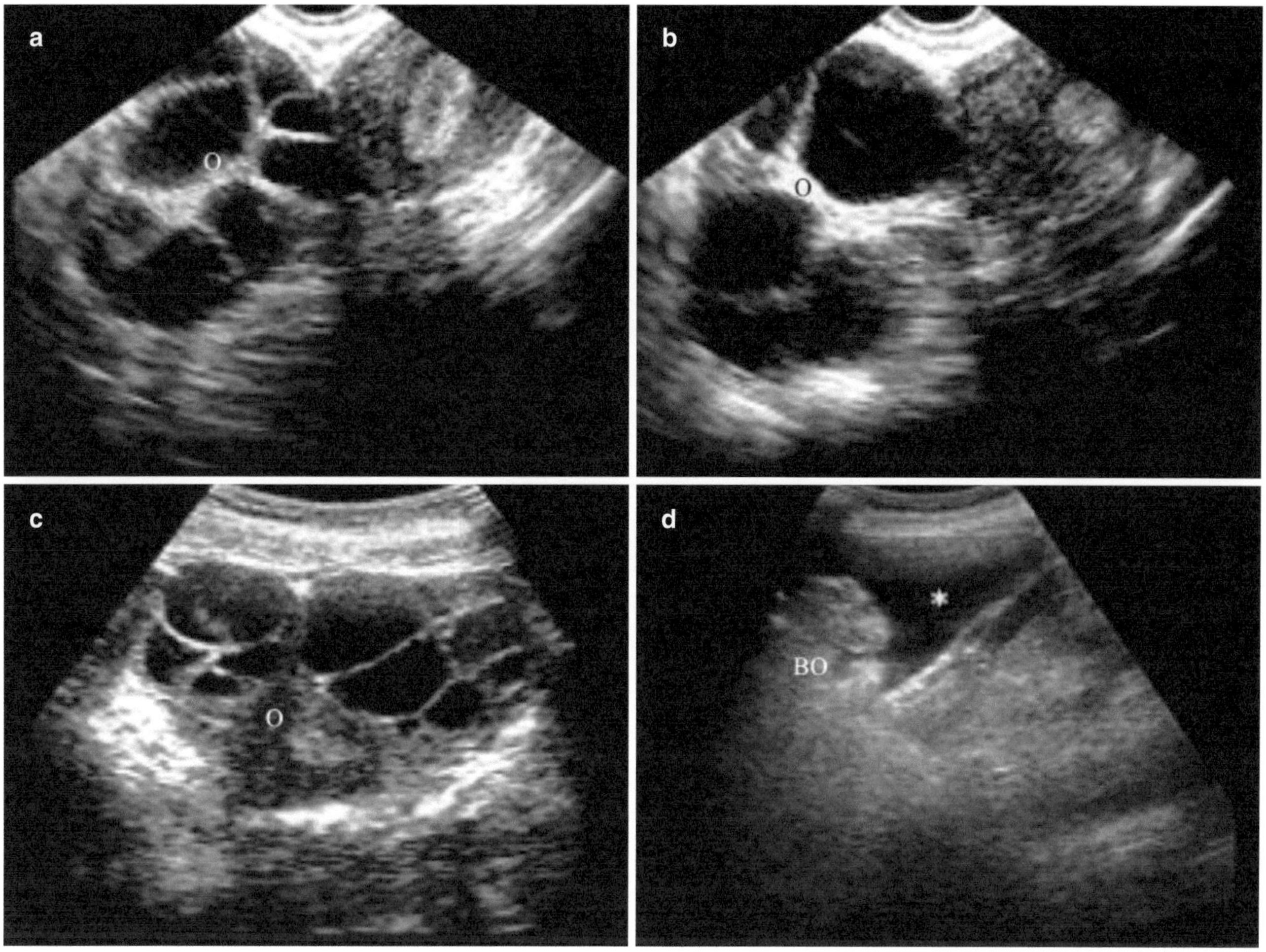

Fig. 6.7 Ovarian hyperstimulation syndrome (**a**, **b**) the bilateral ovaries are significantly enlarged with multilocular cyst after administration of ovulation drug, with the largest cyst diameter of 35 mm. (**c**, **d**) the bilateral ovaries are significantly enlarged with multilocular cyst after injection of ovulation drug, combined with hydrothorax and ascites

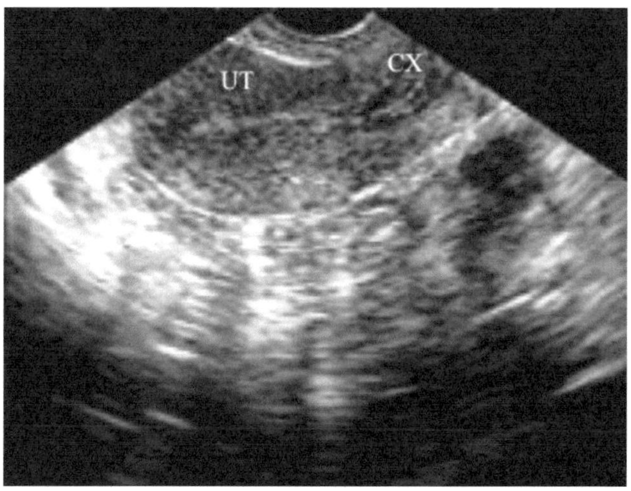

Fig. 6.8 Early stage of hyperplasia. Sonogram shows the endometrium as a thin hyperechoic line

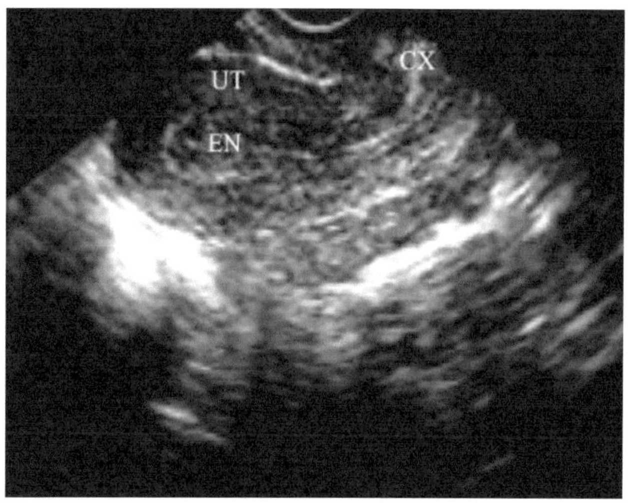

Fig. 6.9 Triple-line sign of endometrium before ovulation

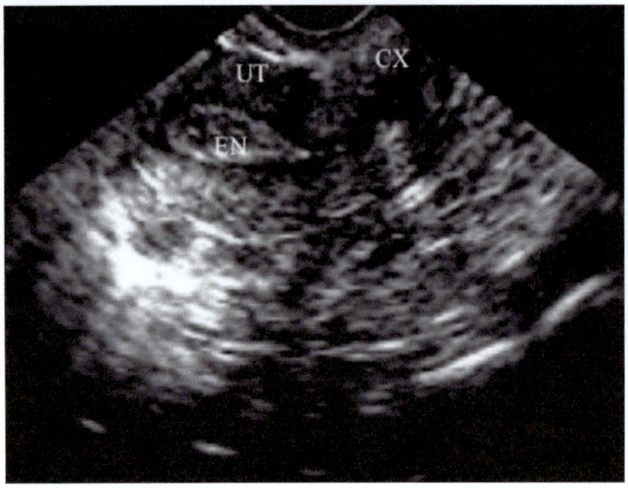

Fig. 6.10 Hyperechoic and fusiform endometrium during late ovulation

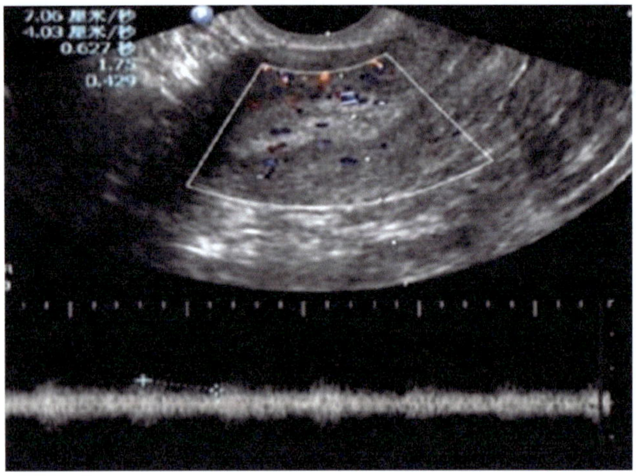

Fig. 6.11 Blood flow is visible in the endometrium on the 21st day of menstruation period

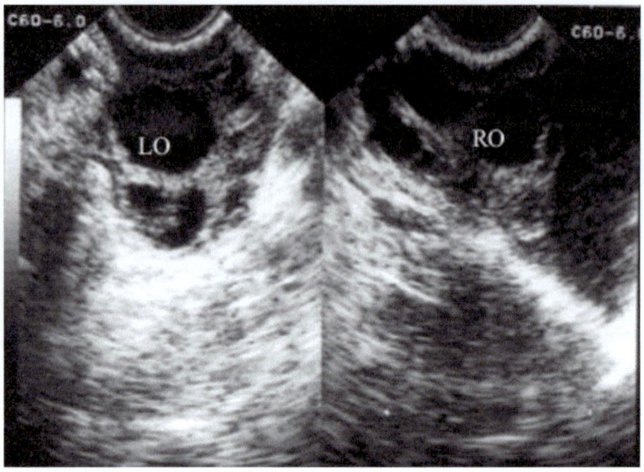

Fig. 6.12 The image shows more than three dominant follicles after medical ovulation treatment

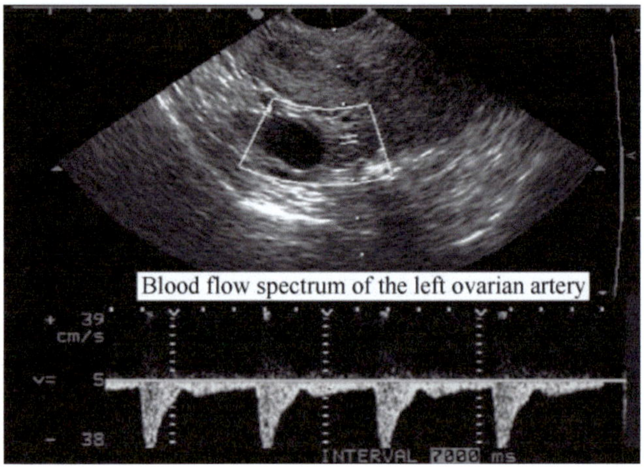

Fig. 6.13 Blood flow spectrum around the follicle

uterine blood perfusion. In this condition, the success rate of embryo implantation is high.

- Under Doppler examination, the diastole velocity of the follicle artery is relatively slow in the early stage of follicle development. There are abundant new blood vessels surrounding the corpus luteum and mature follicles. The decrease of blood resistance means luteal function formation.
- In the natural ovulation cycle, the resistance of artery in the ovary without follicle formation is much higher than that with follicle formation. In the induced ovulation cycle, when the diameter of follicle is more than 15 mm, the blood resistance drops down.
- The velocity of the follicle artery is slow, with increased blood resistance, in the cases of follicular dysplasia, luteal dysfunction, and unruptured follicle luteinization.

6.2 Ultrasound Diagnosis of Intrauterine Device

1. Basic conception

Intrauterine device (IUD) is the common method of birth control, with the characteristic of efficient, simple, reversible and economic. There are various IUDs in clinical application, which are displayed in Fig. 6.14.

- Partial ectopic refers to that part of IUD inserts into the myometrium, while the rest part is still in the cavity. It usually occurs when the IUD is placed improperly or placed for too long, the uterus shrinks after menopause, or the IUD is relatively too large.
- Complete ectopic

- Complete ectopic is characterized as the IUD is completely inserted into the myometrium and cannot be found inside the cavity. Both partial ectopic and complete ectopic all belong to IUD incarceration.
- Extrauterine ectopic
- Extrauterine ectopic is defined as the IUD is completely outside the uterus.
- Ultrasonography is utilized to identify the existence and type of IUD, as well as the location and form of IUD. The displacement, incarceration, perforation, and pregnancy with IUD can be found by ultrasonography.

2. Ultrasonic diagnosis
   - Intrauterine device
     - Different kinds of IUD with different materials show different sonographic characteristics (Figs. 6.15, 6.16, 6.17, 6.18, 6.19, and 6.20). Most tail wire of the IUD shows a hyperechoic line under ultrasonography (Fig. 6.21).
     - There are two common methods to judge whether the IUD is in the right location. (1) On the longitudinal section of uterus, the top of IUD is less than 2 cm away from the exterior periphery of uterine serosal layer. (2) On the longitudinal section of uterus, the superior extremity location of IUD is above the bisector point of the line between the uterine fundus and internal cervical os.
   - Downward IUD. The criteria stated above is used to measure whether the IUD is downward. Significant downward IUD can be totally located in the cervical canal (Figs. 6.22 and 6.23).
   - Ectopic IUD
     - Partial ectopic: IUD is not located in the center of uterine cavity, partially inserted into muscular layer or close to serosal layer, partially in the uterine cavity.
     - Complete ectopic: ultrasound examination shows the depth of IUD inserted into muscular layer and no IUD in the uterine cavity (Fig. 6.24).
     - Extrauterine IUD
     - Ultrasound shows that IUD is in the para-uterine organs, Douglas pouch, or vesicouterine pouch. If the ectopic IUD is far from uterus and covered by the surrounding intestine or above the pelvic cavity, ultrasound examination cannot accurately locate its position, and further examinations such as X-ray, CT, or MRI are necessary.
   - Pregnancy with IUD
   - Pregnancy with IUD mostly happens with ectopic IUD. Both the IUD and gestational sac are shown in

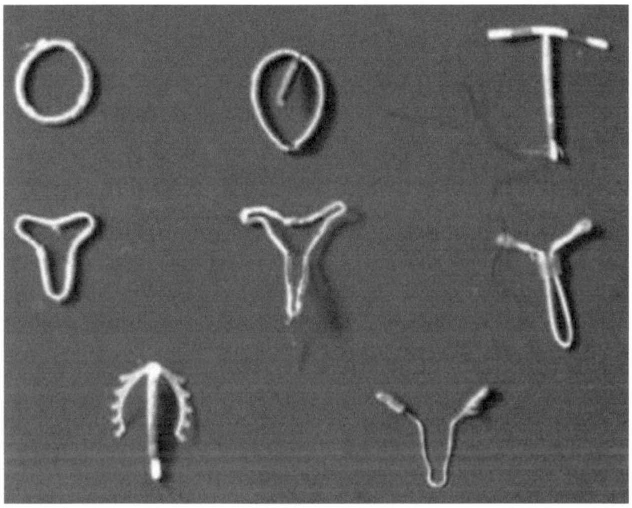

Fig. 6.14 Various kind of IUD. Ectopia of IUD includes partial ectopic, complete ectopic, extrauterine ectopic

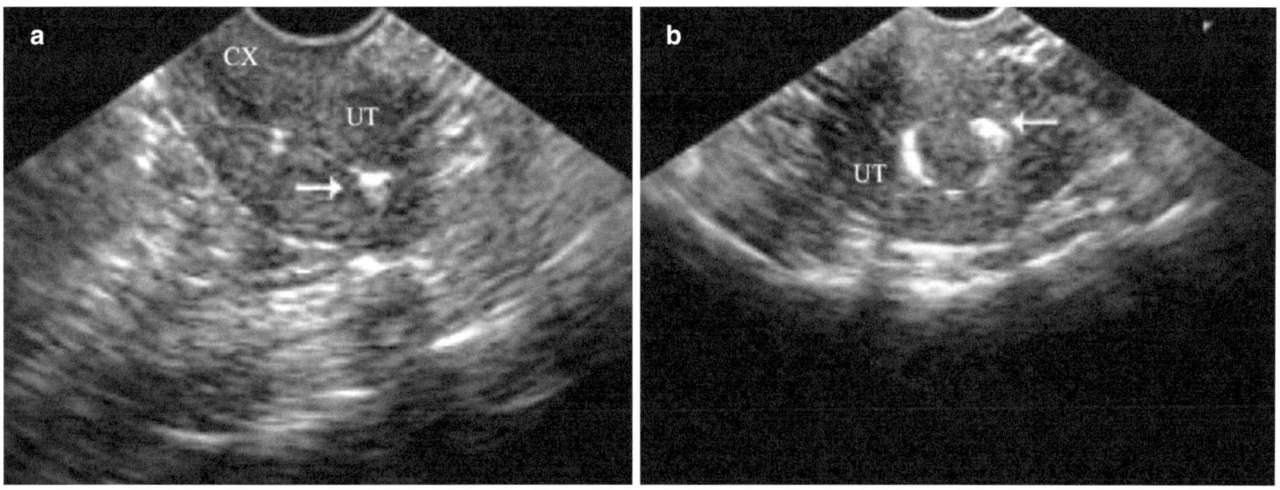

Fig. 6.15 Metal IUD. (**a**) Retroverted uterus. The longitudinal view of the uterus shows two parallel hyperechoic lines in the shape of the Chinese character "二", with posterior comet tail sign. (**b**) The transverse view shows a circle IUD

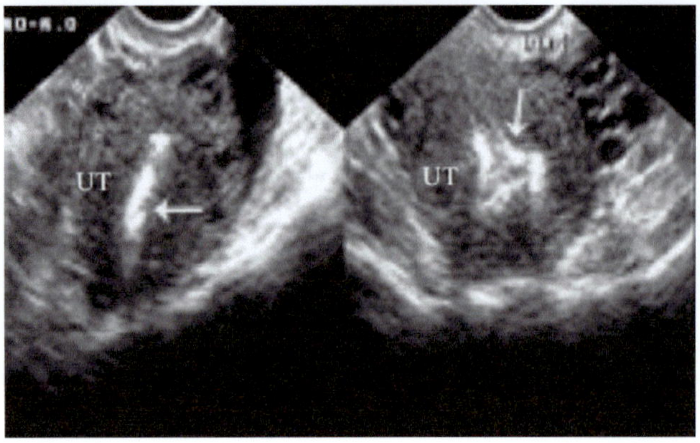

Fig. 6.16 Intrauterine device. Sonogram shows an "I"-shaped hyperechoic IUD in the uterine cavity on the longitudinal view, which shows a hyperechoic triangle on the transverse view

the uterine cavity at the same time. In some conditions, IUD in the normal location could also be combined with pregnancy (Fig. 6.25).

3. Special tips
   - Ultrasound examination is the preferred method to detect the IUD, replacing the X-ray which is commonly used in the past.
   - When sonographer judging the location of the IUD pays attention to the thickness of muscular layer of fundus. If the myometrium is significantly thickened, notice the location relation between the top of IUD and the fundus of the uterus.

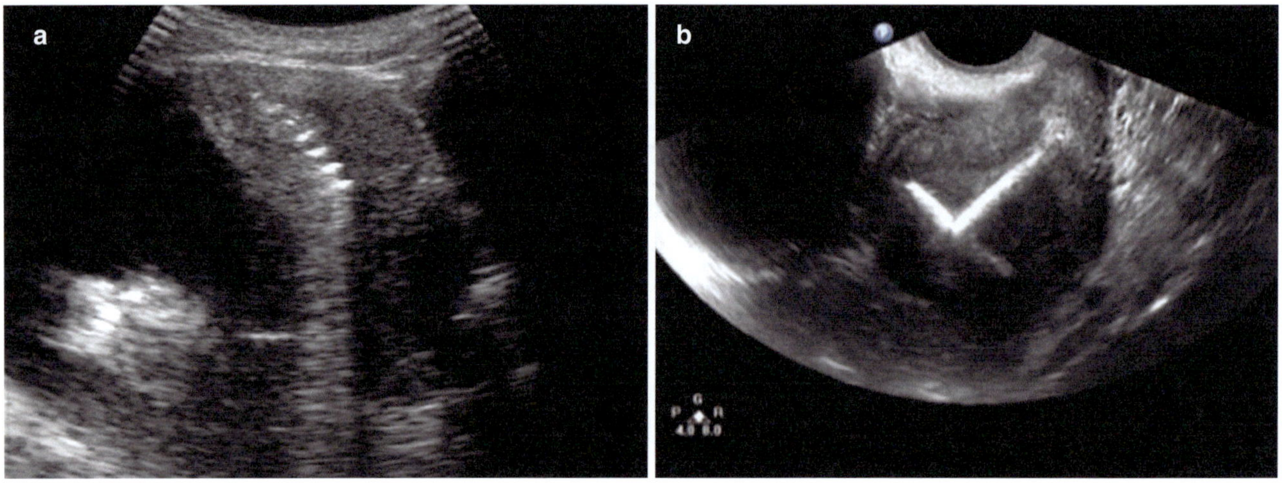

Fig. 6.17 T-shaped IUD. (**a**) Sagittal view shows s beading-shaped hyperechoic IUD. (**b**) Coronal section shows the IUD in a "T" shape

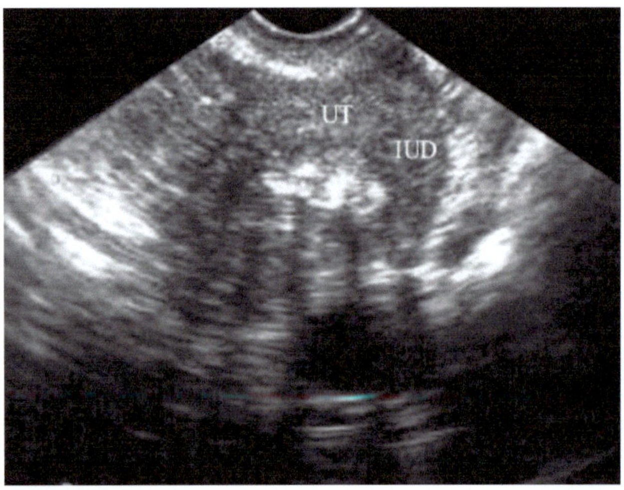

Fig. 6.18 IUD

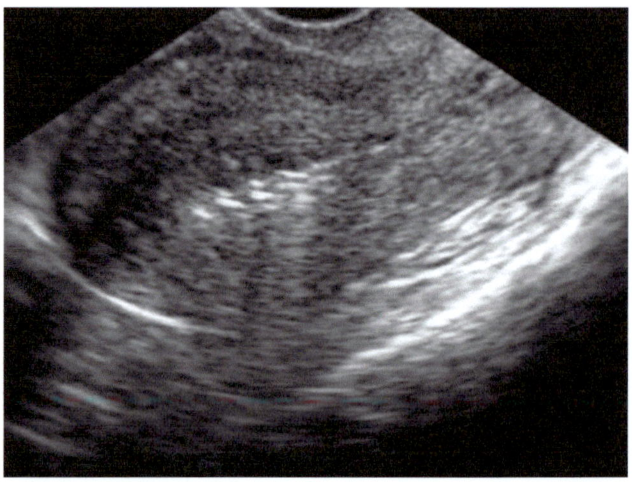

Fig. 6.19 Gyne Fix IUD

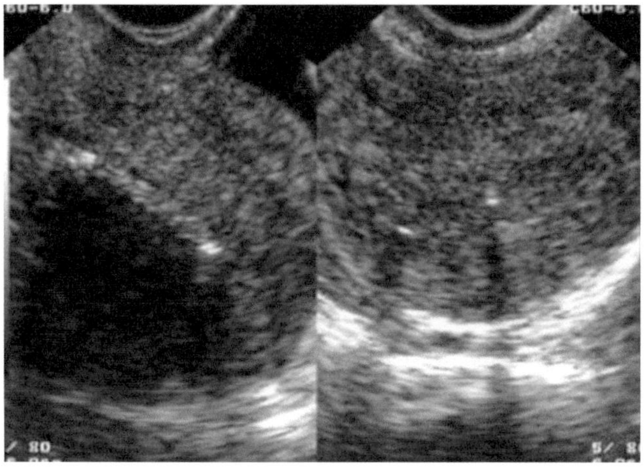

Fig. 6.20 Mirena

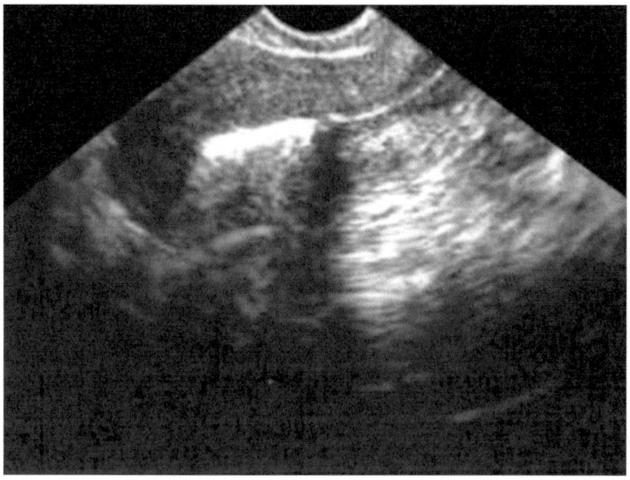

Fig. 6.21 The tail fiber of the IUD shows a bright line

6.3 Ultrasound Diagnosis of Complications of Contraceptive Operation

I. Penetration of uterine

- Basic conception

  Penetration of uterine is the common complication happening during the contraceptive operation. Severe complication is vascular injury, abdominal organs absorbed into the uterine cavity, such as epiploic appendices, omentum, and intestine, resulting in internal hemorrhage, bowel necrosis, inflammation, and even death.

  Common reasons are soft uterus of breastfeeding women, scarred uterus, excessive retroverted or retroflexed uterus, uterine malformation, and unskilled operations.

  Penetration of uterine is divided into incomplete and complete penetration of uterus.

- Ultrasound diagnosis

  – Incomplete penetration of uterus

    Incomplete penetration of uterus refers to the penetration is limited to the myometrium, not involving the serosal layer. The outline of uterus is clearly shown and the echo of serosa is continual. There is no abnormal echo in uterine cavity and only one hyperechoic string is detected in the injured myometrium (Fig. 6.26).

  – Complete penetration of uterus

    Complete penetration of uterine is characterized by the penetration break through the serosal layer, resulting in discontinued serosal layer. The

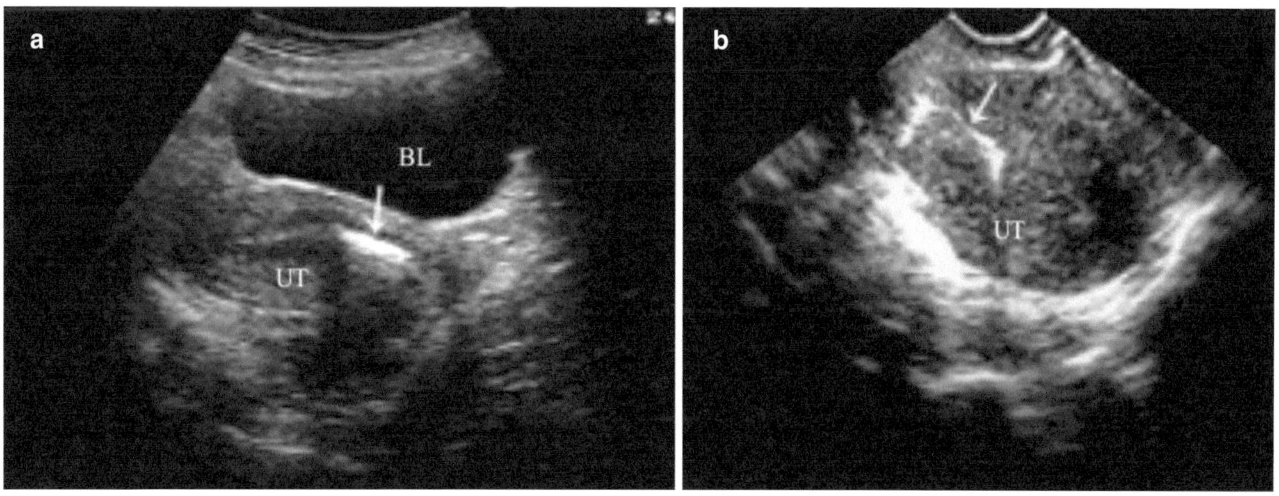

Fig. 6.22 IUD move down to the internal cervical os. (**a**) Transabdominal ultrasound shows that the bottom of IUD reach to the internal os of the cervix. (**b**) Transvaginal ultrasound shows that the bottom of IUD reach to the internal os of the cervix

wide and hyperechoic string echo is visible in the injury with irregular shape. The lesion always protrudes outwards. Intestinal echo can be scanned in the uterine cavity in some cases. Heterogeneous echo is visible around or far from the uterus, and free liquid area is visible in the pelvic cavity (Fig. 6.27).

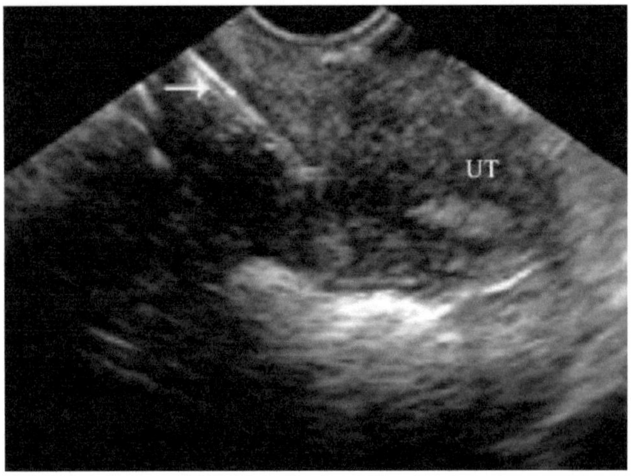

Fig. 6.23 IUD moves down to the cervical canal

- Special tips
  - Pay attention to the continuity of the serosal layer and the completion of the uterine outline in suspected uterine penetration cases.
  - Observe the echo of myometrium and the relationship between the myometrium and the uterine cavity line.
  - Sonographer should be cautious about the abnormal echo in the uterine cavity, parametrial fluid dark area, and masses.
- Typical case

  A 32-year-old patient received uterine curettage because of intrauterine death after 4-month menolipsis and received dilation and curettage three times. She comes to the hospital with the chief complaint of vaginal bleeding. The ultrasonography reports: The size of uterus is larger than normal. The echo of serosal layer is discontinuous. Irregular hyperechoic mass in the size of 20 mm × 16 mm × 23 mm is visible closed to the fundus, partially penetrate through the myometrium and into uterine cavity. The depth of fluid in the Douglas pouch is about 10 mm. The ultrasound manifestation shows suspected penetration of uterus. In the exploratory laparotomy, uterus is found,

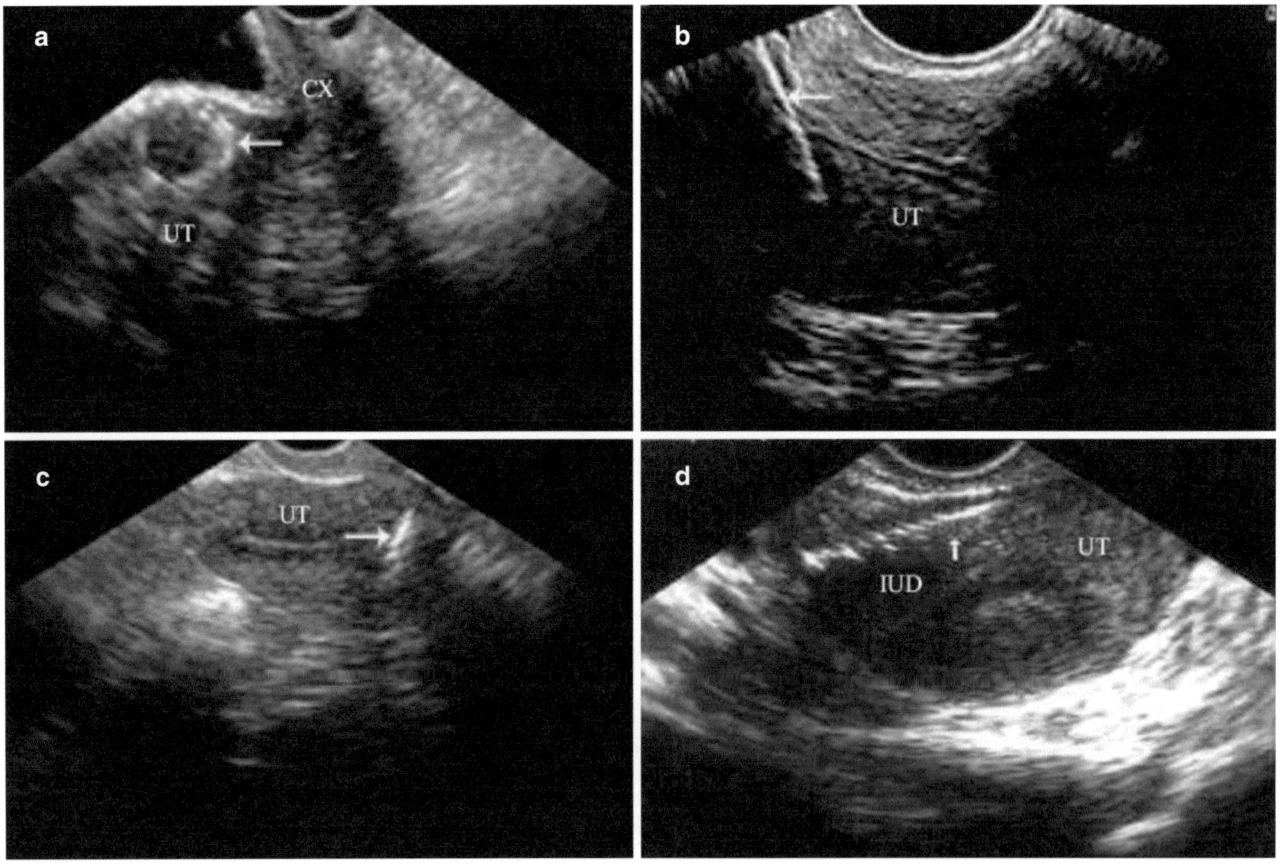

Fig. 6.24 IUD incarceration. (**a**–**d**) IUD inserted into muscular layer partially or completely, representing enhanced echo in the muscular layer

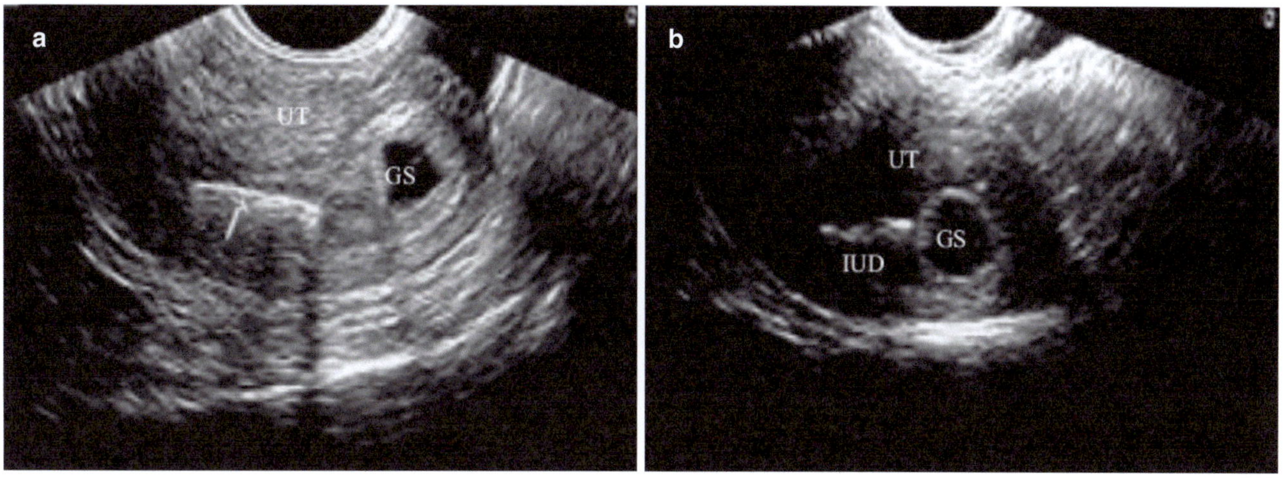

Fig. 6.25 Pregnancy with IUD. (**a**) pregnancy with downward IUD; (**b**) pregnancy with IUD in normal location

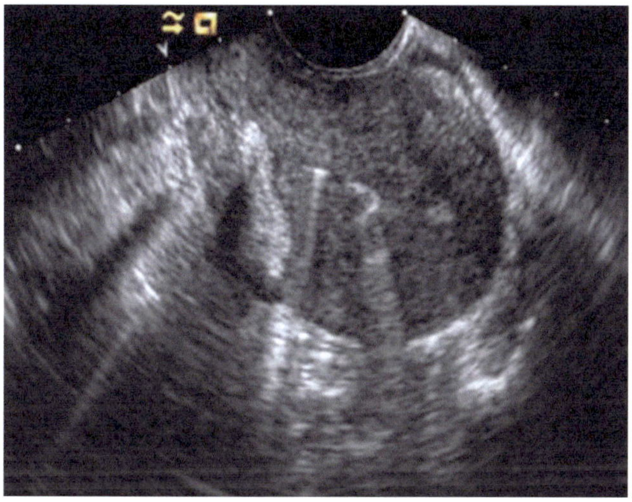

Fig. 6.26 Incomplete penetration of anterior uterine wall, without breaking through to the serosal layer

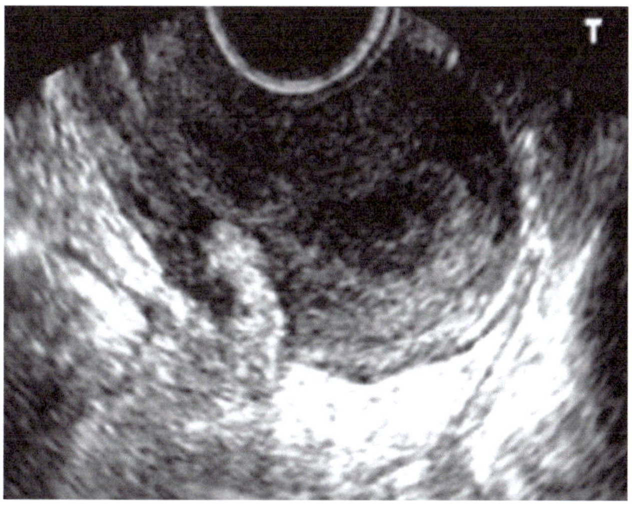

Fig. 6.27 Complete penetration of anterior uterine wall, breaking through the serosal layer

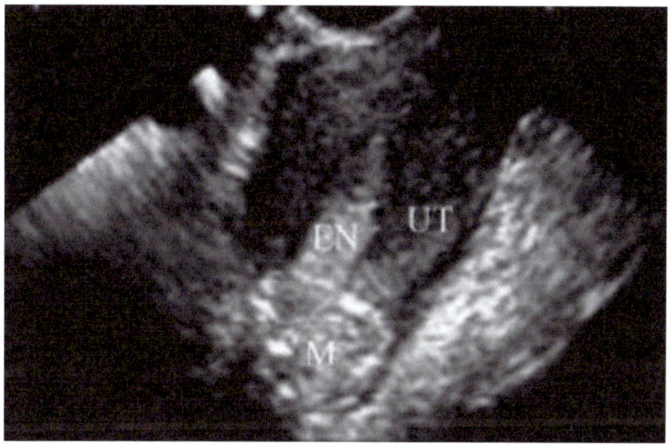

Fig. 6.28 Penetration of uterus. M indicates the mass in the fundus

surrounded with omentum and sigmoid. The mass of 70 mm in size is included with sigmoid, uterine fundus, left ovary fallopian tube, and left pelvic wall, containing fetal scapula and necrotic tissue. The injury is found in the left corner of corpus, which is penetrated with omentum (Fig. 6.28).

II. Intrauterine adhesions and cervical adhesion.
   - Basic conception
     Intrauterine adhesions, also known as Asherman syndrome, is caused by any kind of endometrial injury. The injured endometrium necroses, inflammatory cells infiltrate, and villus or decidual tissue degrades, resulting in fibrous connective tissue and muscular tissue hyperplasia. Even worse, the endometrium is totally injured and fibrous connective tissue or even muscular tissue under it gets exposed and then adheres together. This situation mostly happens after contraceptive operation, curettage, and other intrauterine operation.

The manifestations of Asherman syndrome include: oligomenorrhea, amenorrhea, periodic abdominalgia, infertility, and recurrent abortion. Resistance can be felt during cervical dilatation. In severe cases, the probe fails to go through the cervix to the uterine cavity. After going through the adhered cervix, some dark-red bleed shed out.

According to the location, range, and severity of intrauterine adhesion, the Asherman syndrome is classified as adhesion of internal cervical os, adhesion of uterine cavity, and complex adhesions (Fig. 6.29).

- Ultrasonic diagnosis
  - Simple internal cervical os adhesion: The uterine cavity is separated and fluid dark area is visible in the cavity, with some spotty slight echo. The adhesion lesion of the endometrium is inhomogeneous.
  - Intrauterine adhesion: Adhesion is mostly located in the isthmus uteri. In moderate cases, the uterine cavity is slightly separate, with some scattered echo and hyperechoic line in it. In severe cases, the uterine cavity is obstructed, the cavity line is disappeared, and the endometrium is hypoechoic or anechoic.
  - Complex adhesion
  - Adhesion occurred both in the internal cervical os and uterine cavity. The endometrium is hypoechoic or anechoic, and not clearly identified. The discontinuous endometrium is no more than 2 mm in thickness, and its boundary is not clearly separated from the myometrium.
- Special tips
  - The ultrasonographic feature of intrauterine adhesion is complex. Transvaginal sonohysterography can help to visually show the intrauterine adhesion.
  - Hysteroscopy can evaluate the severity and range of the intrauterine adhesion.

III. Intrauterine pregnancy residual

- Basic conception
  - Intrauterine pregnancy residue is the most common complication of abortion, which could lead to hemorrhage, even hemorrhagic shock.
  - The manifestation of pregnancy residue is vaginal bleeding for more than 10 days after abortion, excessive bleeding, or recurrent bleeding after the bleeding stopped.
- Ultrasonic diagnosis
  - Small amount of intrauterine residue shows a small patchy enhanced echo. Large amount of intrauterine residue shows flaky strong echoes or inhomogeneous echoes, with irregular shapes.
  - Abnormal fluid dark area can be detected in the uterine cavity in patients with bleeding. If observed carefully, flowing slight spotty echo can be captured.
  - If the vaginal bleeding lasts for a long time, the sonogram shows scattered hyperechoic mass in the dark area of separate uterine cavity. Tissue necrosis present as enhanced and disordered echo in the uterine cavity (Fig. 6.30).
  - In some cases, unilateral or bilateral ovarian pregnancy corpus luteum cysts do not disappear.

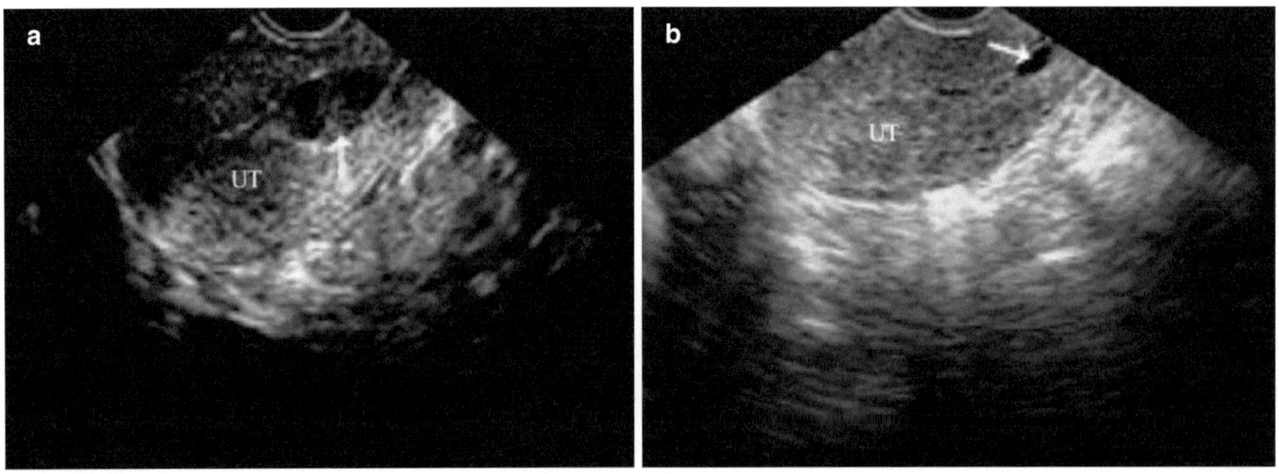

Fig. 6.29 Intrauterine adhesion. (**a**) A 30-year-old patient, amenorrhea 3 months after contraceptive operation. Adhesion is found both in the cervix and uterine cavity. The echo of endometrium is not clear and the mid-down part of uterine cavity is separated by dark area of fluid and slight spot echo. (**b**) Sonogram shows intrauterine adhesion, thin and discontinuous endometrium, and some fluid dark area in the internal cervical os

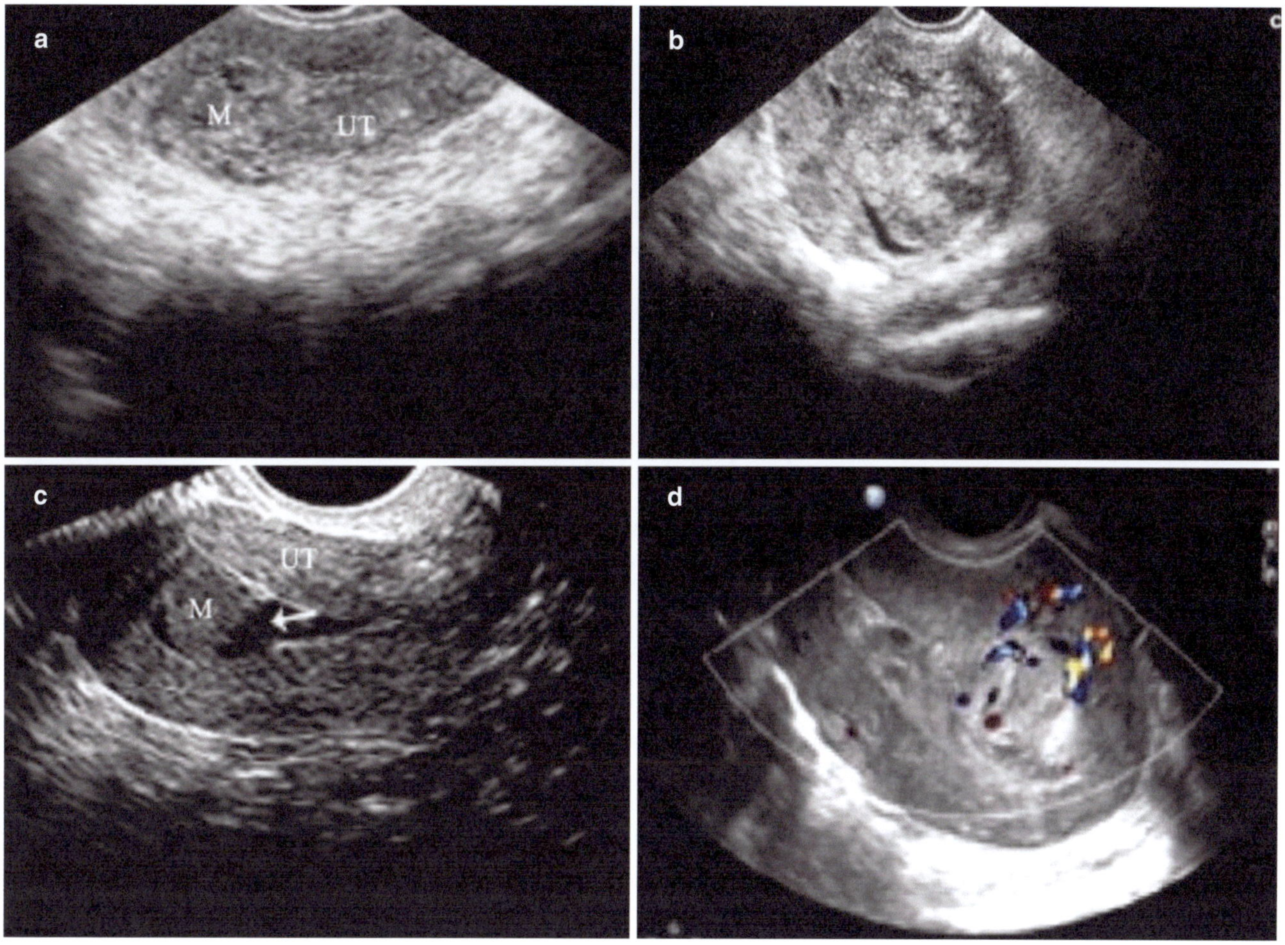

Fig. 6.30 Intrauterine residue. (**a–d**) Images show the intrauterine space-occupying lesions after abortion or induced labor. The curettage was confirmed as residue

– Color Doppler flow image shows the blood flow in the intrauterine occupation, indicating the residue is viable tissue.

IV. Abortion failure

- Basic conception

  Abortion failure is defined as the residual fetus or placental villus in the uterine cavity after abortion.

  The cause of abortion failure includes that the size of embryo sac is too small or too large, excessive uterine flexion, uterine malformation, and operative fault.

- Ultrasonic diagnosis

  – Pregnancy sac is still in the uterine cavity and grows up. Even the embryo and heartbeat are visible (Fig. 6.31).

  – Pay attention to the malformation and abnormal location of the uterus.

V. Pelvic inflammatory disease

- Basic conception

  Pelvic inflammatory disease (PID) refers to the inflammation of female internal genitalia, surrounding connective tissue, and pelvic peritoneum.

  PID caused by contraceptive operation is mostly the result of incomplete suction evacuation and infected operation.

  Fever, abdominal pain, abnormal leukorrhea, and abnormal vaginal bleeding are the main manifestation of PID.

- Ultrasonic diagnosis

  – In mild cases, there are no obvious sonographic features.

  – In severe cases, a sonogram shows the enlarged uterus, thickened and hypoechoic myometrium, and heterogeneous hypoechoic tissue or fluids in the uterine cavity (Fig. 6.32).

  – When inflammation spread to the ovaries and fallopian tubes and forming inflammatory mass, the sonogram shows a cystic mass or hypoechoic mass, with unclear boundary. The patients complain about pain when touching the mass. Fluid is visible around the cyst and in the Douglas pouch.

  – If the pelvic inflammation is not treated in time, it may lead to chronic pelvic inflammation and pelvic cavity adhesion, even pelvic abscess (Fig. 6.33).

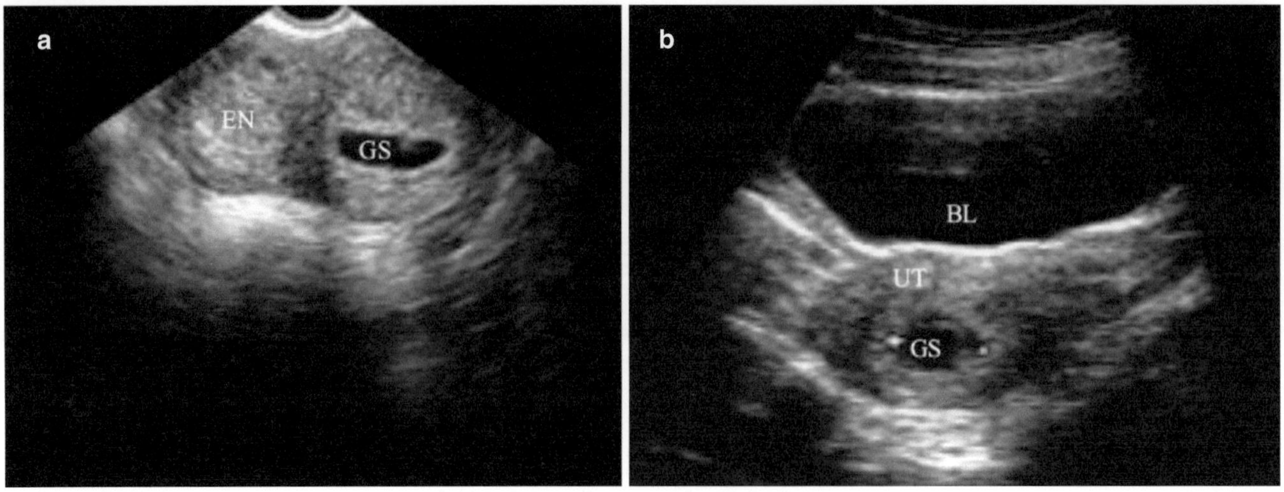

Fig. 6.31 Abortion failure. (**a**) Curettage failure of uterus bicornis. (**b**) After abortion failure, the embryo continues to grow up

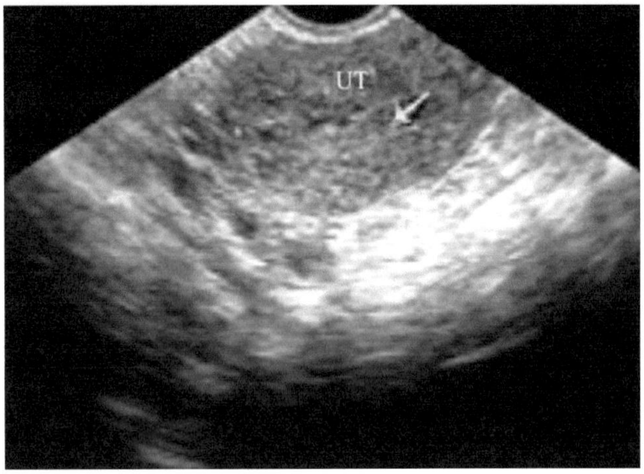

Fig. 6.32 Intrauterine inflammation. A 25-year-old patient, with the complaint of abdominal pain, fever for 1 week after abortion. Sonogram shows inhomogeneous echo in the uterine cavity

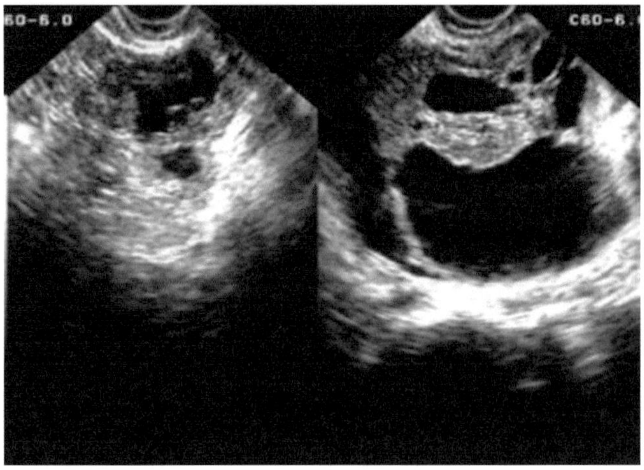

Fig. 6.33 Pelvic inflammatory mass. Twenty days after an induced labor, the patient sees a doctor for lower abdominal pain. The sonogram shows the irregular cystic occupation with septum

Suggested Reading

1. Rollason JC, Outtrim JG, Mathur RS. A pilot study comparing the DuoFertility(®) monitor with ultrasound in infertile women. Int J Women's Health. 2014;6:657–62.
2. Su HW, Yi YC, Wei TY, Chang TC, Cheng CM. Detection of ovulation, a review of currently available methods. Bioeng Transl Med. 2017;2(3):238–46.
3. Nowitzki KM, Hoimes ML, Chen B, Zheng LZ, Kim YH. Ultrasonography of intrauterine devices. Ultrasonography. 2015;34(3):183–94.

Interventional Ultrasound in Obstetrics and Gynecology

7

Hong Luo, Fan Yang, and Min He

7.1 Overview of Interventional Ultrasound

Interventional ultrasound, which is characterized by accurately positioning and minimally invasive, is to complete various biopsies, ultrasonic contrast, aspiration, intubation, and medical injection under the monitor and guidance of real-time ultrasonography, so as to achieve the purpose of diagnosis or treatment.

Interventional ultrasonography has been widely applied in obstetrics and gynecology. For example, it can be used in the process of sampling of prenatal diagnoses, such as chorionic villi biopsy, amniotic fluid extraction, fetal blood sampling, and tissue sampling for biochemical, enzymology, cytogenetics examination. Hysterosalpingography is applied for the diagnosis of the uterine cavity and fallopian tube diseases. Interventional ultrasonography is also used for the intraoperative monitor. In terms of treatment, it is used for puncture biopsy, drainage, and injection of pelvic mass, such as puncture of ovarian endometriotic cyst, encapsulated effusion, and the interventional treatment of ectopic pregnancy. It is also used for follicle puncture, egg retrieval, and fetal reduction during the process of assisted reproduction, as well as intrauterine treatment of fetuses.

At present, three-dimensional ultrasound technology has been used in obstetrics and gynecology. 3-D images can fully and vividly display the spatial relationship and 3-D form of the internal structure of pelvic organs or masses, which helps to accurately locate the lesion for getting biopsies.

This chapter was translated by **Feiran Liu**, Department of Obstetrics and Gynecology, Beijing Shijitan Hospital, Bejing, China

H. Luo (✉) · F. Yang · M. He
Department of Ultrasonography, West China Second University Hospital, Sichuan University, Chengdu, China

7.2 Basic Conditions and Operational Methods of Interventional Ultrasonography

I. Indications and contraindications
- Indications
  - In the purpose of diagnosis: Puncture pump, extraction of umbilical cord blood or amniotic fluid, aspiration cytology, angiography after catheterization, intraoperative monitor, and judgment of tumor nature.
- In the purpose of treatment: Puncture pump, drainage, medical injection (hardeners, antibiotics, hemolytic agents, antitumor drugs and immune preparations, etc.), and nutrients injections (amino acids, blood, etc.)

II. Contraindications
- The images displayed by ultrasound are unclear or unstable or cannot be defined.
- Severe bleeding tendency or impaired coagulation mechanism.
- The approach of puncture cannot avoid essential blood vessels or organs.
- The puncture could lead to the pelvic or abdominal dissemination of lesion.
- The patient is combined with severe systemic diseases, genital inflammation, history of allergy to contrast agents, and related agents.

III. Methods of the operation
- According to the purpose of diagnosis and treatment, choose the supine position, lateral position, prone position, or bladder lithotomy position, and maintained stability.
- Puncture point should be determined under the guidance of real-time ultrasound.
- The puncture area is routinely sterilized and draped.
- After focal anesthesia and locating the targeted lesion, let the patient hold their breath and rapidly

T. Yang, H. Luo (eds.), *Practical Ultrasonography in Obstetrics and Gynecology*,
https://doi.org/10.1007/978-981-16-4477-1_7

puncture the needle into the targeted lesion along the guideline shown on the ultrasound monitor.
- Complete the diagnostic or therapeutic operations such as puncture, biopsy, drainage, and drug injection.
- After the interventional operation, the patients should be observed for 0.5–2 hours, especially paying attention to the vital signs and systemic or local abnormalities such as aggravated abdominal pain, bloody urine, and internal bleeding.

7.3 Application of Intervention Ultrasound in Obstetrics

Under the guidance of real-time ultrasound, the cell, blood, or tissue of the fetus can be obtained accurately for further DNA detection and enzymology examination, which is utilized to diagnose fetal chromosomal abnormalities, hematologic disorders, hereditary disease, and metabolic disease. Interventional ultrasonography is widely applied in the process of amniotic cavity aspiration, fetal blood sampling, and villus sampling. Recently, it is also be used in fetus in utero treatment, egg retrieval, and multifetal reduction. The application of interventional ultrasonography makes the prenatal diagnosis step into the new era of cellular and molecular genetics.

I. Amniotic cavity aspiration.

US-guided amniotic cavity aspiration is to obtain amniotic fluid and gather the cells from the fluid under the guidance of ultrasonography. The analyses of enzyme, protein, metabolite, and karyotype help to diagnose metabolic diseases, neural tube defects, and chromosomal abnormalities. The amniotic injection can also be conducted by interventional ultrasonography. The best time for amniotic cavity aspiration is 18–22 weeks of gestation (Fig.7.1).

- Indications
  - Advanced maternal age (>35 years).
  - In couples with a history of chromosomal disorders and family history, or history of abnormal pregnancy or childbirth.
  - Carriers of X-linked genetic diseases and dominant genetic diseases who require gender identification.
  - Pregnant women with a history of viral infection or radiation exposure; high-risk pregnancy screening or fetal abnormalities detected by routine ultrasonography.
  - Induction of labor by amniocentesis, and intrauterine treatment by injecting drugs and nutrients into the amniotic cavity.

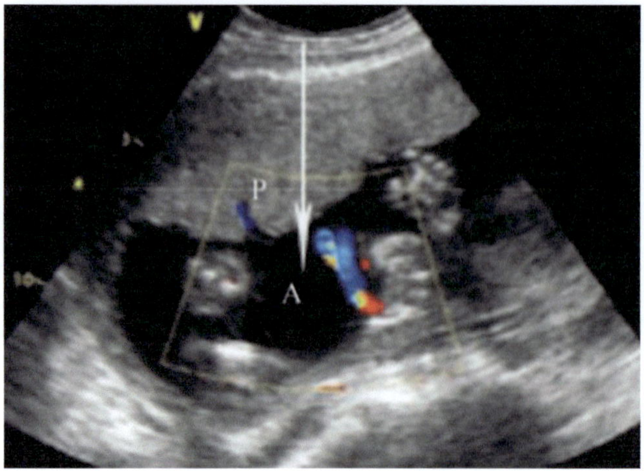

Fig. 7.1 US-guided amniotic cavity aspiration

  - Amniotic fluid was taken for fetal maturity test or bacteriological examination in patients with third-trimester pregnancy or premature rupture of membranes.
- Preoperative preparation
  - Ultrasound equipment. Real-time ultrasound machine is needed and the frequency of the probe is 3.5 MHz, preferably equipped with a puncture guide.
  - Puncture needle. The size of 20-23G is preferable, with a length of 15–18 cm.
  - Medicine. Get preparation for the medicine, according to the purpose of treatment.
  - Others. Tube or culture tube if needed.
- Methods of operation
  - The pregnant woman is placed on the supine position, and routine obstetric ultrasound examination is performed to choose a proper puncture point.
  - After the puncture point is sterilized and draped, determine the insertion route and depth by the ultrasound monitor.
  - The puncture needle reaches into the amniotic cavity, and then removes the needle core. The syringe with the size of 2 ml was used to extract a small amount of amniotic fluid. If blood contamination is excluded, a syringe with the volume of 20 ml is replaced, and extract about 20 ml amniotic liquid for further examination.
  - Inject the medicine into the amniotic cavity if needed.
  - Insert the needle core and pull out the needle.
  - After the operation, check the fetus's heart, fetal movement, and conditions like whether there is active bleeding in the injection point for at least 30 minutes.

- Notes and complications
  - The fetal loss rate of amniotic cavity aspiration is between 0.2% and 1.2%, and the infection rate is 0.3%–2%. The rate of rupture of membranes is about 1%. Other complications include placental abruption, internal bleeding, and leakage of amniotic fluid.
  - The risk of amniocentesis in small gestational age is higher than that in larger gestational age, which can increase the incidence of fetal malformation and strephenopodia may occur.
  - The placenta and fetal body should be kept away as far as possible, and choose the largest amniotic fluid pool. If the placenta is located on the anterior wall, choose the edge or the thinner part of the placenta to inject.

II. US-guided fetal blood sampling

Ultrasound-guided fetal blood sampling can be used to diagnose blood system diseases, such as fetal immune hemolysis, thalassemia, hemophilia, abnormal function, or number of the platelet. It is used to analyze the karyotype of the fetal chromosome to diagnose congenital diseases and metabolic diseases. It can also be used to diagnose viral, bacterial, and toxoplasmosis infections in fetuses. Methods to obtain fetal blood include ultrasound-guided umbilical cord blood sampling, intrahepatic venipuncture, and cardiac puncture (Figs. 7.2 and 7.3).

At present, ultrasound-guided umbilical cord blood sampling has become a standard method to collect fetal blood samples and conduct fetal intravascular transfusion or transfusion therapy. The time of umbilical cord blood sampling is usually after 18 weeks of gestation, with a higher success rate and fewer complications.

Fetal blood can be extracted by ultrasound-guided intrahepatic venipuncture when umbilical vessel puncture is difficult. Ultrasound-guided fetal heart puncture is only used in the condition that umbilical vessel puncture and intrahepatic vein puncture are failed.

- Indications
  - Rapid karyotype analysis is required.
  - Prenatal ultrasound revealed abnormal fetal development or abnormalities. The karyotype analysis of the fetus is needed for further diagnosis.
  - Fetal chromosomal karyotype analysis is required for pregnant women with a history of genetic disease in pregnancy, delivery, or family history of genetic disease.
  - Chromosomal abnormalities found in amniotic fluid cell culture after amniocentesis, such as chimera, needs to be further confirmed.
  - Teratogenic factors, such as fetal toxoplasmosis and history of virus infection.
  - Prenatal diagnosis of TORCH in the fetus.
  - To know about the acid-base equilibrium in the fetus with intrauterine growth restriction.
  - Administration of medicine and blood transfusion through an intravenous umbilical infusion.
  - Diagnosis of hematologic diseases, such as congenital fetal thrombocytopenia, hemoglobin disease, leukocyte disease, hemophilia A, hemophilia B, or other clotting factor diseases.
  - Immunodeficiency disease.
  - Congenital metabolic disorders.
- Preoperative preparation
  - Ultrasound equipment

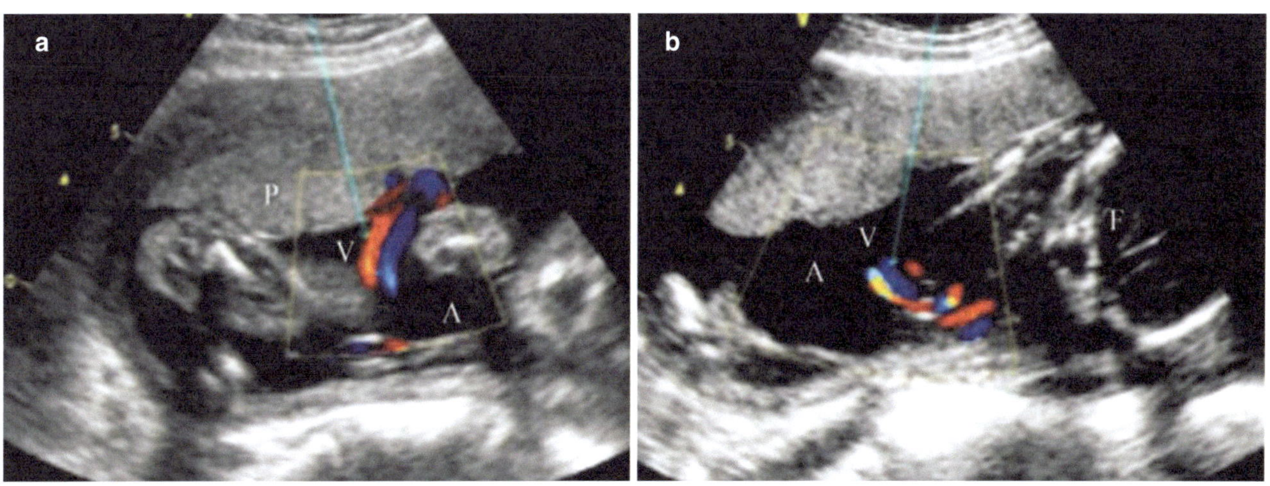

Fig. 7.2 Ultrasound-guided umbilical cord puncture. (**a**) Puncture is performed on the side of the placenta. (**b**) Puncture is shown on the free segment of the umbilical cord

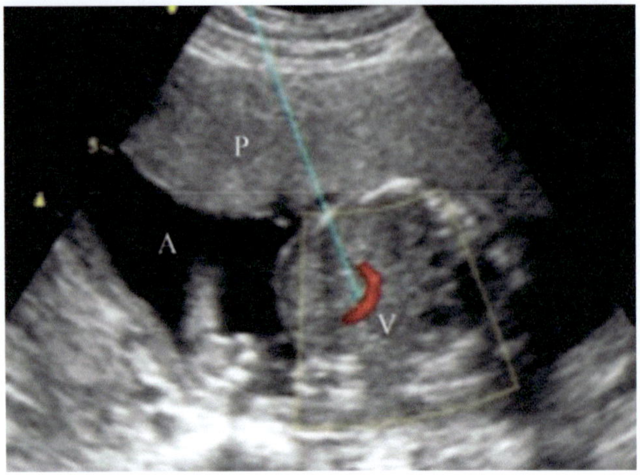

Fig. 7.3 fetal intrahepatic venipuncture

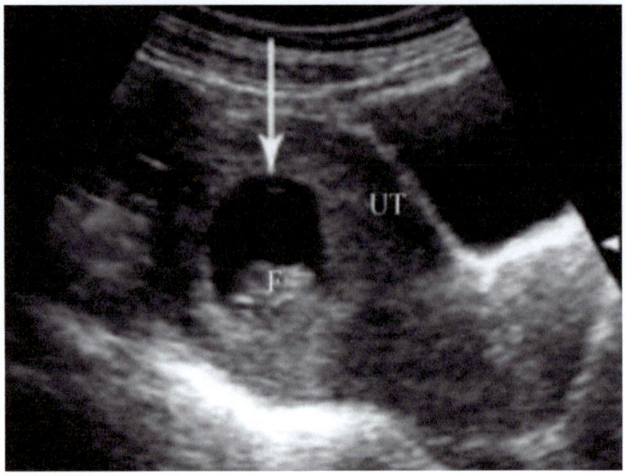

Fig. 7.4 US-guided villus sampling

– Real-time ultrasound equipment is required, and the frequency of the probe is 3.5 MHz. Get preparing for the puncture guidance equipment.
– Puncture needle
– The preferable size is 20-23G, with a length of 15–18 cm.
– Medicine
– Get preparation for the medicine, according to the purpose of examination and treatment.
– Others
– Tube or culture tube if needed.

- Methods of operation
  – The pregnant woman is placed in the supine position, and routine obstetric ultrasound examination is performed to choose a proper puncture point.
  – After the puncture site is sterilized and draped, determine the insertion route and depth under ultrasound guidance.
  – Insert the puncture needle into the puncture site, and then remove the needle core. Fetal blood is extracted for examination.
  – Insert the needle core and pull out the needle.
  – After the operation, check the fetus's heart, fetal movement, and conditions like whether there is active bleeding in the injection point for at least 30 minutes.
- Notes and complications
  – Color Doppler ultrasonography is helpful to detect fetal blood flow, accurately distinguish umbilical vein, hepatic vein, cardiac chamber, and other structures, as well as blood flow, and guide accurate positioning of the puncture needle.
  – For heart puncture, 17G puncture needle can be firstly used in fetal thoracocentesis, and then 23G puncture needle can be used to puncture fetal heart through 17G syringe and then to extract fetal heart blood. Blood can also be obtained directly with a 23G needle.
  – Select a straight and relatively fixed umbilical cord segment for puncture.
  – The rate of fetal loss is 0.8% ~ 5%; the incidence of umbilical cord hemorrhage is 23% ~ 37%. The incidence of fetal bradycardia is about 5%.
  – The success rate of umbilical vessel puncture is closely related to gestational week.
  – The success rate in the second and third trimesters is higher than that in the first trimester.
  – Ultrasound-guided fetal heart puncture may lead to fetal pericardial hemorrhage, bradycardia, and even cardiac arrest.

III. US-guided villus sampling

US-guided villus sampling is one of the early prenatal diagnosis methods to puncture villi and obtain villi tissue under ultrasound guidance for cytogenetic examination to diagnose congenital fetal diseases and metabolic diseases.

- 10 ~ 12 weeks gestation is more suitable for sampling the villi.
- There are two methods to obtain villi tissue under ultrasound guidance: one is to draw villi tissue through the vagina; the other is the aspiration of villi through the abdominal wall. The sampling route is determined according to placental implantation location and uterine location (Fig. 7.4).
- Notes and complications
  – Incompatibility of Rh blood type between mother and child is an absolute contraindication to this examination.
  – The literature reports that the rate of fetal loss is 0.6% ~ 3%. The incidence of vaginal bleeding is 13.6%. The rate of pregnancy sac rupture is about

0.3%. It can also increase the incidence of fetal malformation, such as fetal limb loss.
– Villi sampling should be performed with accurate positioning, gentle operation, and precise actions to minimize complications.

IV. US-guided fetal tissue biopsy

Ultrasound-guided tissue biopsy is to obtain specific tissues of fetus under the guidance of real-time ultrasonography, which is often used for prenatal diagnosis of some deadly diseases.

Main application and precautions of fetal tissue biopsy include:

- The fetal liver tissue is biopsied to diagnose autosomal recessive glucose metabolism disorder and p-carbamate invertase deficiency.
- Hereditary bullous epidermolysis disease is diagnosed by fetal skin biopsy.
- Perform fetal muscle biopsy to diagnose some kind of inherited muscle disease.
- Fetal tissue biopsy should be performed at 20–24 weeks of gestation.

V. US-guided intrauterine fetal therapy

With the continuous improvement of the equipment and technology of interventional ultrasound and minimally invasive surgery, fetal surgical treatment has developed rapidly, and fetal intrauterine treatment under ultrasound guidance has been gradually recognized and applied.

- Main characteristics of US-guided intrauterine fetal therapy.
  – Real-time display of intrauterine conditions makes it possible to timely adjust the direction of puncture.
  – Accurate positioning to avoid blind puncture.
  – No X-ray radiation.
  – Compared with open fetal surgery and fetal endoscopic surgery, it has the advantage of less trauma, fewer complications, and lower cost.
- Application range of US-guided intrauterine fetal therapy.
  – Administration in amniotic cavity, such as dexamethasone to promote lung maturation, amino acid treatment of fetal intrauterine growth retardation.
  – Artificial amniotic fluid is injected into the amniotic cavity for the treatment of oligohydramnios, premature rupture of membranes, variation deceleration of the fetal monitor, and fecal contamination of the amniotic fluid.
  – Amniotic fluid reduction should be carried out for those with excessive amniotic fluid.
  – Transumbilical blood transfusion for fetal with anemia.
  – Subcutaneous or intraperitoneal administration of medicine.
  – Intrauterine therapeutic drainage for a fetus with hydrocephalus and hydrothorax.
  – Ultrasound-guided fetal endoscopic surgery.
- Notes and complications
  – Restricted by fetal position and fetal appendages, the operation is complicated and easily combined with complications.
  – Complications such as amniotic fluid leakage, premature delivery, fetal loss, amniotic cavity infection, and fetal membrane dissection may occur during intrauterine treatment.

VI. The application of interventional ultrasound in assisted reproduction

- Needle aspiration under transvaginal ultrasonography

  At present, there are many methods of egg retrieval under ultrasound monitoring, including transabdominal wall-bladder route, transurethral route, and transvaginal vault route under abdominal ultrasound guidance; transvaginal vault puncture route under vaginal ultrasound guidance.

  Compared with other methods, transvaginal egg retrieval guided by transvaginal ultrasonography has the advantages of simple operation, little trauma, low cost, and fewer complications, which is more comfortable for patients to accept.
- Notes
  – If the distance between the ovaries and the probe in vagina is greater than 4 cm, it is more difficult to puncture the follicle.
  – For the ovary with high activity, if the follicle does not protrude from the surface or the follicle wall is too thick, the needle needs to be inserted quickly to reduce ovarian activity.
  – When the puncture needle inserts into the follicle, the negative pressure needs to be opened to prevent the follicular fluid from flowing into the abdominal cavity.
  – Complications
  – Bleeding and infection may occur during and after the operation.
- Ultrasound-guided multiple pregnancy embryo reductions

  There are two routes of ultrasound-guided selective multiple pregnancy embryo reductions: transabdominal and transvaginal. Transvaginal ultrasound guidance for embryo reduction in early pregnancy is a method of accurate positioning, simple and easy to operate, safe and effective, which can minimize the occurrence of complication.

VII. Fetoscopy

Fetoscopy is composed of transvaginal or transabdominal fiber-optic endoscopes. Under ultrasound guidance, after local anesthesia, the transabdominal or transvaginal fetoscopy is directly inserted into the amniotic cavity, and the fetus and its surrounding environment are observed under direct vision. The fetoscopy can also extract umbilical cord blood and obtain tissue sampling, as well as intrauterine administration and intrauterine surgery. Fetoscopy has the functions of diagnosis and treatment, and its clinical application has a history of 40 years. It has been now widely applied in obstetrics clinics. Perinatal medical professionals from various countries have promoted its indications, the timing and site of puncture, the size of the tube diameter, and the method of taking the specimen. Nowadays, fetoscopy has developed into an effective way that can diagnose more than 70 congenital abnormal diseases.

- Indications

  The indications for fetoscopy are women who require a prenatal diagnosis of cell and/or molecular genetics with less than 22 weeks of pregnancy, including (1) Observe whether the fetus has apparent external anomalies, such as cleft lip and palate, finger (toe) deformity, external genital deformity, spina bifida, gastroschisis, and cerebral hernia, which are found by ultrasound and AFP examination but cannot be certainly diagnosed; (2) The fetal blood is extracted to assist in the diagnosis of fetal genetic hemoglobin diseases such as thalassemia, sickle cell anemia, and chronic granuloma. (3) A family history of inherited skeletal and muscular system diseases; (4) Hereditary skin diseases diagnosed by fetal tissue biopsy; (5) Certain chromosomal abnormalities are found in the amniotic fluid cell culture but cannot be ruled out as mutants happened in vitro.

  In addition, it is also suitable for intrauterine treatment including (1) Intrauterine blood transfusion; (2) Complicated single chorionic twin disease: twin-to-twin transfusion syndrome, single chorionic twin selective intrauterine growth restriction, twin reversed arterial perfusion sequence; (3) Congenital diaphragmatic hernia; (4) Congenital lower urinary tract obstruction; (5) Amniotic band syndrome; (6) Sacrococcygeal teratoma; (7) Placental villous hemangioma; and (8) Medical administration will not be diluted by maternal blood circulation by fetoscopy.

- Contraindication
  - The indication is not clear.
  - Threatened abortion or threatened preterm labor.
  - Intrauterine infection.
  - The placenta is located in the anterior wall of the uterus or fibroid is located in the puncture site, without a suitable puncture site.
- Time selection of fetoscopy

  The timing of fetoscopy is generally determined based on the volume of amniotic fluid, fetal size, the thickness of the umbilical cord, and the purpose of the examination. Within 15 to 17 weeks of gestation, the volume of amniotic fluid is relatively sufficient, and the fetus is relatively small, which is suitable to observe its appearance. From 18 to 22 weeks of pregnancy, the volume of amniotic fluid is increasing, and the umbilical cord is getting thickening, making it easy to extract fetal blood for prenatal diagnosis. After 22 weeks of gestation, the transparency of amniotic fluid decreases, which is not conducive for the observation of fetal appearance. In the third trimester, the uterus becomes more sensitive to mechanical stimulus, during which fetoscopy could induce preterm delivery. If amniotic fluid embolism occurs, it is more severe than that in the second trimester.

- Equipment of fetoscopy

  Fetoscopy is mainly composed of three parts: camera system, light source and lens, and equipment. The most commonly used fetoscopy is 18 cm in length, 112 to 315 mm in diameter, and 0° to 30° in the angle of the mirror. There is a xenon light source conducted by fiber and digital image enhancement facilities. Various length and angle adjustments make it easier for the instrument to enter and exit the cannula and insert into the amniotic cavity. The trocar is rhombic with the needle hidden in the sheath, which prevents uterine bleeding and separation of the membrane. Ultrasonography, radiofrequency knife (cutting tumor), tracheal clamp, perfusion device, Nd-YAG laser (coagulated blood vessel), and other accessories are also equipped within the fetoscopy.

- Operating steps
  - Preoperative preparation

    Conduct routine skin preparation as lower abdominal surgery before surgery, as well as tell the patient to empty the bladder. 50 mg pethidine is injected intramuscularly 10 minutes before the operation. Surgeons routinely wash their hands, wear sterile gloves, regularly sterilize the puncture site, cover with sterile towels, and strictly abide by the aseptic principle.

  - Selection of puncture point

    The puncture point is selected under the guidance of ultrasound. When the cannula is inserted into the uterus, it is necessary to avoid the placenta attachment region. The puncture position should be chosen as the one facing the ventral side of the fetus, under which there is enough amniotic fluid to facilitate puncture. The anterior, lateral wall, or bottom of the uterus without placenta attachment area can be chosen as a puncture site when the operator decides to insert the needle from the abdominal wall. But do not select the lower uterine segment. Because of its poor contractility, the wound is not natural to heal, possibly causing amniotic fluid leakage.

- Local anesthesia and puncture

  After selecting the puncture point, the local incision is subcutaneously infiltrated with lidocaine for anesthesia. Use a sharp blade to make a 2-mm long incision deep into the skin. During the puncture, there are two senses of emptying, one is to penetrate the anterior fascia of the rectus abdominis and the abdominal muscle layer, and the other is to penetrate the peritoneum and the uterine wall into the amniotic cavity. The assistant should make the uterus stable when the needle is penetrating the peritoneum. After the cored cannula has inserted into the amniotic cavity, the core is withdrawn with amniotic fluid pouring out. And then fix the fetoscopy instead.
- Fetoscopy

  Install a cold light source to observe the fetus. The assistant should fix the fetus on the abdominal wall of the pregnant woman or inject a transvenous sedative to control fetal movement. In the single view of the fetoscopy, the entire fetus may not be observed ultimately, but the surface structure of the fetus may be clearly seen. The operator must move the fetoscopy repeatedly to observe the fetus in detail.
- Postoperative notes

  After the operation, the fetoscopy and the cannula are withdrawn together. The puncture site of the abdominal wall needs to be pressed by sterile gauze for at least 5 minutes. After bandaged, the patient needs to lie supine for 3 to 5 hours, under the close monitor of maternal pulse, blood pressure, fetal heart rate, and whether there is a uterine contraction, amniotic fluid or blood leakage, etc. Salbutamol, magnesium sulfate, and other drugs that inhibit uterine contractions are generally not applied, because relaxation of the uterine muscle is not conducive to the closure of wound on the uterine wall, and may lead to amniotic fluid leakage. Ultrasonography is performed on the second postoperative day to check the fetal survival status and volume of amniotic fluid.

- Complication
  - Premature rupture of membranes.
  - Placenta and fetal injury.
  - Abortion and premature delivery.
  - Amniotic fluid leakage and amniotic cavity infection.
  - Maternal pulmonary edema and organ damage.

7.4 Application of Interventional Ultrasonography in Gynecology

Interventional ultrasonography can not only perform needle biopsy and cytohistological examination of pelvic masses, but also can play a therapeutic role by aspiration of fluid and injection of drugs. At present, interventional ultrasound techniques have been carried out in gynecology include needle biopsy of pelvic masses, drainage and injection, hysterosalpingography, and intrauterine monitoring.

I. Needle biopsy, extraction, and treatment of pelvic mass guided by ultrasound

   The puncture, drainage, and medicine injection of pelvic mass under the guidance of interventional ultrasonography avoids unnecessary laparoscopy or open surgery.

   Pelvic mass puncture (US-guided pelvic cyst aspiration) can be processed in two ways: transabdominal and transvaginal, depending on the location, nature of the pelvic mass, and the actual condition of the patient. Observe the patients' uterus and adnexa to know about the relationship between the mass and the pelvic cavity by preoperative ultrasound. The real-time position of the puncture needle is provided to the surgeon by intraoperative ultrasound monitor. The condition of internal bleeding and residual mass is observed by postoperative ultrasound. The puncture needle shows a hyperechoic line in the ultrasound image, followed by an acoustic shadow (Fig. 7.5).

   - Indications
     - The effect of medication administration is not satisfied.
     - After a recurrence of pelvic mass, laparoscopy or open surgery should not be performed again.
     - Patients with pelvic masses who are unsuitable or unwilling to undergo open surgery.
     - Patients with pelvic mass who need a biopsy to confirm the nature of mass.
   - Preoperative preparation
     - Choose a transvaginal probe with the frequency of 5 ~ 7.5 MHz or a transabdominal probe with the frequency of 3.5 MHz. The probe is with a puncture or is equipped with a puncture guide device.
     - Model of puncture needle: Transvaginal puncture needle 16 ~ 17G, with the length of 30 ~ 40 cm; transabdominal puncture needle 20 ~ 22G, 20 cm in length.
     - Atropine is injected into the cervix or intramuscularly before surgery, which can prevent abortion syndrome. The regularly used medicine in surgery are sterile saline, sclerosing agents, such as abso-

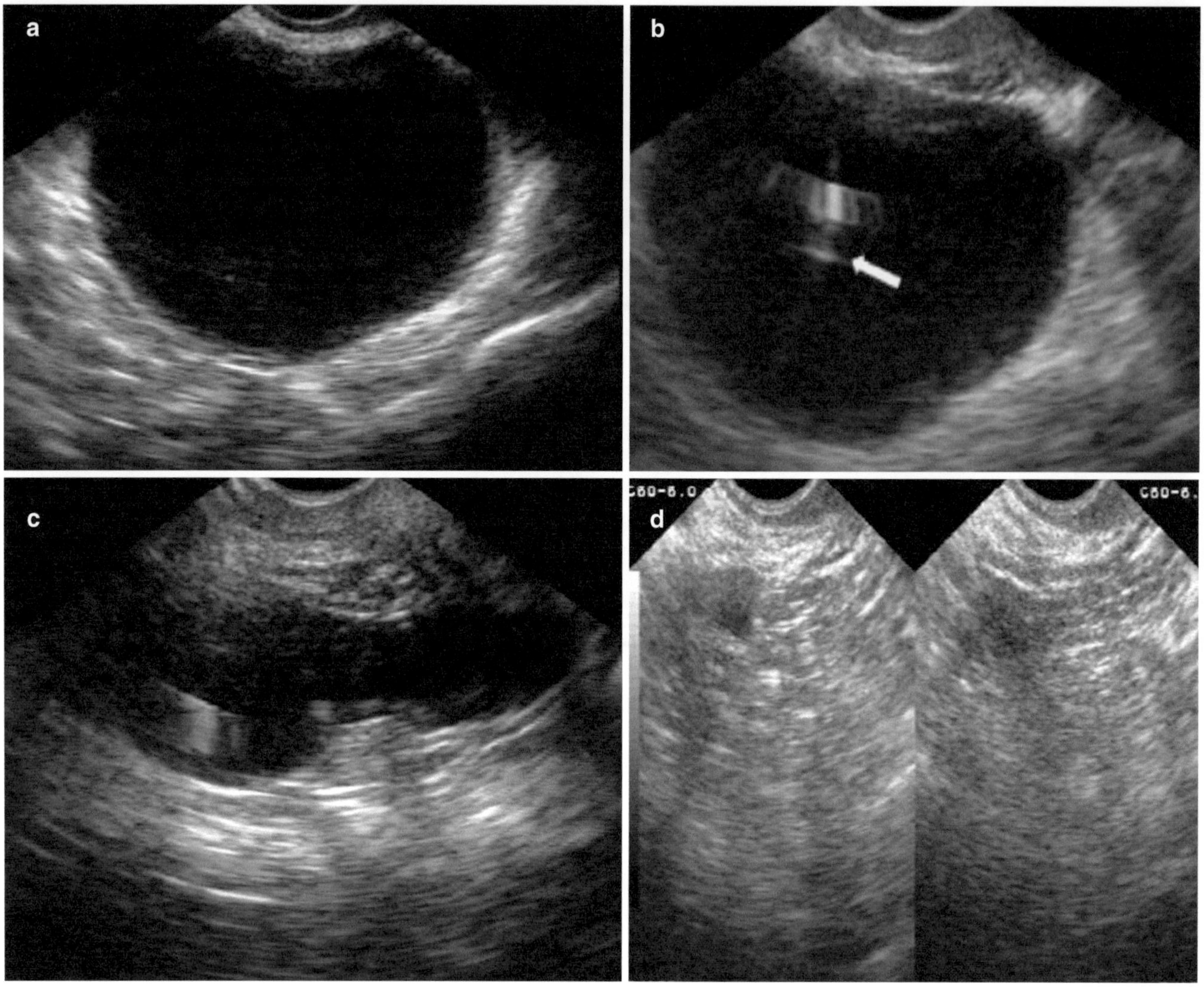

Fig. 7.5 Puncture, extraction, and medicine injection of the pelvic cystic mass. (**a**) The patient is 45 years old, with chief complaint of hysterectomy for 1 year and adnexal cyst for four months. Preoperative transvaginal ultrasound shows a cystic mass of 9.1 cm × 8.5 cm × 7.9 cm in the pelvic cavity without septum. (**b**) About 200 ml of limpid yellow liquid is drawn out during the operation, and the arrow pointed out the tip of the needle in the mass; (**c**) The injection of ethanol to rinse the cavity; (**d**) No recurrence of cyst in the pelvic cavity after one month

lute ethanol, etc.; gentamicin, hydrocortisone, Chymotrypsin, etc. to prevent inflammatory and adhesion. Methotrexate or potassium chloride is applied to kill embryos in the treatment of fallopian tube pregnancy.

- Operative method
  - Preoperative ultrasound is performed to observe the location and boundary of pelvic cysts, the echo characteristics of mass, whether there is septum or adhesion in it, and the relationship with surrounding organs, etc. It also helps to determine the site of puncture to avoid vital organs and vessels.
  - During transabdominal puncture, disinfect and drape the puncture site. Before transvaginal puncture, patients should take bladder lithotomy position, and disinfects and drape the vulva and vagina.
  - Under the guidance of ultrasonography, the needle is inserted along the puncture line into the cyst.
  - Perform puncture biopsy, drainage, and medicine injection according to different purposes.
  - Observe 0.5 to 2 hours after the operation to observe the patient's vital signs and other abnormal conditions.
- Notes and complications
  - Multilocular cysts often need to be punctured multiple times. The cystic fluid should be extracted from each chamber as much as possible, and then ethanol or other sclerosing agent is injected into the cyst.
  - Generally, choose pelvic cyst with the size of above 5 cm to puncture. Before surgery, combined with clinical conditions, the level of CA125 and color Doppler ultrasonography should be taken into consideration. For those suspected of malig-

nant tumor, the puncture is not suitable. Extracted fluids are sent for cytological examination and bacterial examination.
- Anti-inflammatory drugs and sclerosing agent are injected into the capsule to reduce the rate of relapse.
- After interventional puncture treatment for tubal pregnancy, the blood level of hCG should be reviewed regularly.
- Properly apply pressure to the abdominal wall or vaginal fornix with the probe, so that the mass adheres to the abdominal wall or fornix and make it easy to puncture.

- Sonohysterography

Sonohysterography is to inject liquid into the uterine cavity and make use of the expanded uterine cavity to increase the contrast of ultrasound imaging and facilitate the observation of uterine cavity and muscle wall lesions.

Injection of liquid into the uterine cavity and the expansion of the uterine cavity to increase the contrast of ultrasound imaging and facilitate the observation. After the fluid is injected into the uterine cavity, with the pressure increasing, the liquid flows to the fallopian tube to check the obstruction status of the fallopian tube (Fig. 7.6).

II. Indication
- Endometrial diseases, including endometrial polyps, endometrial thickening, and endometrial atrophy.
- Uterine myoma, mainly used for the submucosal myoma and intermuscular myoma protruding to the uterine cavity.
- Intrauterine foreign bodies, including intrauterine residual after surgery and abnormal IUD, such as incarceration, rupture, ectopic, and residual.
- Uterine adhesion, oligomenorrhea, or amenorrhea after uterine cavity operation, suspected cervical or uterine cavity adhesion.
- Suspected uterine malformation.
- Unexplained infertility or habitual abortion.
- Unexplained abnormal uterine bleeding.

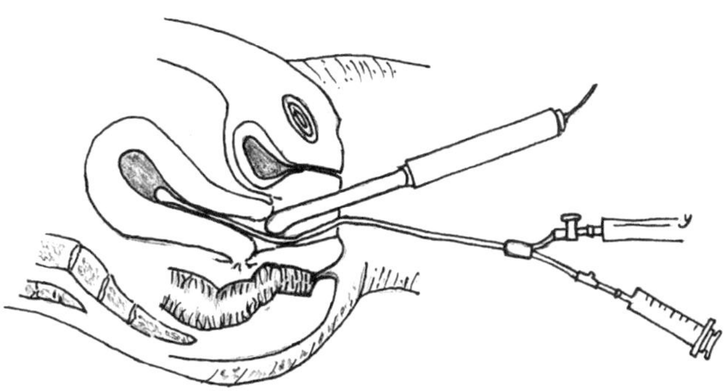

Fig. 7.6 Schematic diagram of Sonohysterography

- Transabdominal or transvaginal ultrasound imaging is unsatisfactory, and further evaluation is required.
- Infertile women who are allergic to iodine need to be known about the situation of the fallopian tubes.

- Preoperative preparation
  - Transvaginal probe with the frequency of 5 ~ 7.5 MHz, or transabdominal probe with the frequency of 3.5 MHz.
  - Sterilized double-lumen radiography tube and related gynecological equipment.
  - Cervical or intramuscular injection of atropine can prevent the occurrence of abortion syndrome; acoustic contrast agents, such as ultrasound microbubble contrast agent (SonoVue), saline and hydrogen peroxide; anti-inflammatory and anti-adhesion drugs, such as gentamicin and chymotrypsin.
- Operative method
  - Before the operation, conduct ultrasound examination to detect the location and the size of uterus and adnexa.
  - The patient takes the bladder lithotomy position. After disinfecting and draping the vulva, expose the cervix with a dilator, then disinfect the vagina and cervix, and probe the depth of the uterine cavity with a probe.
  - Insert a sterile double-lumen radiography tube into the uterine cavity in about 1 cm in depth through the cervix, and inject 1–2 ml of saline into the capsule of the double-lumen tube. After a water sac have been formed to block the inner mouth, it was clamped with vascular forceps, and remove the vaginal dilator.
  - Place the probe with the cover of condom and coupling agent into the vagina, and inject the contrast liquid slowly and continuously into the main catheter of the double-lumen radiography tube. At the same time, ultrasonography should be applied to observe the intrauterine cavity in real time and make a diagnosis.
- Notes and complications
  - The amount of injected contrast agent should be determined according to the size of the uterine cavity, the purpose of the examination, the patient's tolerance, and the clarity of the ultrasound image, which is generally 5–30 ml.
  - The water bladder of the double-lumen tube should not be too large or too small to avoid the missed diagnosis of cervical lesions.
  - The common complications of hysterosalpingography are abortion syndrome and infection.
  - The time of sonohysterography examination should be from 3 to 7 days after the menstruation. And sex life is forbidden in the three days before the examination. The acute phase of genital inflammation and systemic diseases must be

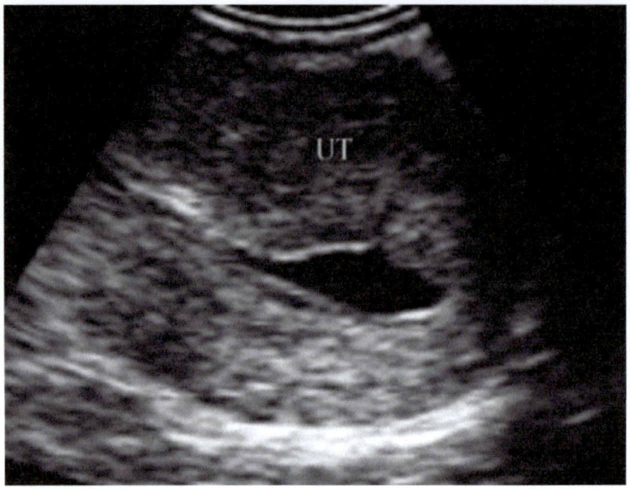

Fig. 7.7 Standard image of sonohysterography. Sagittal plane of the uterus under transvaginal ultrasound examination: after injection of contrast medium, the uterine cavity dilates, the endometrium is regular, and there is no abnormal echo in the uterine cavity

excluded. It is recommended to take antibiotics after the operation and do not have a sex life and tub bathing until two weeks after the surgery.

- Contrast agents can be divided into positive and negative agents. In general, one kind of contrast agent is chosen for each examination. The microbubble contrast agent is a positive contrast agent, which often shows high echo on the sonogram, such as Sonovue and hydrogen peroxide. The negative contrast agent, which often shows anechoic on the sonogram, includes normal saline. Negative contrast agents are commonly used for uterine cavity, and positive contrast agents or negative contrast agents can be used for fallopian tube ultrasound.

- Ultrasonic diagnosis
  - Normal performance of sonohysterography (Fig. 7.7). The uterine cavity is an anechoic area with relatively smooth endometrium.
  - Endometrial polyps: Sonohysterography can clearly show the type, location and number of endometrial polyps (Figs. 7.8, 7.9, 7.10, 7.11, 7.12 and 7.13).
  - Uterine myoma: Sonohysterography improves the accuracy of submucosal myoma positioning and shows the thickness of the pedicle and its relationship with the muscular layer (Figs. 7.14, 7.15 and 7.16).
  - Endometrial carcinoma: Sonohysterography shows the contour and focal morphology of the endometrial carcinoma, as well as the evaluation of muscular penetration, which helps to make the decision on the type and scope of surgery.
  - Endometrial atrophy: The endometrium is thin, showing a slight light echo; the single layer thickness is often less than 2.5 mm (Fig. 7.17).
  - Endometrial hyperplasia: Sonohysterography shows the degree of endometrium thickening, and the interface between endometrium and muscular layer (Figs. 7.18, 7.19 and 7.20).
  - Uterine malformation: The sonohysterography can clearly show the shape of the uterus and uterine cavity, measure the length and thickness of the uterine mediastinum, observe the relationship between the septum and the fundus. It is helpful to determine the kind of uterine malformation, such as residual angle uterus (Figs. 7.21 and 7.22).
  - Intrauterine foreign body: Foreign body represents irregular hyperechoic mass floating with the contrast agent, which is not attached to the inner wall of the uterus. Sonohysterography can show the shape and length of the residual IUD, as well as the incarcerated location, which helps to clinically position (Figs. 7.23, 7.24 and 7.25).
  - Intrauterine adhesions: Sonohysterography shows the small uterine cavity, stiff uterine wall, and the adhesions in the intrauterine cavity. During operation, there may be vaginal bleeding (Fig. 7.26).

    The cases were examined by the West China Second University Hospital of Sichuan University and confirmed by surgery or pathology.
  - Special tips
    - Sonohysterography cannot diagnose polyps that less than 2 mm in diameter.
    - Lesions located in the lower part of the uterine cavity may be poorly displayed due to the balloon.
    - The endometrial carcinoma has no specific ultrasound performance, and pay attention to distinguish it from submucosal myoma, endometrial hyperplasia, and polyps.
    - Ultrasound is limited to identify focal endometrial hyperplasia, polyps, small intrauterine myoma, and endometrial cancer.

III. Salpingography

- Assessment of patency of fallopian tube (positive contrast agent).
  - Unobstructed fallopian tube: There is no resistance and no reflux when injecting the contrast agent. The fallopian tube runs naturally and softly. The ring-shaped hyperechoic area is around the ovary, with the microbubbles in the rectouterine pouch and intestinal space evenly (Fig. 7.27).

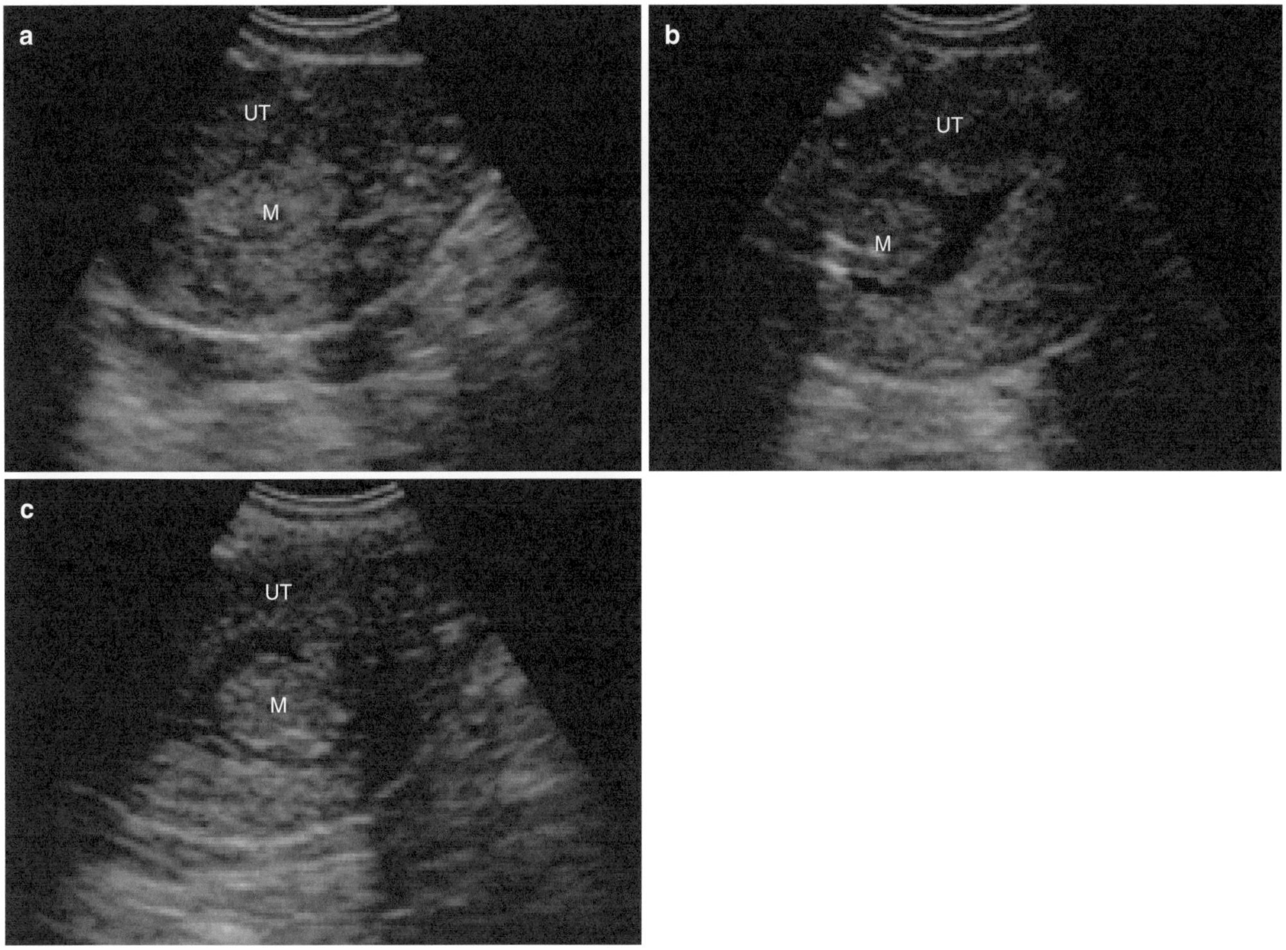

Fig. 7.8 Sonohysterography of single endometrial polyp (I) (**a**). The patient is 41 years old and have menorrhagia for more than one year. Transvaginal ultrasound examination of the uterine cavity shows a hyperechoic mass. (**b**). After injection of contrast agent, a hyperechoic mass about 1.5 cm in diameter is seen attached to the left anterior uterine wall near the fundus, the attachment surface is about 0.8 cm in width. (**c**). Intrauterine cavity findings after injection of contrast agent

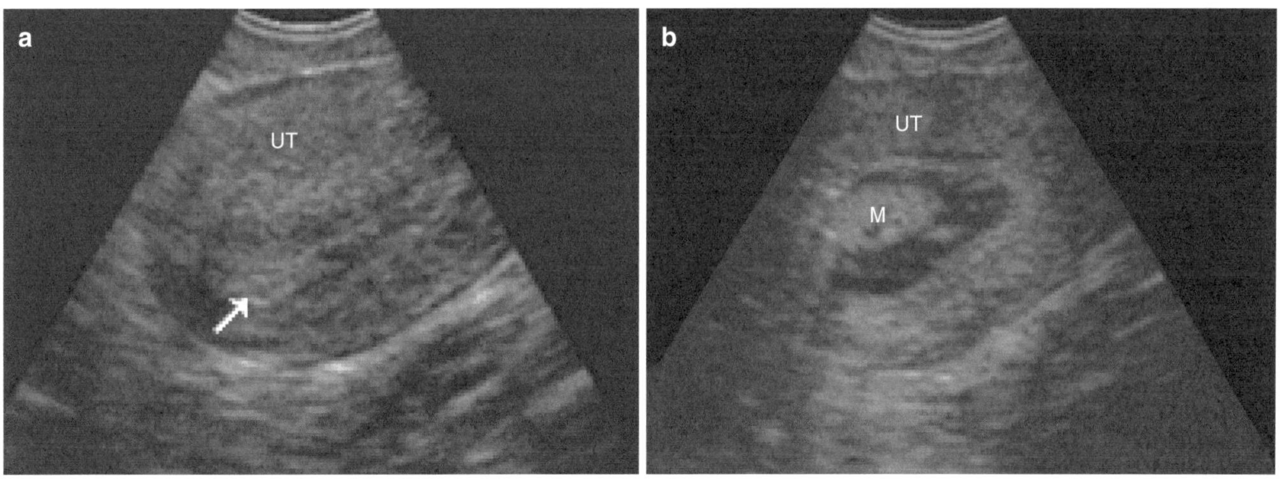

Fig. 7.9 Sonohysterography of single endometrial polyp (II) (**a**). A vaginal ultrasound examination of a 33-year-old woman shows thickening and inhomogeneous endometrium, (**b**). After injection of contrast agent, a hyperechoic mass of 1.5 cm × 1.6 cm × 1.0 cm is observed, and the mass is attached to the anterior wall of the uterine cavity near the fundus, with a 1.1 cm width of attachment surface.

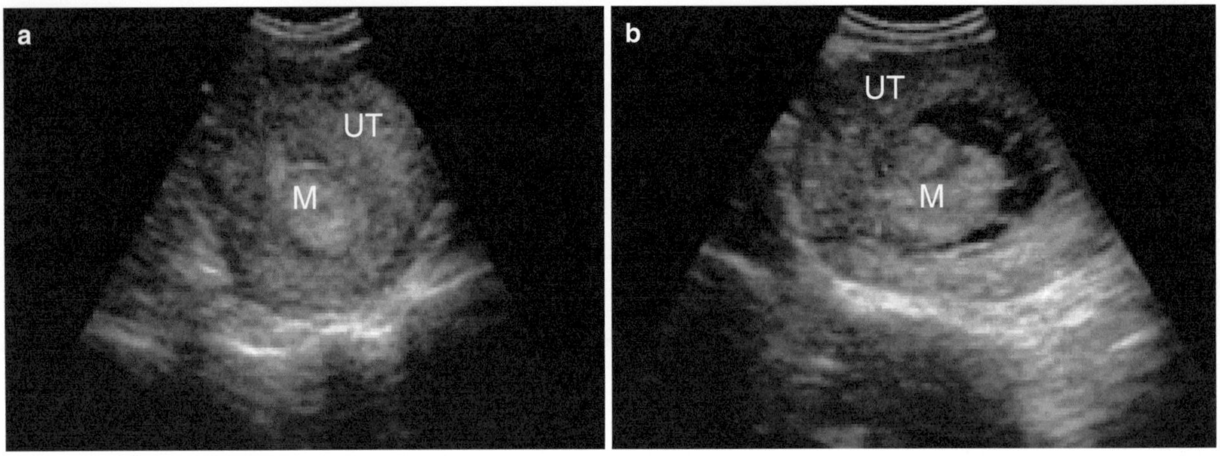

Fig. 7.10 Sonohysterography of single endometrial polyp (III) (**a**). A 29-year-old patient has a hyperechoic mass with a diameter of 2.0 cm in the uterus by vaginal ultrasonography. (**b**). After injection of contrast agent, a hyperechoic mass is shown, which is attached to the right lateral wall with a 1.0 cm width of attachment surface.

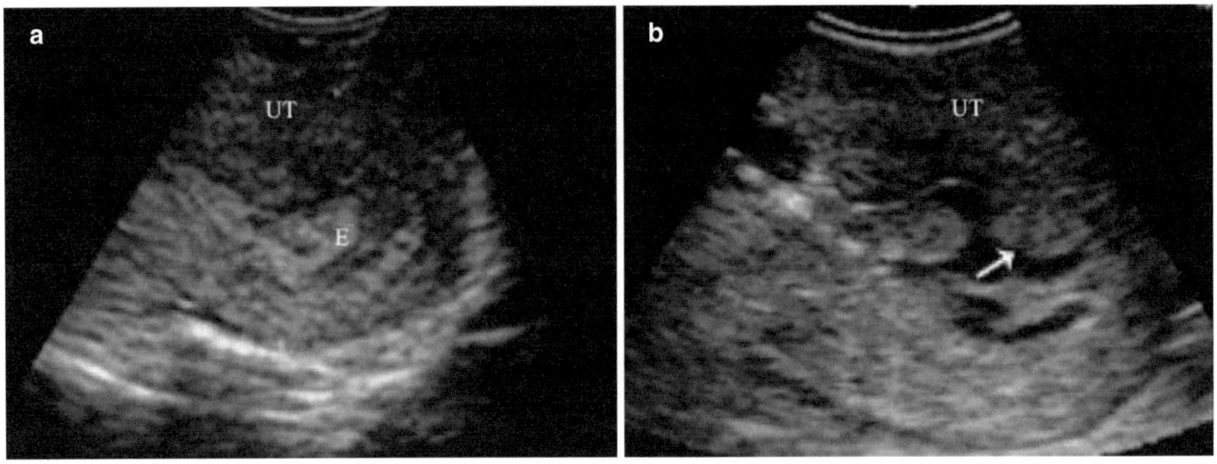

Fig. 7.11 Sonohysterography of multiple endometrial polyps (I). (**a**) The patient is 28 years old, with history of menorrhagia and blood clot bleeding for eight months. Transvaginal ultrasound shows thickened and inhomogeneous endometrium. (**b**) After injection, a number of slightly hyperechoic mass are found on each wall on the uterine cavity, with relatively regular shape and a maximum diameter of 1.2 cm

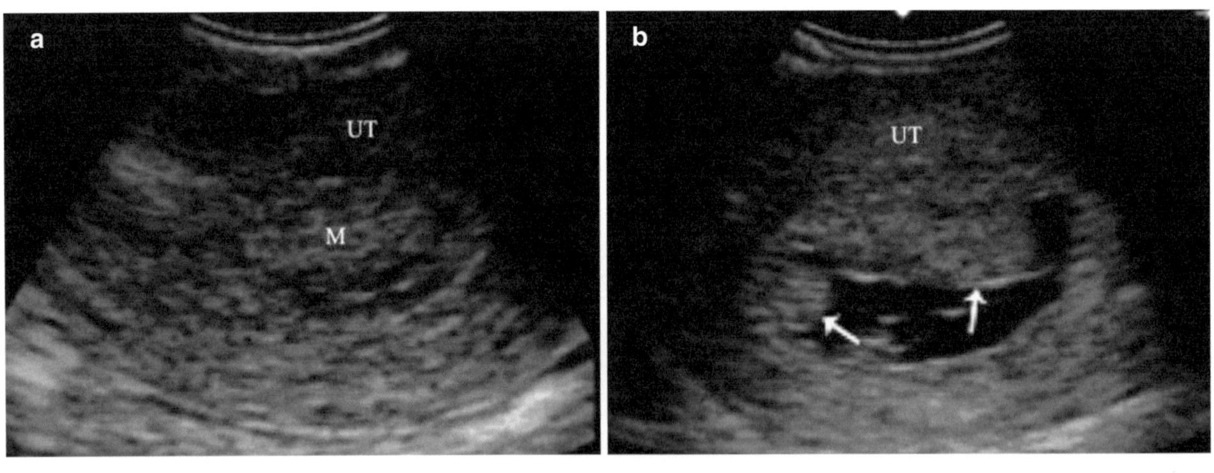

Fig. 7.12 Sonohysterography of multiple endometrial polyps (II). (**a**) The patient is 34 years old, and the ultrasound found "occupation disease in uterine cavity". (**b**) After injection of the contrast agent, multiple slightly hyperechoic masses are found in each wall of the uterine cavity, with the largest one located in the back wall of the cavity with 2.0 cm in diameter, and the attachment surface is about 2.0 cm in width. Whereas the smallest is approximately 0.7 cm in diameter

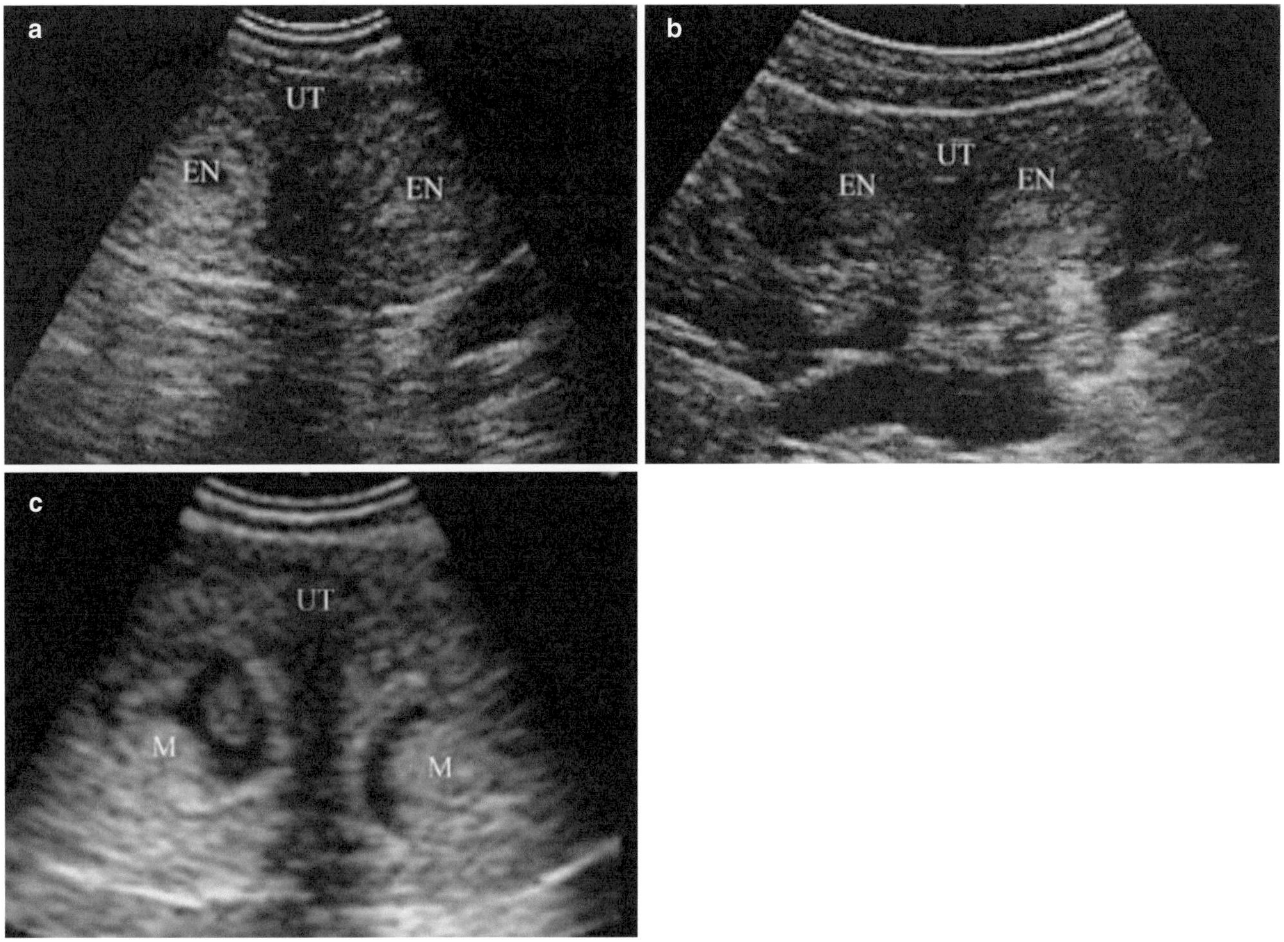

Fig. 7.13 Sonohysterography of multiple endometrial polyps combined with incomplete uterus septum. (**a**) The patient is 27 years old, who was diagnosed with primary infertility. The manifestation of ultrasound shows two separate uterine cavities, with thickened and inhomogeneous endometrium. (**b**) The transverse view of the uterus shows two uterine cavities. (**c**) After injection of contrast agent, the right uterine cavity is observed to be separated by 1.0 cm, and left uterine cavity separated by 1.1 cm. Several slightly hyperechoic masses are found on each wall in each uterine cavity. The shape is smooth, the boundary is clear, the maximum diameter of the mass is 1.5 cm

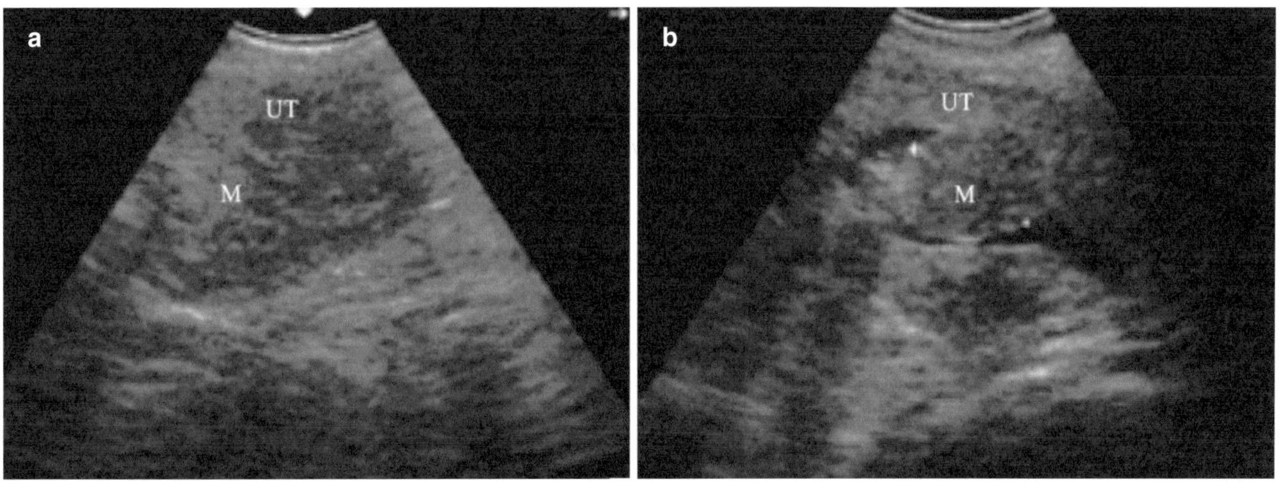

Fig. 7.14 Sonohysterography of submucosal uterine myoma (I). (**a**) The patient is 60 years old. Sonogram shows the slightly hypoechoic occupation in the uterine cavity, with unclear boundary. (**b**) After the injection of contrast agents, the hypoechoic mass in the size of 2.2 cm × 1.7 cm × 1.5 cm is attached to the posterior wall of the uterine cavity. And the width of attachment surface is 1.5 cm

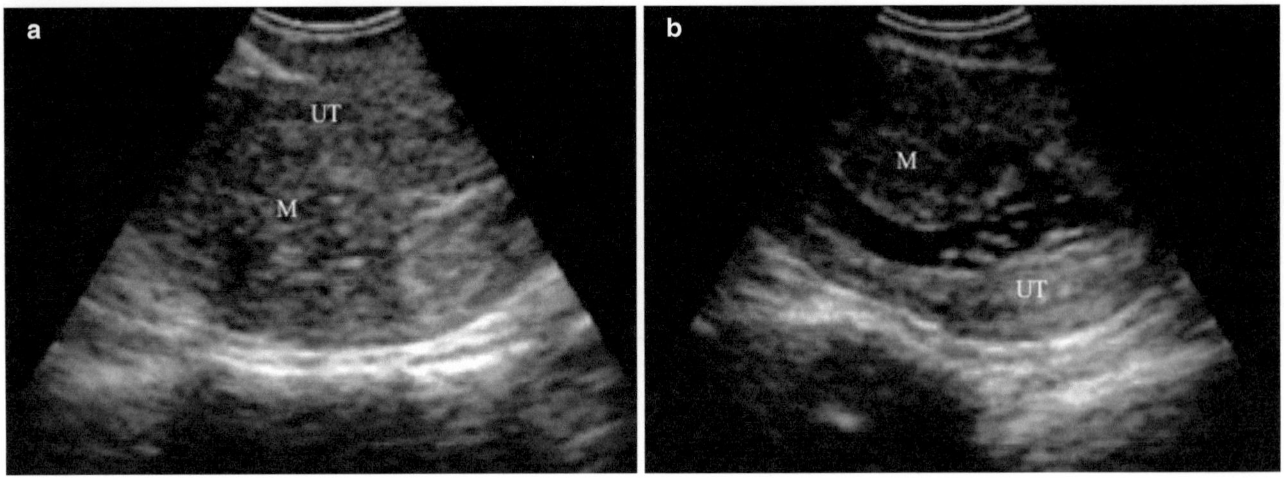

Fig. 7.15 Sonohysterography of submucosal uterine myoma (II). (**a**) The patient is 45 years old and has a history of menorrhagia with blood clots. Sonogram shows the slightly hypoechoic mass in the uterine cavity with the diameter of about 3 cm. (**b**) After the injection of contrast agents, the hypoechoic mass in the size of 2.7 cm × 2.5 cm × 1.7 cm is attached to the anterior wall of the uterine cavity, with inner attenuation

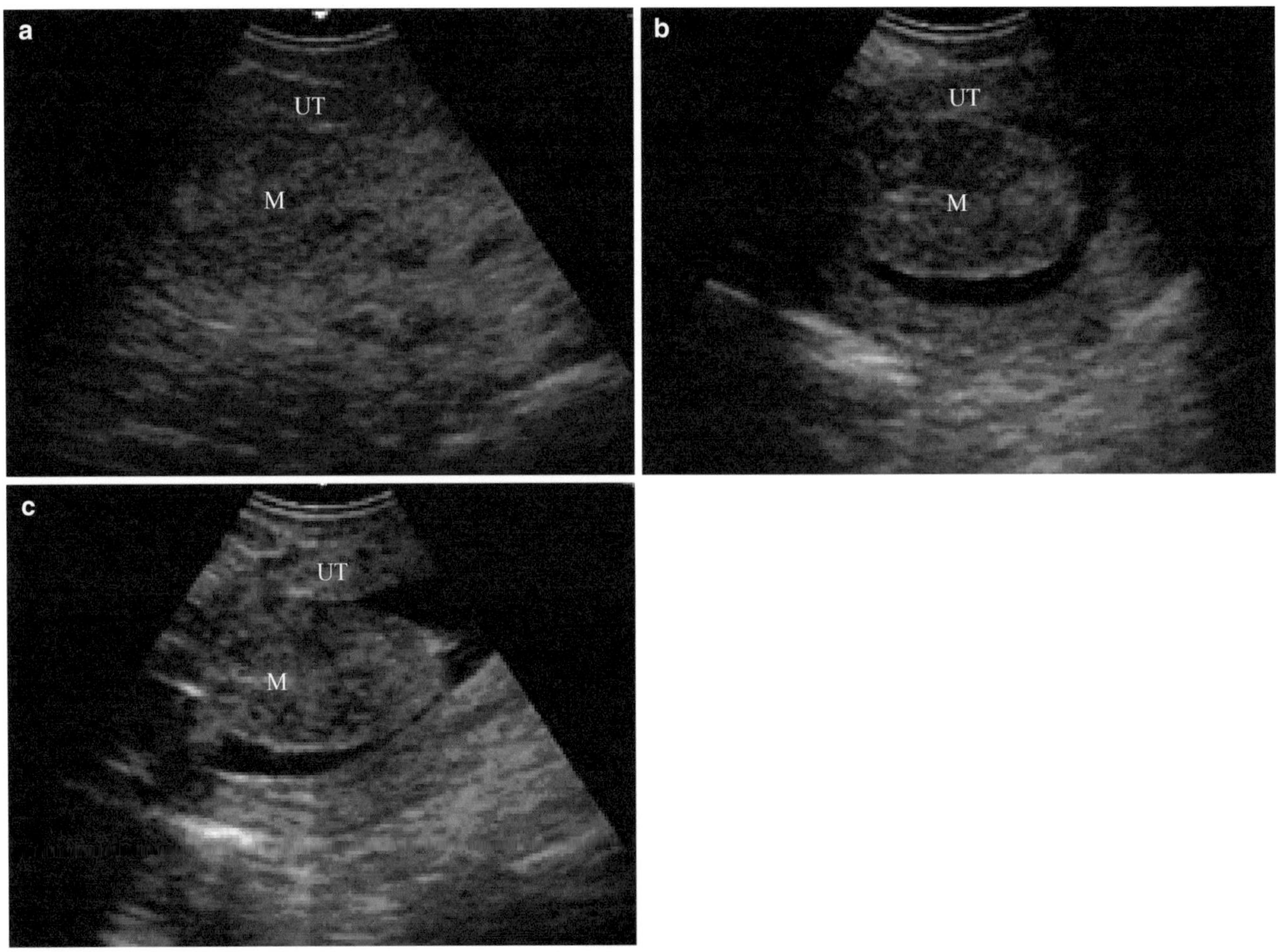

Fig. 7.16 Sonohysterography of intramural uterine myoma extruding to the cavity. (**a**) The patient is 34 years old, and the sonogram shows the occupation in the uterine cavity. (**b**) After injection of the contrast agent, the hypoechoic mass in the uterine cavity is attached to the right anterior wall, near the fundus; (**c**). About two-third of the mass is protruding into the uterine cavity, and one-third is located in the muscle wall

- Obstructed fallopian tube: When injecting the contrast agent, the resistance is large, and the reflux will happen when the injection stops. The fallopian tube is absent or partially displayed. There is no strong echo around the ovary and no microbubble echoes in the pelvic cavity (Fig. 7.28)
- The fallopian tube is partially obstructed: There is resistance when injecting contrast agents and a small amount of reflux. The fallopian tube is locally slender or nodular, and runs in the tortuous and angled way. There is half a circle of strong echo around the ovaries and a small amount of microbubble in the rectouterine pouch and intestinal space (Fig. 7.29).

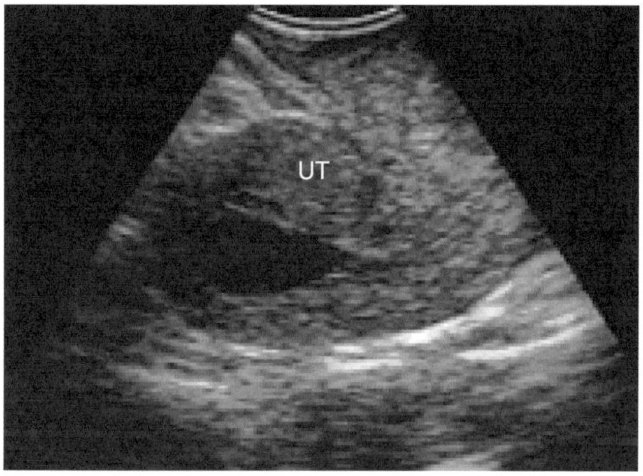

Fig. 7.17 Endometrial atrophy. Sonohysterography shows the thin endometrium, only 1mm in thickness

- patency assessment of the fallopian tube (negative contrast agent),
  - The fallopian tube is unobstructed: After injection, the contrast agent quickly flows out from the bilateral fallopian tubes, and the ultrasonography shows a hyperechoic band around adnexa. Liquid display in the rectouterine pouch and there is no resistance during injection (Fig. 7.30).
  - Obstructed fallopian tube: After injection of contrast medium, the contrast medium forms a vortex at the corner of the uterus, and no contrast medium passes through the fallopian tube. There is no band-like hyperechoic flow seen in the adnexa area, and no obvious liquid dark area in the rectouterine pouch. The resistance is high, and the patient feels abdominal pain or bloating. In hydrosalpinx cases, the injected contrast agent flows in the dilated fallopian tube (Fig. 7.31).
  - The fallopian tube is partially obstructed: After the contrast medium is injected, the contrast medium slowly passes through the fallopian tube, and there is no obvious banding hyperechoic flow around the adnexa, and a little liquid in the rectouterine pouch. When injecting, resistance can be felt.

IV. Intraoperative monitoring during intrauterine surgery.

With the extensive development of uterine cavity surgery, complications have also increased. Application of ultrasonography as intraoperative monitoring can help to ensure the safety of surgery and reduce the occurrence of complications. In the past three years, 676 cases of various difficult transvaginal operations have been con-

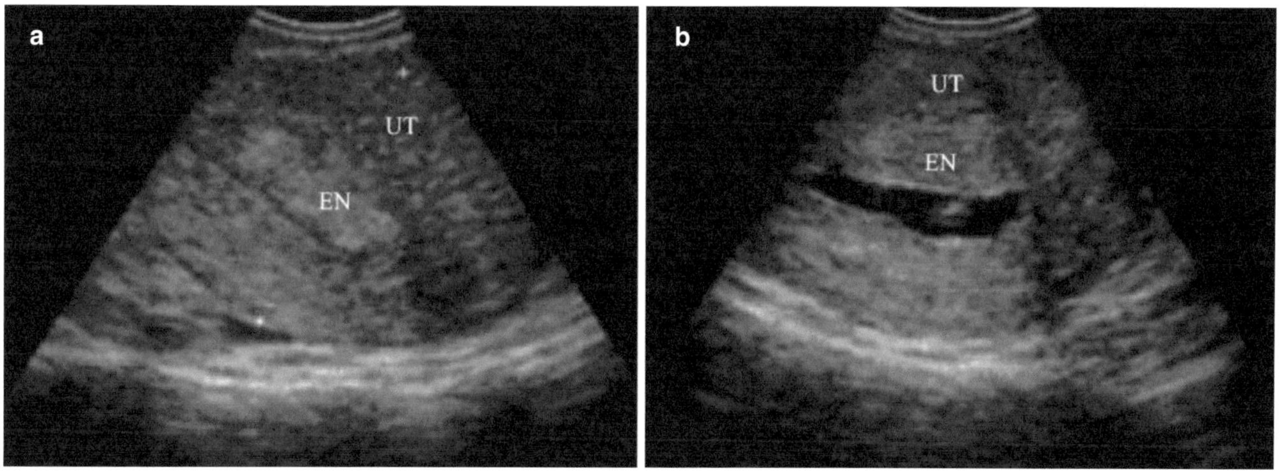

Fig. 7.18 Sonohysterography of endometrial hyperplasia (I). (**a**) The patient is 40 years old, and occupation lesion is suspected in the uterine cavity. (**b**) After injecting the contrast agent, sonogram shows the endometrium is uneven, and the posterior wall is locally thickened by 1.0 cm, with a range of 1.9 cm × 1.6 cm, which is homogeneous and clearly demarcated from the myometrium

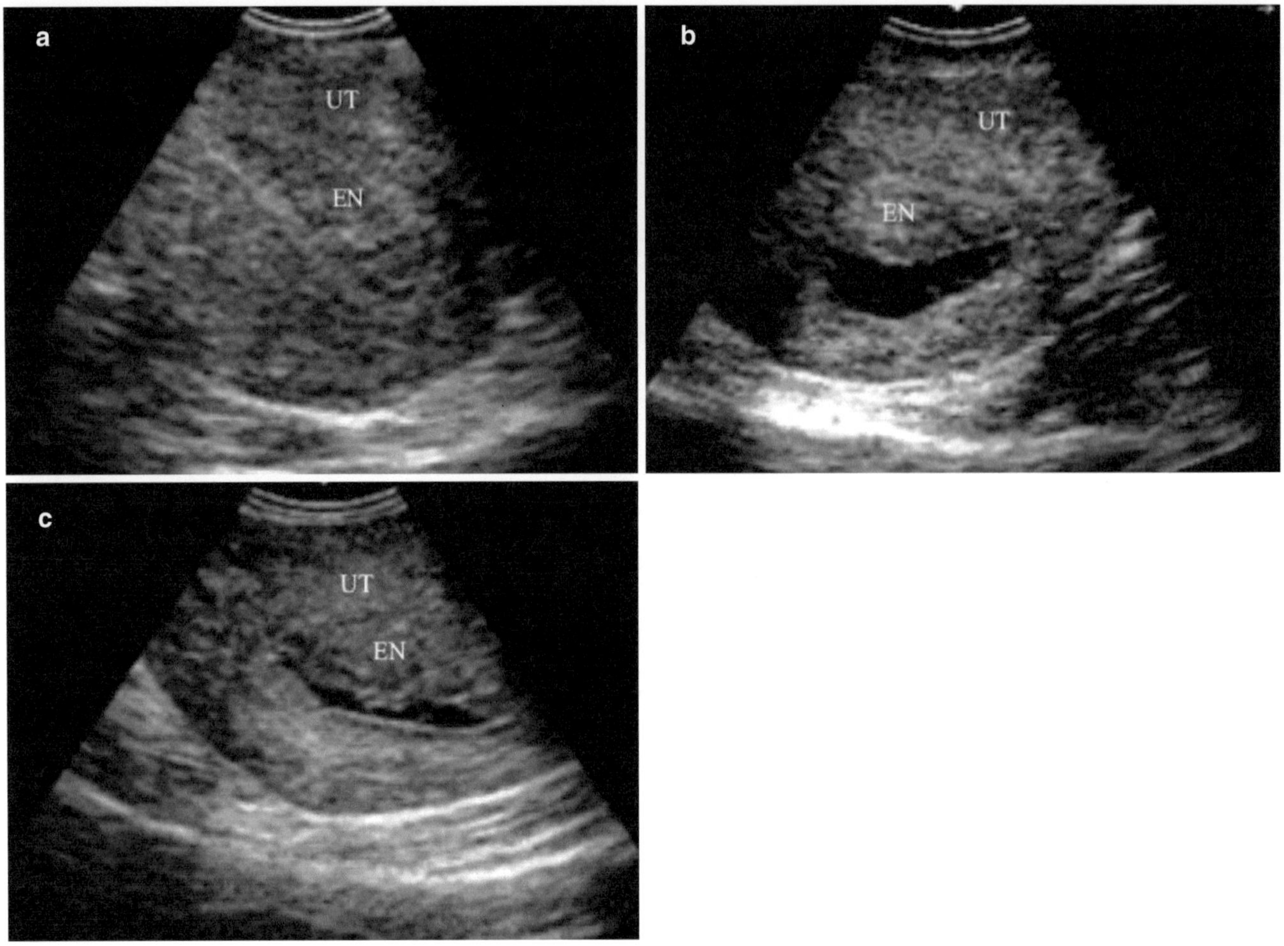

Fig. 7.19 Sonohysterography of endometrial hyperplasia (II). (**a**) The patient is 36 years old and has a history of menorrhagia for 6 months. The endometrium is thickened and inhomogeneous. (**b**) After injection of contrast agents, the thickness of the posterior endometrium is 1.1 cm. (**c**) Sonogram shows the irregular surface of the endometrium after injection of contrast agent

ducted by the monitor of ultrasonography, in our hospital with a success rate of 97.7%, no serious complications occurred. Ultrasonography has been used as a routine monitoring technique in intrauterine surgery.

- Indications
  - Difficult uterine cavity surgery, such as abnormal uterine position, uterine malformation, abnormal pregnancy, and various kinds of uterine cavity surgery that need to be performed again after failure.
  - Hysteroscopy surgery.
- Operation process

  The transabdominal approach is often chosen as ultrasound monitoring for intrauterine surgery.
  - Require the patient to properly fill the bladder before surgery. The patient took the bladder lithotomy position, routinely get disinfected and draped.
  - Ultrasound monitoring is processed in the longitudinal section. Before surgery, observe the position of the uterus, intrauterine gestational sac, villi attachment, and the relationship between occupation disease, uterine cavity, and muscle wall.
  - During the operation, the probe moving up and down, guiding the surgical equipment, and ensures the operation of equipment is within the track.
  - Observe whether there is an abnormal situation in the pelvis cavity after the operation.
- Notes
  - Pay attention to prevent the occurrence of uterine injury and perforation, track the position of the device, and constantly inform the surgeon of the direction and location of the device.
  - Intraoperative ultrasound images show that the operating instruments are strongly echoed with

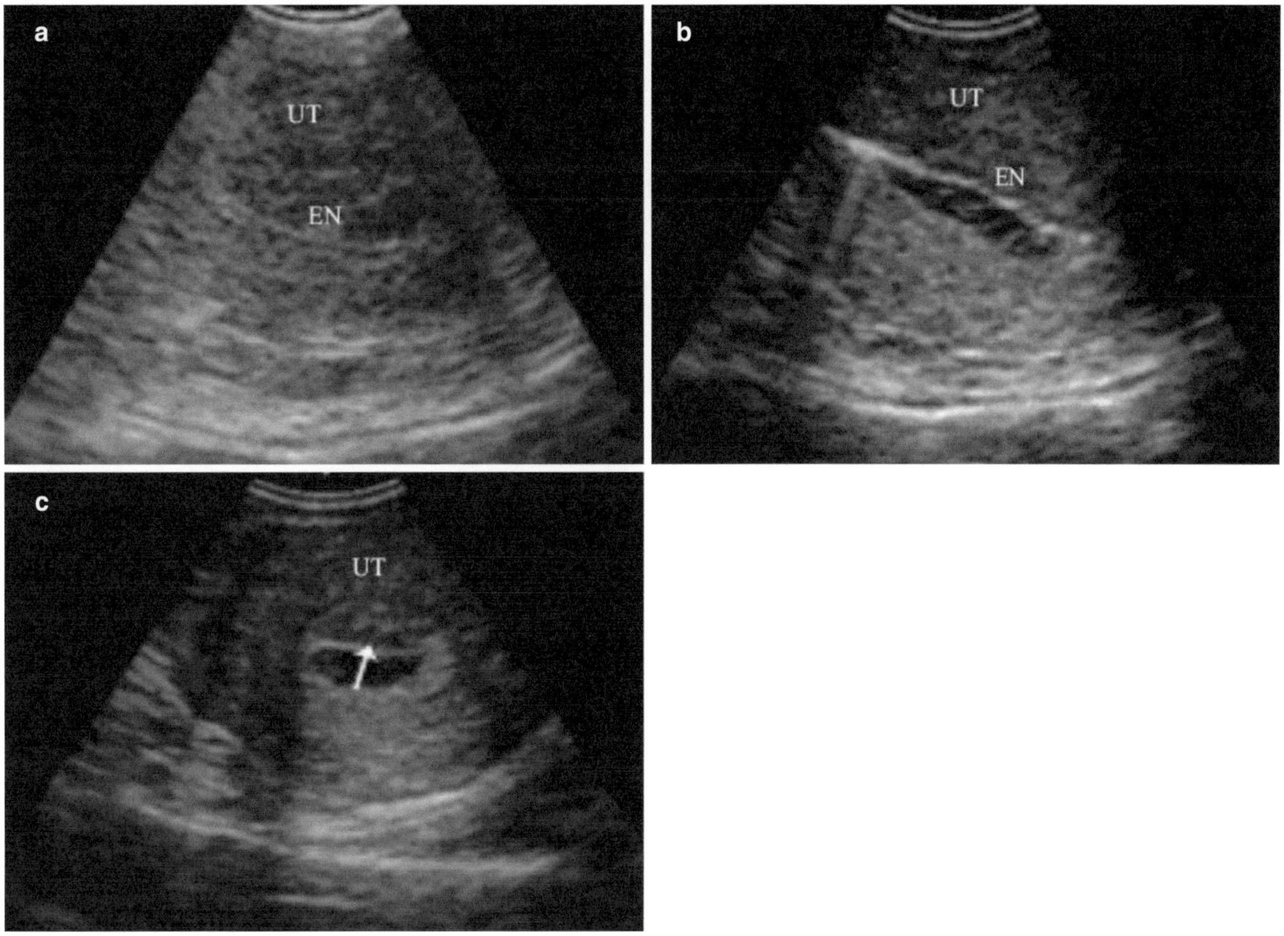

Fig. 7.20 Sonohysterography of endometrial hyperplasia (III). (**a**) The patient is 29 years old, and occupational disease is suspected in the uterine cavity. (**b**) After injection of contrast agent, the thickness of the endometrium is uneven. The endometrial thickness of the anterior wall is 0.3 cm, whereas that of the posterior uterine wall is 0.8 cm. (**c**) After the injection of the contrast agent, sonogram shows the focal thickened endometrium

metallic shadows and pay attention to identify artifacts (Fig. 7.32).

V. Contrast-enhanced ultrasonography

Contrast-enhanced ultrasonography (CEUS) is noninvasive functional imaging of blood perfusion. Ultrasound contrast microbubbles enter the blood circulation after injected into the peripheral vein, and the microbubbles form nonlinear signals in the sound field under the action of ultrasound. Due to the weak signals of the surrounding tissues and blood, and the signal to noise is improved by ultrasound contrast imaging technology, the visualization of blood perfusion in microcirculation has been greatly improved. Contrast microbubbles can flow and distribute along with the blood system throughout the body. It is an excellent blood imaging agent. CEUS is now used in many clinical disciplines.

- Indications
  - Gynecological diseases such as ovarian tumors, uterine myoma, adenomyosis, endometrial cancer, and residual in the uterine cavity.
  - It can be used to understand the blood supply of lesions.
- Preoperative preparation

  Transvaginal probe with the frequency of 5 ~ 7.5 MHz or transabdominal with the frequency of 3.5 MHz.
  - Contrast agent: SonoVue contrast agent produced by Italian Bracco company, each contrast agent contains hexafluoride Sulfur (SF6) gas encapsulating 59 mg of phospholipid. Before usage, mix with 5 ml of normal saline and shake to extract 4.8 ml of white milky microbubble suspension.

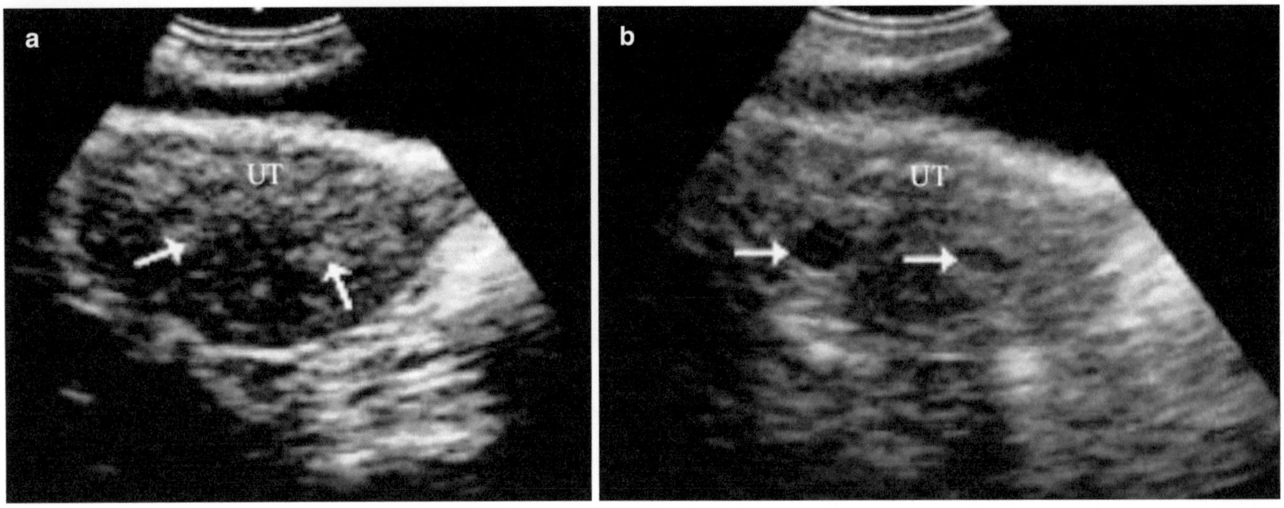

Fig. 7.21 Sonohysterography of the incomplete uterus septum. (**a**) The patient is 30 years old, and uterus septum is suspected by ultrasound examination; (**b**) After injection of contrast agent, the left uterine cavity is separated by 0.7 cm, and the right uterine cavity is divided by 0.8 cm. No specific occupation is found in the uterine cavity on both sides. The width of the septum is about 1.0 cm

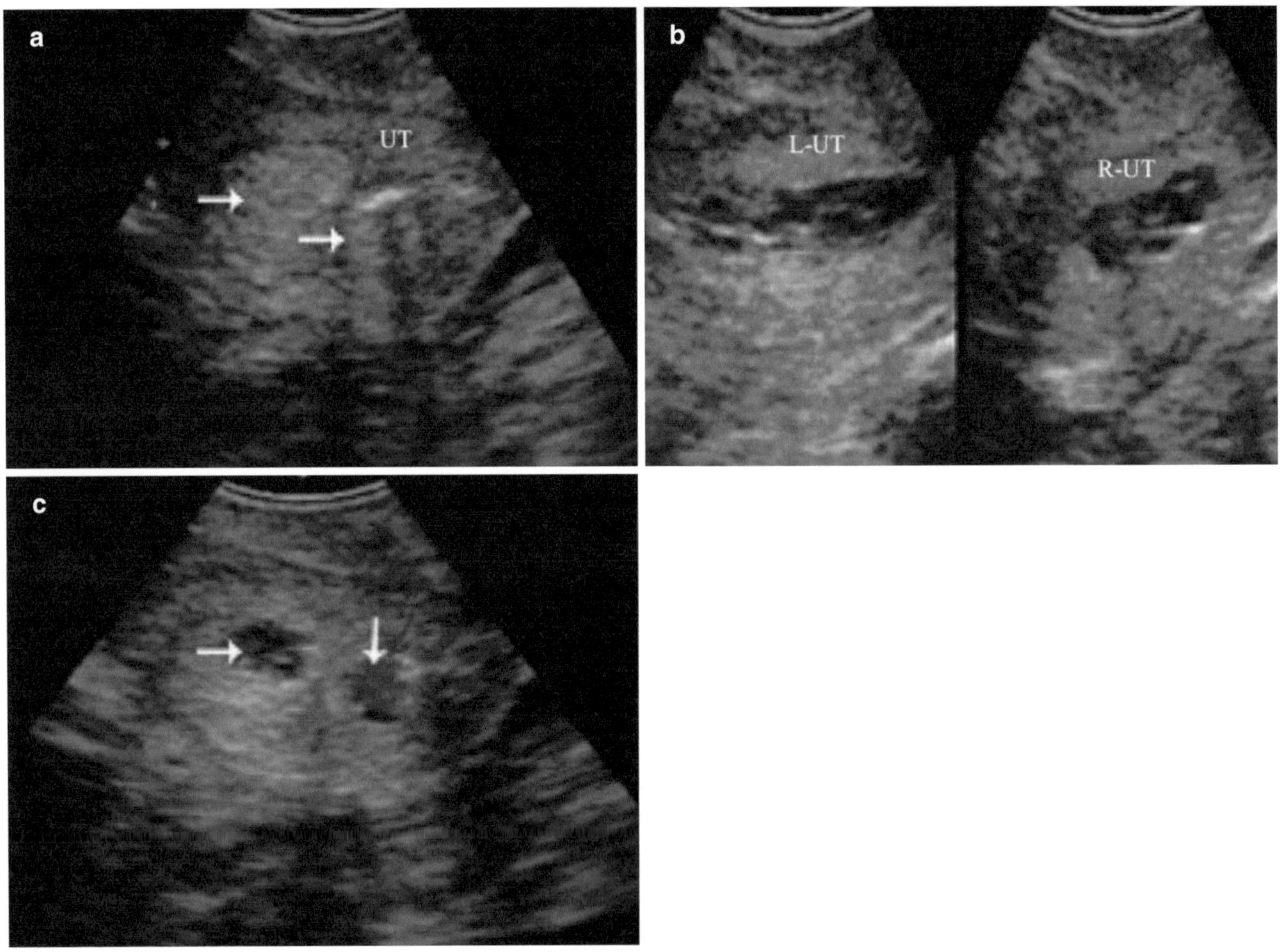

Fig. 7.22 Sonohysterography of complete uterus septum. (**a**) The patient is 26 years old, and uterus septum is suspected. (**b**) After injection of contrast agent, two uterine cavities separate from the cervix to the fundus of the uterus. (**c**) After injection of contrast agent, the septum is approximately 0.6 cm in width and about 3.2 cm long

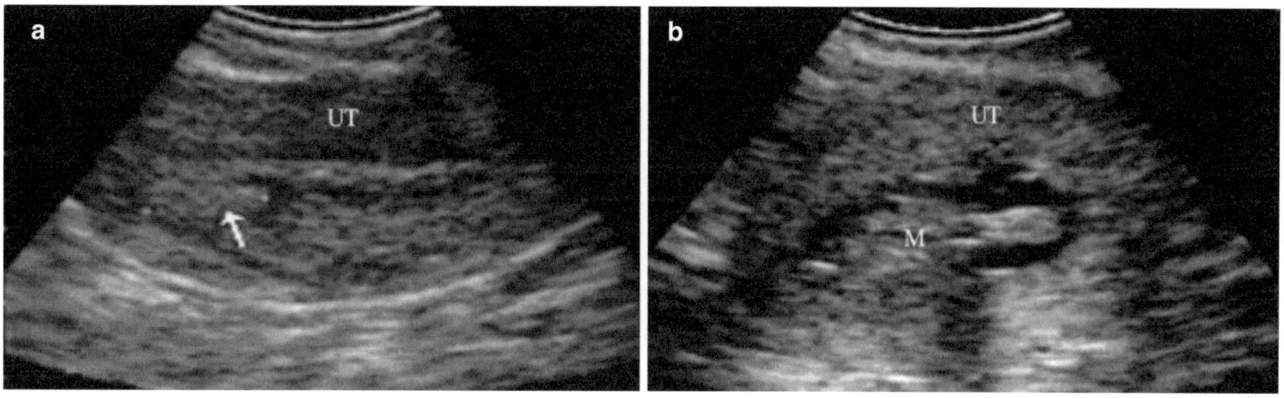

Fig. 7.23 Sonohysterography of intrauterine residues (I). (**a**) The patient is 26 years old and had a miscarriage 2 months ago. Ultrasonography shows a slightly hyperechoic mass with a diameter of about 2.0 cm, located in the right uterine corner; (**b**) After injection of contrast agent, a slightly hyperechoic mass of 2.1 cm × 0.9 cm × 1.8 cm is visible at the right corner of the uterine cavity, with irregular shape and floating in the contrast agent

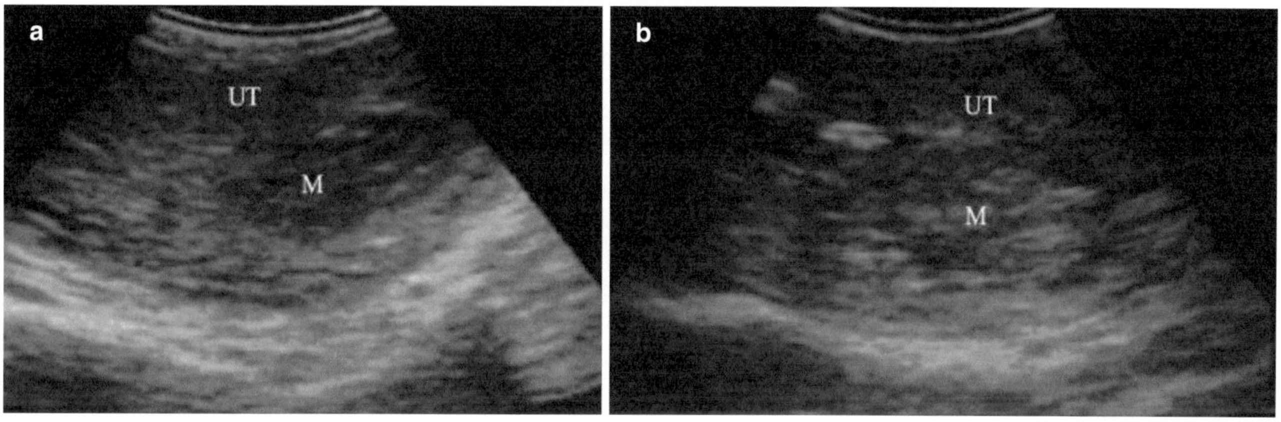

Fig. 7.24 Sonohysterography of intrauterine residues (II). (**a**) The patient is 26 years old and developed amenorrhea after a miscarriage 2 months ago. The ultrasonography shows the posterior uterus, and the hypoechoic mass in the uterine cavity; (**b**) After injection of contrast agent, sonogram shows a slightly hypoechoic mass of 2.1 cm × 1.8 cm × 2.2 cm on the left side of the uterine cavity. The mass is irregular and inhomogeneous, with surrounding irregular echoless area (contrast agent)

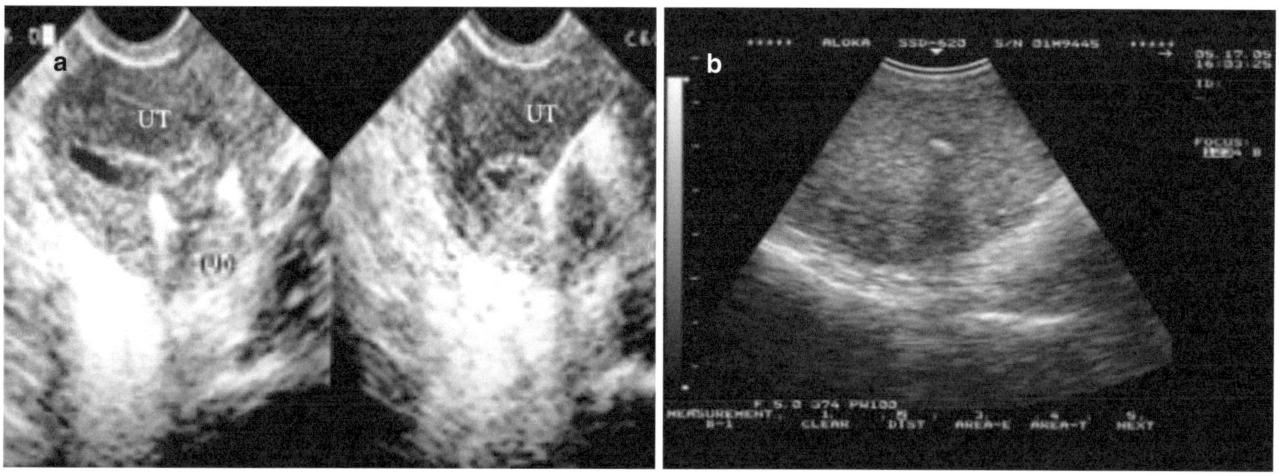

Fig. 7.25 Sonohysterography of incarcerated IUD. (**a**) The patient is 46 years old and failed to take the IUD out of the uterine cavity for 2 months. (**b**) Sonohysterography shows part of the IUD is embedded into the myometrium

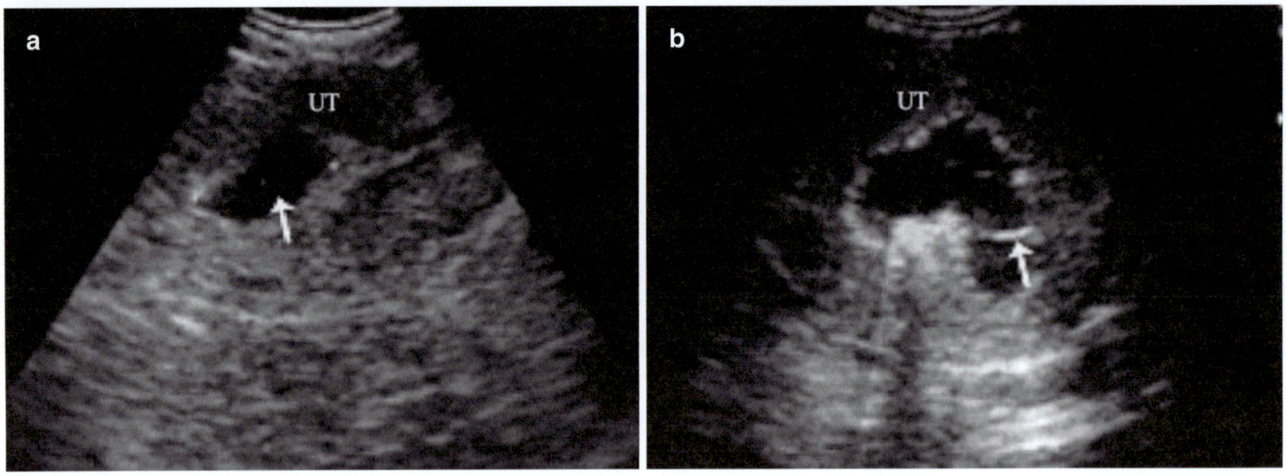

Fig. 7.26 Sonohysterography of intrauterine adhesions. (**a**) The patient is 28 years old and has amenorrhea for three months after the abortion. Before the sonohysterography, ultrasound examination shows that a dark area of 2.1 cm × 2.5 cm × 1.4 cm in the uterine cavity; (**b**) After dilating the cervical ostium, about 3 ml of old hemorrhage flows out. After injection of the contrast agent, the uterine cavity is separated by 1.5 cm, and the hyperechoic adhesion of about 1 cm is found in the uterus

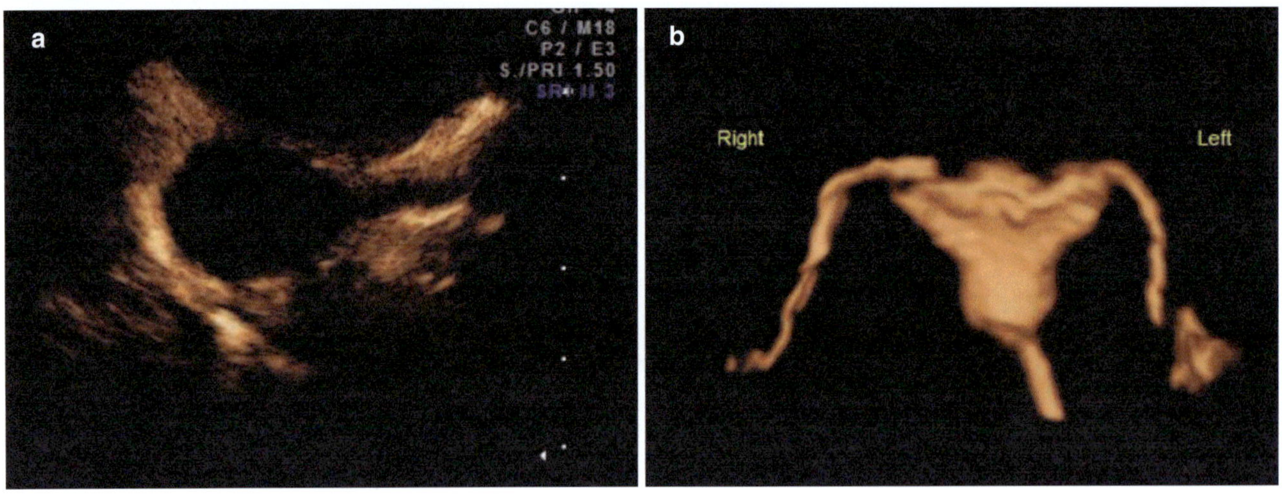

Fig. 7.27 Salpingography of the patent fallopian tube (positive contrast agent). (**a**) The contrast agent is around the ovary in the pelvis; (**b**) Three-dimensional ultrasound shows that the fallopian tubes are unobstructed

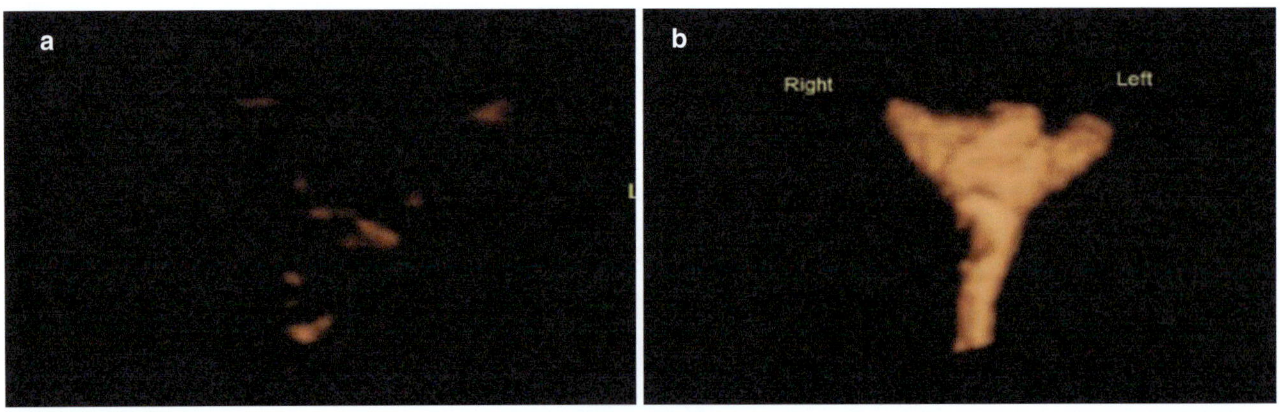

Fig. 7.28 Salpingography of the obstructed fallopian tube (positive contrast agent). (**a**) There is almost no diffusion of contrast agent in the pelvic cavity; (**b**) 3-D ultrasound shows the obstructed proximal end of the fallopian tube

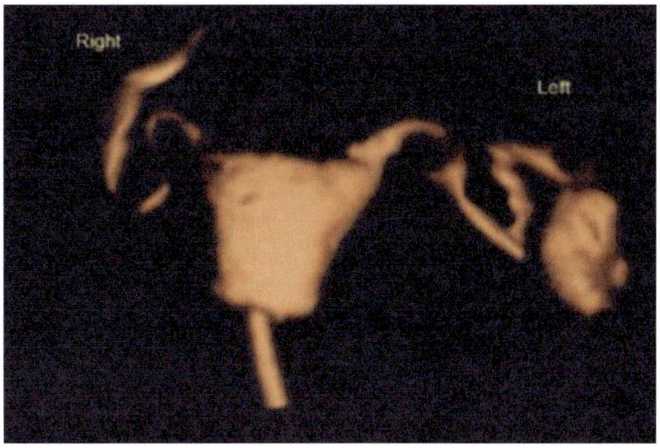

Fig. 7.29 Salpingography of the partially obstructed fallopian tube (positive contrast agent). 3-D ultrasonography shows the partially obstructed right fallopian tube, and the left fallopian tube hydrops

- Operative process (taking ovarian tumor as an example)

  CEUS can be taken in two ways: transabdominal and transvaginal.

  – Routine ultrasound examination

    Transabdominal and transvaginal ultrasonography is applied to observe uterus, adnexa, and pelvic cavity in multiple views to detect the lesion, as well as observe the location, shape, size, nature, boundary, and the internal echo. Color Doppler is used to observing the blood flow condition. Do not forget to store the images.

  – CEUS examination

    2.4 ml of Sonovue microbubble suspension was injected into the left elbow vein within 3 s, and then a bolus of normal saline was injected. The

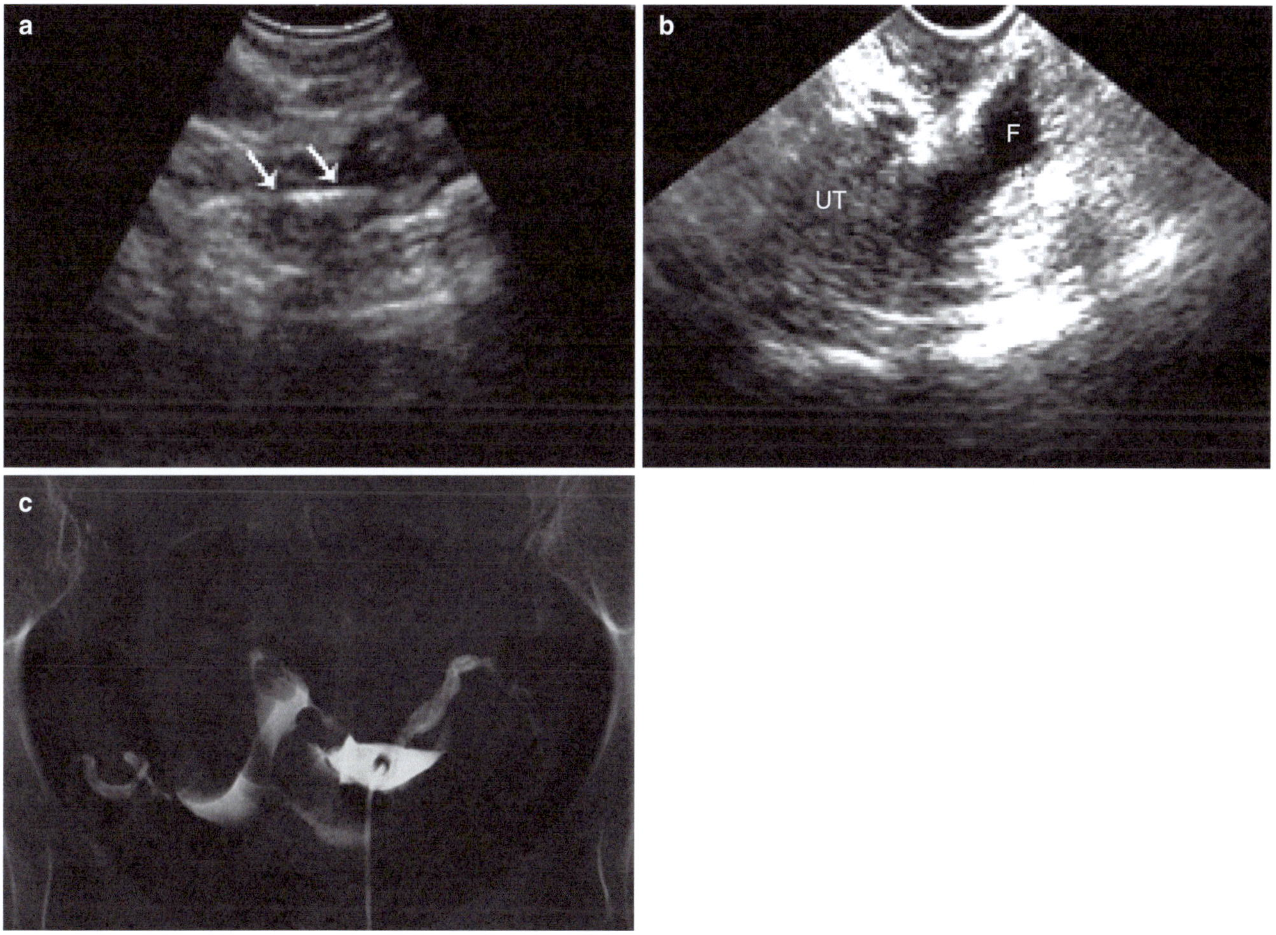

Fig. 7.30 Patency of fallopian tube (negative contrast agent). (**a**) After the injection of the contrast agent, the hyperechoic flowing column of water is visible around the adnexa, indicating that the patient's fallopian tube is unobstructed. (**b**) After the salpingography, there is a free anechoic area in the rectouterine pouch, indirectly indicating that the patient's fallopian tube is unobstructed. (**c**) Hysterosalpingography shows that the patient's bilateral fallopian tubes are unobstructed

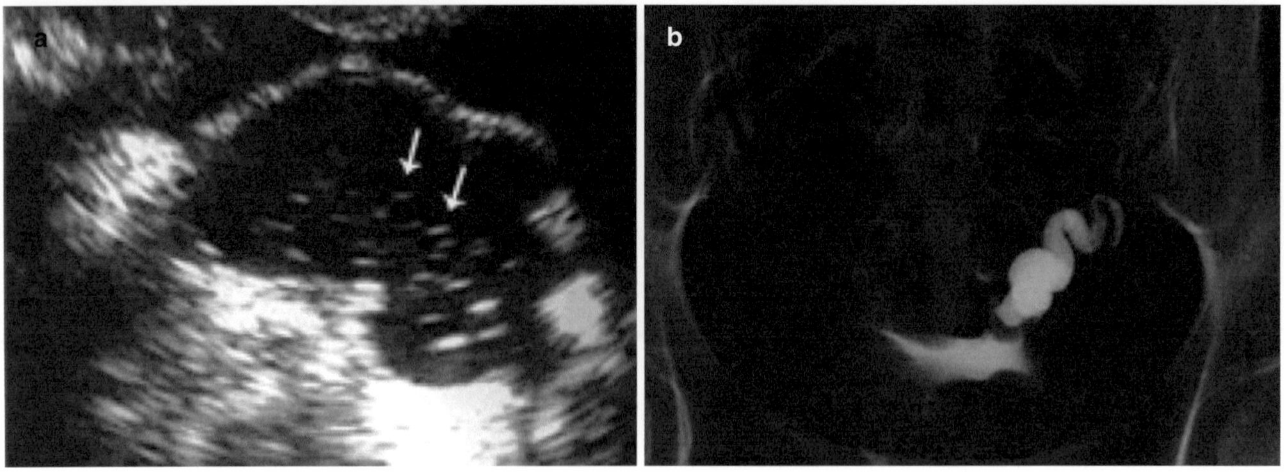

Fig. 7.31 Hysterosalpingography of hydrosalpinx. (**a**) When the contrast medium is injected, there are moving dot echoes in the dilated fallopian tube; (**b**) Hysterosalpingography shows hydrosalpinx

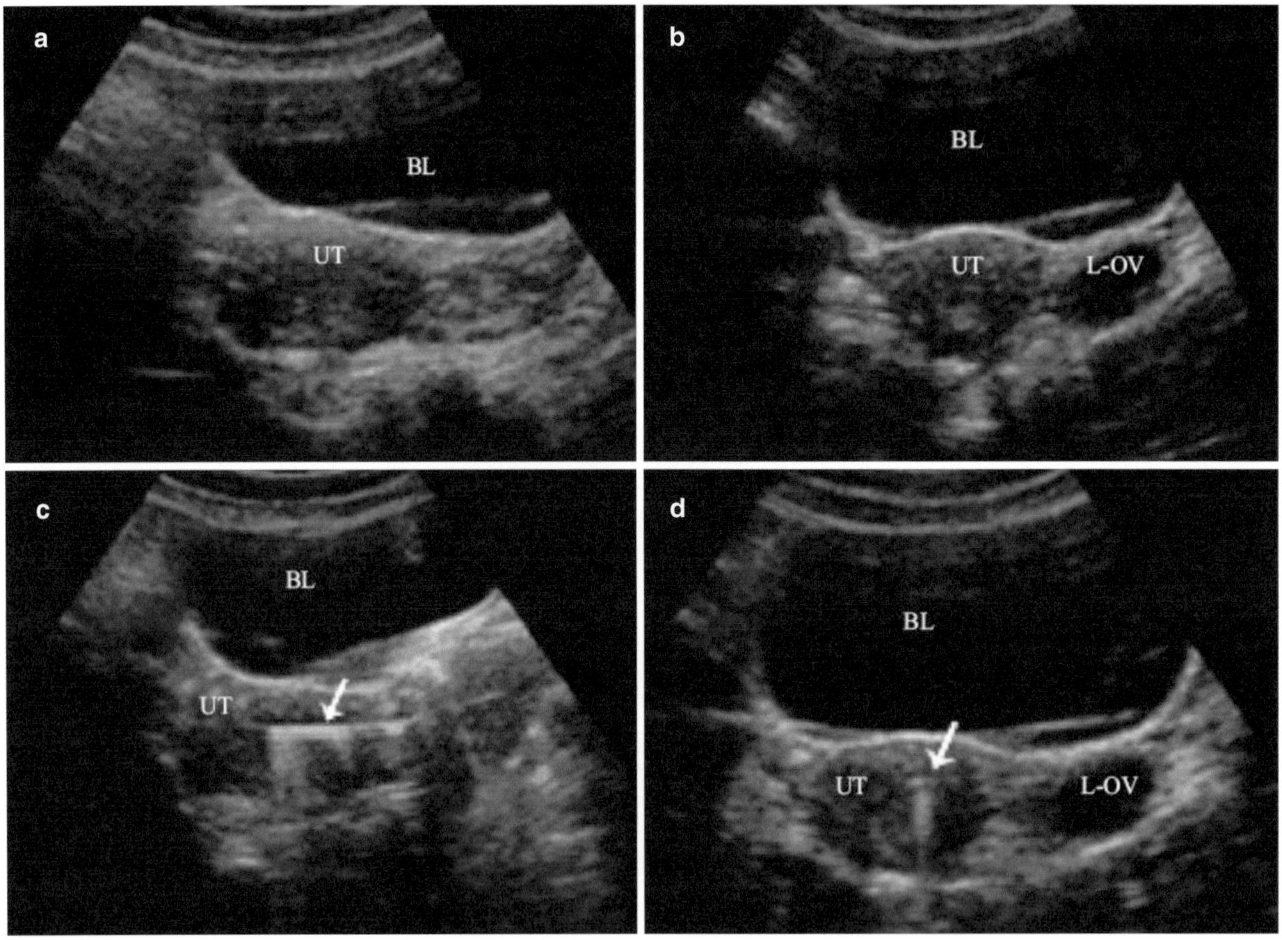

Fig. 7.32 Sonogram of ultrasound monitoring during intrauterine surgery. (**a**) Before the surgery, the sagittal view of the uterus. (**b**) Before the surgery, the transverse section of the uterus. (**c**) During the surgery, in the sagittal view of the uterus, there are hyperechoic bands, followed by "comet tail sign" in the uterine cavity. (**d**) During the surgery, in the transverse section, there is a strong spotty echo in the uterine cavity, followed by "comet tail sign"

imaging technique of PHILIPS iU22 nonlinear imaging-pulse inversion harmonic technology and energy modulation technology are used. Firstly, observe the characteristics of the echo under routine ultrasound. And then switch to the contrast mode. Observe the lesion under the fundamental wave state, and select the largest cross-section of the lesion. Patient's uterus is displayed at the same time, and the fixed section is enabled with a low mechanical index contrast double-amplitude mode (harmonic and fundamental states) and displayed simultaneously. While bolus injection of contrast agent, start the timer and store the dynamic image to 3 min after the injection of contrast agent. Continue to observe the contrast image and save the dynamic image on the hard disk.

- Notes
  - Let the patient breathe as smoothly as possible during the examination and keep the position fixed.
  - Contraindications: Patients with a history of significant allergies; patients with significant abnormal lung function.
  - Images should be analyzed by an experienced physician.
- Ultrasound diagnosis
  - Morphological analysis of CEUS.

    Taking ovarian tumors as an example, based on the observation of perfusion of contrast agent, according to the distribution of the contrast agent in the mass, the ovarian mass can be divided into three types: no enhancement type, no contrast agent enters into the mass; surrounding type, contrast agent is only distributed around the periphery of the mass; extension type, contrast agent enters and distributes inside the mass. According to the intensity of the contrast agent of the mass, it can be divided into three types. For comparison, if the enhancement intensity is lower than that of the uterus, it is a low enhancement; if it is close to or equal to the enhancement intensity of the uterus, it is an equal enhancement; if the enhancement intensity is higher than that of the uterus, it is high enhancement (Fig. 7.33).

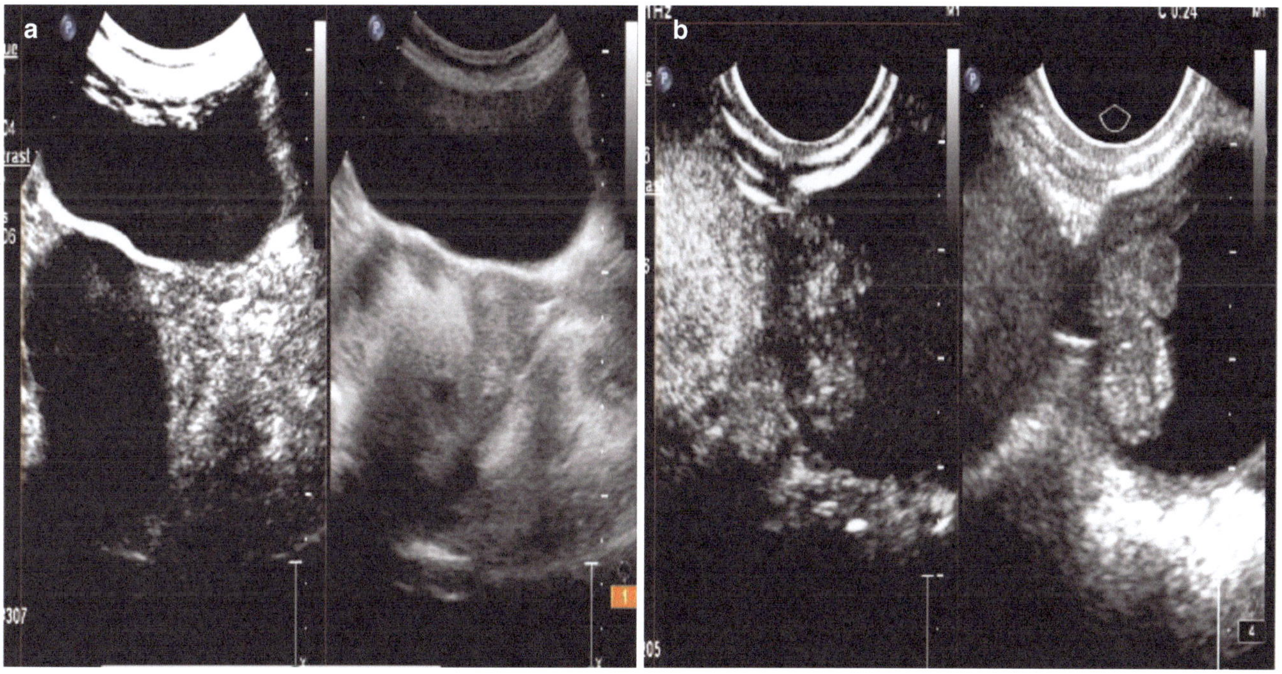

Fig. 7.33 CEUS of ovarian tumors. (**a**) The patient is 26 years old with a right ovarian mass, which is a kind of no enhancement; (**b**) The patient is 46 years old, with a left ovarian mass, which is a kind of extension type and low enhancement; (**c**) The patient is 43 years old with a left ovarian tumor, which is a kind of extension type and equal enhancement; (**d**) The patient is 42 years old with a pelvic mass, which is a kind of extension type and high enhancement

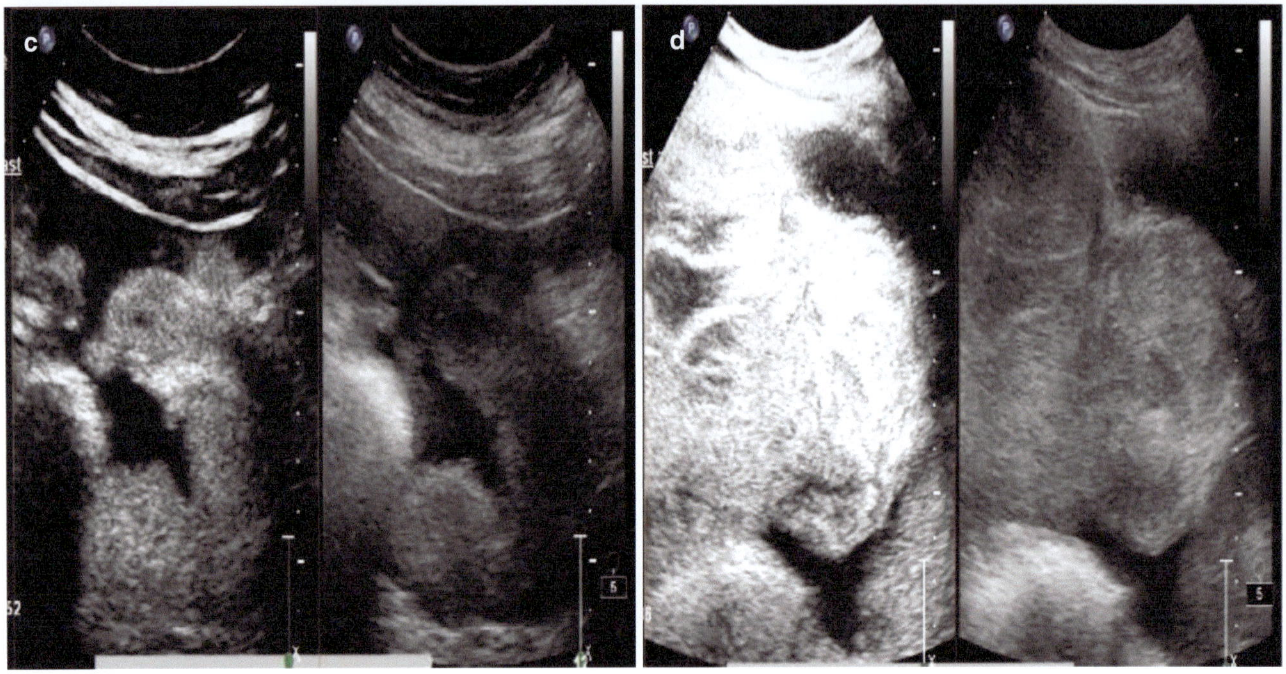

Fig 7.33 (continued)

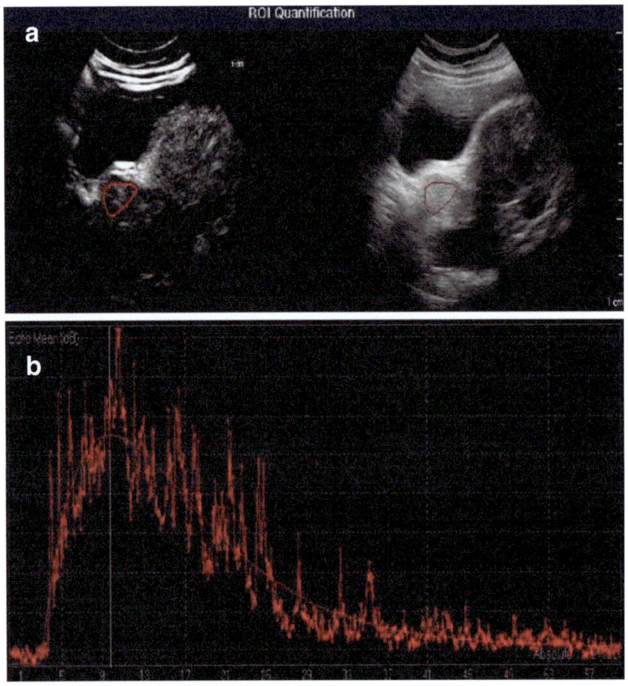

Fig. 7.34 Time–intensity curve analysis of CEUS of ovarian tumors. (**a**) Under contrast harmonic-fundamental double imaging, select ROI in the largest longitudinal section of the ovarian tumor; (**b**) Process curve fitting to the time–intensity curve with gamma fitting function

– Time–intensity curve analysis of CESU.

The obtained dynamic images are analyzed by Qlab-ROI software. Select the area of the lesion; then the time–intensity curve (TIC) is obtained. Select a gamma fitting function suitable for bolus injection to perform gamma curve-fitting on the TIC; obtain contrast perfusion parameters of the lesion site, including rising time (RT), peak intensity (PI), Area under the curve (AUC), time from peak to one half (TTH), and time to peak (TTP) (Fig. 7.34).

Suggested Reading

1. 张美琴, 周彩云, 罗红. 纳米级超声造影剂的技术进展, 华西医学, 2012, 27(10):1585–1587 (无英文摘要).
2. ZHOU Cai-yun, LUO Hong, Ultrasonic contrast's application and development in ovarian tumor, Technical Acoustics. 2010, 29(4):476–478.
3. Fan YANG, Tai-zhu YANG, Hong LUO, et al. Diagnostic value of contrast-enhanced ultrasonography in ovarian tumors. J Sichuan Univ (Med Sci Edi). 2013;44(003):424–8.
4. Fan YANG, Tai-zhu YANG, Hong LUO, et al. Preliminary study of contrast-enhanced ultrasonography in the evaluation of angiogenesis in ovarian tumors. J Sichuan Univ (Med Sci Edi). 2014;45(06):964–9.

Applications of 3D Ultrasound in Obstetrics and Gynecology

8

Taizhu Yang, Jiao Chen, and Houqing Pang

8.1 Introduction of 3D Ultrasound Modes

3D ultrasound, a significant breakthrough of the ultrasonic fields, opens an entirely new visual space. 3D ultrasound technology collects a volume database containing numerous 2D plans, and displays the region of interest (ROI) using various modes, providing new methods of volume measurement without mathematical simulation formula. 3D ultrasound has a considerable clinical influence on obstetrics and gynecology. The advantage of 3D ultrasound is fully reflected because of its increasing popularity.

3D ultrasound provides several display modes, including multiplanes mode, niche mode, surface mode, and transparent mode, etc.

I. Multiplanar mode

Three mutually perpendicular planes, the sagittal plane, transverse plane, and coronal plane, are simultaneously visualized, which can be shifted and rotated arbitrarily. It is convenient to continuously observe the lesion and define the spatial relationship between the lesion and the tissues surrounding it.

II. Niche mode

Observe the internal morphology of the organs or lesions and determine lesion involvement.

III. Surface mode

Visualize the structures surrounded by hypoechoic or anechoic hierarchically and dimensionally. The surface mode is utilized to demonstrate the features of the surface organs or tissues.

IV. Transparent mode

There are three different display modes according to the algorithm of different echo data. Among them, the maximum mode facilitates the study of the fetal skeletal system, the minimum mode is mainly used for the evaluation of vessels and hollow viscera, and the X-ray mode is utilized for the tumor areas and similar-echo structures. Inversion mode inverts the gray-scale information based on the minimum mode. This mode transforms original anechoic structures into hyperechoic structures, and vice versa.

V. B-flow mode. A stereoscopic way to display the blood flow, evaluate the perfusion, and observe the relationship between blood vessels and tissues.

VI. Glass body mode. Highlight the location and distribution of vascular structure, usually with 3D color or power Doppler ultrasound.

VII. Tomographic ultrasound imaging (TUI)

TUI, a relatively new 3D ultrasound imaging mode, obtains multidirectional tomographic images with the collected volume data, facilitating the study of the fetal structure from a new perspective. After scanning with a 3D/4D probe, it generates a 3D database containing multiple continuous 2D plans, allowing for the simultaneous display of several parallel slices in three planes that are orthogonal to each other. It is facilitated to show the structural changes on the same screen by adjusting the slice distance and image rotating, equivalent to CT and MRI, with relatively convenient operation.

VIII. Spatiotemporal image correlation (STIC)

STIC is a feature of real-time 3D technology that is utilized for the fetal heart and great arteries. Volume datasets for fetal echocardiography, composed of sequential 2D plans, are acquired with an automated scan of the volume probe. Combined with time information, the volume datasets of multiple cardiac cycles can be displayed in the same cardiac cycle.

This chapter was translated by Mingchun Zhi, Miaoqian Wang Department of Obstetrics and Gynecology, Beijing Hospital, National Center of Gerontology, Beijing, China

T. Yang (✉) · J. Chen · H. Pang
Department of Ultrasonography, West China Second University Hospital, Sichuan University, Chengdu, China

T. Yang, H. Luo (eds.), *Practical Ultrasonography in Obstetrics and Gynecology*,
https://doi.org/10.1007/978-981-16-4477-1_8

8.2 Application of 3D Ultrasound in Obstetrics

With 3D ultrasound, stereoscopic imaging of the fetal surface and internal structures can be obtained to observe the overall fetal morphology and structure. 3D ultrasound is utilized to demonstrate the normal and pathological morphology during gestation and improve the prenatal diagnosis rate of fetal malformations.

I. Embryo and fetal activity

3D ultrasound is used to observe embryos and fetuses in different gestational weeks. In early pregnancy, the embryo sac is oval or round, covering chorion. The yolk sac is usually spherical; the curved embryo is in a "C" shape, the upper and lower limb buds are spoon-shaped, and the umbilical cord is linear. During the mid and late pregnancy, 3D ultrasound shows the intrauterine fetal movement visually and vividly, including the motion of the fetal head, mouth, arm, trunk, and lower limbs (Figs. 8.1, 8.2, and, 8.3).

II. Fetal biological measurement

TUI technique, utilizing for the measurement of fetal nuchal translucency, postnasal triangle, hard palate, and alveolar bone at 11 ~ 14 weeks of gestation, has been one of the hotspots in early detecting of fetal abnormalities.

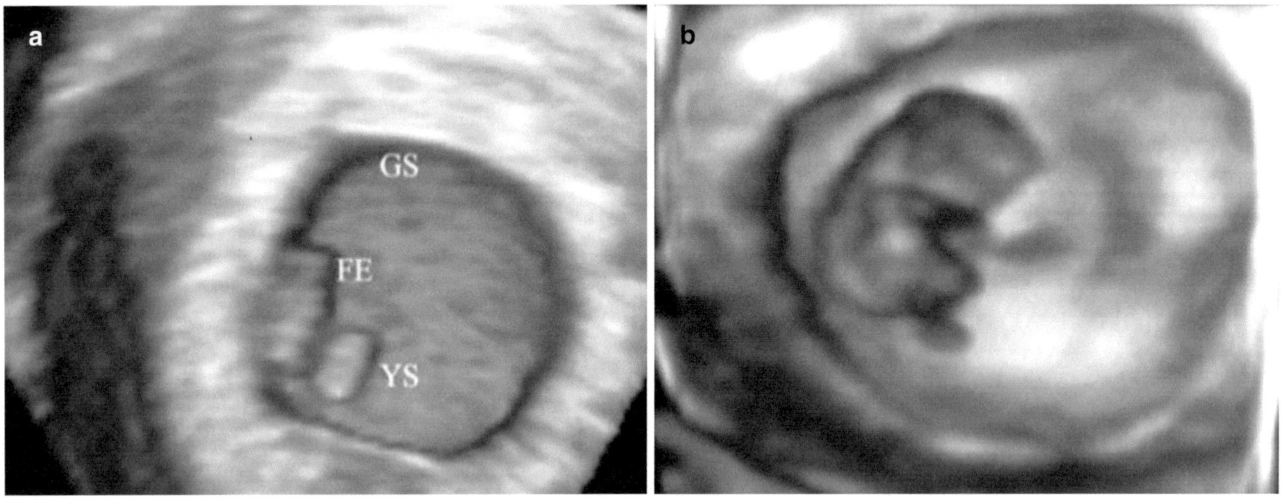

Fig. 8.1 Embryo and fetal activity. (**a**) Six weeks pregnancies. The elliptic gestational sac and the spherical yolk sac are identifiable. (**b**) Ten weeks pregnancies. The bending embryo in the gestational sac is in a "c" shape

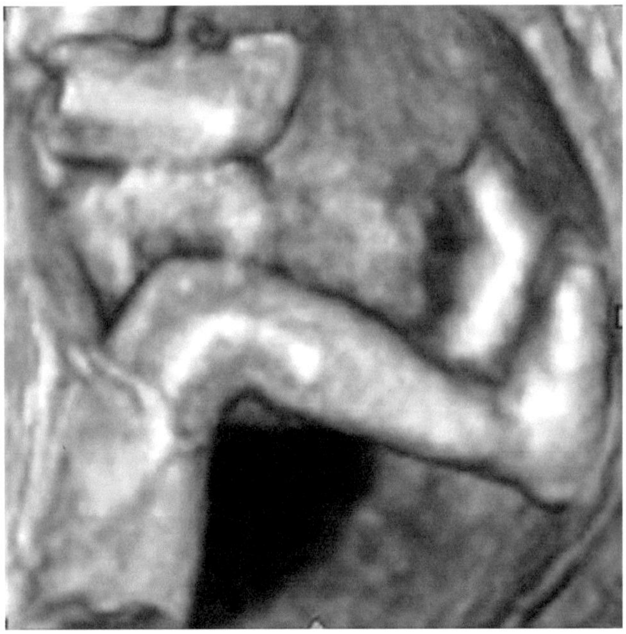

Fig. 8.2 Image of normal fetal lower limb

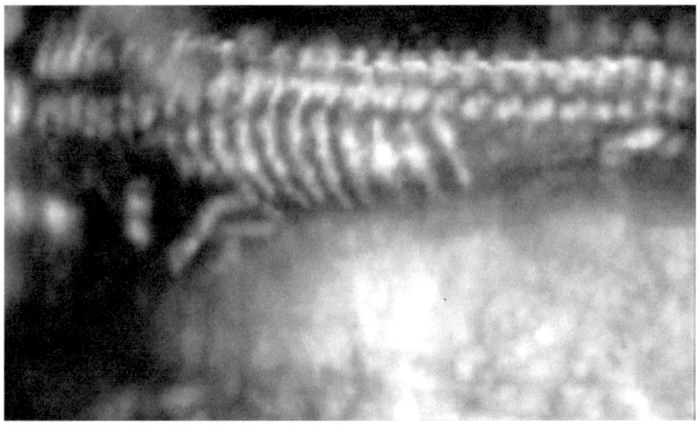

Fig. 8.3 Image of a normal fetal spine

3D ultrasound is used to accurately measure fetal growth indexes, including the diameter of the fetal head, length of the long bones, and the volume of the brain, internal organs and limbs, for the evaluation of fetal development (Figs. 8.4 and 8.5). As 3D technology develops, it is facilitated to observe the structure of fetal corpus callosum, cerebellar vermis, hard palate, and so on. The volume of fetal organs, such as cerebellomedullary cistern, cerebellum, corpus callosum, lung, thyroid, stomach bubble, bladder, are measured accurately. Moreover, 3D is utilized to evaluate the stomach bubble development and the fetal urine production rate, etc.

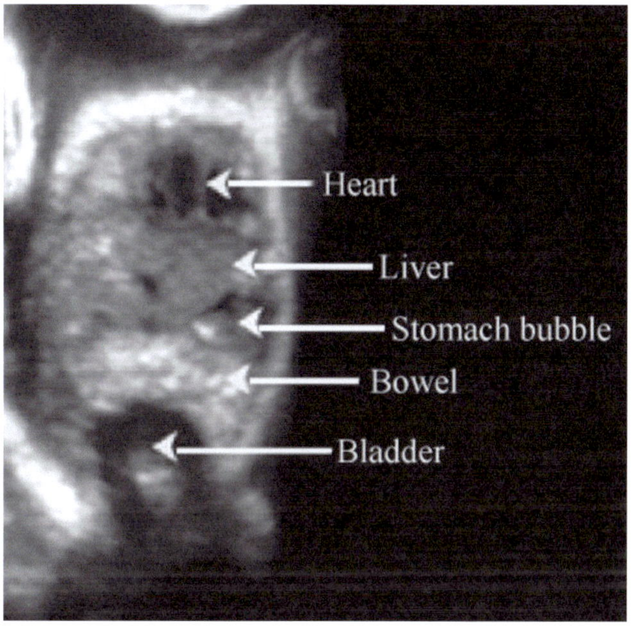

Fig. 8.4 3D Image of normal fetal internal organs

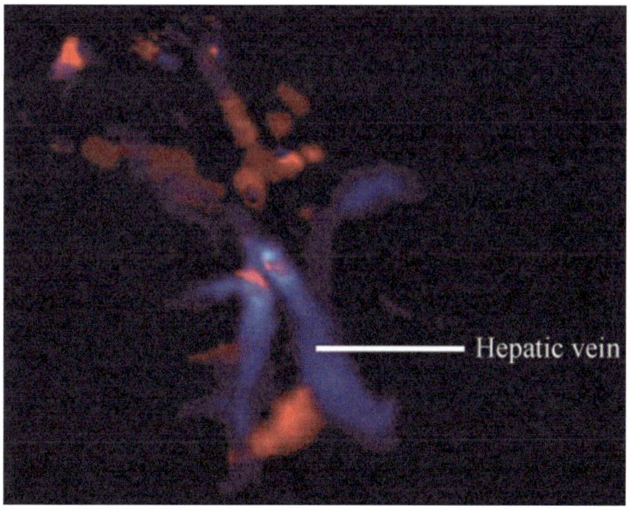

Fig. 8.5 3D color Doppler sonography demonstrates normal fetal liver blood vessels

III. 3D ultrasound diagnosis of fetal malformation

- Fetal facial abnormalities

  3D ultrasound facilitates to show the full view of the fetal face, providing a stereo image to explore facial anomaly. Cleft lip, cleft palate, arhinia, proboscis, collapsed nose bridge, cyclopia, low ears, micrognathia are the most frequently observed abnormalities (Figs. 8.6 and 8.7).

- Fetal skeletal malformation

  The transparent mode of 3D ultrasound is the best way to illustrate the appearance of the fetal skeleton from different angles, especially for evaluating spine development. It contributes to the diagnosis of hemivertebra, scoliosis, spina bifida, and other spinal deformities. 3D ultrasound has an integral role in the diagnosis of local fetal limb deformities, such as the absence of radius, wrist varus, wrist eversion, acheiria finger absence, cleft hand, cleft foot, apodia, and clubfoot (Figs. 8.8 and 8.9).

- Malformation of fetal central nervous system

  3D ultrasound was used to diagnose Dandy–Walker syndrome, corpus callosum dysplasia, and meningocele, etc. 3D color Doppler ultrasound has a significant impact on the diagnosis of vascular mal-

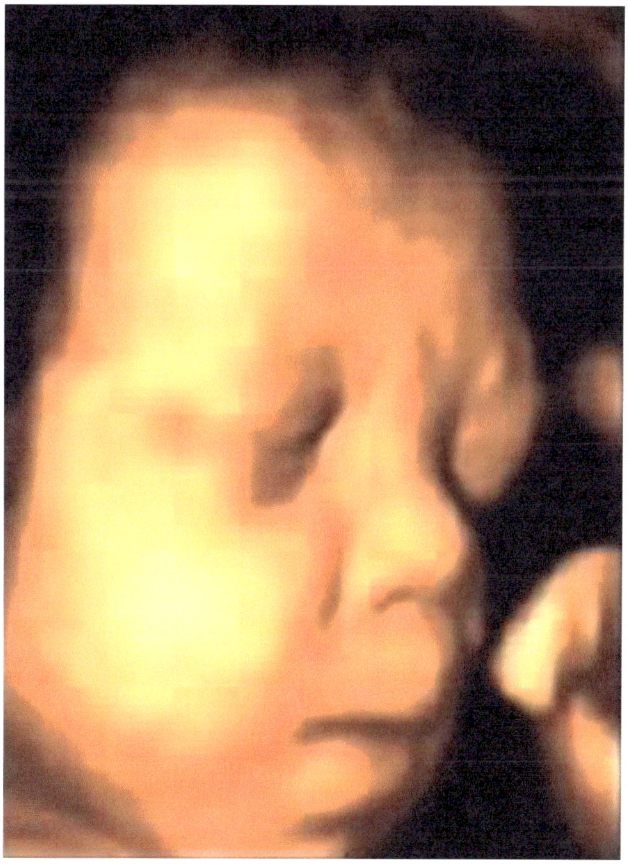

Fig. 8.6 Image of normal fetal face

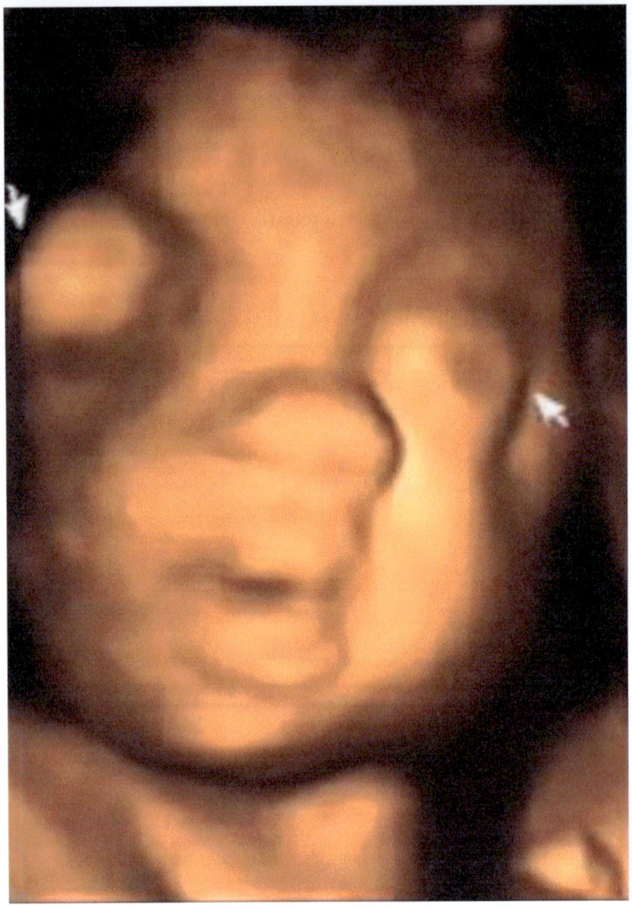

Fig. 8.7 Fetal bilateral exophthalmos image

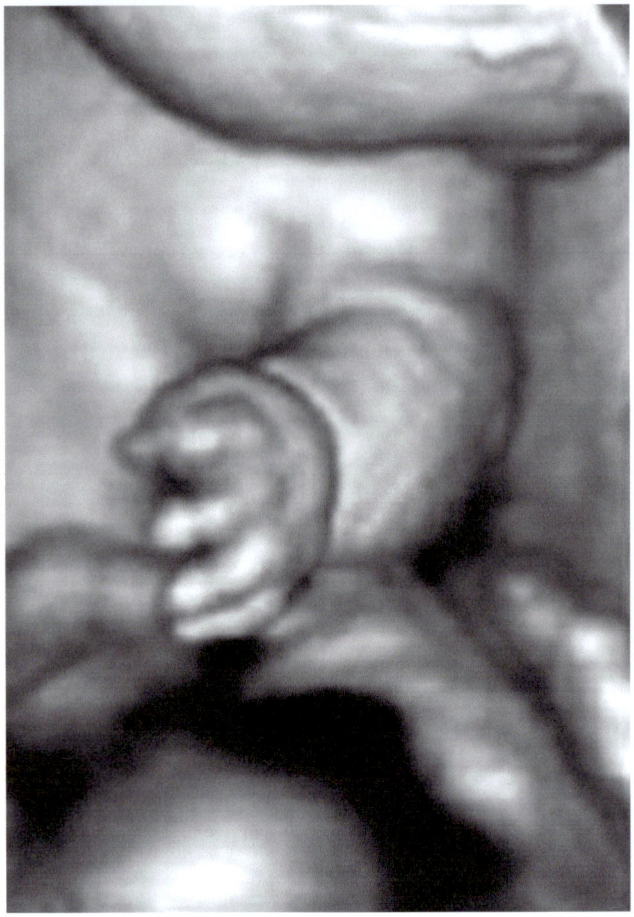

Fig. 8.8 Image of fetal phocomelia

formation by visualizing the circle of Willis intuitively (Figs. 8.10 and 8.11).

- Fetal Abdominal Wall Defect and Abdominal Organ Malformation

  The three orthogonal plans of 3D ultrasound facilitate to simultaneously observe the continuity of the abdominal wall and the spatial relationship of the attached part of the umbilical cord from all angles, which is helpful for the differential diagnosis of umbilical hernia, omphalocele, gastroschisis, and other malformations. Besides, it can quantitatively evaluate the volume of the sac, providing more efficient clinical information (Figs. 8.12 and 8.13).

- Fetal heart and blood vessels

  STIC technology can visually display the spatial structure of the fetal heart and great arteries and obtain plans that are challenging to be acquired or observed in 2D imaging. STIC has significant advantages in the diagnosis of complex congenital cardiac malformations. 3Dtechnology, an objective method for fetal cardiac function measurement, can accurately calculate the fetal cardiac volume, ejection fraction, and cardiac movement. With the use of STIC, volume datasets of the fetal heart are acquired with a single quick sweep of the probe, effectively and time-saving.

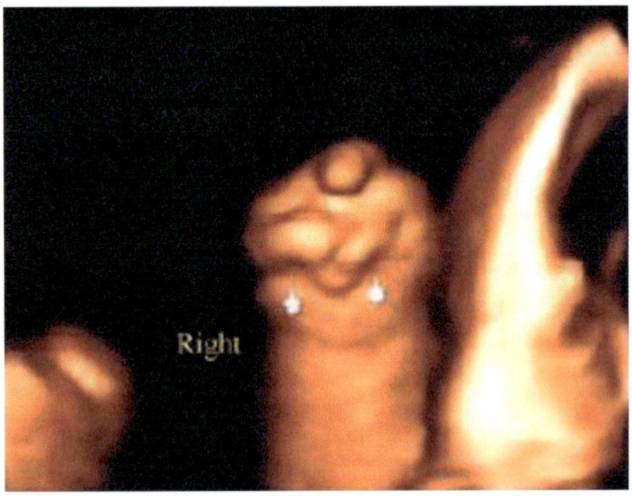

Fig. 8.9 Fetal overlapping finger of the right hand

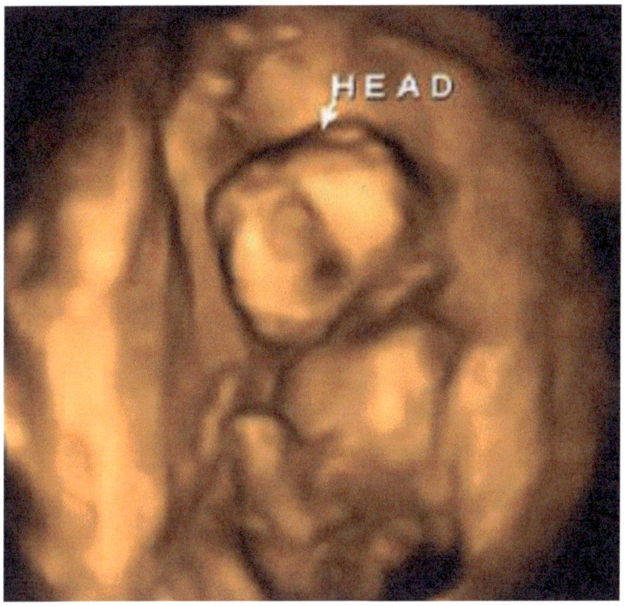

Fig. 8.10 Image of anencephaly

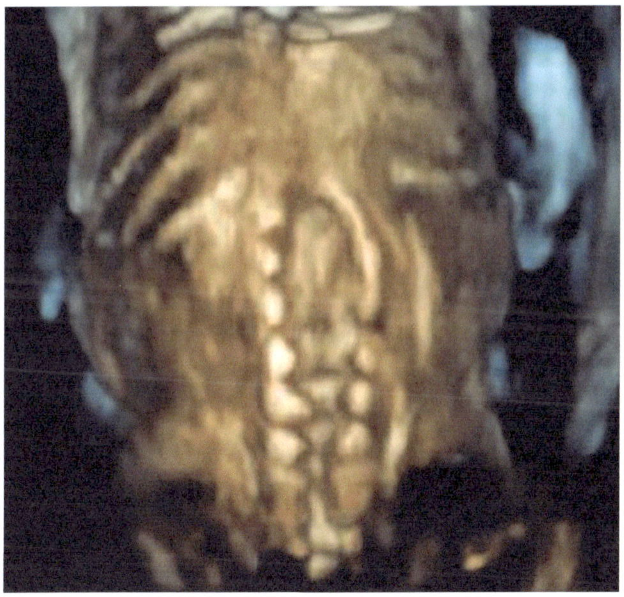

Fig. 8.11 Image of fetal spina bifida

- Urogenital system

  The 3D multiplanar mode can clearly show the polycystic kidney, renal dysplasia, and other diseases. B-flow imaging facilitates the display of renal vascular abnormalities, the diagnosis of congenital renal artery stenosis, and the evaluation of renal blood perfusion. The 3D morphology of the fetal external genitalia, which is of great value for the diagnosis of hermaphroditism and hypospadias, is intuitively displayed with the surface mode (Fig. 8.14).

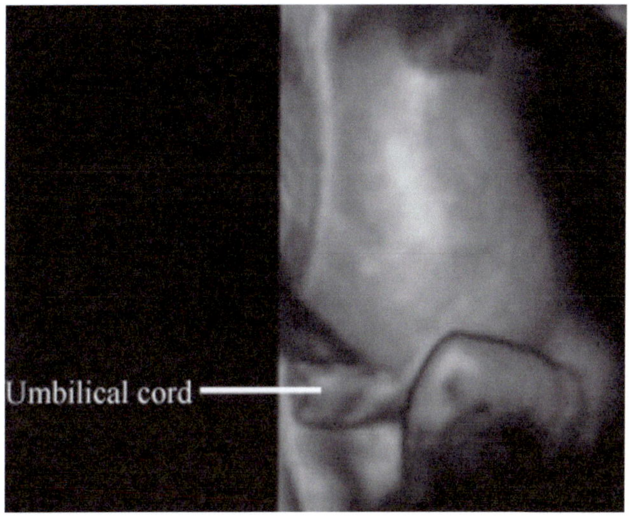

Fig. 8.12 Image of normal fetal ventral wall

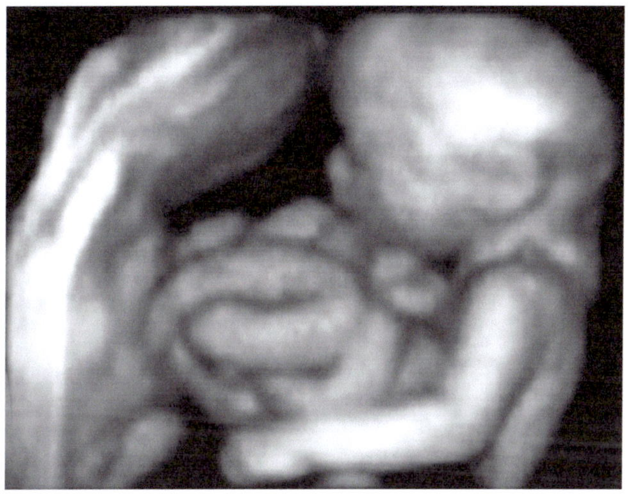

Fig. 8.13 Fetal visceral herniation

- Umbilical cord and placenta

  With 3D ultrasound, it is beneficial to show the number of umbilical arteries and veins, the twisting direction of the cord, the number of the cord around the neck, and true knots in the cord (Figs. 8.15 and 8.16). The 3D power image contributes to evaluate the placental vascular bed, quantitatively calculate the placental blood flow, and monitor the placental blood perfusion. 3D B-flow imaging is suitable for assessing the placental infarction, twin-twin transfusion, and circumvallate placenta, etc. 3D ultrasound facilitates to distinguish the chorionicity by evaluating the intervening membrane in the second and third trimesters, with high sensitivity, specificity, and accuracy.

Fig. 8.14 Urogenital system. (**a**) Fetal external genitalia (female) (**b**) Fetal external genitalia (male)

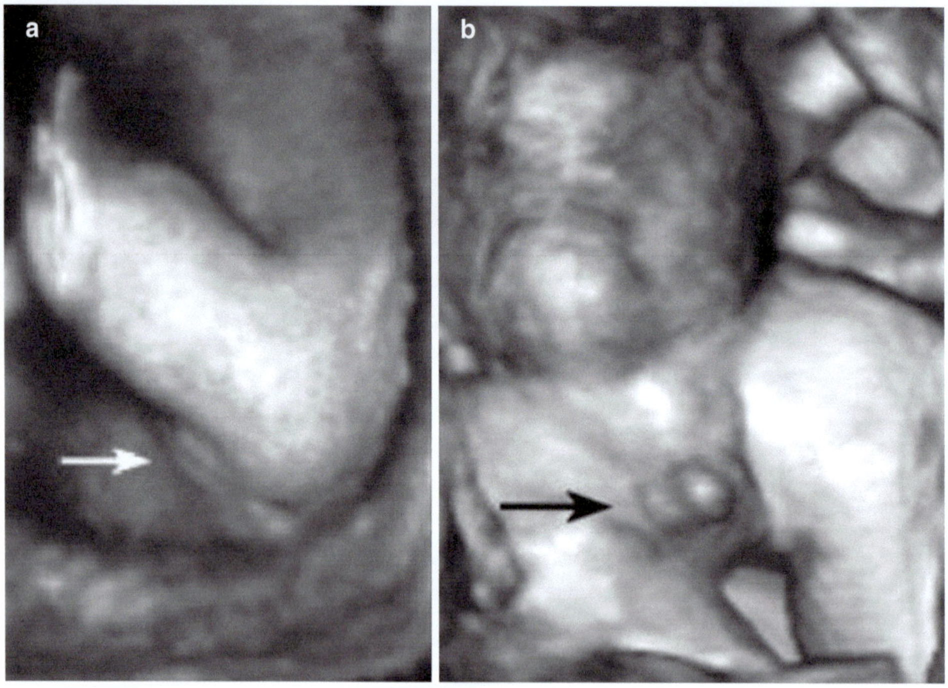

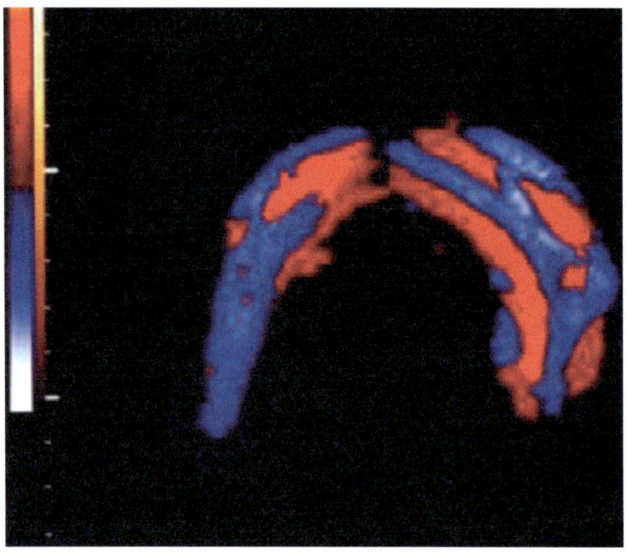

Fig. 8.15 3D B-flow image of fetal umbilical cord

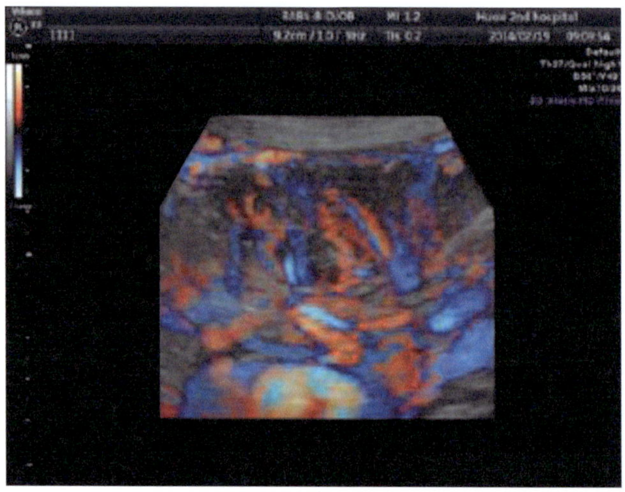

Fig. 8.16 3D image of placental hemangioma

8.3 Application of 3D Ultrasound in Gynecology

3D ultrasound, showing the longitudinal, transverse, and coronal views of the uterus simultaneously, reveals a new technique and provides more accurate information, which makes it possible to simulate the preoperative surgical path. 3D ultrasound is the optimal noninvasive method for all-around observation of the uterus and adnexa, accurate diagnosis, timely treatment, and prognosis evaluation of diseases (Fig. 8.17).

I. Uterine diseases

3D ultrasound can acquire the true coronal view of the uterus that cannot be obtained using 2D ultrasound. By parallel shifting and spinning the anatomic planes of the 3D ultrasound, make a comprehensive analysis of the interested structures, such as uterine malformation, endometrial polyps, and submucous myoma, etc.

- Uterine malformation

  By freely rotating planes, a standard 3D plan can be obtained to measure the depth of the uterine fundal indentation and the length of the intrauterine septum. It is often recommended for definitive diagnosis of the

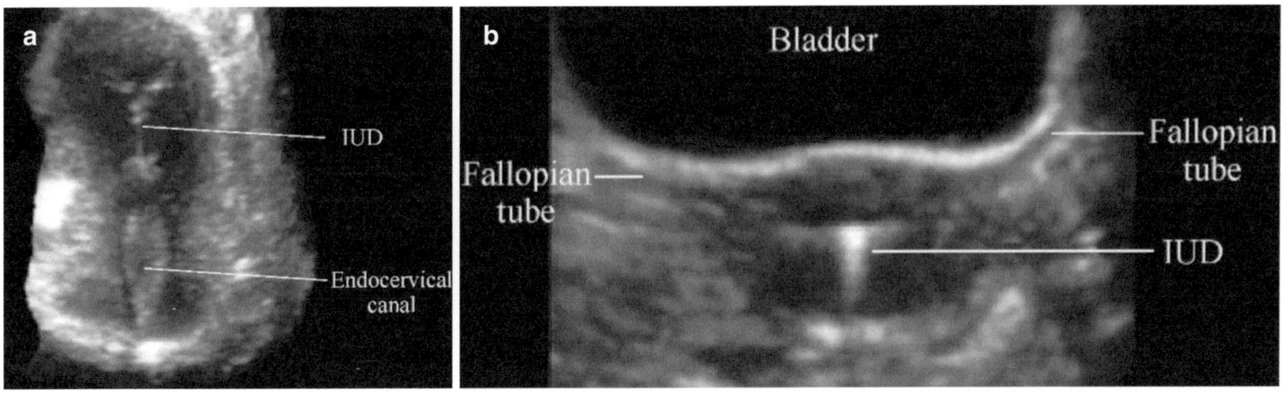

Fig. 8.17 (**a**) Longitudinal view of normal uterus; (**b**) coronal view of normal uterus

Fig. 8.18 Uterine malformation. (**a**) Partial septate uterus; (**b**) Complete septate uterus

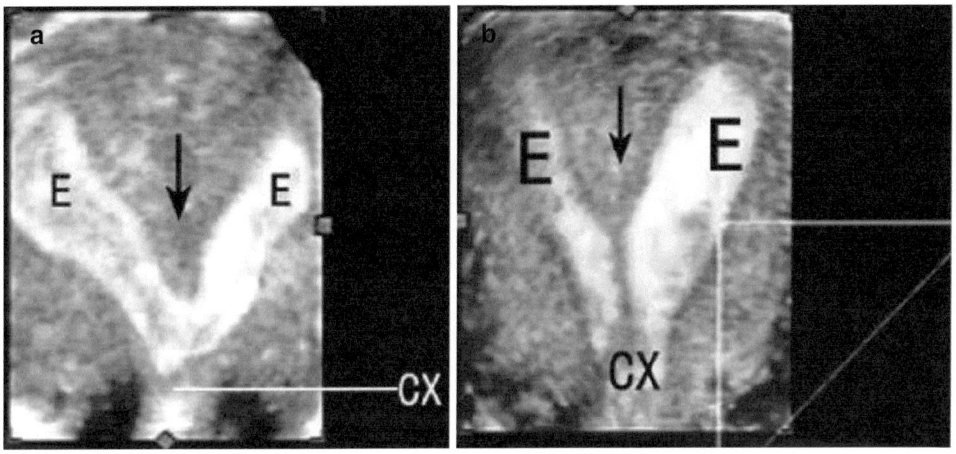

arcuate uterus, septate uterus, and bicornuate uterus, with high sensitivity and specificity (Fig. 8.18).

- Uterine myoma

  3D ultrasound facilitates to accurately measure the size of uterine myoma and distinguish the positional relation with the endometrium, which is conducive to the follow-up (Fig. 8.19).

- Endometrial lesion

  3D ultrasound is utilized to definitively measure the endometrial volume, which can predict and diagnose endometrial cancer. The intrauterine cavernous changes of hydropic chorionic villi and abnormal rich blood flow in hydatidiform mole lesions are stereoscopically demonstrated using 3D ultrasound (Fig. 8.20).

- Intrauterine Space-Occupying Disease

  3D ultrasound can provide the optimal view to show the uterine cavity, evaluate the size, number, and position of the space-occupying lesion.

  The availability of 3D ultrasound combined with sonohysterography has a positive impact on the differential diagnosis of intrauterine residues, endometrial polyp, and other lesions (Fig. 8.21).

- Cervical disease

  In cervical cancer cases, the rich cervical blood flow is fireworks-like displayed. 3D B-flow imaging provides more detailed information for the overall estimation of the cervical cancerous lesion and extent (Fig. 8.22).

II. Intrauterine device (IUD)

With the availability of 3D ultrasound, the shape, size, and type of the IUD are visually displayed. It is possible to precisely ascertain the location of IUD for the detection of slipped IUD using 3D ultrasound (Fig. 8.23).

III. Monitoring follicular development

3D ultrasound can more clearly observe.

The delineation and maturity level of the follicle is visible by 3D ultrasound.

It is utilized to accurately measure the volume of the ovary and follicle for further follicular monitoring, guiding clinical medication, and infertility treatment.

IV. Ovarian diseases

3D ultrasound can intuitively show the spatial relation between the pelvic space-occupying lesion and adjacent organs, such as uterus, ovary, bladder and rec-

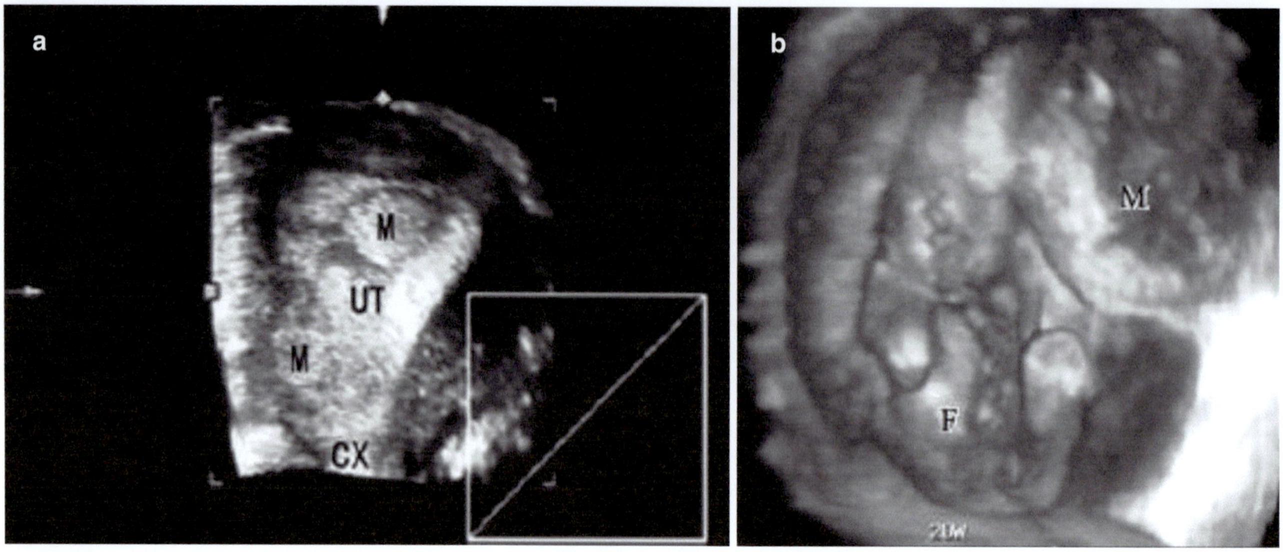

Fig. 8.19 Uterine myoma. (**a**) Submucosal myoma; (**b**) Uterine myoma in middle pregnancy

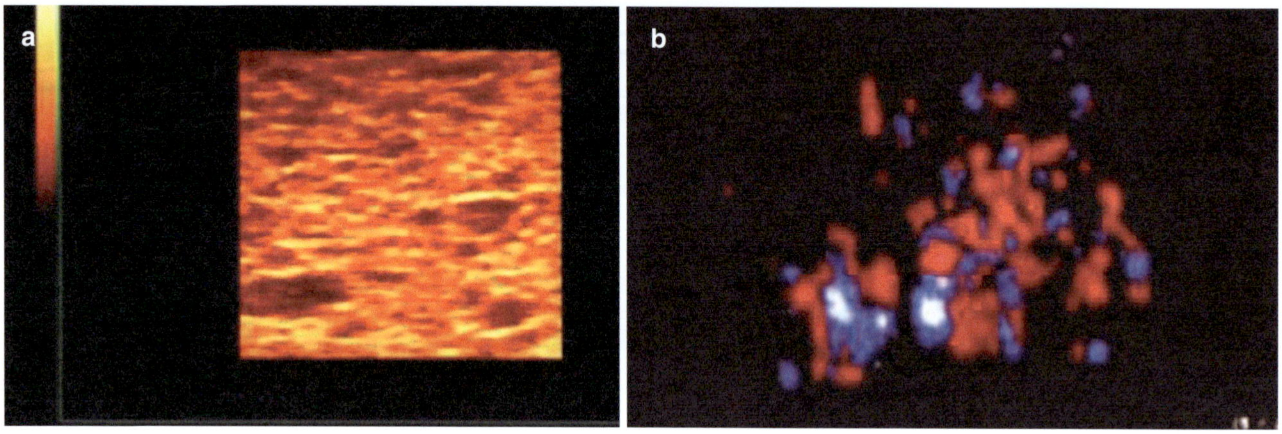

Fig. 8.20 Hydatidiform mole. (**a**) 3D image of hydatidiform mole; (**b**) 3D B-flow imaging of hydatidiform mole

Fig. 8.21 Intrauterine space-occupying lesion. (**a**) Intrauterine residues after abortion; (**b**) Endometrial polyp

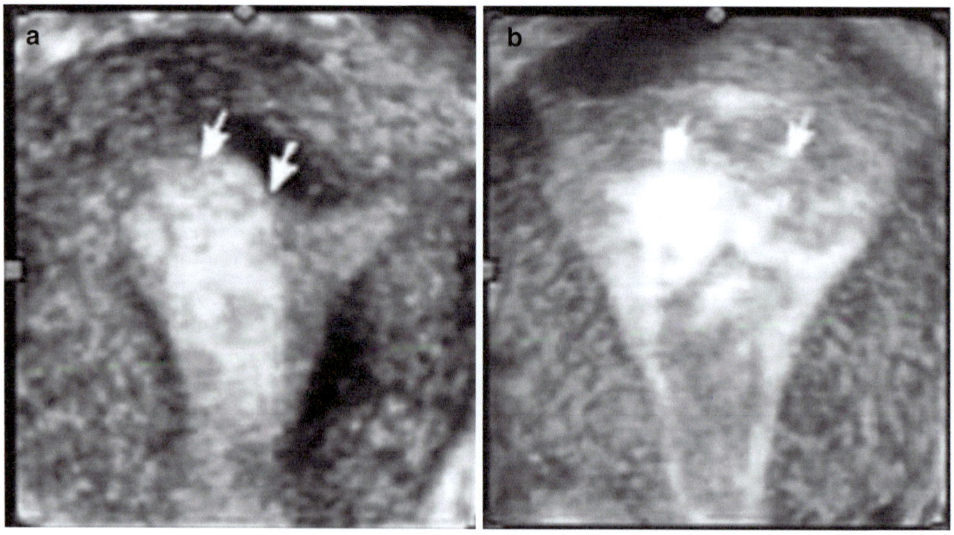

tum, accurately evaluate the volume and infiltration. It facilitates the comprehensively internal observation of the cystic lesion in the pelvic cavity: (1) the thickness, smoothness, and neoplasm of the diaphragm in the cyst; (2) the size and number of the papillae in the cyst, and the relationship with the capsule wall; (3) distinguish the character of cyst contents, such as blood clots and granulated sebum fluid; (4) demonstrate the size and surface morphology of the solid lesion in the cyst, which has an integral role in differentiating the benign from the malignant lesions (Fig. 8.24).

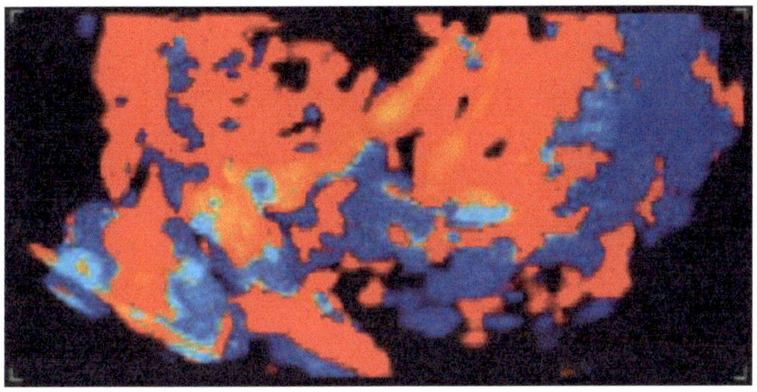

Fig. 8.22 3D B-flow imaging of cervical cancer

V. Pelvic floor ultrasound

3D ultrasound can show the anatomic structure of the pelvic floor in all directions, especially the morphology and direction of the pelvic diaphragm hiatus and levator ani muscle in axial planes. 3D ultrasound is utilized to evaluate the function of the pubic visceral muscles, showing the pelvic organ prolapse. Following are the specific anatomic relationships: The levator ani muscle is a "U"- or "V"-shaped hyperechoic band, bilaterally symmetric, and angulate. The urethra, vagina, and rectum are in a straight line from front to back, and the rhombus structure is symmetrical with this line. The urethra wall presents ring echo, and the anechoic central part represents the urethral cavity. The vagina is next to the back of the urethra wall, with a clear outline, and the typical case is in an "H" shape. The pelvic floor connective tissue connects the levator ani muscle from both sides of the vagina wall. The circular rectum sits behind the vagina, and the muscle and mucous layers of the intestinal wall can be distinguished by high-frequency ultrasound. 3D pelvic diaphragm hiatus plane demonstrates the anatomical structure of the pelvic floor, especially the shape, direction, and continuity of the levator ani muscle in the axial view. A series of parameters are measured in the standard pelvic diaphragm hiatus plane to quantitatively evaluate the pelvic floor volume (Figs. 8.25 and 8.26).

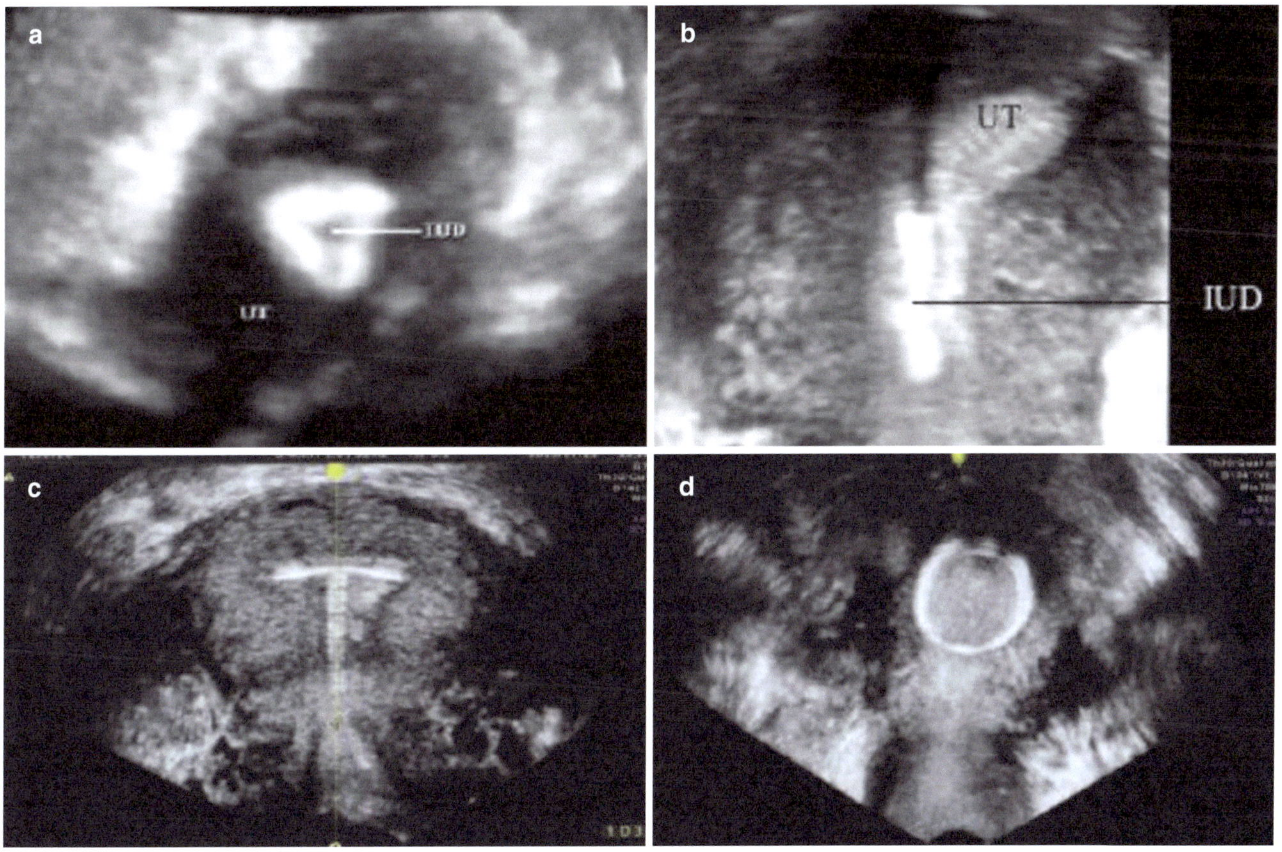

Fig. 8.23 IUD. (**a**) Normal IUD; (**b**) An IUD that slipped into the endocervical canal; (**c**) T-shaped IUD; (**d**) annular IUD

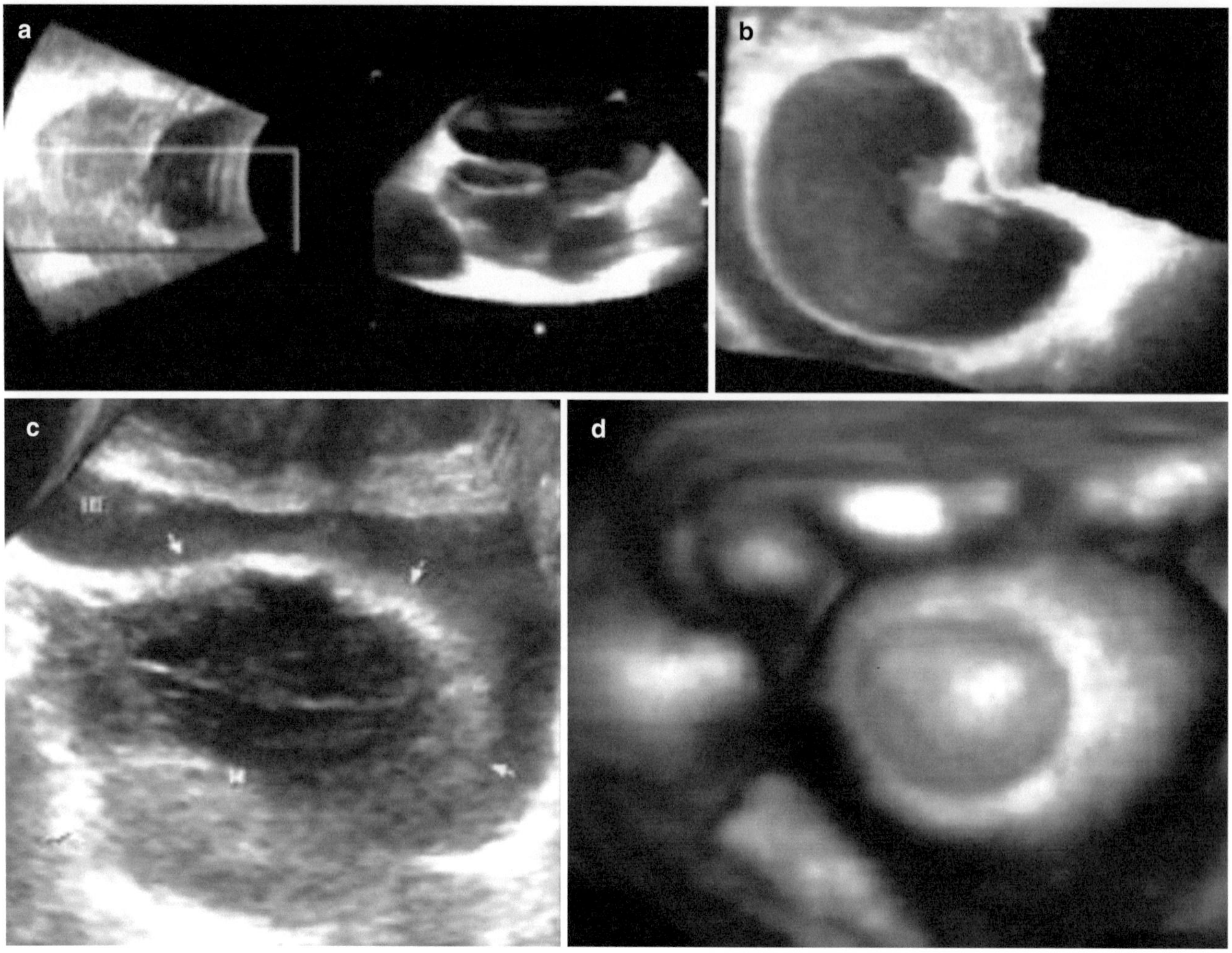

Fig. 8.24 Ovarian diseases. (**a**) 3D image of adnexal cystadenoma; (**b**) 3D image of cystic teratoma; (**c**) Ovarian cancer; (**d**) Pelvic metastasis of gastric cancer

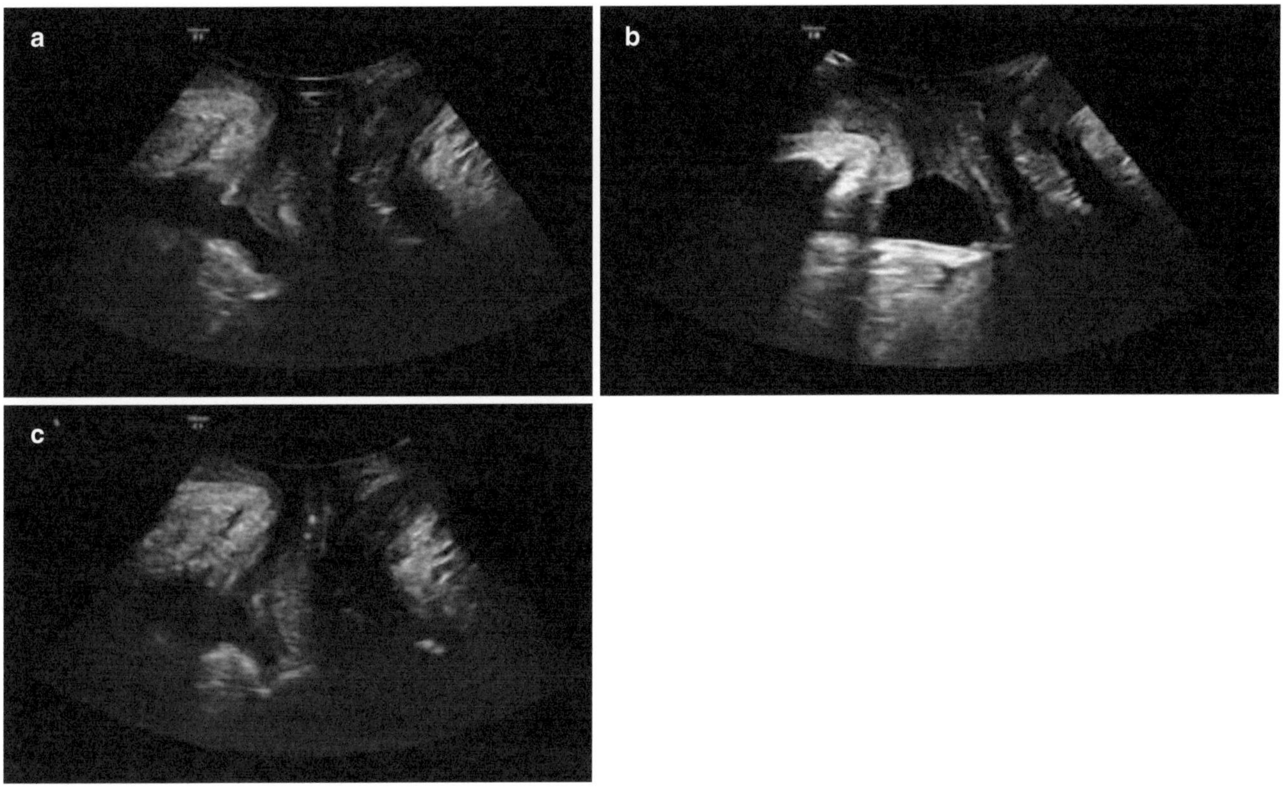

Fig. 8.25 Pelvic floor ultrasound. (**a**) 2D sagittal plane of lower urinary tract at rest; (**b**) 2D sagittal plane of lower urinary tract on Valsalva; (**c**) 2D sagittal plane of lower urinary tract at maximum levator constriction

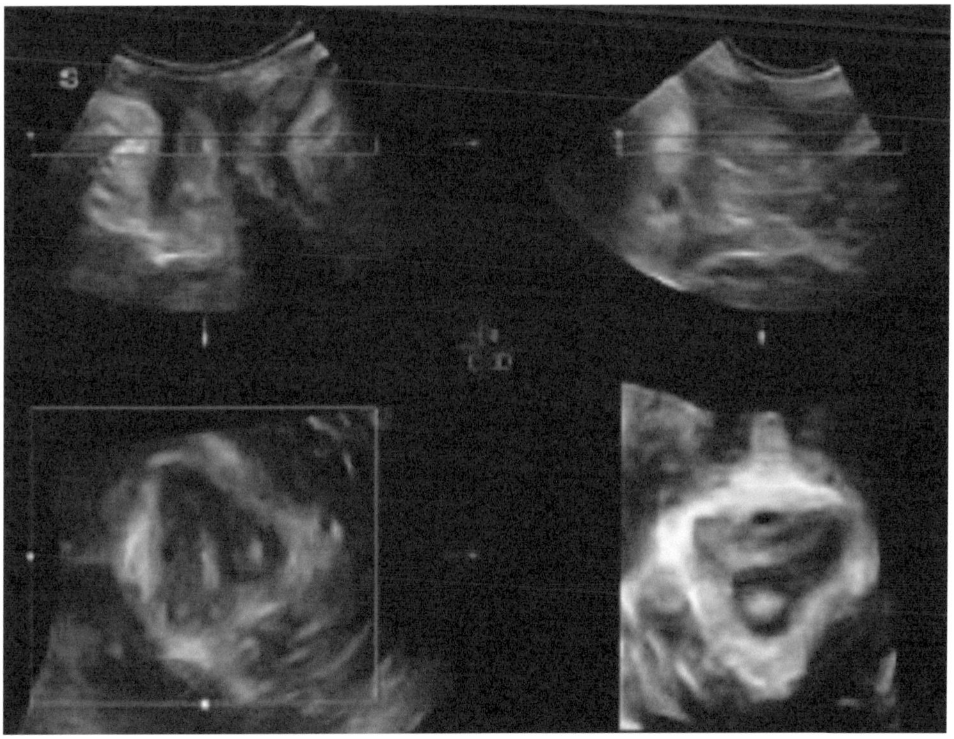

Fig. 8.26 3D ultrasound of the pelvic floor showing the plane of the pelvic diaphragmatic hiatus

Suggested Reading

1. Wong L, White N, Ramkrishna J, et al. Three-dimensional imaging of the uterus: the value of the coronal plane. World J Radiol. 2015;7(12):484–93.
2. Grob ATM, van der Vaart LR, Withagen MIJ, et al. Quality of reporting of diagnostic accuracy studies on pelvic floor three-dimensional transperineal ultrasound: a systematic review. Ultrasound Obstet Gynecol. 2017;50(4):451–7.
3. Wanyan OU, Ping LIN, Ruifang CHEN, et al. Diagnostic value of three-dimensional ultrasound on fetal skeletal malformation. Modern Hospital Dec. 2013;13(12):60–2.
4. 韩瑾 甄理 潘敏等.三种三维超声成像方法在胎儿唇腭裂诊断中的比较. 中华医学超声杂志(电子版), 2014,01:52–54.(无英文摘要).
5. 侯艳琼,罗红. 三维超声在不孕症诊治中的应用研究. 现代妇产科进展, 2013,12:1007–1009.(无英文摘要).
6. 邹娅芳,林小影,孟卓,张彦华,徐英. 二维及三维超声成像在胎儿脊柱病变诊断中的应用. 中华医学超声杂志(电子版), 2013,12:1023–1026. (无英文摘要).
7. Yuqin Z, Xiang L, Xuemei W, et al. The value of efficacy evaluation of cervical cancer radiotherapy by three-dimensional power Doppler. J of Chin Med Univ. 2013;42(9):836–8.
8. Yong-mei WANG, Li CAO, Wen ZHA, et al. Clinical value of quantitative three-dimensional power Doppler ultrasound monitoring normal late pregnancy placental blood flow. J Chin Med imaging. 2013;24(11):818–20.
9. Yanqiong H, Luo H. The value of Three-dimensional power Doppler ultrasound for prediction of pregnancy during frozen-thawed embryo transfer in hormonally controlled cycles. J Sichuan Univ. 2014;35(4):428–30.

9 The Application of Endosonography

Taizhu Yang and Fan Yang

Hysteroscopic examination and hysteroscopic operation are two main compositions of hysteroscopic technology, which is minimally invasive, economical, easy to handle, and directly viewed. Nowadays, hysteroscopic examination is a common method to diagnose intrauterine disease. Hysteroscopy is the primary method to diagnose abnormal uterine bleeding and also the best operative ways on the treatment of uterus septum and endometrial polyps. However, there are still some limitations of hysteroscopy. The application of hysteroscopy is limited to intrauterine disease. During the hysteroscopic operation, the vision is too narrow to figure out the relationship between leisure and surrounding tissue. Electrical conduction is difficult to estimate, leading to complications such as uterine perforation. The combination of hysteroscopy and sonography can help to make up the above shortcomings, also provide evidence of intrauterine lesions to open up the novel method of gynecologic diagnosis and treatment.

9.1 Ultrasound Combined with Hysteroscopy

I. Indication of Hysteroscopic Examination
- Abnormal uterine bleeding
- Biopsy of endometrial polyps and submucous myopia
- Evaluate the situation of the endometrium
- Evaluate the range and stage of endometrial cancer
- Evaluation of IUD
- Evaluation of uterine or cervical factors of infertility, habitat abortion and pregnancy failure
- The intrauterine evaluation before IVF and transplantation

II. Contraindication of Hysteroscopic Examination
- Absolute Contraindication
  - Acute endometritis
  - Acute appendicitis
  - Acute pelvic inflammatory disease. The operation of hysteroscopy is likely to cause the spread of inflammation, so pelvic organ inflammation is the absolute contraindication of hysteroscopic examination.
- Relative Contraindication
  - Massive uterine bleeding
  - Pregnancy
  - Chronic pelvic inflammation

III. Indication of the Combination of Sonography and Hysteroscopy
- The indication of hysteroscopy
- Fallopian tube obstruction
- The decision of surgical option of uterine myoma

IV. Method of Combined Sonography and Hysteroscopy
- The patient performs a bladder lithotomy position. Preoperative preparation: keep the bladder moderately filled. The volume of the bladder varies among people. Patients without a history of pelvic surgery are not necessary to excessively filled in the bladder. Pull the cervix downward to expose the fundus and the top half of the corpus. For patients with a previous history of surgery and pelvic cavity adhesion, the volume of the bladder is advisable when the fundus is fully exposed, as the adhesion limits the movement of the uterus.
- Before the surgery, 2-D ultrasound is applied to evaluate the size, location, thickness of the muscular wall, the location of the line of the uterine cavity, the thickness of the mucosal layer, the situation of bilateral

This chapter was translated by **Feiran Liu**, Department of Obstetrics and Gynecology, Beijing Shijitan Hospital, Bejing, China

T. Yang (✉) · F. Yang
Department of Ultrasonography, West China Second University Hospital, Sichuan University, Chengdu, China

T. Yang, H. Luo (eds.), *Practical Ultrasonography in Obstetrics and Gynecology*,
https://doi.org/10.1007/978-981-16-4477-1_9

ovaries and fallopian tubes, as well as the location, size of pelvic lesions.

- After the evaluation, under the monitor of sonography, the hysteroscopy was conducted into the uterine cavity, which is filled with 5% glucose solution. During the hysteroscopic examination, the ultrasound probe is conducted above the symphysis pubis to scan horizontally and longitudinally, with distention media and filled bladder as reference.
- Sonography scan during the hysteroscopy examination
  - The thickness of the uterine wall and the location of the hysteroscopic probe should be paid attention to avoid uterine perforation. The sonographic features of uterine perforation include:

    There are not specific sonographic features of uterine perforation made by needle because the injury is too small for distention media to infiltrate.

    Sonographic feature of uterine perforation made by cervical dilator is discontinued echo in the muscular layer.

    Sonographic features of uterine perforation made by electrothermal damage include that strong echo, as the result of electrothermal damage, breaking through the whole muscular layer, and the echo of the muscular layer is discontinued.
  - Observe the location and size of the lesion in the uterine cavity and its relationship with the muscular wall or the relationship between intramuscular lesions with the uterine cavity.
  - Monitor the removal process of the lesion.
  - To make further diagnosis.
  - Observe the pressure of distention media and put surveillance on the volume of distention media flowing into the peritoneal cavity through the fallopian tube.
  - During the electrocution, ensure the depth and range of electrosurgical lesion in the uterine wall according to the variation of echo of the endometrium and muscular layer.
  - When the hysteroscopy probe is drawn back, pay attention to whether the distention media infiltrate into a muscular wall or the alteration of sonograph before and after the distention of the uterus.

V. Common Diseases

- Submucous Myoma

  Submucous myoma in the diameter of less than 2 cm is shown as a thickened echo in the uterine cavity. Within the contrast of distention media and bladder, the lesion can be clearly shown as a round or oval mass, surrounded by the anechoic distention media. The diameter of the submucous myoma is more than 2 cm, which is displayed as a hypoechoic mass in the uterine cavity. The size, number, location and whether the myoma is with peduncle can be measured in the combined examination (Fig. 9.1).
- Endometrial Polyp

  Hysteroscopy is a preferable method for the diagnosis and treatment of endometrial polyp. Single polyp and multiple polyps are not easily found by transabdominal examination, which is only displayed as a thickened endometrium. In the combined examination, polyp represents a middle hyperechoic mass with peduncle and not fixed in the uterine cavity by the contrast of distention media and bladder (Fig. 9.2).
- Endometrial Hyperplasia

  The ultrasonic manifestation of endometrial hyperplasia is thickened endometrium with a honeycomb-like anechoic area ranging in size. And the boundary between the endometrium and muscular wall is clear. Sometimes it is difficult to differentiate clumped endometrial hyperplasia from the endometrial polyp and submucous myoma. In the

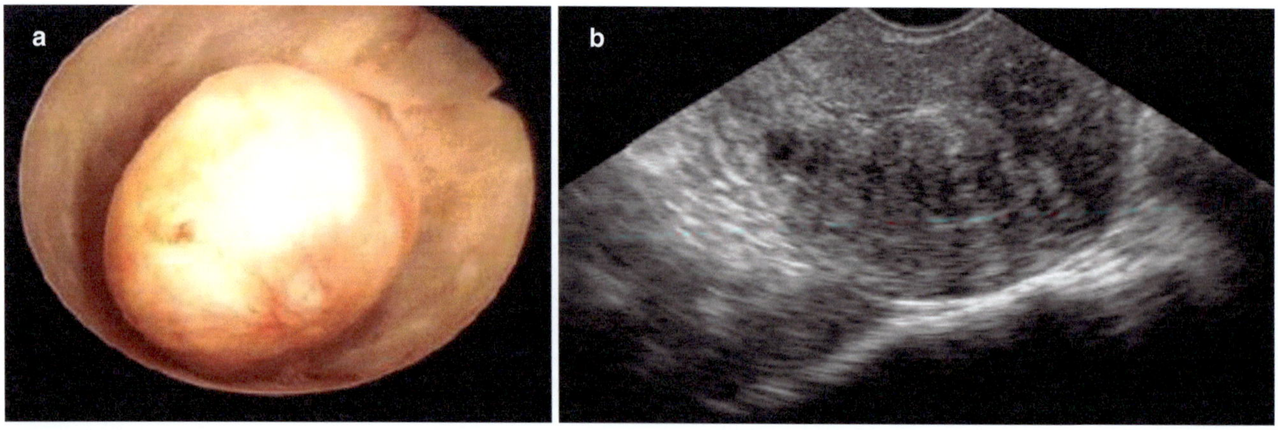

Fig. 9.1 Submucous myoma. (**a**) Hysteroscopy shows the submucous myoma. (**b**) Ultrasonography shows the submucous myoma

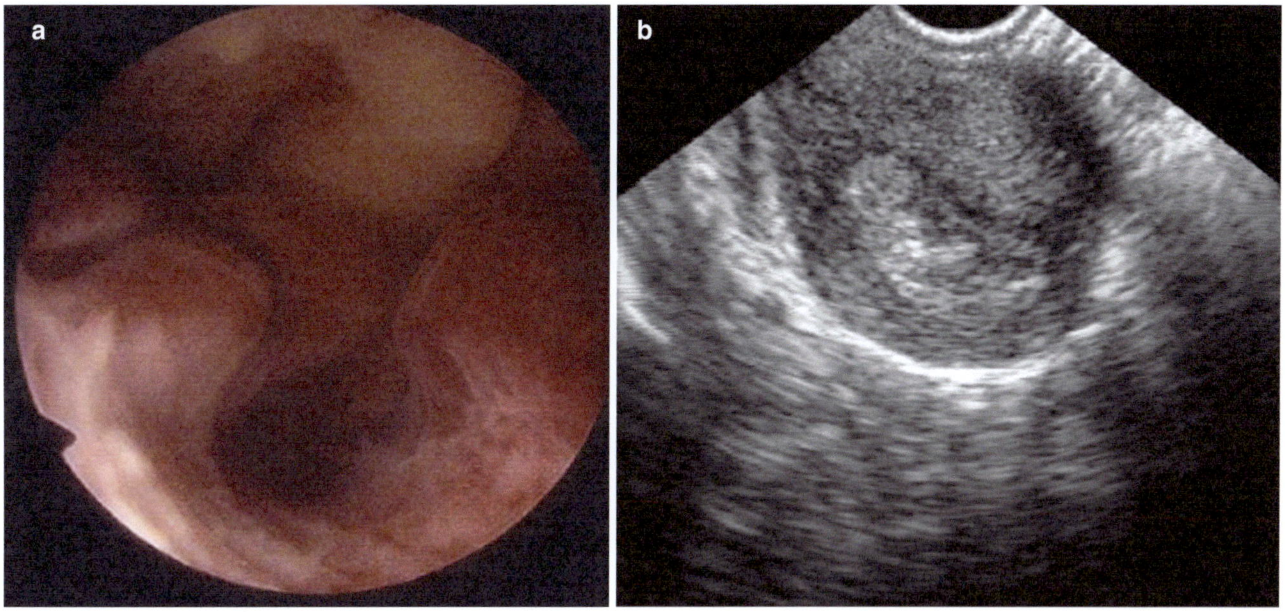

Fig. 9.2 Endometrial polyp. (**a**) Multiple polyps displayed by hysteroscopy. (**b**) irregular thickened endometrium shown by ultrasound

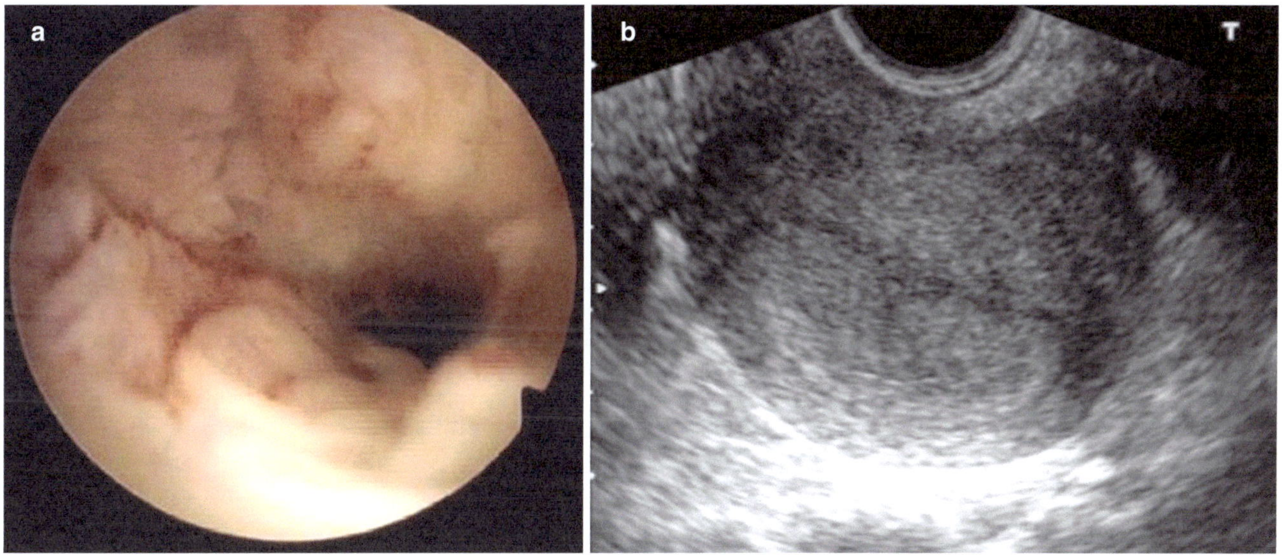

Fig. 9.3 Endometrial hyperplasia. (**a**) The endometrium is clearly showed by hysteroscopy. (**b**) thickened endometrium is displayed by ultrasound

combined examination, when conducted increased distention pressure, the endometrium gets thinner, the honeycomb and hyperechoic mass may disappear. So the endometrial hyperplasia should be differentiated from other diseases (Fig. 9.3).

- Uterine Malformation

  Uterine malformation usually causes infertility and recurrent abortion. It includes fusion defects and absorption defects of bilateral paramesonephric ducts. The uterus septum is a common type of uterine malformation. In the ultrasound examination, a complete uterus septum with communicating area is usually mistaken for an incomplete uterus septum. However, it is usually mistaken for a double uterus, in the diagnosis of hysteroscopy. The observation of the shape of fundus uteri is the key point to differentiate between uterus septum and double uterus. The combined examination help to increase the accuracy rate of diagnosis, which could give guidance to clinical treatment. Ultrasound examination can show whether the outline of the fundus uteri is depressed, and the depth of depression of the uterus septum is less than

10 mm, which is partly reversible. While in the condition of uterus bicornis, the depth of depression of fundus uteri is more than 10 mm and is not related to uterine contraction. Hysteroscopy is not a suitable way for the treatment of uterus bicornis. In the cases of incomplete uterus septum, the bilateral uterine cavity besides septum can be detected after the injection of distention fluid (Fig. 9.4).

- Asherman Syndrome Combined with Uterine Haemorrhage

Hysteroscopy could only discover the uterine adhesion, fails to detect the structures above the adhesion bands. Two-dimensional transabdominal ultrasound examination cannot find the uterine adhesion, only if the adhesion combined with hemorrhage, represents a fluid area in the uterine cavity. The combined examination is able to clearly find out the location, range of the uterine adhesion, and whether there is a hemorrhage or hydrops (Fig. 9.5).

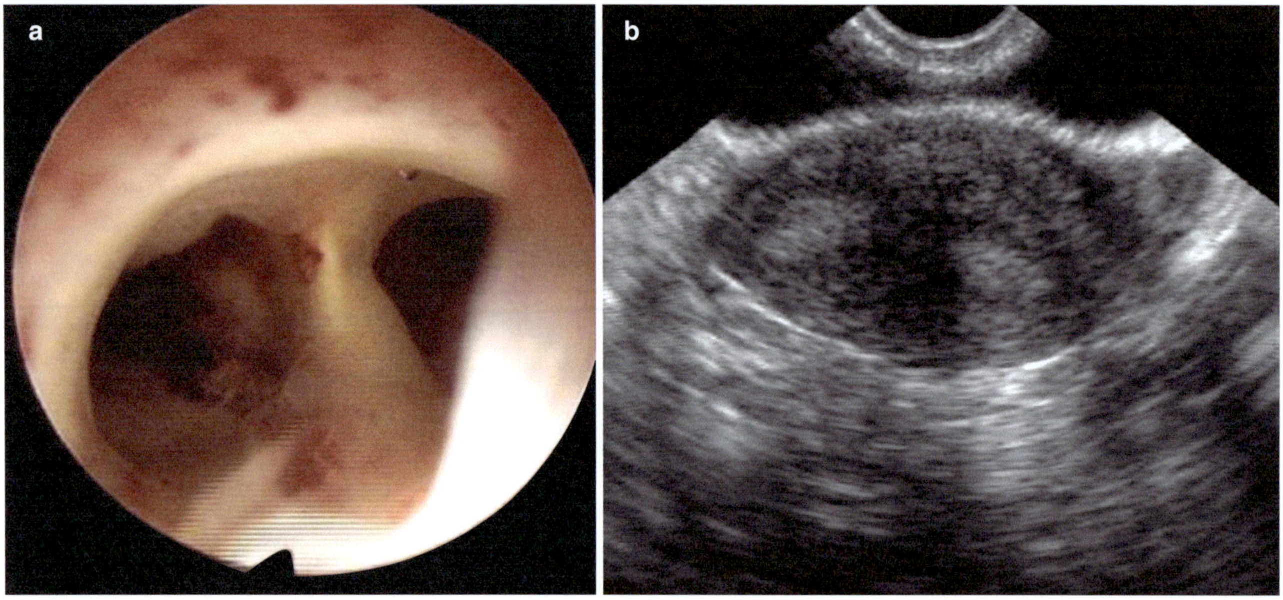

Fig. 9.4 uterus septum. (**a**) The incomplete uterus septum is displayed under the hysteroscopy examination. Two uterine cavities are shown in the fundus uterus. (**b**) Ultrasound examination shows the endometrium in the shape of the Chinese character "八" in uterus septum cases

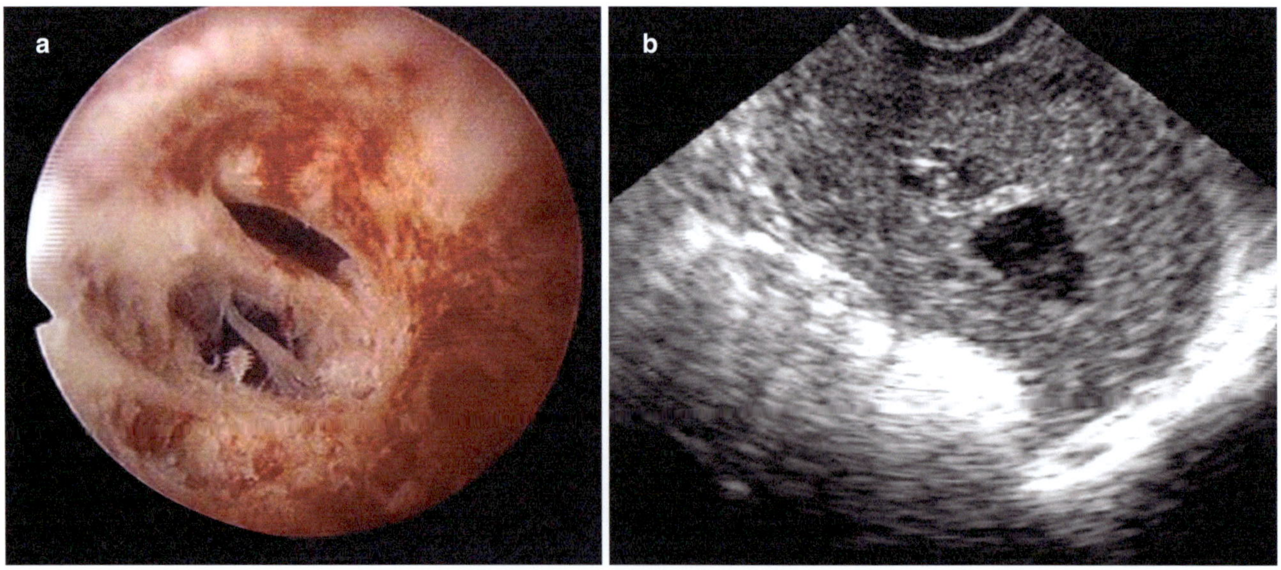

Fig. 9.5 uterine adhesion combined with hematocele. (**a**) hysteroscopic image of uterine adhesion. (**b**) ultrasonography shows the adhesion bands and hematocele in the uterine cavity

- Intrauterine Foreign body

  The insertion of IUD, remained fragments of IUD and intrauterine pregnancy residues are common intrauterine foreign bodies, which can be diagnosed by hysteroscopy. The ultrasound can detect the depth and location of the insertion to the muscular layer. A combined examination can confirm the adhesion of residues (Fig. 9.6).
- Intramural Myoma

  Intramural myoma is usually mistaken for submucous myoma without peduncle under the examination of transabdominal ultrasound. In the hysteroscopy, under the pressure of distention fluid, the intramural myoma which protrudes inside tends to retract to the muscular layer and is not easy to be diagnosed. Combined examination help to clarify the relationship among myoma, uterine cavity and uterine wall and confirm the surgical method (Fig. 9.7)
- Adenomyosis

  Typical adenomyosis can be diagnosed by ultrasonography. Atypical cases should be diagnosed with the combined examination. Under the pressure of distention fluid, some fluid infiltrates into the uterine wall, which represents inhomogeneous cloud-shape

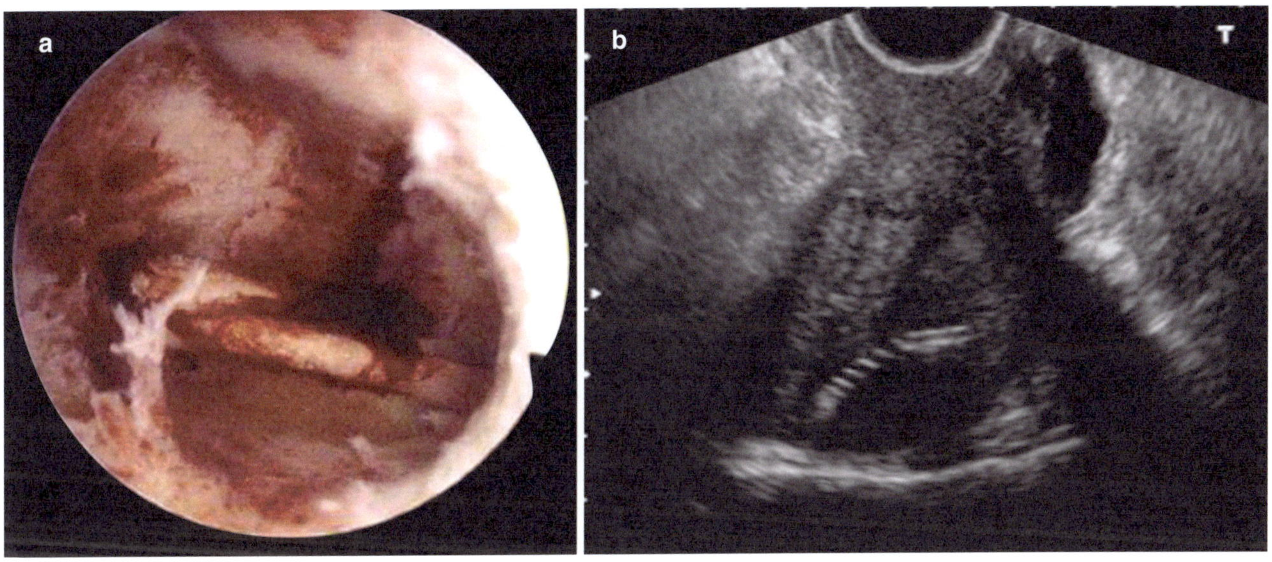

Fig. 9.6 incarceration of IUD. (**a**) Only part of IUD is shown in the uterine cavity under the examination of hysteroscopy. (**b**) Ultrasound examination shows that part of the hyperechoic IUD is inserted into the muscular layer

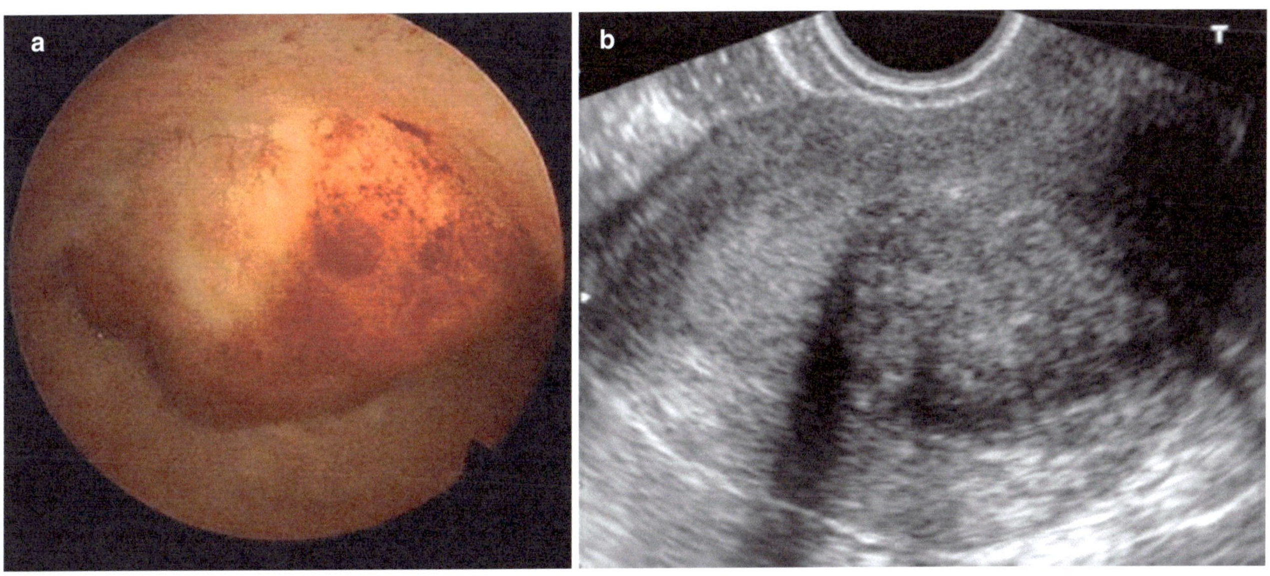

Fig. 9.7 intramural myoma. (**a**) Hysteroscopy shows the myoma partly extrudes into the uterine cavity. (**b**) Intramural myoma is displayed by ultrasonography

hyperechoic under ultrasound. Under the hysteroscopy, the opening of the gland duct or the purple-blue dot hidden under the mucosa can be seen in the mucosal layer.

- Endometrial Carcinoma

  Ultrasound examination, especially TVS, color Doppler ultrasound, and 3-D ultrasound, plays an important role in the diagnosis and staging of endometrial carcinoma. Hysteroscopy examination is practical for the diagnosis. The special appearance of the bulge can sometimes be used to diagnose endometrial cancer under hysteroscopy. Some lesions can be presumed about their pathological type and grade of differentiation. It can also be used to determine the location of the disease and make a biopsy under direct vision to avoid blind curettage, as well as to detect whether there is cancer invasion in the cervical canal and the stage of cancer.

9.2 Ultrasound Examination inside the Uterine Cavity

Transvaginal ultrasound can clearly show the uterine cavity and muscular layer compared with transabdominal ultrasound. However, it has limitations in the preparation evaluation of the endometrium. The high-frequency probe in the uterine cavity can clearly detect the intrauterine lesion compared with transvaginal ultrasound. And it can observe the endometrium thickness, minor lesion, and invasion depth of intrauterine cancer.

9.3 Laparoscopic Intraoperative Ultrasound

In the examination of intraoperative laparoscopic ultrasonography, the ultrasound probe is directly conducted into the pelvic cavity and then to the surface of the uterus. In the other way, the probe of laparoscopy is conducted to the distention fluid of the pelvic cavity to clearly show the intrauterine image, avoiding the effects of intestinal gas, which not only observe the appearance of the uterus but also give guidance to the intrauterine operation. The high-frequency probe (5.0 MHz, 6.0 MHz, 7.5 MHz), which clearly shows the tissue, makes it possible to observe adhesion tissue and a dead cavity formed after adhesion。 It can differentiate calcification and residual fetal bone to distinguish the strong echo made by electrocution, residual fetal bone, and residual IUD. It contributes to the diagnosis as well as the guidance of operation, making it possible for the completion of hysteroscopic, which is difficult to complete under the transabdominal ultrasound. It can also display the depth of invasion, the range and the lymph node involvement of carcinoma, which helps to determine the staging and the operation plan. Whereas laparoscopic intraoperative ultrasound is still micro-trauma examination and only applied in patients who cannot be diagnosed with ultrasound and need laparoscopic examination. That is why laparoscopic intraoperative ultrasound is not the common monitor method.

Suggested Reading

1. Yu H, Nian Y, Qi F. Clinical significance of hysteroscopy and ultrasonography in diagnosis of endometrial lesions. J Nanchang University (Med Sci). 2014;54(3):32–6.
2. 程建英, 王新忠, 左绪磊. 宫腔镜联合超声检查诊断149例绝经后妇女宫内病变临床分析[J]. 中国妇幼保健(19):134–136.(无英文摘要).
3. 曹士红.经阴道彩色多普勒超声诊断黏膜下病变与宫腔镜对照探究[J].实用妇科内分泌杂志(电子版),2016,3(17):51–52.(无英文摘要).
4. 金云兰.超声结合宫腔镜用于内突型壁间子宫肌瘤治疗价值评价[J].实用妇科内分泌杂志(电子版),2016,3(15):132–133.(无英文摘要).

Chinese-English Glossary

A

安全性	Safety

B

白内障	Cataracts
瘢痕妊娠	Cesarean scar pregnancy
半侧巨脑畸形	Hemimegalencephaly
鼻骨	Nasal bone (NB)
鼻骨发育不良	Hypoplastic nasal bone
鼻骨缺如	Absent nasal bone
鼻泪管囊肿	Dacrocystoceles
闭经	Amenorrhea
边缘轮状胎	Circummarginate placenta
边缘性脐带入口	Marginal insertion
边缘性前置胎盘	Marginal placenta previa
部分性前置胎盘	Partial placenta previa
变形	Deformation
标准差	Standard deviation (SD)
表观分布系数	Apparent diffusion coefficient (ADC)
不孕	Infertility
部分型肺静脉异位引流	Partial anomalous pulmonary venous connection (PAPVC)
部分性葡萄	Partial moles
部分容积效应	Partial volume effect

C

彩色多普	Color Doppler
残角	Rudimentary horn
侧裂	Sylvian cistern
侧脑室	Lateral cerebral ventricles
侧壁声影	Edge shadow
超声	Ultrasound
超声波	Ultrasonic wave
超声成像	Ultrasonic imaging
超声断层显像	Tomographic ultrasound imaging (TUI)
产后	Postpartum
产褥期	Puerperium
肠疝	Enterocele
肠管回声增强	Hyperechoic bowel
肠系膜上动脉	Superior mesenteric artery
常染色体显性遗传多囊肾病	Autosomal dominant polycystic kidney disease (ADPKD)
常染色体隐性遗传多囊肾病	Autosomal recessive polycystic kidney disease (ARPKD)
成骨不全	Osteogenesis imperfecta (OI)
成人型多囊性肾病	Adult polycystic kidney disease
尺骨	Ulna
重复肾	Duplex kidney
出生缺陷	Birth defects
出血	Hemorrhage
出血性囊肿	Hemorrhagic cysts
处女膜	Hymen
处女膜闭锁	Imperforate hymen
串珠征	String of pearls sign
唇裂	Cleft lip (CL)
磁共振成像	Magnetic resonance imaging (MRI)
雌二醇	Estradiol
促卵泡激素	Follicle-stimulating hormone (FSH)
错构瘤	Hamartoma
Cantrell 五联征	Pentalogy of Cantrell

D

大脑后动脉	Posterior cerebral artery
大脑前动脉	Anterior cerebral artery
大脑中动脉	Middle cerebral artery (MCA)
大血管转位	Transposition of the great arteries (TGA)
单角子宫	Unicornuate uterus

T. Yang, H. Luo (eds.), *Practical Ultrasonography in Obstetrics and Gynecology*,
https://doi.org/10.1007/978-981-16-4477-1

单脐动脉	Single umbilical artery (SUA)
单心房	Single atrium (SA)
单心室	Single ventricle (SV)
单纯性囊肿	Simple cyst
Dandy-Walker畸形	Dandy-Walker malformation (DWM)
胆囊	Gallbladder
道格拉斯窝	cul-de-sac
低置胎盘	Low-lying placenta
动静脉畸形	Arteriovenous malformation (AVM)
动静脉瘘	Arteriovenous fistulas (AVF)
动脉导管未闭	Patent ductus arteriosus (PDA)
短肢骨发育不良	Short limb skeletal dysplasia
多囊卵巢综合征	Polycystic ovary syndrome (PCOS)
多囊性发育不良肾	Multicystic dysplastic kidney (MCDK)
多普勒	Doppler
多普勒频谱	Doppler waveform
多普勒频移	Doppler shift
多普勒效应	Doppler effect
多胎妊娠	Multiple pregnancy
骶骨	Sacrum

E

恶性	Malignant
腭裂	Cleft palate (CP)

F

发育不全	Hypoplasia
法洛四联症	Tetralogy of Fallot (TOF)
帆状胎盘	Velamentous cord insertion
房间隔缺损	Atrial septal defect (ASD)
房室间隔缺损	Atrioventricular septal defect (AVSD)
分娩	Delivery
腓骨	Fibula
腹部	Abdomen
腹围	Abdominal circumference (AC)
腹腔异位妊娠	Abdominal ectopic pregnancy
腹壁	Abdominal wall
腹膜炎	Peritonitis
腹痛	Abdominal pain
腹裂	Gastroschisis
腹腔干	Celiac axis
腹主动脉	Abdominal aorta
腹水	Ascites
腹部肿块	Abdominal mass
腹部径线	Abdominal diameter (AD)
富于细胞性平滑肌瘤	Cellular leiomyoma
附件	Adnexa
附件扭转	Adnexal torsion
复杂性增生	Complex hyperplasia
副胎盘	Succenturiate lobe

G

肝	Liver
感染	Infection
钙化	Calcification
肛门闭锁	Imperforate anus
肛提肌裂孔	Levator hiatus
肛直肠角	Anorectal angle
膈疝	Diaphragmatic hernia
隔离肺	Extralobar sequestration (ELS)
供血儿	Donor
弓状子宫	Arcuate uterus
弓状动脉	Arcuate arteries
宫内发育迟缓	Intrauterine growth retardation (IUGR)
宫内节育器	Intrauterine devices, (IUD)
宫颈	Cervix
宫颈癌	Cervical cancer
宫颈长度	Cervical length (CL)
宫颈息肉	Cervical polyp
宫颈囊肿	Nabothian cyst
宫颈炎	Cervicitis
宫腔镜	Hysteroscopy
功能层	Zona functionalis
肱骨	Humerus
股骨	Femur
股骨长	Femur length (FL)
关闭不全	Regurgitation

H

后尿道瓣膜	Posterior urethral valve (PUV)
后倾	Retroversion
后屈	Retroflexion
混响伪像	Reverberation
回声失落	Echo drop-out
黄体囊肿	Corpus luteum cyst
横切面	Transverse plane (TP)
横纹肌瘤	Rhabdomyomas
黑质	Substantianigra

红色样变	Red degeneration
壶腹部	Ampulla
华通胶	Wharton jelly
环状胎盘	Ring-shaped placenta
黄体	Corpus luteum
黄体酮	Progesterone
灰阶	Gray-scale

J

肌肉组织	Musculature
基底层	Basalis layer
脊柱裂	Spina bifida
脊髓脊膜膨出	Myelomeningocele
畸胎瘤	Teratoma
畸形	Malformation
激素替代治疗	Hormone replacement therapy (HRT)
脊柱	Spine
脊柱侧弯	Scoliosis
计算机断层扫描	Computed tomography (CT)
经腹部超声超声	Transabdominal sonography (TAS)
经阴道超声超声	Transvaginal Sonography (TVS)
经直肠超声超声	Transrectal sonography, (TRS)
经会阴扫查	Transperineal scan (TPS)
胫骨	Tibia
假骨盆	False pelvis
降主动脉	Descending aorta (DAO)
结肠	Colon
颈项透明层	Nuchal translucency (NT)
颈部淋巴水囊瘤	Nuchal cystic hygroma
静脉导管	Ductus venous (DV)
镜像伪像	Mirror artifact
甲胎蛋白	Alpha fetoprotein (AFP)
交界性	Borderline
脚间池	Interpeduncular cisterns
巨细胞病毒	Cytomegalovirus (CMV)
巨大儿	Macrosomia
巨结肠	Megacolon
巨膀胱	Megacystis

K

颗粒细胞瘤	Granulosa cell tumor
空化效应	Cavitation
扣带回	Cingulate gyrus
阔韧带	Broad ligament

L

阑尾	Appendix
卵巢	Ovary
连续多普勒	Continuous wave Doppler (CW)
良性	Benign
临界值	Discriminatory zone
流产	Abortion
露脑畸形	Exeucephalia
颅内肿瘤	Intracranial tumor
卵巢冠囊肿	Parovarian cyst
卵巢固有韧带	Ovarian ligament
卵巢扭转	Ovarian torsion
卵巢系膜	Mesovarium
卵巢悬韧带	Suspensory ligament
卵巢过度刺激综合征	Ovarian hyperstimulation syndrome (OHSS)
卵泡	Follicle
卵泡膜纤维瘤	Fibrothecomas
卵泡膜细胞瘤	Theca cell tumor
卵巢性索间质肿瘤	Ovarian sex cord-stromal tumor
卵巢囊腺癌	Ovarian cystadenocarcinoma
卵黄囊	Yolk sac (YS)
轮状胎盘	Circumvallate placenta
螺旋动脉	Spiral arteries

M

M型超声	M-mode ultrasound imaging
脉冲多普勒	Pulsed Doppler (PW)
脉络丛	Choroid plexus
脉络丛囊肿	Choroid plexus cyst (CPC)
曼月乐	Mirena
马蹄内翻足	Club foot
梅格斯综合征	Meigs syndrome
迷走左锁骨下动脉	Aberrant left subclavian artery (ALSA)
迷走右锁骨下动脉	Aberrant right subclavian artery (ARSA)
泌尿道	Urinary tract (UT)
末次月经时间	Last menstrual period (LMP)

N

脑膨出	Encephalocele
脑膜膨出	Meningocele

脑膜脑膨出	Encephalocele
脑积水	Hydrocephalus
脑脊液	Cerebrospinal fluid
脑室扩张	Ventriculomegaly
脑穿通畸形	Porencephaly
脑保护效应	Brain-sparing effect
内脏异位综合征	Heterotaxy syndromes
内胚层	Endoderm
内胚窦瘤	Endodermal sinus tumor
能量多普勒	Power Doppler
尿路梗阻	Urethremphraxis
尿道闭锁	Urethral atresia
脓肿	Abscess

P

膀胱	Bladder
膀胱外翻	Bladder exstrophy
膀胱子陷凹	Vesicouterine pouch
旁瓣	Side lobe
旁瓣伪像	Side lobe artifact
胚胎	Embryo
胚胎移植	Embryo transfer
盆腔	Pelvic cavity
盆腔炎	Pelvic inflammatory disease (PID)
脾	Spleen
胼胝体	Corpus callosum
胼胝体发育不良	Agenesis of corpus callosum (ACC)
贫血	Anemia
频移	Frequency shift
平滑肌瘤	Leiomyoma
平滑肌肉瘤	Leiomyosarcomas
剖宫产	Cesarean delivery
剖宫产瘢痕妊娠	Cesarean scar ectopic pregnancy
葡萄胎	Hydatidiform mole (HM)

Q

脐带	Umbilical cord
脐动脉	Umbilical artery (UA)
脐静脉	Umbilical vein (UV)
脐带扭转	Torsion of cord
脐膨出	Omphalocele
气管	Trachea
前脑无裂畸形	Holoprosencephaly
侵蚀性葡萄胎	Invasive mole
前置胎盘	Placenta previa
球拍状胎盘	Battledore placenta
丘脑	Thalamus
缺血缺氧性脑病	Hypoxic-ischemic cerbral injury

R

绒毛膜性	Chorionicity
绒毛膜血管瘤	Chorangioma
绒毛膜癌	Choriocarcinoma
双顶径	Biparietal diameter (BPD)
人绒毛膜促性腺激素	Human chorionic gonado-tropin (hCG)
妊娠囊	Gastational sac (GS)
妊娠物残留	Gestational residential
妊娠滋养细胞疾病	Gestational trophoblastic disease (GTD)
妊娠滋养细胞肿瘤	Gestational trophoblastic neoplasia
容积成像	Volume rendering
软骨发育不良	Achondroplasia
软指标	Soft indicator

S

三维超声	Three-dimensional ultrasound
三尖瓣下移	Ebstein's anomaly
三尖瓣闭锁	Tricuspid valve atresia (TVA)
三尖瓣反流	Tricuspid regurgitation
三倍体	Triploidy
三血管切面	Three-vessel view
双顶径	Biparietal diameter (BPD)
双环征	Double decidual sac sign
双胎妊娠	Twin pregnancies
双胎输血综合征	Twin-twin transfusion syndrome (TTTS)
双胎联体畸形	Conjoined twins
双胎反向动脉灌注	Twin reversed arterial perfusion (TRAP)
双子宫	Uterus didelphys
双角子宫	Bicornuate uterus
双泡征	Double bubble sign
上腔静脉	Superior vena cava
生理性中肠疝	Physiologic bowel herniation
深部内膜异位症	Deep pelvic endometriosis
肾脏	Kidney
肾动脉	Renal artery (RA)
肾母细胞瘤	Wilms tumor
肾缺如	Renal absence
肾上腺	Adrenal glands
肾上腺囊肿	Adrenal cyst

声强	Acoustic intensity
声阻抗	Acoustic impedance
声反射	Acoustic reflection
声衰减	Acoustic attenuation
声影	Acoustic shadow
声速	Acoustic velocity
四维超声	Four-dimensional ultrasound
四腔心切面	Four-chamber view
死胎	Fetal death
室间隔缺损	Ventricular septal defect (VSD)
始基子宫	Primordial uterus
十二指肠狭窄	Duodenal stenosis
十二指肠闭锁	Duodenal atresia
时间增益补偿	Time-gain compensation
食管	Esophagus
矢状	Sagittal
受血儿	Recipient
受精卵	Conceptus
水泡状胎块	Hydatidiform mole
速度型彩色多普勒	Color Doppler velocity (CDV)
输卵管	Fallopian tube
输卵管炎	Salpingitis
输尿管	Ureters
衰减	Attenuation

T

胎儿	Fetus
胎儿超声心动图	Echocardiogram
胎方位	Fetal position
胎先露	Fetal presentation
胎儿宫内发育迟缓	Intrauterine growth retardation (IUGR)
胎儿心血管整体评分	Cardiovascular profifile score (CVPS)
胎儿生长受限	Fetal growth restriction (FGR)
胎粪性腹膜炎	Meconium peritonitis
胎粪性肠梗阻	Meconium ileus
胎膜早破	Premature rupture of membranes (PROM)
胎盘	Placenta
胎盘小叶	Cotyledons
胎盘血管瘤	Placental hemangioma
胎盘早剥	Placental abruption
胎盘植入	Placenta implantation
探头	Probe
头臀长	Crown-rump length (CRL)
头臂干	Brachiocephalic artery
头围	Head circumference (HC)
痛经	Dysmenorrhra
体蒂异常	Body stalk anomaly
透明隔	Septum pellucidum
透明隔腔	Cavum septi pellucidi

W

完全型肺静脉异位引流	Total anomalous pulmonary venous connection (TAPVC)
伪像	Artifacts
尾状核	Caudate nucleus
尾骨	Coccyx
纹状体	Corpus striatum
无脑儿	Aneucephalia
无脑畸形	Anencephaly
无鼻	Arhinia
无耳畸形	Anotia
无眼畸形	Anophthalmia
未成熟畸胎瘤	Immature teratoma
无性细胞瘤	Dysgerminoma

X

息肉	Polyps
细胞滋养层	Cytotrophoblast
下颌骨	Mandible
下腔静脉	Lower urinary tract obstruction (LUTO)
小肠	Small intestine
小脑	Cerebellum
小脑延髓池	Cisterna magna
小脑蚓部	Cerebellar vermis
小头畸形	Microcephaly
小耳畸形	Microtia
小下颌	Micrognathia
泄殖腔	Cloaca
泄殖腔外翻	Cloacal exstrophy
泄殖腔外翻序列	Cloacal exstrophy sequence
胸腔	Chest
胸腔积液	Pleural effusion/hydrothorax
先天性心脏病	Congenital heart disease (CHD)
先天性肺囊性腺瘤样病变	Congenital cystic adenomatoid malformation (CCAM)
先天性矫正型大动脉转位	Congenitally corrected transposition of the great arteries (CCTGA)
先天性脊柱侧弯	Congenital scoliosis
先天性畸形	Congenital anomalies

先天性巨结肠	Hirschsprung disease
先天性无子宫	Congenital absence of uterus
先天性食管闭锁	Esophageal atresia
先兆早产	Preterm labor (PTL)
纤维瘤	Fibroma
胸骨	Sternum
心内膜垫缺损	Endocardial cushion defect
心律失常	Cardiac arrhythmias
心房颤动	Atrial fifibrillation
心包积液	Pericardial effusions
心肌病	Cardiomyopathy
心脏内强回声	Echogenic intracardiac focus (EIF)
新生儿	Neonate
新生儿缺氧缺血性脑病	Hypoxic-ischemic encephalopathy (HIE)
漩涡征	Whirlpool sign
血管前置	Vasa previa
血管瘤	Hemangioma
血肿	Haematoma

Y

眼距过宽	Hypertelorism
眼距过窄	Hypotelorism
羊膜	Amnion
羊膜囊	Amnion sac (AS)
羊膜腔穿刺	Amniocentesis
羊膜囊肿	Amniotic cyst
羊膜带综合征	Amniotic band syndrome (ABS)
羊膜性	Amnionicity
羊水	Amniotic fluid
羊水量	Amniotic fluid volume (AFV)
羊水指数	Amniotic fluid index (AFI)
羊水过多	Polyhydramnios
羊水过少	Oligohydramnios
洋葱皮征	Onion skin sign
阴道	Vagina
异位妊娠	Ectopic pregnancy (EP)
异位肾	Ectopic kidney
隐睾	Cryptorchidism
永存动脉干	Truncus arteriosus (TA)
优势卵泡	Dominant follicles
右室流出道	Right ventricular outflow tract (RVOT)
右室双流出道	Double outlet right ventricle (DORV)
右锁骨下动脉迷走	Aberrant right subclavian artery (ARSA)
右位心	Dextrocardia
右心发育不良综合征	Hypoplastic right heart syndrome
幼稚子宫	Infantile uterus
预产期	Estimated due date (EDD)
圆韧带	Round ligament
孕周	Gestational age

Z

早产	Preterm birth (PTB)
早孕期	First trimester
早早孕	Early first trimester
诊刮术	Dilation and curettage (D&C)
枕额径	Occipitofrontal diameter (OFD)
真骨盆	True pelvis
正常变异	Normal variants
正中裂	Median cleft
帧频	Frame rate
支气管闭锁	Bronchial atresia
直肠	Rectum
直肠子宫陷凹	Rectouterine pouch
振铃伪像	Ringing artifact
蛛网膜囊肿	Arachnoid cyst
主动脉	Aorta
主动脉弓	Aorta arch
主动脉瓣	Aorta valve
主动脉缩窄	Aortic coarctation
滋养层细胞	Trophoblast
子宫	Uterus
子宫动脉	Uterine artery
子宫内膜	Endometrium
子宫畸形	Uterine anomalies
子宫内膜癌	Endometrial carcinoma
子宫内膜样腺癌	Endometrioid carcinoma
子宫内膜异位症	Endometriosis
子宫内膜异位囊肿	Endometriomas
子宫内膜炎	Endometritis
子宫腺肌症	Adenomyosis
子宫腺肌瘤	Adenomyoma/ endomettrioma
子宫平滑肌瘤	Leiomyoma
子宫输卵管造影	Hysterosalpingography (HSG)
子宫肉瘤	Sarcoma
子宫切除术	Hysterectomy
致死性侏儒	Thanatophoric dysplasia
纵隔子宫	Uterus septus
纵切面/矢状切面	Sagittal plane (SP)
中央性前置胎盘	Complete placenta previa
中胚层	Mesoderm
中孕期	Second trimester

组织多普勒技术	Tissue Doppler imaging (TDI)	左心发育不良综合征	Hypoplastic left heart syndrome (HLHS)
阻力指数	Resistive index (RI)	21三体综合征	Trisomy 21
左室流出道	Left ventricular outflow tract (LVOT)	18三体综合征	Trisomy 18
		13三体综合征	Trisomy 13
左锁骨下动脉	Left subclavian artery		

MIX
Papier aus verantwortungsvollen Quellen
Paper from responsible sources
FSC® C105338

If you have any concerns about our products,
you can contact us on
ProductSafety@springernature.com

In case Publisher is established outside the EU,
the EU authorized representative is:
Springer Nature Customer Service Center GmbH
Europaplatz 3, 69115 Heidelberg, Germany

Printed by Libri Plureos GmbH
in Hamburg, Germany